Illness and Enlightenment

Illness and Enlightenment

Exploring Tibetan Perspectives on Madness in Text and Everyday Life

Susannah Deane

berghahn
NEW YORK • OXFORD
www.berghahnbooks.com

First published in 2025 by
Berghahn Books
www.berghahnbooks.com

Library of Congress Cataloging-in-Publication Data
A C.I.P. cataloging record is available from the Library of Congress
Library of Congress Cataloging in Publication Control Number: 2024033550

British Library Cataloguing in Publication Data
A catalogue record for this book is available from the British Library

ISBN 978-1-80539-840-0 hardback
ISBN 978-1-80539-841-7 epub
ISBN 978-1-80539-842-4 web pdf

https://doi.org/10.3167/9781805398400

Contents

Figures

Acknowledgements

My huge thanks go to the people in Amdo who made this research possible. During my twelve months conducting ethnographic research in the region, many people kindly agreed to be interviewed. Many more took the time to answer endless questions and explain things to me, often inviting me into their lives in the city and their home towns, sharing knowledge about local life; taking me along to religious and medical institutions and to festivals; and passing me on to friends, colleagues and acquaintances who they thought might be able to assist me in my research. Given the sensitive nature of the topic, people's engagement with my questions was never taken for granted. Those with knowledge of English took time to discuss possible translations of Tibetan terms, and to interpret for me when conversation was too fast for me to keep up in Tibetan. Some of these people became friends, allowing me to become part of their families and communities, and making my time in Amdo enjoyable as well as fascinating. Many thanks too to my Tibetan teacher in Xining. In between patiently encouraging my language learning and helping me translate the Lhasa dialect I knew into the very different Amdo dialect and pronunciation I now needed to learn, she took time to talk about her life in Xining and her hometown in Golok, and gave me endless useful information about navigating the city. While all Tibetan names in this work are pseudonyms, my appreciation of each and every Tibetan interviewee, friend and stranger who helped me with my research and with everyday life in Amdo is heartfelt.

In Amdo, a number of non-Tibetan friends also provided information, inspiration, friendship and support during my time there. Special thanks to Valentina Punzi, Anne Kukuczka, Alex Rhea, Monika Kolodziej and Agnes Conrad for their help in navigating Xining and Rebkong – and for frequently translating Chinese for me. Thanks too to Todd Marek and Monika Budáčová for their introductions to Xining and its medical landscape.

Many thanks go to the British Academy, who funded this project through a postdoctoral research fellowship, including an extension in the face of COVID-19. The fellowship was conducted at the University of Bristol in the UK, kindly hosted by the Department for Religion and Theology, where Rupert Gethin, and also Rita Langer and Benedetta Lomi, provided support. Much thanks too to Minzu University of China in Beijing, who hosted me as a visiting researcher for one year, allowing me to conduct my research in Qinghai.

Many people also provided practical support and encouragement in the writing up of this research, including colleagues both at my own institution and those farther afield. Thanks especially go to David Leech and Pierce Salguero for their interest in my work, and for providing feedback on some of the chapters in this book; and thanks to those who showed interest in my work, inviting me to present my research at seminars and conferences. The thoughtful feedback and discussions that resulted from these events always proved invaluable. Thanks too to my peer reviewers, particularly Colin Millard, whose un-anonymised peer review of the manuscript provided extremely thoughtful comments, queries and suggestions.

Long after their responsibilities as Ph.D. supervisors concluded, both Geoffrey Samuel and Tracey Loughran have continued to provide invaluable support and encouragement – with Geoffrey, as ever, filling some of the blanks in my knowledge from his many years of research. Both of them continue to inspire me with their passion and energy for research.

My sincere thanks to Berghahn Books for all of their work and patient support in getting this to the finish line, particularly the editorial team and the cover designer, who have been a pleasure to work with; their hard work is not underestimated.

And finally, to those friends and family who have offered support during the long process of research and book-writing: thanks go to my parents, Jenny and John Deane; my sister, Alexa Deane; my incredible friends Jessi, Craig and the girls; and the many friends who kept me sane with their good company, listening ears and encouragement.

A Note on Terminology, Transliterations and Translations

For Tibetan words in the text, I have primarily used the Tibetan & Himalayan Library's Simplified Phonetic Transcription of Standard Tibetan devised by David Germano and Nicolas Tounadre.[1] While this does not take into account Amdo pronunciations (which can be significantly different from other Tibetan dialects), it should be accessible to a majority of readers familiar with the Lhasa dialect of Modern spoken Tibetan and/or Classical Tibetan. In addition to this, as written Tibetan does not separate words (only syllables, separated with the *tsek* 'dot'), I have attempted to group together syllables as logically as possible in relation to their English translations to ease reading.

Exceptions to this phonetic transcription include words and Tibetan names (of both people and places) that have become commonly used internationally with particular spellings (for example, the key Tibetan medical text, *The Four Tantras*, usually referred to as the *Gyüshi*). For specialists, I have provided a full Glossary with exact transliterations of Tibetan terms used in this work, using the Wylie system (Wylie 1959). For the names of Tibetan texts that are only mentioned once or twice, I have used standard Wylie transliteration for ease in finding the primary texts for any interested readers. When referencing the key *Gyüshi* medical text, I have simply referred to the specific volume being cited (e.g. *Gyüshi I*, *Gyüshi IV*), with page numbers referring to a 2015 copy of *The Four Tantras* published by the Tibet People's Publishing House (bod ljongs mi dmangs dpe skrun khang) in Beijing (see Bibliography).

Tibetan words are italicized, except where they have come into common usage in English conversation or in the English-language literature (e.g. lama, rinpoche) – here, I have used these common phonetic spellings (unitalicized). This is the same for Sanskrit words that are commonly used in English-language literature (e.g. chakra, karma, Dharma). As Tibetan does not pluralize nouns, to keep things simple, I have used the English plural marker as an unitalicized 's' at the end of Tibetan words where necessary.

Where Tibetan concepts are already commonly translated into specific English terms, I have used Tibetan and English interchangeably in my writing. It is worth remembering that these translations are not perfect: many of these concepts have no English-language equivalents, and the difficulties of translating such terms successfully into English is clear through examples such as *sem* (usually rendered as 'mind', but in fact much broader than this) and *lung* (commonly 'wind', but not equal to English understandings of wind – nor to the Greek humoral concept of 'wind', to which it is often compared). With this in mind, where I have translated Tibetan language conversations into English, I have left the key Tibetan technical terms untranslated to demonstrate how people used these concepts.

In dealing with interview material from my fieldwork in Amdo, I have used people's professional descriptions or titles as they were given to me (e.g. lama, yogi). All those with the title Dr (doctor) are Tibetan medicine doctors. Occasionally I use the term 'Amdo-wa' to refer to Amdo Tibetans, as is common in the region. I have included information on interviewees' ages and home regions to give more context, and where an individual's home town is different from the town in which they were residing at the time of the interview, I have included both (e.g. Nyingyal [33, Golok/Xining] who hailed from Golok, but at that time was studying in Xining).

Note

1. Available online at https://www.thlib.org/reference/transliteration/phconverter.php [retrieved May 2023].

Introduction

In October 2018, a Tibetan friend, Sonam, took me to meet her childhood friend Lobsang, a Gelugpa Buddhist monk, at his monastery in Rebkong, Amdo. She suggested that Lobsang might be able help with my research on Tibetan notions of *nyoné* – 'madness'. We chatted in broken English and Tibetan as we walked from the bright autumn sunshine of the town's busy streets to the shaded narrow lanes that wove between monastery buildings, and Sonam, laughing, joked, 'You should interview Lobsang! We say he is crazy! He is always laughing and telling jokes. He's not like a normal monk!'

Searching for Lobsang, we arrived at one of the main temples and found a hub of activity, as monks and lay people made preparations for an upcoming ritual that had been commissioned by a group of women from a nearby village. Lobsang broke away to talk to us, and Sonam's description of him was proven correct as he laughed loudly and easily as we chatted, and indeed throughout the day, as we continued talking over tea, and then eventually dinner in a local hotpot restaurant. When I explained my research topic, he laughed loudly and playfully slapped my arm, saying,

> There is an old lama here who is *nyoné*! Do you want to see him? He is eighty-three; he has been *nyoné* for a long time – since he was young – as a result of *sok lung* [a form of 'wind' illness]. I can take you to see him if you like . . . He can still practise – he can meditate and read texts. But when you ask a question, he can't answer you; he responds with something completely different, not making sense. He is too old now – there's no way to treat him.

Rather than trouble an elderly monk, Lobsang took us instead to meet Wangyal (62), an older *lama* (teacher), who he said would be able to answer my questions about Buddhist understandings of *nyoné*. We ended up spending the afternoon in Wangyal's monastic quarters, drinking tea and chatting at length about Buddhist notions of mind and madness. Wangyal, like so many of the people I met in Amdo, was generous with his time, patiently answering questions and explaining complex Buddhist concepts as we chatted in a mix of English (of which he had learnt a little while travelling in Europe) and my developing Amdo Tibetan dialect, with Sonam – an English teacher – helping to translate between us. It was a wide-ranging conversation, taking in different types of illness-causing spirits, *nyoné* precipitated by difficult life events, and monks who had apparently 'become mad' following intensive meditation practice.

A few weeks later, over lunch in her uncle's restaurant, Sonam too would tell me about a case of madness – this one a relative of hers, who 'suddenly went crazy', as she described it. The family took her to a 'Chinese [i.e. biomedical] hospital', where doctors 'did body tests and couldn't find anything wrong with her', and so the family turned to religious means, consulting multiple Buddhist ritual specialists in search of diagnosis and treatment, and finally her condition had improved somewhat. I asked Sonam what she thought caused this kind of 'madness', and she told me, 'I don't know . . . some people say *nying* [heart], and some people say *dön* [spirits] . . . I think both of them are connected.'

*

This short vignette illustrates some of the different ways in which 'madness' is understood and talked about in Tibetan communities, from describing a person's unusual behaviour to a serious condition from which they may or may not be expected to recover, as in Lobsang's description of the elderly monk in his monastery or Sonam's narrative about her own relative. Here, explanations of *nyoné* take in multiple Tibetan notions of mind and body. For example, concepts of *nyoné* as an illness reference the three factors of *lung* (wind), *tripa* (bile) and *béken* (phlegm) (see for example Epstein and Topgay 1982; Dorjee and Richards 1985: 22), as well as notions of *nying* (heart) and *don né* (spirit afflictions) (cf. Day 1989; Clifford 1984; Rapgay 1985; Samuel 2007) – all of which are described in Tibetan medical texts. And in Tibetan Buddhist texts we can read about *nyoné* caused by Tantric practices 'gone wrong' (see, for example, Epstein and Lieff 1981), as Lobsang described in the case of the elderly Rebkong monk. As a result, we find remedies for treating *nyoné* described in both medical and Tantric texts. In addition, the well-known figure of the *lama nyonpa* ('mad lama/yogin') is sometimes said to represent a pinnacle of Buddhist enlightenment: finally having seen beyond dualistic notions of good and bad, purity and impurity, he behaves in strange ways – appearing 'mad', but actually enlightened (cf. DiValerio 2015; Ardussi and Epstein 1978; Pitkin 2017).

Across these diverse narratives, Tibetan medical and Tantric notions of mind-body structure and (dys)functioning converge and diverge as we hear about different medical and Tantric representations of the body, and different ways to both understand and experience madness. The aim of this monograph is to conduct an exploration of this multifaceted Tibetan concept of *nyoné* across these spheres of medicine and religion, in both historical and contemporary perspectives. The work brings together material from interviews conducted during a 2018/19 period of fieldwork in the Tibetan region of Amdo in northwest China, with an examination of some Tibetan historical and contemporary medical and religious texts. This allows us to explore the ways in which key Tibetan medical and religious conceptions of mind-body – including notions of heart, 'wind' and spirit–human relationships – are implicated in different manifestations of 'madness'.

*

The Tibetan term *nyoné* (also *nyonpa*) is usually translated – by both Tibetan and non-Tibetan medicine practitioners and scholars – into the English terms madness, insanity or psychosis. Used in a vernacular way, it may refer to someone behaving oddly, or eccentrically, without denoting illness of any kind, as it is in English (and as we saw above, in reference to Lobsang's apparently unusual behaviour for a monk). Used to refer to illness, Tibetan notions of *nyoné* show significant similarities with biomedical concepts of psychosis (Millard 2007).[1] For example, Tibetan medical texts list symptoms of the illness of *nyoné* including confusion, distortions of perception, a focus on sadness, excessive talking and/or crying, and anger/aggression (*Gyüshi III* 2015: 383–85) – and ethnographic research has demonstrated similar findings (Jacobson 2002: 261; Deane 2014a: 451).[2] In addition, madness may play a key part in the process of becoming a recognized spirit-medium in many Tibetan and Himalayan communities (Day 1989; Rösing 2006).

The illness of *nyoné* is described clearly in key Tibetan medical texts such as the twelfth-century *Gyüshi* (*Four Tantras*).[3] However, many discussions of Tibetan perspectives on mind, mental health and illness[4] will also take in Tibetan religious concepts of mind, body and cosmos. Some of these understandings are included in the medical literature (for example, descriptions of illness-causing spirits in the *Gyüshi*, where 101 illnesses caused by spirit intervention are listed). Others are more localized, such as diverse concepts of pollution or impurity (Tib. *drip*, *mi tsangwa*) in different Tibetan communities. These understandings of the individual and his/her relationship to the wider world derive not just from Buddhism but also from pre-Buddhist ideas – some of which have been adopted into Buddhist theory and practice to a greater or lesser extent, others of which remain at the margins of Buddhist culture. Thus, following extensive work on healing in Tibetan communities, Schrempf has described 'a cultural logic of healing in which "medicine" and "religion" are intertwined' (2011: 162), and I would argue that this is exemplified in Tibetan understandings of madness.

Pertinent here too is the Bon tradition. The categorization 'Bon' is currently used to refer to three intertwining but distinct traditions across a broad range of time periods (Kvaerne 1995: 9),[5] including diverse healing practices within contemporary Bon communities.[6] The question of Bon's history, origins and whether it can be classed as a school within Tibetan Buddhism is complex. Contemporary relations between Buddhism and Bon communities can be 'strained' (Dhondup 2011a: 51); Samuel reports significant stigma of Bonpos from many Buddhists (2013b: 79), and Millard describes Bonpos as having 'historically been marginalised and vilified by mainstream Buddhist Tibetan culture' (2013b: 144). Moreover, texts and traditions have been copied, shared and claimed as 'original' on both sides, and practitioners conducting near-identical practices often declare themselves entirely different from each other, with different histories and lineages attributed.[7]

For our purposes here, the only Bon tradition I am referring to is contemporary scholastic Bon, as this was what I encountered through my interviews in Amdo – a tradition described by Sihlé as a 'Tibetan quasi-Buddhist religion, which is very close to the Nyingma order, both sociologically and in terms of religious content' (2018: 163). This represents an 'organized religion' usually referred to as Yung Drung Bon, which developed in Tibet in the tenth and eleventh centuries 'alongside various forms of Buddhism' (Millard 2013b: 145). Its founder, Tonpa Shenrab, while said by his followers to have lived many centuries before Sakyamuni Buddha, and to have come from an area west of Tibet named as sTag gzig, is also described as having been born into a royal family before embarking on his path towards realization.[8]

During my time in Amdo, the vast majority of Tibetans that I got to know were members of the various Buddhist communities in the area – predominantly Gelug and Nyingma. Indeed, Samuel has described the Amdo region as dominated by large Gelugpa monastic institutions, with – particularly around Rebkong – a 'well-established tradition' of smaller Nyingmapa institutions, which are 'associated with a network of local lay Rnying ma pa village temples and tantric practitioners', alongside a 'parallel tradition of Bon po monasteries, village temples and lay tantric practitioners' (2013a: 7). As a result, all but one of my interviewees were Buddhist, and therefore the resulting narratives are almost entirely from Buddhist perspectives. However, as we shall see, key Tibetan medical and religious concepts of mind-body and related Tantric practices explored in these pages are found in both Buddhist and Bon traditions, associated 'primarily with the highest yoga (*annuttarayayoga*) tantric texts such as the Kalachakra Tantra (*Dus 'khor rgyud*) and the Bon's Mother Tantra (*Ma rgyud*)' (Millard 2005 and 2006: 12).

In this work, then, I will talk broadly of 'Dharmic' and 'Tantric' traditions and practices. These are orientations that are shared across the Tibetan Buddhist and Bon religious traditions relevant to our discussion here. Similarly, references to Tibetan medical texts are focused on the *Gyüshi*, attributed to the Medicine Buddha, but might usually equally be made about the Bon *Bumshi* medical text. While the latter is attributed to the founder of the Bon tradition, Tonpa Shenrab, the contents of the texts are 'essentially the same' (Millard 2005 and 2006: 8). As Millard has asserted, this situation is not necessarily a problem for Bon doctors; he and others have described Bon Tibetan medicine doctors studying the *Gyüshi* (Millard 2013a, Schrempf 2007: 96), or using these Buddhist and Bon medical texts 'interchangeably' (Millard 2005 and 2006: 15).[9] In addition, a doctor's specific medical lineage is often key in their community, with the 'knowledge and experience of the teacher' valued more than a particular religious affiliation (Millard 2013a: 376).[10]

Ultimately, as will become clear in the following chapters, the boundaries between these different traditions and practices are not always clear cut – particularly between the spheres of so-called 'Buddhist', pre-Buddhist 'folk' religion and 'Bon'.[11] And within these pages, we will see how both practitioners and lay Tibetans often straddle interlinked medical, religious, Dharmic, Tantric and folk-religious explanatory frameworks in reference to *nyoné*. Here, for example, we meet an elderly doctor who works in a state-affiliated Tibetan medicine hospital during the day, and then performs Buddhist ritual activities for his patients at home in the evenings and weekends; description of a Buddhist rinpoche[12] who is said to produce medicinal pills from his own body following successful treatment of a serious illness; and narratives of spirit-caused madness diagnosed and treated by ritual specialists.

Moreover, the history of many of these religious and medical ideas (and related practices) can be traced to a multiplicity of sources and traditions – notably the Indian Tantric, Buddhist and Ayurvedic traditions, which predate the arrival of Buddhism into Tibet, but also influences from Hellenic, Chinese and Persian medical traditions. And in both Tantric and medical understandings, the role of *lung* (wind/energy) is key: said to flow throughout thousands of channels in the body, *lung* is understood to be closely related to the functioning of the mind. Tibetan medicine doctor and author Lobsang Rapgay describes wind as 'the foundation of mental consciousness . . . [it] encompasses the mind but is not limited to the mind' (1984: 50). Thus, when we speak of 'mind' in Tibetan understanding, as Samuel explains, we are not dealing with mind as purely a cognitive process (2014: 33), as we might interpret it in biomedical understanding. Instead, we are looking at complex notions of mind (Tib. *sem*) and consciousness (Tib. *namshé*), which take in specific Tibetan Buddhist, pre-Buddhist and medical notions of mind-body structure and functioning, and are referenced by a number of interrelated Tibetan concepts including *sem* (Skt. *citta*; mind, primary consciousness) and *yi* (Skt. *manas*; intentions, emotions, thought, perception) (Samuel 2014: 33).[13] Related to this too is the concept of *la* – 'life-force' or 'life essence' – a multivarious concept that 'pervades Tibetan and Himalayan folk, literary, medical, astrological and religious spaces' (Gerke 2007: 191).[14] Indeed, Millard reports being told in Dhortapan, Nepal, that the *la* is 'often considered as part of the threefold group' of '*la yi sem sum* [three]'; here, '*[s]ems* is the ordinary mind, *yid* is a deeper layer of the mind in which thoughts circulate, and the *bla* is the vital energy which sets things in motion' (2005 and 2006: 14). The close relationship of mind/consciousness to *lung* is evident in Tibetan medical texts, and also the Tantric Buddhist and Bon texts, where it forms the basis of high-level practices, as we shall see in the following chapters. Moreover, in Tibetan understanding, the individual and the cosmos are also interrelated – with the human body, as microcosm, understood to contain 'all the energies and elements of the universe', the macrocosm (Drungtso 2004: 123)[15] – and the 'influence' of Tantric cosmology on Tibetan medical traditions is particularly evident in the sections on Tibetan medical theory about anatomy in the *Gyüshi* and the *Bumshi* (Chapter 4 of the second volume of both texts) (Millard 2005 and 2006: 12).

However, despite these significant overlaps between medical and religious descriptions of mind-body, in many contemporary Tibetan communities, practitioners and their practices are divided in quite practical terms between somewhat separate 'medical' and 'religious' spheres. Today, medical and religious specialists usually train and work in different places, and study different – if overlapping – descriptions of mind and body elucidated in medical and Tantric texts and practices, as we shall see.

Tibetan Medicine

While there is some diversity in the forms of practice that come under the umbrella of 'Tibetan medicine'[16] across the Himalayan region, key here is the twelfth-century, four-volume medical text, the *Gyüshi* (*Four Tantras*). The text is thought to be a composite work: while much of it is understood to be a translation of a key seventh-century Sanskrit Ayurvedic medical text, the *Aṣṭāṅgahṛdayasaṃhitā* (Ga 2010: 85),[17] it was also influenced by multiple sources including Sanskrit and Chinese texts alongside original Tibetan medical concepts (Emmerick 1977; Ga 2010 – see also Ga 2014; Garrett 2008: 38–41; Gerke 2014; J. Gyatso 2015), and it is thought that much of the *Gyüshi* was codified in the twelfth century by the Tibetan scholar Yutok Yonten Gonpo and his students.[18] The text became the 'root' medical work in Tibet (J. Gyatso 2004: 84), used at the Chagpori medical institution, which was established in Lhasa in the seventeenth century by renowned politician and scholar Desi Sangye Gyatso (Meyer 2003), who also authored multiple works on Tibetan medicine. The *Gyüshi* text covers anatomy and the nosological framework of medicine, as well as diagnostic and treatment methodology (Ga 2010).[19] This text is made up of 156 chapters across four sections:

1. *Tsa Gyü* (*Root Tantra*/*First Tantra*, six chapters): This provides an introduction and outline of the text, including the basis of health and illness, diagnosis, treatment and the use of metaphors in Tibetan medicine.
2. *Shé Gyü* (*Explanatory Tantra*/*Second Tantra*, thirty-one chapters): This includes embryology, anatomy, causes and conditions (or 'secondary causes') of disease, and the principles of diagnosis and treatment (including dietary and behavioural guidance as well as medical treatments), as well as description on the expected personal qualities of a doctor.
3. *Men ngak Gyü* (*Oral Instruction Tantra*/*Third Tantra*, ninety-two chapters): This describes diseases of the three *nyépa* ('energies' or 'faults') and provides a comprehensive explanation of causes, conditions, classification, diagnosis, symptoms and treatments for a broad range of conditions, including several chapters on illness-causing spirits.
4. *Chi mé Gyü* (*Additional* or *Final Tantra*/*Fourth Tantra*, twenty-five chapters): This covers pulse and urine diagnosis and contains descriptions of multiple medicinal compounds and external therapies, including herbal poultices and baths, moxibustion, bloodletting and enemas.[20]

In fact, a multitude of medical texts are necessary for Tibetan medical study and practice, not least the corpus of texts known as 'commentaries' (*nyam yig*, lit. 'writing from experience'). These were authored by medical practitioners on the basis that direct experience was often superior to learning medicine from texts. Chui has described the significant role that these commentarial texts have played in the development of the Tibetan medical tradition (2019: 87); indeed, over time, these commentaries began to supplant the *Gyüshi* text itself (J. Gyatso 2004: 86). And as Chui explains, some of these texts contain 'novel information on the diagnosis and treatment of disease, which reflects perspectives of medical practices within their social, cultural and political contexts' (2019: 87). In addition, with the *Gyüshi* text dense and written in verse, as Janes notes, it is 'open to multiple interpretations', and these commentaries are thus key to much medical practice. And over time, differences in training and practice in different geographical regions have produced numerous medical traditions that may vary significantly 'according to individual teacher-student relationships' (Janes 1995: 13). Indeed, this was likely to be particularly the case when many medical practitioners studied medicine on a one-to-one teacher–student basis rather than in medical colleges or at universities, as is the norm today.

Nonetheless, across different traditions and regions, there are significant similarities, including diagnostic techniques focused on pulse analysis, urine analysis and/or questioning of the patient; the use of medicinal formulae containing plant, mineral and animal-derived ingredients; and external therapies including massage, moxibustion, bloodletting and herbal baths. Practitioners may specialize in different aspects of medicine – for example, only diagnosing through urine analysis, or becoming particularly well-known for moxibustion, or making their own medical formulae – but overall, there is much commonality in medical theory and practice.

Key in Tibetan medical theory – and in any discussions with Tibetan medicine doctors – are the three *nyépa* ('energies' or 'faults'): *lung* (wind), *tripa* (bile) and *béken* (phlegm). These are perhaps best understood as properties rather than literal substances. For example, Epstein and Topgay explain that the qualities of *lung* can be said to be 'roughness, lightness, coldness, mobility, compactness, and subtleness'; the qualities of *tripa*, 'heat, greasiness, sharpness, lightness, purging, and moistness'; and those of *béken*, 'greasiness, coolness, heaviness, bluntness, softness, firmness, and adhesiveness' (Epstein and Topgay 1982: 69–71). They describe the 'dualistic function' of these *nyépa*: 'when kept in balance they maintain physical and mental health; but when disturbed, increased or decreased, they act as causes of disease' (Ibid.: 69). Thus, the *nyépa* are both 'essential for life and for the continuance of the mind-body complex' but are also 'potential causers of harm' (Ibid.: 70). Additionally, a number of factors named as 'secondary causes' or conditions (Tib. *kyen*) may contribute to the causation of illness: season, spirits, diet and behaviour (*Gyüshi I* 2015: 10).

Within this tripartite system, the *lung* is particularly important: described as the 'king' or 'integrating principle' of the mind-body (Janes 1999b: 394), it is particularly linked to the mind and consciousness – and therefore with the (dys)functioning of the mind, as we shall see in the following chapters. We thus find *nyoné* described in two sections of the *Gyüshi* and *Bumshi* medical texts: under the general category of *lung* illness; and in the section on spirit-caused illnesses, where we encounter description of 'spirits that cause madness' (Tib. *nyo jé gyi dön*). Across these sections, we find a number of diagnostic categories where symptoms such as hallucinations or confusion are listed alongside symptoms such as headache and dizziness.

Buddhism, Bon and Tantra

In the Tibetan Tantric traditions of Buddhism and Bon, the role of wind is again key. Here, multiple canonical and commentarial Tantric texts (known as the *Kangyur* and *Tengyur* respectively) prescribe manipulations of this energy through complex mind-body practices, ultimately aimed at attaining enlightenment. A distinction is made here between the coarse body ('the body of which we are ordinarily aware, composed of the four elements and the substances evolved from them'), subtle body (comprising channels, winds and drops) and very subtle body ('the very subtle fundamental wind in the indestructible drop that serves as the mount of the mind of clear light') (Cozort 1986: 95–96).

Variations of this 'energetic' or 'subtle' body exist in multiple Asian and Western religious and esoteric traditions (Samuel 2014: 33).[21] In Tibetan Tantric traditions, as we will see in the following chapters, we can view this as a 'map' of the body, made up of channels, through which *lung* flows, and energy centres (Tib. *khorlo*, Skt. *cakra*; often referred to in English-language spheres as 'chakras') where these channels intersect. I would agree with Samuel's assertion that, rather than a 'straightforward description' of the body, we are looking instead at a 'structuring', where the different Tantric traditions describe 'slightly different modes of visualizing the system' (1993: 237). In other words, we are talking here about an *instructive*, rather than *descriptive*, 'map' of the body, for the purposes of meditative practice.

There are two collections of Tantric texts in the Tibetan Buddhist traditions: the Old (*Nyingma*) Tantras, initially transmitted from India to Tibet in the eighth and ninth centuries, and New (*Sarma*) Tantras, transmitted from India to Tibet in the eleventh and twelfth centuries. The first are relevant to the Nyingma Buddhist tradition; the second to the Kagyu, Sakya and Gelug traditions. Bon has its own Tantric tradition that it claims derives from different sources, but their background is unclear (Samuel 1993: 228–29), and in reality, there is much overlap between the Buddhist and Bon texts.[22]

As we shall see in Part II, some of the key practices described in these texts are based on enlightened Tantric deities known as *bodhisattva*,[23] with many high-level Buddhist and Bon Tantric practices focused on a practitioner evoking this kind of deity within him/herself as a method for attaining realization. However, Tantric practices are not only individual practices aimed at a practitioner's own enlightenment. They may also be ritual activities performed for the broader community, such as dealing with local spirit afflictions. In such cases, ritual deity practices are public performances, conducted either within a monastery or temple or in a person's home. In this context too, we find mention of *nyoné*. Some Tantric Buddhist texts, for example, include much writing on the causes and treatments of *nyoné* (see for example

Lusthaus 2017: 50); others describe how *nyoné* might be caused and treated through meditative practices (see Marek and Oliphant 2017).

And finally, the *lama nyonpa* ('mad yogin' or 'crazy lama') is a well-known Tibetan figure, described by Ardussi and Epstein as '[o]ne of the most fascinating characters that runs through the oral and literary traditions of Tibet' (1978: 327). Historical figures such as the fourteenth–fifteenth-century Madman of Tsang and Madman of Ü may be fondly described by contemporary Tibetans despite behaving in ways very unusual for religious practitioners, such as 'drinking to excess, fornicating, thieving, defying authority, playing magical tricks' (Ibid.). In fact, we are told that these strange men (and occasionally women) were not behaving this way because they were suffering from an illness of madness, but because they were *enlightened*: seeing beyond the samsaric divisions of 'good' versus 'bad', 'pure' and 'impure', they behave accordingly.

Entanglements of 'Medicine' and 'Religion'

The spheres of medicine and religion have long been interlinked in Tibetan perspectives[24] – with, for example, the necessity of ritual treatments for some conditions described in the *Gyüshi* and other medical texts,[25] and various illnesses and their potential treatments described in some of the Buddhist and Bon Tantras. Moreover, in the Tibetan medical tradition, the three *nyépa* of *lung*, *tripa* and *béken* are said to arise from the three 'poisons' (Tib. *duk sum*) of the Dharmic traditions: attachment, hatred/aversion and delusion. In addition, the authorship of the *Gyüshi* was traditionally attributed to the Medicine Buddha, Bhaiṣajyaguru, and its written style suggests a traditional Buddhist teaching between a buddha and the interlocutor, as in Tantric texts (Samuel 2001b: 256; see also Ga 2010: 152–53 and J. Gyatso 2015: 141–91).[26] Equally, the *Bumshi* is said by Bonpos to have been taught by the buddha Tonpa Shenrab to his son Tribu Trishi; the text then passed on 'through the medical lineage in Tazig and Zhang Zhung, eventually to be translated into Tibetan at the time of the second king of Tibet, Mutri Tsenpo', with Yutok Yonten Gonpo said to have 'transformed the *Bumshi* into the *Gyüshi*' (Millard 2013a: 356). Indeed, one Bon medical practitioner Millard spoke to within a Tibetan Bon community in Dhortapan, Nepal, described the *Gyüshi* as a 'Buddhist reworking' of the Bon medical text (2005 and 2006: 7).[27]

However, the relationship between these medical and religious traditions has varied throughout history, and it is clear that discussions and disagreements about the compatibility of the medical and Tantric approaches to mind-body date back centuries (J. Gyatso 2015). For example, Janet Gyatso has described a deliberate process of 'Buddhicization' of the medical tradition, which was assisted by some of the existing commonalities between the two traditions.[28] In the contemporary arena, in some regions we find practitioners who span the spheres of medicine and religion (see, for example, Besch's work in Spiti, India, where he describes several Tibetan medicine doctors who were also renowned ritual specialists [2006], and Millard's description of Bon doctors in Kailash, for whom religion was an 'important component of medical practice' [2013a: 377]). In others, these spheres may be quite distinct in terms of training and practice – with contemporary Tibetan medicine doctors usually studying in universities, and religious practitioners training and working separately in religious institutions.[29]

Therefore, in many contemporary Tibetan communities in both the People's Republic of China (PRC) and beyond, lay people, Tibetan medicine doctors and religious specialists often mediate between multiple explanatory frameworks. Here, we cannot always draw strict boundaries between so-called 'medical' and 'religious' practices, practitioners or approaches to mind-body. J. Gyatso describes 'overlap and fuzzy borders' between the medical and religious systems (2015: 101),[30] and previous field researchers have described a complex picture of interrelationships between religion, Tibetan medicine and biomedicine[31] in contemporary Tibetan communities and institutions. Working in Amdo, Schrempf, for example, described 'variations in the way in which "religion" and "medicine" are either treated separately, overlap or are combined', noting that while there are certainly some healing practices that belong 'exclusively to one of the two different domains of "religion" and "medicine", in training and expertise', these are often combined in diverse ways in healing and health-seeking behaviour (2011: 163).[32] And during my own time in Amdo in 2018–19, I saw how these factors can differ by institution: in state-affiliated Tibetan medicine hospitals, for example, 'religious' practices were not allowed; in contrast, independent medical institutions had more freedom to choose how they were run, and I witnessed one group of Tibetan medicine doctors and nurses starting their work day with their daily recitation of a Buddhist prayer.

Many of those I spoke to in Amdo described consulting multiple healing practitioners, either concurrently or in sequence, and discussed health and illness using a range of concepts from diverse medical and healing systems. Here, traditional Tibetan notions of mind-body, health and illness often sat alongside some biomedical terminology and concepts. This kind of 'pluralistic' approach in health-seeking behaviour is not unusual of course (see, for example, Hepburn 1988), and this was evident in my previous research within Tibetan communities in Darjeeling too (Deane 2018). As Schrempf has described in her own research in the Amdo region, illness can affect 'all levels of the body – the individual, social, environmental and cosmological'.

With this perspective, exploring healing in multiple ways concurrently might simply be the 'most efficacious' approach (2011: 177). Schrempf references Samuel's notion of the 'mind-body-society-environment context' to illness and healing (Samuel 2006: 123). Indeed, we see this in the Tibetan medical texts' descriptions of multiple causative and contributory factors for a case of illness – including, for example, disturbance in the *nyépa* (both causing and contributing to particular mental states) and spirit afflictions (sometimes related to a person's interaction with the environment). This kind of approach is often even more evident 'on the ground' in Tibetan communities, as people navigate their way through an experience of illness.

We will see this in some of the narratives within these chapters, as we hear how lay Tibetans, and religious and medical specialists, discuss cases of *nyoné* and other conditions. And I would argue that this pluralistic approach to illness and healing is perhaps even more likely in the context of a condition such as *nyoné*, which may be hard to make sense of and particularly worrying and/or frightening for an afflicted person and their family – especially if the situation is acute. Moreover, in a medically pluralistic arena such as contemporary Amdo, where individuals and their families may have a plethora of healing practitioners and practices to choose from, health-seeking behaviour will necessarily be complex and nuanced, as we shall see in the following chapters. Here, factors such as reputation and previous experience will sit alongside issues of cost and accessibility – both geographical and practical (for example, in relation to language knowledge)[33] – contributing to decision-making. Thus, Craig describes how, in contemporary China, a combination of the Chinese model of rural cooperative medicine and major developments in transport and other infrastructure has significantly increased access to both biomedical and Tibetan medical services for people in rural areas (2012: 144). In addition, working in the region in 2005–7, Schrempf found that, for some patients, perceived notions of efficacy and trust may be more significant than any thoughts about what tradition or medical system a healer is practising (2011: 159, 165). For example, Nianggajia reported many Tibetan and non-Tibetans preferring to consult private Tibetan medicine clinics, whose (often senior) doctors were seen to be 'more experienced, learned, and easily approachable' (2015: 228), or even 'much more empathetic towards their patients' and 'more approachable after hours' than their biomedical counterparts (Ibid.: 227). There are also questions around the impact of health insurance (specifically the New Cooperative Medical Scheme, instituted in 2003), which were rarely mentioned by my interviewees but which probably influence people's health-seeking behaviours.[34]

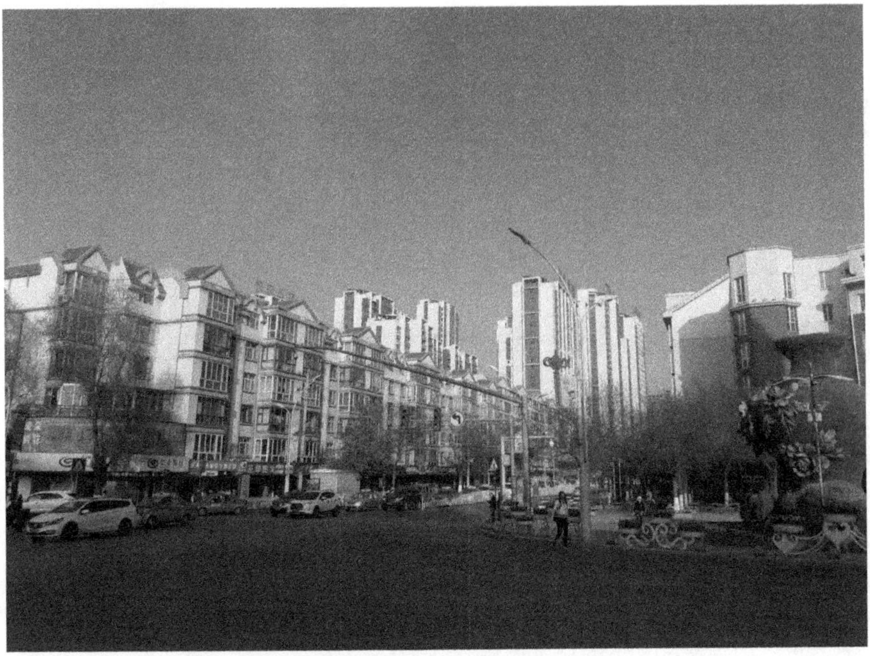

Figure 0.1. Downtown Xining, 2018. © Susannah Deane.

Working in Amdo

I spent twelve months conducting ethnographic research in Amdo in 2018–19. Traditionally one of the three major regions of Tibet (Amdo in the northeast, Kham in the east and U-Tsang in the centre and west), this area now spans parts of Qinghai, Gansu and Sichuan provinces. Granted visiting-researcher status at Minzu University of China in Beijing, I was granted permission to conduct fieldwork in Qinghai, allowing me to base myself in Xining, its capital city, and travel around the region freely on buses, trains, flights and taxis. During this time, I had the opportunity to inhabit multiple spaces and visit diverse medical and religious institutions, among other places, sometimes moving between related roles of 'participant' and 'observer' at locations, events and in clinics as well as conducting a number of in-depth interviews with a broad range of people residing in the area.

Amdo is a particularly interesting region. In Xining, I experienced the busyness and comforts of living in what is a comparably small city in northwest China (see Figure 0.1).[35] Its inhabitants mostly live – as I did – in tall apartment blocks in large residential complexes across the different areas of the city, travelling to school, university or work on the many city buses or

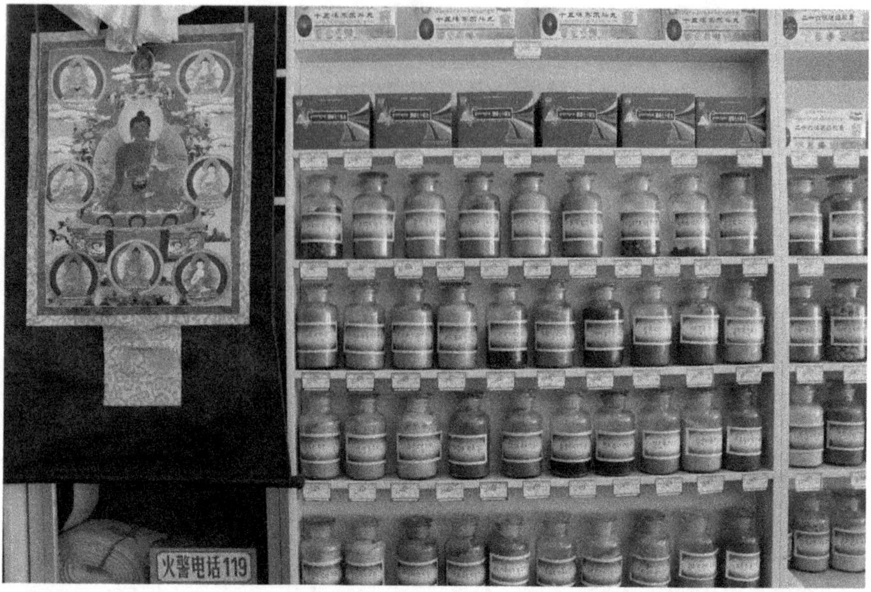

Figure 0.2. Tibetan medicines in a private Tibetan medicine hospital pharmacy in Rebkong, 2019. © Susannah Deane.

taxis; shopping in street markets and the rapidly multiplying, large shopping centres; drinking coffee and tea in local- or foreign-owned cafes; and eating out in the multitude of Chinese, Tibetan and Muslim restaurants.

The Tibetan population makes up a minority of Xining's inhabitants, but Tibetan communities and their traditions are evident across the city – in the large, state-affiliated and private Tibetan medicine hospitals where inpatients and outpatients can receive traditional Tibetan medical formulae (see Figure 0.2), as well as external therapies such as herbal baths;[36] in shops and market stalls selling Tibetan Buddhist statues and temple decorations; on the street stalls where Tibetan men and women sell fresh yak-milk yoghurt every evening. From Tibetan friends, I heard about practitioners working within and across related Tibetan healing traditions. Here, discussions about *nyoné* were not uncommon: almost all of the people I interviewed in Amdo described at least one person – whether a close relative or a member of their local community – who had experienced this, and both friends and interviewees often spoke at length about this topic.

I also spent a lot of my time in the region of Rebkong (Ch. Tongren). Around 180 km or two hours south from Xining, this is the capital of Malho (Ch. Huangnan) Tibetan Autonomous Prefecture. Here, Buddhist monasteries and temples are spread in the main town and out across the Rebkong valley in multiple Tibetan towns and villages. Nianggajia references pre-publication 2015 census data that describes a total population of 89,654 in Rebkong county, of which Tibetans are the predominant ethnic group (72.94%), with smaller populations of Mongour (11.8%), Han Chinese (8.83%), Hui (3.86%), Salar (1.68%), and others (Nianggajia 2015: 223). A majority of this Tibetan population belongs to the Gelug Buddhist tradition (Millard 2013b: 143), with smaller Nyingma Buddhist and Bon populations.

The large Gelugpa Buddhist monastery at Rongwo (Rongwo Gonchen [rong bo dgon chen]) dates to 1342 (Dhondup 2011a), and Rebkong is home to the second largest Bon community in Amdo (Millard 2013b: 147).[37] Millard references a 1996 survey of Bon monasteries in Qinghai by the Tibetan scholar Tsering Thar (2003), which counted '46 Bon villages in the Rebkong area comprising around 691 families with a total population of 4368', in addition to approximately 4,000 nomadic people who are 'connected with the area and who also follow the Bon religion' (Millard 2013b: 148). Easily accessible from Xining by bus, Rebkong's majority Tibetan population meant that it was easy to meet people and recruit interviewees here, as Tibetan friends and acquaintances suggested people they thought might be able to help me in my research, and invited me to visit religious and medical institutions in the town and surrounding area. I thus spent a considerable amount of time there, staying in local hotels, visiting religious sites and getting to know people living and working in the town or in the villages of the surrounding valley.

Notable in Rebkong is its significant *ngakpa* community. In a 2018 paper, Sihlé estimated approximately 2,000 of these practitioners across the Rebkong Nyingma Buddhist and Bon communities (2018: 162). Often referred to locally as *hön*, these Tantric practitioners can trace their history back to the ninth century (Dhondup 2011a: 47–49)[38] and can be identified by their long (often dreadlocked) hair and their white, or red and white, robes. Ritual specialists, *ngakpa* are often consulted by members of the lay community for purposes such as controlling the weather and treating illnesses suspected to be caused by spirits. This is because, while both celibate monastic practitioners and *ngakpa* are trained in the practice of Tantric rituals, the latter are viewed as the 'pre-eminent specialists' for 'powerful and/or violent' ritual forms (Sihlé 2018: 162). Dhondup describes twelve to eighteen years' study for these practitioners, involving 'rigorous training and practice in reciting mantras, meditation, readings, receiving esoteric instructions and transmissions and undertaking solitary retreats' (2011a: 14), and in Rebkong it was common to see many of these practitioners around the town.

Both Xining and the Rebkong valley are culturally and medically pluralistic areas, and the region of Amdo as a whole has for a long time been a place of contact between diverse cultures (Samuel 2013a: 6), with questions of ethnicity rather complex across the different communities of Tibetan, Han,

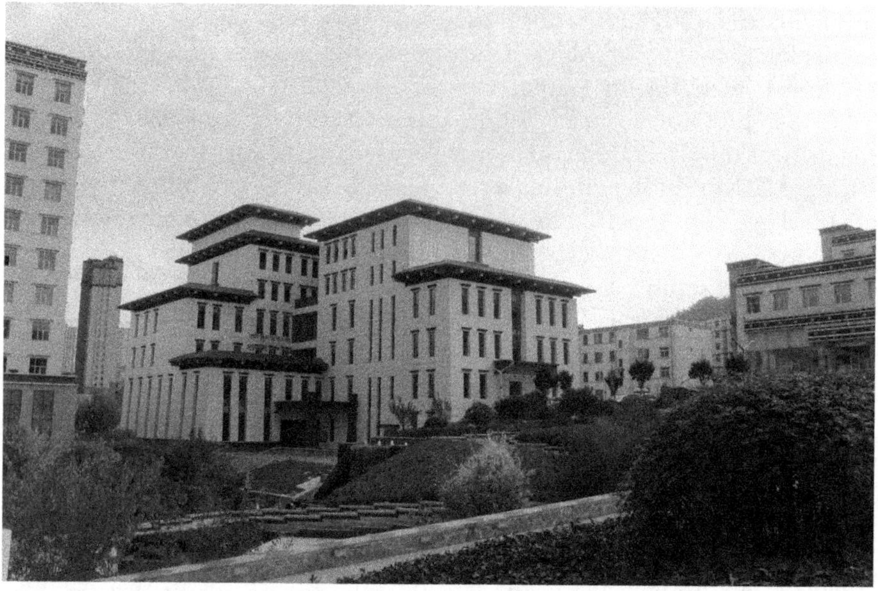

Figure 0.3. Qinghai Province Tibetan Medicine Hospital, Xining 2018. © Susannah Deane.

Hui, Salar, Mongol and Tu populations.[39] In addition, many of the Tibetans I spoke to in the area were notably mobile. Often working and living in different places (for example, living in Rebkong and working during the week in Xining, or vice versa; or spending term time teaching in a school in a small town miles from where they lived the rest of their time in Rebkong), or living in the city but speaking frequently of their 'home town' – often hundreds of miles away in another area of Amdo. In addition, I was also able to spend some time in Golok, staying with a friend who kindly invited me to stay with her in her home town after we initially met in Xining, and also to visit some other towns in the Amdo region, where I was able to conduct several interviews.

Amdo is home to a large number of medical institutions and practitioners. Xining boasts the large state-affiliated Qinghai Province Tibetan Medicine Hospital (Tso ngon Shing chen Bö Men Khang, see Figure 0.3),[40] founded in 1983, as well as a large private Tibetan medicine hospital and numerous smaller Tibetan medicine clinics. Smaller towns and villages were home to smaller Tibetan medicine hospitals and clinics; Rebkong, for example, had several private Tibetan medicine hospitals[41] (including one situated at the main Rongwo Monastery [see Figure 0.4])[42] as well as a state-affiliated Tibetan medicine hospital, the Malho Prefecture Tibetan Hospital. In fact, Rebkong has a rich history of Tibetan medicine, with a number of renowned

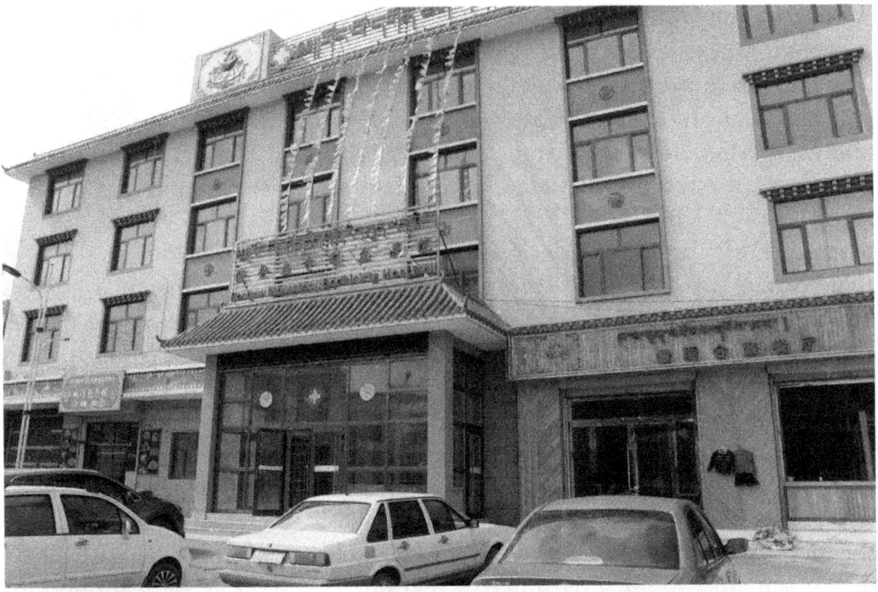

Figure 0.4. Rongwo Monastery Bodhicitta Hospital, 2018. © Susannah Deane.

Tibetan medicine doctors and generations of 'lineage physicians' (Tib. *men gyud*) originating in this region, as well as 'scholar-physicians' who played a key role in 'building up Rebgong as a centre for traditional Tibetan medicine in the late eighteenth and nineteenth centuries' (Nianggajia 2015: 222–24).[43]

There are also multiple biomedical hospitals and clinics in the area. In Amdo, biomedicine was usually referred to by Tibetans as 'Chinese medicine' (Tib. *ja men*) in contrast to Traditional Chinese Medicine (TCM), which was referred to as 'Chinese herbal medicine' (Tib. *ja tsa men*).[44] Among the numerous biomedical hospitals and clinics in Xining, for example, was the Qinghai Province Third People's Hospital Psychiatric Consultation Center – commonly known as the Number Three Hospital – a biomedical psychiatric facility. Moreover, today, many 'Tibetan medicine hospitals' also include a certain degree of biomedicine. For example, use of sphygmomanometers to measure patients' blood pressure is common during consultation with Tibetan medicine doctors, and in the Qinghai Province Tibetan Medicine Hospital, for example, some doctors also used ECG, X-ray, MRI, CT, CRDR, TCD and ultrasound machines. This pluralistic approach to practice can be seen in record-keeping too, where Craig has described, for example, Tibetan language used to record diagnoses and 'specific indications of medicines' and Chinese language used to record prescriptions and lab tests at the hospital (2012: 69). Moreover, sometimes biomedical medications were used in 'Tibetan medicine' hospitals too, as we shall see in Chapter 2. Indeed, Schrempf notes that the administration of biomedical injections and antibiotic drugs is common practice in 'most' Tibetan medicine clinics and hospitals (2015: 279). In these modern hospitals, departments are usually divided up in a way similar to biomedical hospitals (e.g. Department for Stomach Illnesses and Indigestion, and Department for Liver and Gall Bladder Diseases), and patient record-keeping is 'meticulously maintained, as required of a government hospital' (Ibid.: 296).[45]

Particularly interesting in relation to my research topic was the fact that, before my arrival in Amdo, the Qinghai Province Tibetan Medicine Hospital in Xining had had a specific department for severe mental illness, the Department for Wind Illnesses and Impurities (Tib. Lung Né Drip Tsen Khak), operational between 2014 and 2017. It had closed down by the time I arrived in early 2018, but I was able to interview Dr Dechen, one of the Tibetan medicine doctors who had worked there during that time. Dr Dechen explained that the facility had been aimed predominantly at patients with *nyoné*, and had been staffed by six doctors — five Tibetan medicine doctors (of Tibetan ethnicity) and one Han Chinese doctor who specialized in biomedicine – and seven nurses. There had been space for a number of inpatients, who were treated with a combination of Tibetan medicine medicinal compounds and external therapies such as herbal compresses and massage.

During my twelve months in Amdo, as spring turned to summer, and then autumn sun gave way to winter snows, I was able to conduct in-depth, semi-structured interviews with twenty-nine lay Tibetans, aged 20 to 72; eleven religious specialists (Buddhist and Bon monastic and lay practitioners as well as one spirit-medium); and ten Tibetan medicine doctors.[46] A couple of these practitioners straddled the interrelated spheres of 'medicine' and 'religion', trained and practising as both Tibetan medicine doctors and *ngakpa* ritual or monastic specialists. Others spanned these spheres less 'officially', such as a few Tibetan medicine doctors who described studying with Buddhist teachers they knew personally to a greater or lesser degree, out of their own interest to supplement their medical knowledge. Religious specialist interviewees were predominantly from Buddhist Nyingma and Gelug communities, with just one Bon practitioner – a lama at a local Bon monastery – among my Amdo interviewees.

Interviewees were recruited through snowball sampling: starting with three Tibetan and foreign friends/acquaintances, and a few 'cold calls', I was able to meet a diversity of practitioners and lay people through both Tibetan and non-Tibetan formal and informal networks in the area. In addition, aiming to interview male and female Tibetans from urban and rural areas, across a range of ages and occupations, I recruited interviewees situated in a variety of communities predominantly within Xining and/or Rebkong, working in (or retired from) diverse sectors including teaching, technology and business, as well as a few university students studying in the city. I also interviewed a handful of lay people and practitioners in other regions of Amdo, including Golok and Chabcha. This method of sampling is not perfect, of course, and has the potential to lead to some sample bias. However, in initiating my approaches across a variety of communities, I was able to meet, talk to and interview a fairly broad range of people. Indeed, with this kind of exploratory research, where we are not looking for definitive 'answers', this approach allowed me to start building up a picture of the diversity of perspectives on the topic at hand.

All of these people were kind enough to give me their time to discuss this fascinating topic. One Tibetan medicine doctor invited me to sit in on one of his clinics for a morning, chatting about different conditions and his many decades of experience in between patient consultations. Another invited me to try one of the external therapies on offer at his private Tibetan medicine hospital, and I found myself lying in a traditional 'sand bath' alongside a local Tibetan patient on a Saturday morning in November, while nurses and other interested onlookers appeared around the door intermittently to see what a foreigner made of this traditional Tibetan medical treatment.

Some of these Amdo Tibetans – the majority of whom I met and got to know during these twelve months – became friends. They gave their time generously to speak at length not only about my research topic but also about broader aspects of Tibetan culture and their own life experiences, introducing me to colleagues, friends and relatives whom they thought I might be interested to meet – and inviting me along to religious events, friendly teas, lunches and dinners, and to spend time with them and their families in their homes. One Tibetan friend collated groups of her colleagues to answer questions and chat about my research and related topics over endless pots of tea – creating a sort of 'focus group', where I was able to listen as they discussed and debated different ideas about mind, body, health, illness and *nyoné*, observing how my questions could highlight differing perspectives from those hailing from different geographical regions. Here, my role segued from observer to participant, to friend and back again – again and again. I tried to reciprocate this generosity however I could; more often than not, this involved English assistance, helping people with English-language questions, documents and proof-reading whenever asked. I thought often of the privilege of being a native English speaker in this globalized world, and gave assistance to those who asked for it where I could. In Xining, I answered a call out on a local WeChat group to volunteer a couple of hours every other week for a semi-organized English conversation session with a group of Tibetan Masters students at a university campus across the city. I hoped this was useful for them; of course, it also provided another window for me into diverse Tibetan lives in the city.

With my own interdisciplinary background spanning the spheres of psychology, medical anthropology and religious studies, and an awareness of the lack of research on this topic, I did not take a specific disciplinary approach to this endeavour. This allowed me to gather a broad range of perspectives and thoughts on the topics at hand. Indeed, rather than attempting to gain some definitive answer to questions about causes and treatments of madness in Tibetan understanding, for example, I aimed instead to explore the diversity evident in the perspectives of lay people and religious and medical specialists, to start to map out different understandings of the concept of *nyoné*, and to explore the overlapping and diverging threads that run through them.

And as the winds of ethnography change for the better, and we aim to increase reflexivity in our practice, questions of ownership and sharing of knowledge are particularly pertinent when working within Tibetan communities in the PRC. Conducting fieldwork anywhere within contemporary China can be complicated – particularly when focusing on an official minority group. The extra caution needed in this region prevents the naming of those who shared so much of their time, thoughts, knowledge and experiences with me for the benefit of this work. Certainly, this work would not have been possible without the generosity of a network of Amdo-wa who made this project not only *possible* but also enjoyable. Even when conducting research on a subject that is not obviously politically sensitive, it is still wise to take extra care here. In practice, this included my never raising 'politically sensitive' topics in casual conversations or interviews, and being aware of surroundings and navigating conversations carefully if these topics should be raised by those I was speaking to. However, 'being careful' is not always a simple matter – as Hofer has described in relation to her work in the Tibet Autonomous Region (TAR), 'politically sensitive' topics are often 'not clearly defined or openly articulated; rather they have to be figured out and one's behaviors constantly adjusted' (2018: 25). As Yeh has explained, in this kind of environment 'all interactions and relationships are shaped to some extent by wariness of political trouble', undoubtably shaping the research (2006: 97). In this context, she argues, a 'politics of fear' will produce 'subjects who internalize surveillance' (Ibid.). Yeh was working in Lhasa, and while this issue is certainly less pronounced in Tibetan communities outside of the TAR, it still needs to be considered. In Amdo, approaching my field research with care meant always thinking not only about what was safe to talk about – and of course, commit to published material – at the time that I was there, but always also with an eye to the future, and considering how these parameters might shift. One result of this, of course, is the anonymization of all of my interviewees' and friends' names and no reference to specific villages or monasteries with which they were affiliated, except where these were particularly large institutions.[47] And in fact, while Tibetan friends in the area did sometimes discuss sensitive topics including the ongoing political situation within the PRC with me, this was generally not mentioned in relation to mental health in our discussions.[48]

Through these many encounters and experiences, I was able to build up a picture of the multiple ways in which 'madness' can be understood within these contemporary Tibetan communities in Amdo. My position as an interviewer, foreigner and friend no doubt both helped and hindered this exploration in different ways at different times – probably sometimes in a manner invisible to me. As the field started to 'take shape' for me, the field itself was also shaped by my interactions with it, as Rapport suggests (1997: 179). My linguistic shortcomings – having previously studied and worked in the Lhasa dialect of Tibetan, I was now learning the very different Amdo dialect through one-to-one lessons with a local teacher – no doubt impacted on this too. Some conversations were conducted directly between myself and an interviewee or friend – either entirely in Tibetan, entirely in English or a mixture of the two, depending on our mix of language abilities. Many interviews – particularly those with medical and religious specialists – required the aid of an interpreter, which undoubtably impacted on the nature of the encounter. Interviews were usually recorded, with permission, allowing me to re-listen to explanations of Tibetan medical and religious concepts and their complex relationships, and to double-check translations – indeed, my interpreter often described unfamiliarity with some of these religious and medical terms. Where my interlocutor used Tibetan terms like *nyoné* and *nying* (whether in a Tibetan-language conversation or in a predominantly English-language conversation but with Tibetan terms interspersed), I have kept these in Tibetan in these pages. Where they used English terms like 'madness', 'crazy' and 'heart illness', I too have used the English as they did. Dialogues are presented either unedited or edited minimally to aid readability (after translation). We can see, then, how my interlocutors translated or didn't translate these terms themselves. My interview questions developed, expanded and refined as I spoke to more and more people, interweaving data collection, hypothesis construction and theory building, as has been described by Silverman (2000: 143), and taking me back to some interviewees when my growing knowledge led to further questions.

Within this process, I tried to keep my questions as open as possible, to record and translate people's responses in a way that represented the diversity of perspectives I encountered as accurately as possible. As I was not attempting to interview inpatients or outpatients at clinics or hospitals, when speaking to lay individuals about concepts of mind-body, health and illness, information was self-reported outside of any clinical context. I have included interviewees' ages and home towns/residences to provide some context to these different perspectives. It will become clear just how complex this notion of *nyoné* is, informed by multiple medical and religious perspectives of mind-body across different traditions – and sometimes different geographical areas.

In addition, I have explored various descriptions of madness in Tibetan medical and religious texts. With different Tantric traditions focusing on different texts – some shared between the traditions, others exclusive to one in particular – there can be significant differences between them. Thus, rather than attempt to present an exhaustive list of the mentions and discussions across all Tibetan texts (an impossible task!), I have tried to include instead a range of texts from different Tibetan Tantric traditions. With my spoken Modern Colloquial Tibetan much better than my Classical Tibetan, for Tantric texts I have predominantly relied on Tibetan Buddhist and Bon texts that have already been translated into English, and more recent works written in English by Tibetan religious and medical scholars of the last century. Of course, this approach has limitations, but I hope that it allows us to start exploring some of the key ways in which 'madness' is discussed and described by Tibetan medical and religious scholars, and to get a flavour of some of the ideas and themes that recur again and again, as well as some which seem rather more idiosyncratic. Indeed, in drawing from a number of different Tantric historical and recent canonical and commentarial texts, I aim to show a range of perspectives that demonstrate some similarities and differences in how this topic is understood. I hope that future research will build on this initial work to bring more light on this topic through the exploration of more texts and further ethnographic research.

Thus, over the following chapters, we will see how different notions of 'madness' across religion and medicine converge and diverge to illustrate overlapping Tibetan Tantric and medical notions of mind-body structure and (dys)functioning, how this plays out in some contemporary Tibetan communities in the Amdo region, and how these contemporary perspectives sit alongside what we find in some of the multiple medical and religious texts in these interrelated Tibetan traditions.

The book is arranged across two parts, with Part I focusing predominantly on the Tibetan concept of 'wind' and its place in Tibetan medicine and Tantra in the context of *nyoné*, and Part II focusing on Tibetan perspectives on the role of spirits and deities in *nyoné* specifically, and health, illness and Tantric practice more broadly. With this in mind, each part opens with a chapter focused on ethnographic findings from Amdo, aimed at explicating the complex picture in some contemporary Tibetan communities through an exploration of multiple perspectives.

Chapter 1 explores the diverse ways in which notions of 'wind' and 'heart' were discussed in relation to the mind and to madness in Amdo, based on interview material from Tibetan religious and medical specialists as well as lay

Tibetans. Here, overlapping Tibetan Tantric and medical notions of mind-body are brought into play to explain diverse cases of *nyoné*, its causation and treatment by both medical and religious means, encompassing ideas about 'heart illness' (e.g. sadness, depression) and 'wind illness' – caused by factors including Tantric practice.

Chapter 2 focuses on 'wind' in the Tibetan medical tradition, exploring the different ways in which disruptions in its flow can be both a cause and a consequence of illness affecting the mind and/or body, as is described in the *Gyüshi* text and by contemporary and historical Tibetan medicine doctors, including those I spoke to in Amdo. It becomes evident that connections between 'wind', 'heart' and 'mind' are key to understanding the diverse range of causes, symptoms and treatments in different forms of 'wind illness' – including *nyoné* – in Tibetan medical perspectives.

In Chapter 3, we investigate the role of 'wind' in Tibetan Buddhist and Bon Tantra, exploring the key relationship between wind and concepts of *bodhicitta* ('mind of enlightenment'), and examining practices focused on the manipulation of particular winds through the body and mind in pursuit of enlightenment. With such practices often described as highly complex and difficult, I explore textual and ethnographic discussions on 'madness caused by practice', wherein the possibility of achieving enlightenment is counter-balanced by the potential for mental and physical harms – including *nyoné* – that may result from conducting them incorrectly. This chapter also considers the figure of the *lama nyonpa* ('mad yogin'), common in Tibetan historical narratives and contemporary discourse. These individuals – usually described as 'acting crazy' – are, in fact, understood by many to be enlightened – behaving the way they do as a result of their higher realization.

In Part II, Chapter 4 situates us firmly back in Amdo, exploring contemporary Amdo narratives of spirits, deities and 'impurities'/'pollution' and their role in the causation of *nyoné*. Here, we explore Amdo perspectives on interrelationships between lay people, spirits, gods and highly accomplished Buddhist and Bon practitioners, and the treatment of spirit-caused illnesses in medical and religious spheres.

Chapter 5 focuses on Tibetan perspectives on the role of 'uninvited' spirits, deities and impurities in causing madness, and their treatment via medical and/or religious means, according to both textual material and the perspectives of contemporary practitioners. Here, we explore the different kinds of spirits and deities that may be involved – via the inadvertent 'offending' of local deities or family gods or through possession by local spirits, some of which are described in the *Gyüshi*. It becomes evident that the 'madness-causing spirits' described in Tibetan medical texts form only part of the picture, in an arena where ritual treatment may be viewed as more effective than any 'medical' treatment.

In Chapter 6, we explore the role of spirits and deities in Tibetan Tantric practices, and the ways in which these may be implicated in the causation of *nyoné*. There are a number of different ways in which religious practitioners may engage with enlightened and unenlightened spirits and deities in Tibetan religious traditions, and explanations of 'madness' often focus on narratives of a Tantric practitioner conducting practices 'incorrectly' – for example, without proper instruction and/or appropriate initiation. In addition, we briefly explore here the practices of Tibetan figures such as spirit-mediums and oracles, who take possession of unenlightened deities in order to perform ritual services for their community such as divination and/or healing – sometimes also treating cases of madness caused by spirits. Key here are Tibetan notions of 'spiritual power' and the ability of practitioners to overcome any 'doubts' about the practice, or the limitations of the unenlightened mind.

Finally, a short Conclusion draws together the common threads that run through the ethnographic findings from Amdo and the medical and Tantric textual material, to consider a complex picture of Tibetan perspectives on *nyoné*. Bringing these multiple medical and Tantric notions of 'madness' together for the first time, we see that despite the evident diversity of perspectives, there are significant connections between the different manifestations of this condition – and these are related to fundamental Tibetan notions of not only mind and body but also individuals' relationships to the wider world, and the spirits and deities understood to reside within it. It becomes clear how notions of the illness of 'madness' and of 'enlightenment' are interconnected through these longstanding Tibetan medical and religious understandings of mind, body and universe.

Notes

1. See, for example, descriptions in the eleventh edition of the *International Classification of Disease* (ICD-11) (World Health Organization 2018).
2. In addition, in everyday reality, *nyoné* can also be used to refer to a broader range of illness by non-specialists: in Amdo, for example, I encountered a handful people using it to refer to the separate category of *za* illness (usually interpreted as epilepsy) and conditions that sounded like cognitive disabilities.
3. The full title of the text is often given as *bdud rtsi snying po yan lag brgyad pa gsang ba man ngag gi rgyud*, although in practice the title varies somewhat between different editions.
4. A general Tibetan term for this would be *sem né* – literally 'mind illness' or 'illness of the mind' – and it carries broadly similar notions as the English term 'mental illness'.
5. For an exploration of the variety of ways that 'Bon' and related terms are used in ethnically Tibetan and other Himalayan communities across Tibet, India, Nepal and Bhutan, see Samuel 2013b. The situation has also been complicated by early European misinter-

pretations of Tibetan religion, whereby 'Bon' became 'a repository for all the elements of Tibetan religion which did not appear to derive from the somewhat idealized pictures of Indian Buddhism prevailing at that time' (Samuel 2013b: 79), as well as Tibetan Buddhists' prejudice against the Bon community (Norbu 1981: 22).

6. See, for example, work by des Jardins (2009), Helman-Ważny and Ramble (2023), Huber (2020), Orofino (2015), Punzi (2021) and Thar (2008). For general explorations of Bon traditions, see Karmay (1972, 1998 and 2005), Karmay and Watt (2007), Kvaerne (1995) and Snellgrove (1967).
7. For more on Bon history and identity, see Blezer (2011), Karmay (1998 and 2005), Kvaerne (1995, 2000), Thar (2000), Van Schaik (2013).
8. It is worth noting, however, that Tonpa Shenrab is described quite differently in different Bon texts composed in different eras (Bellezza 2010).
9. For in-depth explorations of contemporary Bon medical practitioners, see Millard (2005 and 2006, 2013a) and Schrempf (2007).
10. Interestingly, there are significant Bon medical lineages documented by Schrempf in Nagchu (2007) and Millard in western Tibet and Kham (2013a), although 'very few' Bon family medical lineages in Amdo (Millard 2013a: 370).
11. In Rebkong, for example, Dhondup describes villages where a non-monastic 'Tantric Hall' (*ngak khang*) is used by both Nyingma Buddhist and Bon Tantric practitioners, with Buddhist statues on one side and Bon on the other (2013: 126).
12. Literally 'precious one', this term is used to refer to someone recognized as the rebirth of an earlier, distinguished Dharma practitioner.
13. Samuel notes the use of the term 'heart-mind', for example, which perhaps indicates better the complexity of the concept and the related terms such as *yi*, *sem*, *tuk* (emotions) and *namshé* in Tibetan understanding (2014: 33). Here, I will use the term 'mind' due the differential use of the concept of 'heart' (Tib. *nying*) in this context, as we shall see.
14. In fact, there are three types of *la* said to circulate in the body (Millard 2005 and 2006: 13–14). See Gerke (2007 and 2012) and Karmay (1998) for more on the Tibetan notion of *la*. Gerke describes this as a 'subtle life-essence' that supports the '*sok*' – 'life itself', or 'vital force' (2012: 7). A person's *la* may be lost due to a shock (stories of which I heard occasionally in Amdo) or stolen by spirits. Once lost/stolen, ritual is usually required to bring it back to the person.
15. For example, Drungtso explains, 'The earth element functions to maintain the solidity of the body, Water element functions to maintain the fluid level of the body, Fire element maintains the heat level of the body, Wind element maintains proper flow of the blood and movements of the limbs. The space element is responsible for providing room for further development' (2004: 141).
16. Often referred to as Sowa Rigpa (lit. 'science/knowledge of healing'), this term is a commonly used name for Tibetan medical traditions as they are practised across the Himalayan region. However, in Amdo, Tibetans generally referred to this simply as 'Tibetan medicine' (*bö men*), and so this is how I will refer to the tradition in this work. In the People's Republic of China (PRC), Tibetan medicine officially comes under the umbrella of Chinese medicine (http://lv.china-embassy.gov.cn/eng/zt/zgxz/200605/t20060509_2913740.htm [retrieved 14 May 2023]). In exile, the main medical authority is the government-in-exile-affiliated Men-Tsee-Khang Tibetan Medical & Astro Institute based in Dharamsala, India (https://mentseekhang.org/ [retrieved 14 May 2023]), although there are also a number of other, independent Tibetan medicine institutes. Since 2010, the Government of India has officially recognized Sowa Rigpa as an 'Indian

system of medicine' (Kloos 2016: 20; see also https://www.ccimindia.org.in/sowa-rigpa/ [retrieved 14 May 2023]) and there is also a political dimension to this naming in India, as described by Kloos (2010: 248–50).

17. See Ga for a description of the translation and dissemination of this text, the translated Tibetan version of which spawned a number of teaching lineages in Tibet and which was used as a textbook in numerous medical schools throughout the eleventh to thirteenth centuries (2010: 75–85).
18. As Millard has described, while the standard Buddhist view is that the *Gyüshi* is a translation of a Sanskrit original first taught by the Medicine Buddha and then passed on to Yutok Yonten Gonpo the Younger in the twelfth century, in fact there was also another Tibetan historical tradition started by one of Yutok's disciples, which claimed that the text was in fact *composed* by Yutok Yonten Gonpo the Younger himself (2013a: 355–56).
19. Parts of the *Gyüshi* have been translated into English and German (for example, see Clark 1995; Donden 1997 and Clifford 1984). The Men-Tsee-Khang Documentation and Publication Department's Translation Section has produced translations of the First, Second (Men-Tsee-Khang 2008) and Fourth Tantras (Men-Tsee-Khang 2011), and is currently translating the large Third Tantra in several sections, with the first part published in 2017 (Men-Tsee-Khang 2017).
20. See Millard for a comparison with the four-volume *Bumshi* text, which – with 'the exception of sections dealing with history' – is almost identical (2013a: 357).
21. Note that the term 'subtle body' is not ideal but, due to its common usage across the English-language literature on Tibetan medicine and Tantra, I will continue to use it here. While the term 'subtle body' is often used by Western scholars in the context of Tibetan medical notions of the body, Gerke points out that it does not in fact feature in the *Gyüshi* and argues that it is generally *not* used in this manner by Tibetan doctors, some of whom discuss the 'Vajra body' (Tib. *dorjé lü*, or *ku dor jé*) instead – although this term is also absent from the *Four Tantras.* She asserts instead that there can be said in the Tibetan medicine tradition to be 'several subtle aspects of the body' (2013: 85–86, 95). In addition, as Samuel and Johnston note, the term 'subtle body' became established in English usage in the nineteenth century through those associated with the Theosophical Society, initially as a translation of the Vedantic term *sūkṣmaśarīra* (2013: 2), and therefore remains rather problematic.
22. See Samuel (1993: 228–32) for more on the history and classification of the Tibetan Buddhist and Bon Tantric texts.
23. As Pitkin describes, the status of these figures is actually rather ambiguous: the term *bodhisattva* may refer to 'a supermundane, cosmic Buddha figure personifying an aspect of enlightenment', an 'ordinary human being who has committed to the bodhisattva path through taking vows and is working through the stages of Buddhist practice' or 'an enlightened being who has already perfected the result of the Buddhist path'. In addition, these 'supermundane' beings can incarnate as human – for example, in the case of the Dalai Lama, who is understood to be an incarnation of the Tantric deity Avalokiteśvara (Pitkin 2017: 15).
24. This is not only the case, of course, for the Tibetan traditions; for some examinations of the connections between various Asian Buddhist and medical traditions, see Salguero (2017, 2019) and Salguero, Cheung and Deane (2024).
25. These include, for example, rituals that should be performed to cure diseases caused by spirits, rituals aimed at returning a person's *la* (life-force), and an emphasis on the importance of ritual intervention for some conditions in the section on pulse diagnosis near the

end of Chapter 1 of the *Fourth Tantra* (*Gyüshi IV* 2015: 561). As Millard notes, while the *Gyüshi* and *Bumshi* texts do not describe any healing rituals in detail they *do* 'identify the types of sickness where such rituals should be performed' (2005 and 2006: 26).

26. In reality, it has long been known to many Tibetan scholars that large parts of the *Gyüshi* are translations of the Ayurvedic *Aṣṭāṅgahṛdayasaṃhitā* text (Ga 2010: 85).
27. Where these differ, then, is in their descriptions of medical history and lineage; see Millard (2005 and 2006) for more on this. For a comparison of the titles of the four volumes of the *Gyüshi* and *Bumshi*, see Millard (2013a: 362). As Millard notes, this Bon perspective on Tibetan medical history was 'little known outside Bon communities until recently' as a result of state suppression of the Bon tradition over centuries in Tibet (Ibid.: 256).
28. Gyatso describes, for example, how the historical Buddha's teachings were often 'characterized as a remedy for both the physical and spiritual ailments' – a theme that can be traced from the Pāli Canon, through the developments of the Mahayana tradition, which included texts focused on the Medicine Buddha (J. Gyatso 2015: 98).
29. I explore this topic in more detail in Deane (2024).
30. Janet Gyatso provides a fascinating and very comprehensive exploration of the complex relationship between Tibetan medicine and Buddhism in this 2015 work, which I highly recommend.
31. For more detail on the history of biomedicine in Tibet, see McKay (2007, 2011). Adams and others have explored the complex relationship between Tibetan medicine and biomedicine, and the various factors that have influenced medical training and practice within the PRC in depth (Adams 2001, 2007; Adams, Dhondup and Le 2011; Adams, Schrempf and Craig 2011; Janes 2001) and exile (Gerke 2011). In addition, Hofer's highly important 2018 work explores the narratives of Tibetan medical practitioners' experiences during and after the Cultural Revolution, and the ways in which Tibetan medicine was transformed during that time under government regulations.
32. See also work by Adams (2001), Gerke (2011, 2019) and Deane (2018, 2024) for work exploring this situation in different Tibetan communities.
33. Craig has related, for example, the difficulties that one Tibetan woman from Huangnan described in not understanding Xining hospital doctors' Chinese, coupled with the significant expense of travelling there, which demonstrate some of the barriers to accessing healthcare for many Tibetans in the region (2012: 122).
34. For more information on this scheme, see Nianggajia (2011), Nianggajia and Fjeld (2017), and You and Kobayashi (2009).
35. In 2015, Nianggajia numbered the population of Xining at approximately 1,267,600 inhabitants (2015: 242).
36. See Craig for a wonderfully evocative description of the medicinal baths division at the Qinghai Province Tibetan Medicine Hospital in Xining, where she also details some of the costs and financial aspects of receiving this and other treatments there (2012: 62–65).
37. In fact, as Dhondup has pointed out, Rebkong is 'the main centre of the Bon religion in the Kokonor area', where a Bonpo monastery was built during the reign of Trisong Detsan (790–844) (Dhondup 2011a: 51). For more on Bon in the Rebkong area, see Millard (2013a and 2013b), and for an in-depth exploration of the varieties of religious practices and practitioners in Rebkong and surroundings, see Dhondup, Pagel and Samuel's 2013 edited volume.
38. For more detail on the history of this tradition, see Dhondup (2011b, 2013) and Stoddard (2013).

39. Moreover, as Samuel asserts, how these ethnic groups are now defined by both insiders and outsiders is the result of a 'long historical process' (2013a: 6).
40. See Craig (2012) for descriptions of daily life at this institution based on her ethnographic research in the region.
41. Nianggajia and Fjeld reference a 2014 Tongren Country Health Bureau description of 'sixteen registered private Tibetan medical clinics in Rebgong', and note that this figure also does not include the many 'unregistered practitioners based in their homes' (2017: 51).
42. In fact, Nianggajia and Fjeld note the historical importance of this monastery, which 'has hosted and trained outstanding physicians' for centuries, and which was instrumental in the revival of Tibetan medicine in the aftermath of the Cultural Revolution (2017: 47–48).
43. See Nianggajia (2015) for more information of the history of Tibetan medicine and some of the key figures who have worked in the medical sphere in this area.
44. There are also a number of Traditional Chinese Medicine hospitals and clinics in the city, but they were not discussed at all by my Tibetan interviewees in reference to this topic, and so I shall not include them here.
45. See Schrempf for a description of prescribing practices for inpatients and outpatients at the Xining Tibetan Medicine Hospital (2015: 296). Notable in Xining too is the Arura Tibetan Medicine Co., and its well-known museum displaying Tibetan *materia medica*, medical instruments and medical *thangka* (traditional silk or cloth paintings) on the outskirts of the city (see Saxer 2013 for more on this organization and its changing relationship to the state).
46. In conversation, these practitioners were usually referred to as *menba* (*sman pa*, 'medicine person), but there are a range of terms used across different Tibetan communities to refer to Tibetan medicine doctors, including the common term *amchi* in central Tibet, Nepal and India, as well as the terms *bon lha* (*dbon lha*), *lha je* (*lha rje*) and *tso je* (*'tsho byed*) in Tibet (Soktsang and Millard 2013: 480).
47. Ethical approval for the research was sought and gained from the University of Bristol Faculty of Arts Ethics Committee. In addition, before leaving for China, I spoke to other researchers who had recently conducted research in the Amdo region to get information and advice on undertaking such a research project, as well as the respect and safety of my interviewees and others in the Amdo communities that I engaged with.
48. This is in sharp contrast to research conducted in other Tibetan communities, where certain diagnoses related to mental health have been politicized – see, for example, Adams (1998) and Janes (1999b) in Lhasa, and Prost (2006) and Jacobson (2000, 2007) in India.

Part I

Wind

Chapter 1

HEART, WIND AND MIND

Discussions on *Nyoné* in Contemporary Amdo

> *One woman in my husband's hometown became* nyoné. *I don't know what the cause was . . . maybe it was because she was so sad – because her son and her husband both died . . . Maybe* nyoné *is caused by being very sad – some* nyoné *is related to your* nying *[heart] – it's* nying né *[heart illness].*
>
> —Yeshe (80, Xunhua)

In Amdo, discussions on the illness of *nyoné* predominantly focused on three main factors: *nying né* ('heart illness'), 'incorrect' religious practice and *dön né* (spirit affliction). In Part I of this book, we will examine the first two of these causative factors – exploring Tibetan conceptions of heart and mind, and the particular role that *lung* (wind) plays in Tibetan medical and religious traditions and practices. In this first chapter, we will explore some Amdo narratives of *nyoné* focused on 'heart illness', and *nyoné* attributed to high-level Tantric practice within Buddhist and Bon traditions. Here, we will see how Tibetan medical and religious notions of mind and body converge and diverge in their connections to both *nyoné* as an illness and the Dharmic goal of realization.

As we shall see, across these narratives of *nyoné*, discussions of its symptomatology were fairly consistent among the lay Tibetans, religious practitioners and medical specialists I spoke to in Amdo. Here, descriptions mostly focused on afflicted individuals behaving 'strangely' – for example, displaying strange or nonsensical speech, aggression or even violence – as well as disturbance(s) in the senses, such as hearing or seeing things that no one else could see/hear. For example, Dr Pema (40), a Tibetan medicine doctor and professor in Xining, described to me common symptoms of individuals suffering from *nyoné*:

> Behaviour change is the main symptom – the [afflicted] person can't control their own behaviour, and they don't know what they are talking about . . . They don't know how to control themselves – including bodily behaviour, speech behaviour, and of course mental behaviour – for example, they don't know what they should say, or what they should *not* say.

Similarly, his colleague Dr Tangun (50), explained: 'There are many different kinds of symptoms, but the most common *nyonpa* behaviour is to speak differently – the person says something strange. Also some people see strange colours or something like that – the doctor cannot see [this], but just the *nyonpa* can see'. Dr Tenpa (36, Rebkong/Xining) summarized:

> For *nyoné* patients, it is primarily mind, body, and speech: all of these things will experience a change. In terms of body, the way of moving and walking around becomes disturbed. In terms of speech, the things that are said will be strange, unusual, [for example,] speaking languages one doesn't understand or know, like Sanskrit or English. In terms of mind, their mood will be disturbed easily and change easily. For example, before getting sick someone didn't often cry, but after becoming affected they cry frequently.

Such descriptions were echoed in the narratives of lay people and religious specialists I spoke to. For example, I interviewed Yeshe (80), from Xunhua county, while she was staying with family in Xining city over the winter. She described how people with *nyoné* 'talk to themselves', or 'do something strange – they cannot control themselves'. Similarly, Nyingma Buddhist lama Namgyal (32) in Chabcha (Ch. Gonghe), several hours south of Xining in Tsolho Autonomous Prefecture, told me, '*Nyoné* patients can be immediately identified by doctors' because 'they are talking nonsense, and doing really strange things'.

In contrast, there were some differences in the ways in which lay people, Tibetan medicine doctors and religious specialists discussed the *causation* of *nyoné* – particularly in relation to the notions of *nying* ('heart') and *lung* ('wind'), and their roles in mind-body functioning. The *Gyüshi* medical text delineates causes of illness including diet, behaviour, poison and spirits, but primary here are the three *nyépa* – 'energies' of *lung* (wind), *tripa* (bile) and *béken* (phlegm). In other words, one or more of the *nyépa* are *always* involved to some extent in any kind of illness, amongst a number of causes (or primary causes, Tib. *gyu*) and conditions (or secondary causes, Tib. *kyen*) that may be involved in any one case of illness. And in terms of mental illnesses, it is *lung* that tends to be predominant due to its close relationship with the mind.

While *lung* is integral to Tibetan medical and Tantric notions of mind-body, as will become clear, in reality many of my Tibetan interviewees in Amdo did not mention it at all. Indeed, as we shall see here, in many of these narratives from Amdo – particularly lay narratives – explanations focused instead on stories of sadness, trauma or everyday stress, and their impact on heart in the causation of madness. However, on further exploration with Tibetan medicine doctors, the key role of wind – and its relationship to the heart and mind – starts to become clear. Equally, in cases of religious practitioners understood to have become *nyoné* as a result of their practice, lay interviewees mostly spoke of practitioners 'spending too much time alone' or 'not following their teacher's instructions'. In contrast, Tantric specialists described how such problems can arise from errors in the manipulation of wind in the mind-body – activities that form a key part of many Tibetan Tantric practices.

As we examine a range of narratives from lay individuals and medical and religious specialists based in different parts of Amdo, we will find commonalities and diversities in these explanations of *nyoné*, its causation and treatment. As I mentioned briefly in the Introduction, for approximately three years between 2014 and 2017, the Qinghai Province Tibetan Medicine Hospital in Xining in fact had its own department for illnesses related to the mind – named the 'Department for Wind Illnesses and Impurities' (Tib. Lungné Drip[1] Tsen Khak). I was told that the department had received thirty inpatients during that time. However, it was notable that amongst my cohort of lay interviewees – many of whom lived and/or worked in Xining – few mentioned this department; indeed, apparently only a minority of lay interviewees had been aware of its existence. Given that all those I spoke to were very familiar with this hospital in general (and discussed it in very positive terms), I was rather surprised by this. However, as we explore lay and medical perspectives on causation and treatment of *nyoné* through the various chapters of this book, the reasons for this will become clearer. Here, we will see how longstanding Tibetan religious and medical concepts of mind, body, health, illness and medicine are engaged to explain and understand cases of *nyoné* in ways that often leave little space for certain types of 'medical' treatment.

As I mentioned in the Introduction, in contemporary Amdo I encountered discussions about health, illness and healing encompassing a plurality of explanatory frameworks. Here, Amdo-wa often referenced a range of medical and religious concepts in relation to heart or wind illness, sometimes mentioned alongside biomedical or Western notions such as 'stress'. Through an exploration of these narratives, we can start to build up a picture of the ways in which 'heart', 'mind' and 'wind' are understood within these Amdo Tibetan communities, and their various roles in the causation and treatment of *nyoné*, before moving on to explore Tibetan medical and Tantric notions of wind, and their presentations in medical and religious texts, in more detail in Chapters 2 and 3.

Nying né: Discussing Heart Illness in Amdo

During my time in Amdo, in the many discussions on *nyoné* referencing *nying* ('heart') and *nying né* ('heart illness'), I heard numerous narratives of 'sadness' and difficult life events leading to a person developing *nyoné*. The condition of *nying né* was discussed often by lay interviewees as well as Tibetan medical and religious specialists, with many people describing cases within their own family or community. How can we understand these Tibetan concepts of *nying* and *nying né*? In Amdo, those who spoke English translated these terms literally, discussing 'heart illness' and/or 'heart disease'. On more than one such occasion, we had to clarify the difference in meaning between biomedical notions of 'heart disease' (as related to a range of physical conditions which affect the heart organ), and the Tibetan concept of *nying né*, where people were usually referring to some kind of emotional pain or difficulty. Key here are differential perspectives on the mind (Tib. *sem*), and its location: for Tibetans, the mind is located in the heart, and therefore thinking, emotions, upset, trauma and so on are all related predominantly to the *heart* rather than to the head (Tib. *go*) or brain (Tib. *lépa*). Thus, Dr Nyima (38), a Tibetan medicine doctor and professor in Xining, asserted that the terms *nying né* (heart illness) and *sem né* (mind illness) are, in fact, one and the same – in other words, what we would probably describe in English as 'mental illness'. However, in Amdo, I rarely heard this term '*sem né*', with the vast majority of interviewees discussing *nying né*. For example, when I asked Khandro (22, Mangdzong/Xining, about these terms, she was unsure, responding, in mixed Tibetan and English: 'Are *sem né* and *nying né* different, or the same? . . . I think it's the same . . . *sem né* is heart disease, *nying né* is also heart disease . . . Because *sem* and *nying* in Tibetan are the same – heart'.

In contrast, Wangchuk (31, Golok/Xining), was more familiar with this term, asserting that: '*Sem né* is actually [about] the *emotions*; the mind is normal – just like everyone else – but if the person experiences something painful, then they become worried . . . And if they worry for a long time, then their mind can become *nyoné*'.

Indeed, this kind of explanation of *nyoné* – describing sadness, worry and other emotions, often related to specific events – was common among interviewees. I discussed this with Dr Ngawang (72), a retired Tibetan medicine doctor from the Golok area, who was staying with family in Xining when we met in December 2018. He described three causes of *nyoné* related to the mind, referencing loss, anger and sadness:

> The first cause is because the person's belongings have been stolen, and so he/she will *slowly* become *nyoné*. The second one is when the person is very angry, and *suddenly* becomes *nyoné*. The third one is because of anxiety [Tib. *sem trel*], and the person can't think about bigger things, and then the person *slowly* becomes *nyoné* . . . [In this case,] you can't control your *sem* [mind] – you are thinking too much.

Similarly, Tibetan medicine doctor and Nyingma Buddhist *ngakpa* Dr Sonam (69, Rebkong/Xining) described how someone might become afflicted with *nying né*: 'The first cause [of *nying né*] is because of suffering – for example, suffering as a result of the death of one's relatives, such as one's parents. After this suffering, the heart cannot tolerate it, so it suddenly turns to illness'. Similarly, in her own research in this region, Bassini found *nying né* often 'connected to discourses of bereavement' (2013a: 239). I heard this kind of explanation – some kind of upset or trauma leading to *nying né*, followed by *nyoné* – many times from lay interviewees in Amdo, with references to close bereavements, loss of property and stresses related to work or school exams being common. However, while initial discussions on *nyoné* with Tibetan medicine doctors also frequently focused on *nying né*, more detailed explications on the topic referenced complex understandings of mind-body, health and illness. Integral to these is the notion of *lung* (wind) – a key factor in mind-body functioning, and particularly important in illnesses related to the mind.

Understood to flow through thousands of channels (Tib. *tsa*) throughout the body, and described as 'inseparable' from the mind and consciousness (Rabgay[2] 1984: 47–48), wind is intimately connected to mental and emotional activity as well as the physical state and functioning of the body. Thus, any kind of emotional state will likely affect the 'flow' of *lung* through its channels; similarly, the flow of wind affects the mind and consciousness, as Dr Nyima (38, Rebkong/Xining) explained to me using a mix of English and Tibetan terminology:

> If someone has *sok lung né* [life-sustaining wind/life wind illness] which is severe, and lasts for a long time, then this may lead to *nyoné* . . . Sometimes people get depressed for a long time, and if it's severe, then they could get *nyoné* – [this is] caused by *lung*. For example, sometimes when people get *nyoné* – there is a really specific cause, like . . . the patient's partner or children passed away, or something really, really bad happened to them. Then the patient becomes very sad – very sad for a very long time – and they get depression. So, because of this – if many bad things happened to them, and they experienced many stresses – that could cause *nyoné*.

I have described in more detail elsewhere this somewhat 'circular' relationship between wind and mind in relation to the mind and mental health, where the functioning of each affects the other, and mental and emotional states may be described as both cause and symptom of any disruptions in wind (Deane 2019b). However, key here too is the role of *nying* – also intimately related to the mind and emotions, as we heard above. This is in part related to the Tibetan conception of the very *location* of wind inside the body, whereby *lung* may become 'disturbed' in the region of the heart. Thus Dr Ngawang (72, Golok) described someone from his village, whom he explained had suffered from *nyoné* as a result of very difficult experiences during the Cultural Revolution, and his resulting feelings of loss:

> There is a Mongolian *nyonpa* in our village. People say that he's from a rich family . . . During the Cultural Revolution, all the rich people's properties were given to others, and then he became *nyonpa* – because of *nying né* from this situation. He was attached to his property . . . These kinds of people [in such a situation] will *slowly* get the symptoms of *nyoné*. . . He was too worried about his property, and then the *lung* [wind] went inside his *nying* [heart] and they became mixed, and then slowly he became *nyoné* . . . Sometimes he is ok – normal . . . But then suddenly when the *lung* is disrupted, he will become violent to other people.

Similarly, Samdrup (27, Ngawa/Xining) narrated a story about a neighbour of his, which he said had occurred two years previously:

> This man had many yak . . . All of his yak were stolen . . . and after some days, he saw one of his yak with another family, and he told them, 'This is my yak!'. But that family said, 'It is not your yak'. Then he became *nyoné*. Every day, he said, 'This is my yak . . . this is my yak . . . this is my yak'; then after forty days, he died. He was going around everywhere, talking nonsense, repeating 'This is my yak, this is my yak', wandering everywhere, and hitting people – *nyoné*.

Thus, we start to see the ways in which Tibetan conceptions of 'heart', 'wind' and 'mind' are understood to be connected, with some disruption in the flow of wind, perhaps resulting from emotional upset, potentially affecting the heart and leading to a condition known as *nying lung (né)* (wind in the heart [illness/disorder]).[3] This disruption – particularly if left untreated – may then escalate, potentially leading to *nyoné*. In addition, one particular wind 'current' known as *sok (dzin) lung* (life-sustaining wind) is often implicated here, in part due to its especially close connection to the mind. In Xining, Tibetan medicine doctor Dr Dechen (39) described the 'most common' causation of *nyoné* as '*sems kham*' (psychology/state of mind), explaining how emotional states can lead to *nying lung né* (heart-wind illness), which in turn (particularly if not successfully treated) may lead to *sok lung (né)* (life-sustaining wind [disorder]) and then *nyoné*:

> If a person is scared or frightened, and then a further frightening situation leads to anxiety, then anxiety may cause *nying lung* and *sok lung* instability . . . *Sok lung [né]* is a state between *nying lung* and *nyoné*: first you have *nying lung*, and then you have *sok lung*, and then maybe you will become *nyoné* . . . If you reach that level of illness, it's hardly cured.

As I have described here, discussions with lay Amdo-wa on this type of *nyoné* predominantly focused on heart and heart illness, rather than wind. For example, Rinchen (26, Rebkong/Xining) told me in a mixture of English and Tibetan, 'If someone can't control their emotion, then they get sickness, or they become *nyoné*'. He described the case of a man from his village who had become *nyoné* after his mother had died: 'I think that that man became *nyoné* because he got more pressure [stress] – he felt *very* sad, so he became *nyoné*'. I asked Rinchen whether this might be related to *lung* or *sok (dzin) lung*, but he replied that he had never heard of *sok lung* before.

Other lay interviewees in Amdo had a little more knowledge of *lung* and *sok lung*, but I encountered diverse perspectives on its connection to *nying né* and/or *nyoné*. For example, Dhondup (25, Labrang/Xining) asserted, '*Sok lung* can really increase if you've been studying a lot, and then people get angry really easily – get into fights really easily – but this is something that's quite common, so I think it's something quite separate from *nyoné*'. His classmate Dawa (30), from Trika, disagreed, telling us, 'Maybe some cases of *nyoné* might be caused by *lung* or *sok lung*'. In addition, several interviewees in Amdo described 'too much study' as a cause of *nyoné*, sometimes referencing the role of wind here. Dawa (30), for example, told me that 'reading too many books can disturb your *lung* . . . This has a connection with *sok lung*, which can cause *nyoné*'.

Occasionally, Tibetan medicine doctors and lay Tibetans in Amdo also referenced biomedical concepts in their explanations of *nyoné*, sometimes combining biomedical and Tibetan medicine terms and concepts. For example, retired Dr Ngawang (72) gave an example of *nyoné* caused by 'anger' (Tib. *lung lang*): 'Perhaps a person becomes very angry, and their heartbeat becomes raised very fast, and then their blood pressure rises too high,[4] and maybe this goes to the channel [Tib. *tsa*].[5] In Tibetan maybe we'll say this [*nyoné*] is related to the *sok lung*'. Here again, we see the 'heart' discussed in the causation of *nyoné*, but this time in a rather different way with reference to biomedical notions of blood pressure. Nonetheless, there is still a connection made to the notion of *sok lung* and its role in the causation of *nyoné*.

Practice-Related Wind Illnesses and *Nyoné*

Another cause of *nyoné* commonly discussed in Amdo was religious practice – in relation to both Buddhist and Bon traditions. I encountered a variety of explanations about how and why this might occur, including descriptions of 'too much study' and 'incorrect practice'. Such narratives were common: almost all of the lay people I spoke to in Amdo described at least one practitioner they had heard of who had become *nyoné* in this manner, and several religious specialists also described this as a common problem. In Rebkong, for example, Bon lama Tsering (57) told me: 'I have seen this many times – of course, many times . . . This occurs in perhaps one out of every one hundred practitioners'. Similarly, Nyingma Buddhist *ngakpa* and Tibetan medicine doctor Aku Wangchuk (72, Rebkong) asserted, 'Most of these practitioners with *nyoné* did something wrong in their practice – this happens a lot', and Gelugpa Geshe Dhondup (50, Rebkong) described this as an 'inside' cause of *nyoné*, telling me: '*Nyoné* can be divided into different types, and the main cause can be from outside or inside . . . The *inside* causes usually result from incorrect [religious] practices, with the practitioner not having the proper guidance or teachings from teachers'.

Indeed, such 'complications' of meditation practice are discussed in Tibetan Tantric texts, as we will see in Chapter 3. Here, the focus is often on *tsa lung* ('channel-wind') practices, which are aimed at manipulating the flows of *lung* through the channels throughout body, and it is well known that such practices can go awry, particularly in relation to the *sok lung* (life-sustaining wind current). In such cases, the *lung* may become 'blocked' in a certain area of the body or may 'increase', causing psychological and/or physiological symptoms. In Xining, Tibetan medicine professor Dr Rinchen (55) described *nyoné* caused by *sok lung* disturbance resulting from such practice as 'common', and Dr Nyima (38, Rebkong/Xining) explained in a mix of English and Tibetan: 'Some practitioners practise their Tantra alone [– working with] their *lung*. If they make some mistake, then there may be an increase [in *lung*] or the *lung* may go in some wrong direction . . . Then, you may get *lung né*, or *nyoné*'. Dr Pema (40) agreed, explaining in English: 'In Buddhist practice, meditation is very complicated – if you don't do [it] the very correct way, it causes so many mental problems. There are many possible side effects, for example the *sok lung* may become blocked – [we call this] *sok lung* or *nyoné*'.

With such 'risks' – particularly regarding high-level practice – well known by practitioners, several interviewees described the high responsibility religious teachers hold for ensuring that their students have the correct preparation for practice. This includes providing not only instruction but also initiation into each particular practice. Thus, Bon lama Tsering (57) explained:

> Before you go for retreat in the mountains, your lama will give you some teaching and guidance, including preliminary practices and things like that, to prepare you for the retreat . . . But if someone doesn't have a teacher to give this guidance, and they go on retreat, then sometimes their heart may become uncontrolled. This can cause *nyoné* through *nying lung né*: if you cannot control your heart, then you cannot control your mind.

Aku Wangchuk (72) also explained the responsibility religious teachers have for ensuring that students are aware of possible problems related to these kinds of practice:

> At the beginning of teaching, the teacher usually tells the students, 'You have to be careful; you have to follow the instructions, otherwise the *lung* can go in the wrong way, and you can become *nyoné* – usually they will give this speech . . . These practices are related not only to wind – also to the channels and drops [Tib. *tiklé*][6] – so you have to work to control all of these . . . This is really complicated and very difficult – that's why many people make a mistake when they practise – at *that* level – the level of these three . . . This practice is really complicated and very difficult, so people can make mistakes.

The importance of such initiation for Tantric practice was well known among lay people too – discussed by many of those I spoke to. For example, Rinchen (26, Rebkong/Xining) told me (in English):

> I heard about a monk who became crazy because he read a Buddhist text . . . You can't read that text by yourself before the lama gives you initiation. If you don't have this kind of permission, and you read that text, then you can become *nyoné* . . . He disrobed – because he became crazy . . . When people do meditation, if they can't find the correct method, *then* they can become *nyoné* – this is what I think.

Here, even reading a Tantric text – as opposed to conducting any practice – is understood to be risky for someone who has not had the correct initiation, and this kind of causation was sometimes also ascribed to those thought to be lacking a solid foundational knowledge of the Dharma. Both foundational knowledge of Buddhism or Bon through study of the texts, and Tantric 'preliminary practices' are understood to be necessary foundations for the more advanced practices described in high-level Tantric texts. I thus heard several narratives about people 'jumping too fast' into advanced Tantric practices, whether through arrogance or enthusiasm – as Dr Rinchen (55) explained:

> Sometimes, some monks straightaway just study the Tantras – they didn't study the Sutras first. First, you *must* study about the Sutra – the Sutra is the foundation of Tantra. If you just study about Tantra, this method is just wrong

> . . . Because of this you cannot control your *sok lung* or do that kind of meditation, and you can't control your mind, so you become *nyoné.*

In Rebkong, Tamdrin (26) told me about a relative of his:

> One of my uncles was trying reach the high level of Tantric practice, and he became *nyoné.* Now he has recovered, but he was *nyoné* for almost twenty years . . . You know, the Buddhist texts are very difficult to understand – for example it is especially difficult to understand emptiness. So if a particular text is trying to explain emptiness, we might say that not *everyone* should be reading that book, because we vary from person to person – people are different. So sometimes, people say this book is good for *you*, but not good for *me.* For example, maybe a book is trying to explain emptiness, and when a person reaches the meaning of this book, the knowledge is too big for them, and they can't understand the meaning of this. Maybe they will get *namtok* [doubt, discursive thoughts] – sometimes experiencing suspicion, sometimes trust. Between these, they lose their mind, and become *nyoné.*

These various explanations of practice-related *nyoné* thus encompass a broad variety of concepts, ranging from 'misdirected' wind affecting mind-body functioning and a lack of requisite knowledge for advanced Tantric practices, having doubts or misconceptions about the practice, or perhaps even just glimpsing the very idea of emptiness, to some apparently rather more prosaic notions of afflicted practitioners conducting 'too much study' or spending 'too much time alone'. In fact, these latter explanations were also discussed in relation to non-religious descriptions of causation too, where I heard stories of students becoming *nyoné* from spending too much time 'in their head' studying at school or university, without enough social contact with family and/or friends, and/or experiencing 'stress' caused by study and exams. From a medical perspective, wind is very clearly implicated in such explanations too – particularly in notions of someone spending a lot of time doing mental activity, such as book study, leading to an increase in wind. Lay interviewees had varying levels of knowledge of this process. Thus, some people described 'too much study' as a cause of *nyoné* but reported uncertainty about why this might be the case, sometimes describing it in quite general terms about people needing more social interactions. In contrast, Nyingma lama Namgyal (32, Chabcha) clearly explained the role of *lung* here – referencing both the general understanding that a lot of mental activity can affect the wind, as well as the possibility of a practitioner conducting their practices 'incorrectly', as described above:

> Those lamas who focus too much concentration on their studies or Buddhist teachings may experience *sok lung né* [life-wind illness]. There are many lamas with *sok lung né*; this is no different from lay people with *nyoné* related to *sok*

> *lung* – it is probably caused by studying too much, days and nights of studying: those lamas have spent too much time on their studying, or too much concentration on their studies . . . Alongside that, maybe they have conducted key Tantric practices incorrectly. This second type of cause is when the meditation is wrong, or [has] been conducted incorrectly, then this has caused *sok lung né.* Not all kinds of meditation will lead someone to go astray, or go wrong, but the methods for conducting the practice are important – if they are done incorrectly, then this may lead to some kinds of difficulties.

Moreover, in some of these explanations, there was also often another layer of causation referenced: the notion of *namtok* – conceptual/discursive thoughts or doubts/hesitations.[7] For example, above we heard Tamdrin's mention of 'suspicion' in his explanation of the causation of his uncle's *nyoné.* I discussed this topic with Migmar (30, Golok/Xining), who was partway through a postgraduate degree in Buddhist Studies at university in Xining. He told me that if practitioners – particularly those who are younger and/or less experienced – have 'anxiety' while they are practising, then this may cause *nyoné.* In Rebkong, I asked Gelug lama Wangyal (62) about this, and he described practitioners afflicted in this way:

> A person who is affected like this will want to stay in a dark room. This is a preliminary state: first, they stay alone too much in the dark, and then they want to stay alone and go deeper into their practice – wanting to avoid all their friends and acquaintances, every day staying there alone . . . They may become paranoid, for example, thinking that others are talking about them. If that continues for some time, they may get a rash [Tib. *dzé,* often translated as leprosy] on the skin of the upper part of their body, and then their heart and their general health may become unstable. When the heart is unstable, then the person may have much *namtok.*
>
> When someone is doing meditation or reading, firstly, they want to seclude themself from the busy world to study; they want to increase their knowledge and wisdom. In that state, many people can accumulate much wisdom, but some people become trapped, because their way of meditating is not really good. For example, perhaps a monk realises he doesn't have as much knowledge as he thought he had. Maybe he even gave some teachings to others, and this could be why he thinks he has a high knowledge, but perhaps those students didn't address him as they should address a teacher, and many people didn't recognize or acknowledge his great knowledge. When he thinks about this situation too much, then he may become angry, and envious [of others] – in that state, he may become *nyoné.* Once a person has become *nyoné,* if someone doesn't try to take care of them, it can escalate . . . If a person becomes *nyoné,* it is hard to control: like a fire, when it increases significantly, it is very difficult to extinguish it. Then help may be in vain, or it may even cause some further problems.

These diverse narratives of practice-caused *nyoné* from Amdo clearly illustrate some common Tibetan perspectives on the complexities and potential complications of Tantric practice. Said to be highly effective in the pursuit of enlightenment (particularly in comparison with *non*-Tantric religious practices), these kinds of high-level practices are also understood to be difficult and potentially dangerous – particularly for those not correctly prepared, due to a lack of knowledge, experience and/or initiation. Many of those I spoke to in Amdo emphasized the importance of the student–teacher relationship – something that has been central to Tibetan Buddhist and Bon traditions and their transmission from the earliest days until now. It was clearly understood that a student could not simply be handed a text of instructions and sent on his/her way, but must be taught, one-to-one, by an experienced teacher – one able to assess the student's readiness for each stage of practice and instruct him/her accordingly. The perils of Tantric practice without this kind of teaching were frequently noted by all those I spoke to in Amdo, even while there was a diversity in explanations of exactly *how* 'incorrect' Tantric practice might lead to *nyoné*.

Lama Nyönpa: The Figure of the 'Crazy Lama'

A rather different, but relatively common, reference to *nyoné* in Amdo was in relation to the so-called *lama nyonpa* (crazy lama/mad yogin). This figure is well known in Buddhist historical narratives:[8] a practitioner who appears to be *nyoné* – doing strange, usually transgressive, things such as eating dirt, dressing in strange clothes and/or engaging in transgressive sexual or violent behaviours. However, these figures are not seen to be experiencing illness in the ways that we have explored above. Instead, they are perceived to be enlightened – acting the way they do as a result of their higher realization. We often hear the renowned eleventh-century Buddhist teacher, practitioner and poet Milarepa described as one such figure. Thus, yogi Lodro (42),[9] a Tantric specialist whom I interviewed in Chabcha, explained, 'In the Buddhist philosophical understanding, there are two different kinds of *lama nyonpa*. One is the *tokdenpa* [realized one] who is enlightened, and the other is a monk who has *nyoné* caused by *sok lung*'. Indeed, yogi Lodro told me that there were 'many *lama tokden* [realized lamas]' in the Nyingma Buddhist tradition to which he belonged. These practitioners, he asserted, have attained realization: 'They are enlightened'.

These 'mad yogin' figures were referred to by a number of different terms in Amdo, including *lama nyonpa* (mad lama), *tokdenpa* (realized person) and *lama tokden* (realized lama), with some suggesting '*lama nyonpa*' to be rather derogatory and others describing it as a most usual term.[10] In Amdo,

I heard several narratives of contemporary *lama nyonpa*/*tokdenpa*, including this description from Dawa (30, Trika/Xining) about a figure far away in the Kham region:

> There is this well-known lama from a monastery near Derge, and it's like, is he *nyonpa*, or not *nyonpa*? He has a very high level of attainment . . . but sometimes he'll go and destroy shops in the area, or he'll throw stones at things, or he'll walk around or sit on the ground totally naked . . . But people go to see him, and a lot of lay people really have faith in him. He is still alive today – he is fifty now . . . Sometimes he'll read, and sometimes he'll throw stones, and do unpredictable things. But he really is a *druptop* [*siddha*] . . . He actually has a lot of Chinese followers, who are patients who go to get cured by him . . . This man is *definitely* one of those people. You can tell he's *tokdenpa* and not *nyonpa*: firstly, because the public has a lot of faith in him, and they interpret a lot of his actions as being things he is doing to *help* them. For example, on WeChat, he smokes and drinks, and if beautiful girls come by, he says 'I'm going to kiss you!', and he'll do crazy things, but most people are interpreting these behaviours as something guiding [them], or to prevent obstacles for them. So from one side, he's kind of crazy, but from the other side, because of the way people are interpreting his actions, he's highly realized.

Similarly, Khandro (22, Trika/Xining) told me about a Buddhist practitioner in her home town: 'There is a *ngakpa* in my village. One day we invited him to our home to chant some scriptures. He was in another room, and at midnight, I heard a loud noise, and so my father went up to see what the *ngakpa* was doing, and he was [she mimes levitating] – flying! . . . Maybe one meter off the ground! It's so strange'. In fact, the narrative became even more astounding, as Khandro told me what she had heard about this *ngakpa*'s behaviour on another occasion, while he was staying in his tent just outside the village:

> One year, he was near our village, and he put up a tent, and lived there for five months . . . He lived there, and he didn't talk to anyone – he was on retreat. And when some villagers went to see him, they looked through the door of the tent, and they said that he had pulled out all of his intestines – pulled them out! Yes – they say that! They were very afraid of that at that time.[11]

The practitioner was apparently seen by villagers some time later, with no outward signs of harm. Khandro told me, in English, 'This is crazy!', but she was equally clear to emphasize: 'This is not *nyonpa* – in Tibetan culture, we say it is *trül* [magic, illusion] . . . It's about religion . . . high level practice'.

Others too described practitioners with incredible abilities. For example, Samdrup (27, Ngawa/Xining) also asserted that some such individuals can 'levitate' and also 'go underground'. And his classmate Rinchen (26, Rebkong/Xining) had an even more incredible story, about a '*tokdenpa*' mastering the forces of life and death: 'I haven't seen this, but, not many years ago, my grandfather said that when he was a child, one of the lamas in my village looked very crazy. And if someone got sick, he would take a gun and shoot them – really! It looked like he killed them, but after he had done this, the patients recovered'.

However, while a number of interviewees mentioned such practitioners to me, they were nearly always described second hand – few people spoke of having seen or met such individuals themselves. Equally, it was common in such discussions for interviewees to mention well-known examples of *lama nyonpa* from the past, but less common to hear of any contemporary practitioners still alive at that time. I asked my interviewees whether there are many – or even *any* – such practitioners today, and received mixed responses. Samdrup (27, Ngawa/Xining), for example, said that *lama nyonpa* usually 'live in the mountains – doing retreat . . . They stay there doing meditation, trying to become enlightened . . . They stay alone for a long time'. I asked whether either he or Rinchen (26), who we were also talking to, thought there were still some of these people alive today, but they were both unsure – Rinchen saying simply, 'I don't know', while Samdrup instead referenced the well-known historical example: 'I don't know . . . You know Milarepa? He was a *tokdenpa*'. And, reflecting the comments I heard from many of my interviewees – often living and studying or working in Xining city having grown up in a smaller town, village or nomadic area – Wangyal (40, Rebkong/Xining) told me, 'In the village we hear many stories like this, but people like us, we are living in the city, so we hear fewer stories like this'. And Dhondup (25, Labrang/Xining) told me, 'There probably are some *tokdenpa* [alive today], but I don't know any'.

An obvious question, perhaps, is how one might determine whether an apparently '*nyoné*' religious practitioner is such a figure – a high-level *lama nyonpa*/*tokdenpa* – or simply a practitioner (or even *non*-practitioner) who has become 'mad' – whether through their practice or from some other cause(s). I put this question to yogi Lodro (42, Chabcha), after he told me a mind-bending story about a *tokdenpa*'s altercation with a dragon. He asserted that through questioning a practitioner acting in such a *nyonpa* fashion we can assess their condition: 'The difference is in the way they explain their reasons [for their actions]'. A *lama tokden*, he told me, 'is all-knowing, and can predict everything, before seeing a situation'. I asked whether there was any chance that such a practitioner might be mistaken for someone suffering from 'ordinary' *nyoné*, and taken to hospital for treatment, but Lodro said no: 'If a *lama tokden* goes to hospital, that is probably a sign that he is *falsely* claiming to be *tokden*'. Indeed, he insisted, 'If you are able to be controlled by other people and forced to go to hospital, then that means that you are not *tokden*'.

Treating *Nyoné* in Amdo

For those who *are* seen to require intervention – i.e. individuals understood to be suffering from the illness of 'madness', rather than realized practitioners – much of the treatment focus is on the intertwining factors of heart and wind described above. In this section, then, we will explore the various treatment approaches that were discussed in relation to *nyoné* caused by 'heart illness' and disordered wind (including that related to Tantric practice) by those I spoke to in Amdo.

In October 2018, I interviewed Dr Dechen (39, Rebkong/Xining), a Tibetan medicine doctor who had worked in the Department for Wind Illnesses and Impurities within the Qinghai Province Tibetan Medicine Hospital in Xining. Dr Dechen told me that that this department had been set up predominantly to treat patients suffering from *nyoné*, and she described 'four [Tibetan medicine] treatment steps' for patients whose *nyoné* was caused by *sok lung* or *nying lung*, explaining in some detail the treatments that had been available to patients with *nyoné* in that department. These were divided into 'soft' treatments, such as *numjuk* (massage of the hands and/or feet with melted butter/fat[12] mixed with herbs) and *hormé* (medicinal poultice); and 'hard' treatments, such as *mé tsa* (moxibustion) and *telpal telwa* (a pair of metal instruments used to apply extreme heat to specific points on the body – see Figure 1.1).

Over the approximately three years that it had been operational (2014–17), this department had had thirty inpatients with *nyoné*, seventeen of whom, she reported, had responded very well to treatment. However, Dr Dechen also recounted some practical difficulties the doctors had encountered in terms of dealing with a number of patients with *nyoné* simultaneously, describing initial concerns doctors had over how to control patients' behaviour well enough to be able to administer Tibetan medicine treatments to them. In fact, as she explained, the answer came not from Tibetan medicine but instead from biomedicine:

> At the beginning, patients were very *nyonpa* – [for example] they used long sticks to frighten the doctors away . . . The doctors were really afraid of the patients, because they were violent! Because of this, we [doctors] went to the Chinese Number Three [psychiatric] Hospital to find solutions – to see their methods for controlling patients – such as injections of sedatives or painkillers. The doctors [from our department] went there to find out how they [doctors at

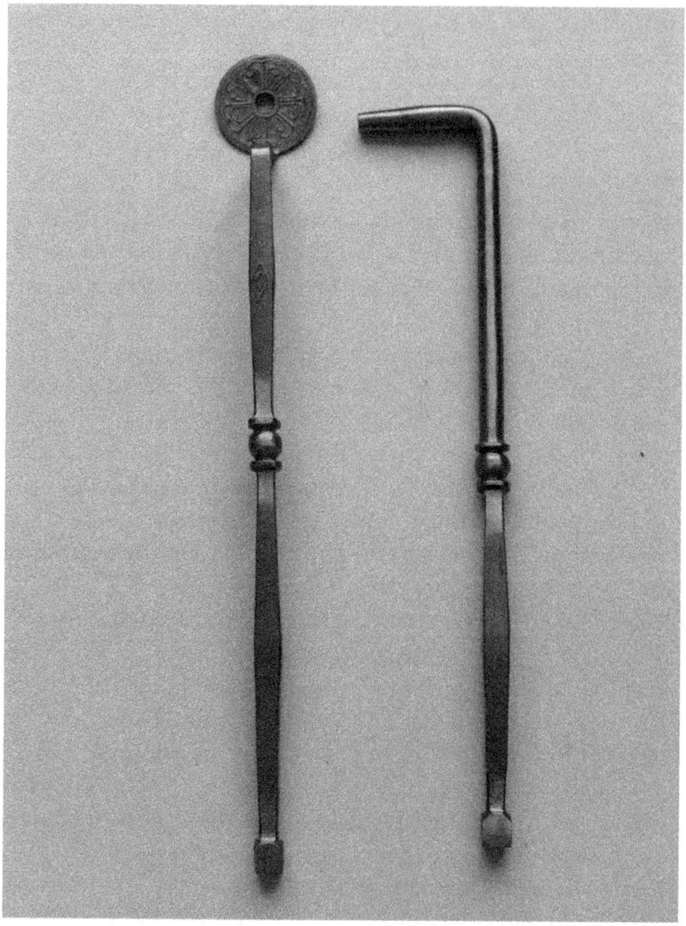

Figure 1.1. *Telwa* medical instruments, Qinghai Province Tibetan Medicine Hospital, Xining 2018. © Susannah Deane.

Number Three Hospital] managed this type of behaviour. Then they returned, and also added their own ways of treating these patients.

Of course these patients [with *nyoné*] were hospitalized: because of the instability in *nying lung* they had to be hospitalized . . . First of all, when a patient arrived at the hospital, normally no Tibetan medicine could treat them – some of them were restrained [in their beds], and stayed like this for two weeks or more, and some of the patients were yelling and screaming and even chasing people, hitting things, or running around very boisterously. Physically, they were healthy, but some of them didn't eat for days; some of them didn't speak for a long time. That's why, when the patients first arrived at the hospital, we injected them with some [biomedical] sedative, and that calmed them down.

Dr Dechen explained that, having sedated patients presenting with *nyoné*, it was then possible for the doctors in the department to administer Tibetan medicine treatments to them, including the external therapies described above and a variety of medicinal compounds. And, like many other doctors and lay people I spoke to, she was clear that it is far preferable to treat such patients as early as possible, explaining that once *nying lung né* (heart-wind illness) has led to *nyoné*, it can be much more difficult – if not impossible – to treat. Of course, chosen treatment methods will vary depending on the presumed cause(s) of the condition, with causation usually determined through various traditional means, such as pulse diagnosis.[13] Thus, Dr Rinchen (55) gave the example of one medicine named simply '*sok lung men*' (life-sustaining wind medicine) that may be used in the treatment of *nyoné* related to *sok lung (né)*.

Discussing *nyoné* with Dr Nyima (38, Rebkong/Xining), a well-known doctor and professor of Tibetan medicine, he told me that in fifteen years of medical practice he had seen only two patients with *nyoné*: one Tibetan and one Han Chinese. Dr Nyima recounted how he had prescribed some medicine for wind disturbance for one of these patients, alongside the recommendation that she also consult a religious specialist. However, he was unsure if this advice had been followed, as the patient had not returned. Retired Dr Ngawang (72, Golok) – who had described *nyoné* and *sok lung né* caused by anger (above) – asserted that it was 'easy' to treat those people who have become *nyoné* 'very suddenly from anger' with a combination of religious and medical intervention. In fact, even where he referenced the (sometimes related) biomedical notion of 'high blood pressure', he described the efficacy of Buddhist activities, explaining that such patients used to consult his father-in-law, a Nyingma Buddhist lama, for this kind of illness. The lama would chant and conduct rituals on the patient's behalf, he explained – treatment that he said was often successful. Dr Ngawang then related the story of a previous patient of his of around 38 years old, who had been taken to a Buddhist lama by family members after becoming *nyoné* some years previously:

> This woman got *nyoné* after arguments. Two people were restraining her because she was out of control, and then they went to the lama, but she wouldn't do the [usual] prostrations – and she was very strong. They pushed her to sit near the lama, and the lama was chanting, and he also hit her with a Buddhist text, and chanted. And slowly, she became better . . . This lama is also a [Tibetan medicine] doctor too, so he also gave her some medicine, and also gave her some moxibustion – just on two points . . . So they did the ritual on the first day, and then she had two or three days of medicine, and then she came back and she had moxibustion again: one on the front of her body, and one on the back, and when they did the one on her back, she fainted. And when she woke up, she was better – recovered. The medicine they gave her over those two or three days was given to her like for a child – putting it in her

> food, or giving it with sweets – otherwise she wouldn't take it. And then after the second round of moxibustion, she was totally normal again, and she was taking the medicines herself, and she recovered. She continued to come back and see the lama-doctor, but she didn't have the symptoms again.

Several interviewees in Amdo described taking this kind of approach to the treatment of many different kinds of illness – i.e. combining medicine and/or external therapies alongside some form of religious intervention. Indeed, as mentioned in the Introduction, with many cases of illness seen to involve multiple causes and contributary factors, it often makes sense to employ multiple healing modalities to address these multiple components. This is evident, for example, in Tibetan medicine approaches to spirit affliction, where medicine to treat disrupted wind may be used alongside any religious intervention(s) aimed at the spirit itself (see Part II for more on this). Thus, in Amdo, those who *did* discuss the utility of Tibetan medicine treatment for *nyoné* or related conditions spoke quite pragmatically about potentially utilizing a number of diverse treatment approaches for *nyoné*, either simultaneously or in sequence, for this kind of illness. For example, Khandro (22, Mangdzong/Xining) told me: 'Tibetan lamas have some ways to treat *sem né* and *nyoné* through ritual, but we also use Chinese medicine [i.e. biomedicine], and we also use Tibetan medicine – either . . . It depends, I think – whichever medicine is helpful for you, you should use that one', and Namgyal (32) suggested, 'If medical treatments don't work, then you can take a Buddhist approach and you can visit a lama'.

Similarly, Wangchuk (31, Golok/Xining) described the sad case of Dekyi, a woman in his home town in Golok who had apparently become *nyoné* following two abusive marriages (the first of which he described as a case of forced marriage implemented by the woman's family). He explained that Dekyi had been treated with both biomedicine and Buddhist rituals, staying in the Number Three (psychiatric) Hospital in Xining for around fifteen days, where she was given medicine that 'helped a lot'. Wangchuk explained that Dekyi had also had some rituals done on her behalf by lamas at her local monastery: 'I don't know if this helped or not; I *think* it helped . . . Now she recovered a little – her behaviour is not like it was before, so she is better – but only a little bit better'.

Nonetheless, for many of my lay interviewees in Amdo – and, indeed, some of the Tibetan medicine doctors I spoke to – religious intervention was described as the predominant treatment option for *nyoné*. This was also evident in the fact that, as I noted above, the Department for Wind Illnesses and Impurities at the Qinghai Province Tibetan Medicine Hospital had seen only thirty patients across the three years that it had been operational, and many of the lay Tibetans I spoke to in and around Xining appeared to be entirely unaware of the prior existence of this department – despite the hospital as a whole being very well known and well regarded.

Given that several of my interviewees in Xining city were in fact students or workers from other parts of the province – who had therefore not been in the city more than a few months or years, and/or spent only part of the year living in it – it is perhaps unsurprising that they might not be entirely familiar with such medical facilities, either Tibetan or biomedical. But it was interesting to hear so many people describe 'medicine' (Tibetan *or* Western) as entirely irrelevant for treating many cases of *nyoné* – even those clearly described in the Tibetan medical texts. For example, when I mentioned the Number Three Hospital to Dhondup (25, Labrang/Xining), he exclaimed, surprised, 'I've never heard of someone going to the [biomedical] hospital for having *nyoné*!'. Others had heard of such facilities for patients with *nyoné*, but described them as probably unhelpful, if not downright harmful, for someone with this condition. Indeed, many interviewees – particularly the older Tibetans I spoke to – had a poor view of biomedical treatments for mental illnesses in general, and the facilities at biomedical psychiatric hospitals in particular. Such negative views on the utility of 'Chinese medicine' [i.e. biomedicine] for treating *nyoné* (or other conditions related to the mind) was sometimes ascribed to the conditions in the hospital – particularly the belief that being around a significant number of other people in various states of mental distress would be entirely unconducive to any kind of recovery – especially for a patient suffering from *nying né*. For example, Sonam (27, Rebkong), told me: 'Some people said that if the people with *nyoné* go to the *nyoné* [psychiatric] hospital, it is not good – it's very *bad* . . . Maybe some people go there and they get worse. I don't know why – maybe because there are so many *nyonpa* there, so their heart gets very heavy . . . they get upset, and so they get worse. I heard this, but I don't know'.

Moreover, many times (in the context of both mental and physical illnesses), I heard the common refrain that biomedicine 'only treats the symptoms' of an illness and not the underlying cause(s). This was often contrasted with Tibetan medicine – and, indeed, religious rituals – which were frequently described as being able to treat the 'root cause of an illness'. As Wangchuk (31, Golok/Xining) told me: 'Western medicine stops the illness quickly, but it doesn't treat it *deeply* – it stops the *symptoms*. But if you take Tibetan medicine for a long time, it treats the sickness deeply, and you never get that sickness again'. Indeed, this reflects what I had often heard from Tibetans in Darjeeling too – delineating biomedicine as a fast-acting treatment for 'acute' conditions in contrast to Tibetan medicine, often described as a slower-acting, longer-term treatment for 'chronic' conditions (Deane 2018: 120), and this has also been reported by others working in Tibetan contexts (see, for example Samuel 2009; Schrempf 2011; Wangda 1996).[14]

Thus, resorting to such biomedical treatment(s) for this illness was described by some as a result of a lack of faith in Buddhism and/or Tibetan medicine. For example, Dr Ngawang (72) told me:

> If you have a very good family, then they will take you to see a lama, and they will get Tibetan medicines for you, and then you will slowly be cured. If you go to the Number Three [psychiatric] Hospital, you will never be completely cured . . . If a family really takes care of the person with *nyoné*, and if they have a strong belief in Tibetan Buddhism, they will never put them inside that kind of hospital. Those who don't have much faith, and who don't really pay much attention to taking care of that person – they will take them to [this kind of] hospital, and they will not be cured . . . Even if you get a little bit better, you still won't be cured.

In addition, some interviewees mentioned *rinchen rilbu* ('precious pills') here. These multi-ingredient medicinal pills, which span the overlapping spheres of medicine and religion, are prepared ritually by lamas. I often heard them described as having the ability to cure all kinds of illnesses – especially those which are often hard to treat. For example, Dawa (30, Trika/Xining), described the importance of such pills in contrast to biomedicine for treating many kinds of *nyoné*:

> There are some medicines, known as *rinchen rilbu* – the way that they are prepared means that they are very helpful for problems of *nying* and *sem* . . . But I don't think there is a Chinese medicine [i.e. biomedicine] which is helpful [for these kinds of illness] . . . If it's the kind of *nyoné* that relates to your *sem kham* [psychology/state of mind] or being affected by a spirit, then what can be done for you at the Number Three Hospital?

However, he added, if the *nyoné* is caused by 'something related to your brain' – if a person has '*this* type of *nyoné*' – then it 'probably makes sense' to go to the hospital.

Despite the commonly expressed view that biomedicine is inappropriate for treating many kinds of *nyoné*, a small number of people in Amdo did describe to me the use of biomedical facilities for such patients. For example, Dr Dechen described a patient with *nyoné* who had been brought to the Department for Wind Illnesses and Impurities, before her family changed their mind and said that they would take her instead to the Number Three Hospital. In Rebkong, Norbu (30) told me about attempting to have his father's *nyoné* treated at a biomedical hospital (although not a psychiatric hospital) in Xining several years previously. However, this had not helped, and his father had then instead been successfully treated with a combination of Buddhist rituals, after it was determined via divination that the illness had been caused by a family connection to a particular kind of deity known as a *gyalpo*.[15] Others described visiting a biomedical hospital for 'body checks' (i.e. scans, blood tests, etc.) as a way to rule out certain kinds of causative factors. In such cases, an absence of positive results from these kinds of tests was often taken as indication that the cause must therefore be something 'untestable' via biomedical equipment. For example, in Rebkong, Sonam (27) described how a relative, who had suddenly become *nyoné*, had been taken by family members to a biomedical hospital: 'Her family took her to a Chinese [i.e. biomedical] hospital, but they did body tests and couldn't find anything wrong with her . . . They said that there was no sickness in her body'. Thus, it was determined that the cause was probably a spirit affliction and the woman was taken to see a high-level lama instead, who performed Buddhist rituals, which Sonam reported had helped to some extent. In such cases, causation – and, thus, treatment – is often determined through a process of elimination, with biomedical tests understood to have ruled out certain causes, leaving 'religious' explanations likely.[16]

In discussions on *nyoné* specifically related to Tantric practice, biomedicine was again described as irrelevant by a majority of interviewees. However, some of the Tibetan medicine doctors and religious specialists I spoke to explained that Tibetan medical treatments could in fact be useful. They spoke of the utility of medical treatments designed for wind increases, decreases and disturbances – alongside religious practices designed to manage and remedy disordered wind. It was here again that the importance of a knowledgeable and skilled Tantric teacher was often highlighted – not least because, as Bonpo lama Tsering (57) explained, 'Usually you need to get help from the lama or Rinpoche . . . because while you are experiencing *nyoné*, your mind is unclear'. *Ngakpa* and Tibetan medicine doctor Aku Wangchuk (72) asserted that 'practitioners can rarely treat this by themselves'; instead, practitioners 'often go to the [Tibetan medicine] doctor for treatment, and sometimes they will change their practice' – usually on the guidance of their teacher. Dr Nyima (38) also emphasized the importance of religious intervention in such cases, explaining that 'in this case, you need a more knowledgeable practitioner to teach you to practise correctly, and recover slowly, slowly'. In addition, he said, Tibetan medicine could also help to 'bring the wind down'. Similarly, Dr Rinchen (55) asserted:

> Sometimes we should take Tibetan medicines [for this condition], but medicine is not that important . . . You should [follow] the way of Dharma. Religious activities are the best way to deal with these kind of problems – not medicines . . . We can take medicine [for this], but it's not so important.

Indeed, Bon lama Tsering (57) explained that such wind problems related to Tantric practice are clearly described in Bon texts, as they are in their

Buddhist counterparts, with a number of texts describing wind disturbances that may result from *tsa lung* practices, as well as their appropriate treatments. He gave some examples of suitable treatments:

> Most of this kind of knowledge [on practice-related *nyoné*] is in the texts, but some of it comes from practitioners' own experience . . . When different people have this kind of *nying lung* [from practice] during retreat, there are many ways of treating this. For example, in the Tibetan sense, it can be treated by mixing *tsampa*[17] and butter and rubbing this on the body – this can ease the *nying lung*. Another way to treat this is for the person to lie down with the sunshine on the lower half of their body. Also, if someone has *nying lung*, you can bury an onion in ashes in the fire until it is half burnt, and then you eat it . . . We also have another way of treating the *nying lung* – by practising *tsa lung* [channel-wind practices].

From Tibetan medical and religious perspectives, then, a combination of medicines, external therapies, diet and further practices aimed at manipulating the wind within the body may be effective in treating such problems. However, the importance of early intervention was also often mentioned here, and it was well understood that not all cases could be successfully treated. Indeed, as I described in the Introduction, in Rebkong, Lobsang (30) described an elderly lama in his monastery who had apparently been *nyoné* for many years as a result of his practice. Unfortunately, Lobsang said, the lama had had *nyoné* for a long time, and it would be impossible to treat him successfully.

And finally, amongst the multiple causes and conditions of *nyoné* and other illnesses discussed in Amdo, there was also some mention of karma. This was often referenced in cases where illness remained despite the application of a variety of treatments. For example, in Xining, Dr Tangun (50) explained: 'According to Tibetan Buddhism, *nyoné* may also be related to other causes, such as the previous life – *lé* [karma, action] . . . If it is caused by the previous life, then the medicine won't work for your *nyoné*, so you need to read religious texts . . . do ritual(s) . . . practise Buddhism . . . do meditation – all of these kinds of things'. In such cases, I was told – by lay Tibetans, Tibetan medicine doctors and religious specialists – ultimately there might be no cure in this lifetime. The best option for such a patient is simply to conduct Buddhist activities aimed at improving the next lifetime.

*

Exploring these narratives from lay people and medical and religious specialists in contemporary Amdo, we can start to build up a picture of the multiple ways in which *nyoné*, its causation and treatment are understood in relation to Tibetan medical and religious concepts of 'heart', 'mind' and 'wind'.

Much commonality between lay people's and practitioners' perspectives was evident here, with many lay interviewees describing causation and treatment through 'simplified cognates' of complex medical and religious terminology and theory, as Jacobson also described in Darjeeling (2007: 231–32). Here, disturbances to heart, mind and/or wind – for example, through life stresses or religious practice – were implicated in many cases of *nyoné*. Amongst the doctors and religious specialists I interviewed in Amdo, this was usually explicated through the concept of *lung* – reflecting, as we will see in the following two chapters, what is to be found in both medical and religious texts. Among the lay people I spoke to, there was often less clarity around how these facets of mind-body (dys)functioning were interrelated and involved in the manifestation of *nyoné*. However, common understandings of the relationship between difficult life circumstances, negative emotions, 'heart illness' and *nyoné* were evident – even if the underlying mechanisms and the key role of wind here were less well understood by non-specialists. Similarly, the notion that Tantric practice can lead to *nyoné* when conducted 'incorrectly', or without proper instruction, was well known by lay interviewees, even if there was disagreement over the train of causation here – for example, whether the problem was 'too much time alone', 'too much study' or some effect of wind in certain Tantric practices.

These complex connections between various aspects of mind-body structure and functioning are integral to understanding Tibetan medical and religious perspectives on *nyoné*, its causation and treatment. In the next two chapters, we will examine the key concept of wind and its role in the causation of *nyoné* in more depth, through an exploration of medical and religious textual materials alongside the work of previous researchers in these related spheres. While commonalities between medical and Tantric perspectives will become clear – with concepts of mind-body structure and (dys)functioning shared by many lay individuals and medical and religious specialists across diverse Tibetan communities – clear differences will become evident too. We will see how medical and Tantric notions of the body diverge, and how practitioners and scholars – both historic and contemporary – have attempted to make sense of differing descriptions and understandings. Next, then, in Chapter 2, we will explore *lung* in the context of Tibetan medicine, examining medical concepts of mind and body, and the interrelated concepts of 'heart' and 'mind' in relation to *nyoné*. Following on from this, in Chapter 3, we will examine the notion of *lung* in Tibetan Tantric traditions, where successful manipulations of its flow through the bodily channels are key to attaining enlightenment. However, as we have heard here, missteps and mistakes in practice have the potential to lead to all kinds of problems in mind and/or body – including, potentially, *nyoné*. It is not for nothing that many Tibetan Tantrists view their approach as a highly efficacious, but also complex and difficult, path towards realization, as we shall see.

Notes

1. The Tibetan term *drip* is generally translated as impurity, contamination or defilement, and is often said to result from being in proximity to things such as dead bodies, others' clothes or belongings, or 'impure' objects. In Amdo, such concepts were often discussed through the related concept of *mi tsangwa* – literally, 'unclean' – with many lay individuals, particularly, connecting it to notions of spirits (Tib, *dön*). We will explore these interlinked concepts in Part II.
2. Note the differential spelling of Lobsang Rabgay/Rapgay's name in different publications.
3. In Tibetan, such conditions may be referred to in full, or a shortened form that omits the '*né*' (illness/disorder) – for example, '*lung (né)*', '*nying lung (né)*', '*sok lung (né)*'. '*Lung*', then, may refer to 'wind' but also to 'wind illness'; similarly '*sok lung*' may refer only to the life-sustaining wind itself, or to the condition resulting from its disorder – the meaning is usually evident from the context.
4. With most consultations at provincial Tibetan medicine hospitals including the use of a sphygmomanometer by Tibetan doctors, the notion of 'blood pressure' was very familiar to all of my Tibetan interviewees. In fact, the Tibetan term *trak lung* ('blood wind') is usually translated as 'blood pressure', and often said to be roughly equivalent in terms of symptoms. Moreover, research conducted in Golok by Bassini highlights some overlaps between the different Tibetan and biomedical notions of 'heart illness', when she lists a number of physical symptoms of *nying né* described by her Golok interviewees, including a feeling of the heart 'pushing up', a 'piercing pain in the heart', the 'heart being squeezed' (2013a: 240).
5. As we will see in the next chapter, this Tibetan term, while usually translated quite generally as 'channels', in fact refers to a variety of circulatory and non-circulatory structures in the body including energetic channels through which the *lung* flows, and blood vessels – as he seems to be referring to here.
6. Related to the notion of *bodhicitta* – 'mind of enlightenment' – the control of these drops is integral to Tantric subtle-body practices, as we will explore in some detail in Chapter 3.
7. This term has a range of meanings, both technical and colloquial (see, for example, the Tibetan and Himalayan Library translation from the Wylie transliteration *rnam rtog* [https://ttt.thlib.org/] for a broad range of translations). It is usually translated as something like 'conceptual/discursive thoughts' or '*mis*conceptions' (DiValerio 2015: 7) in literary Tibetan and classical Buddhist and Bon literature. In this context, *namtok* refers to the incorrect understandings of the nature of reality that result from our lack of realization – i.e. the misapprehension that things have intrinsic existence, on the basis of which we – as unenlightened beings – create the ego. However, in Modern Colloquial Tibetan it is often used to mean something akin to 'doubt', and was usually translated as 'doubt' or 'suspicion' by Amdo Tibetans with a good knowledge of English; Ardussi and Epstein describe it as 'hesitation' or 'scruple' (1978: 330). In this context, it was sometimes discussed by lay Tibetans in Amdo in the context of a practitioner not having sufficient 'faith' (Tib. *dépa*) in Buddhist teachings, and therefore experiencing doubt

and/or fear when conducting complex high-level practices, which consequently led to problems for them. This concept will be explored in more detail in Chapter 3, and will also crop up again in Part II, when we find it referenced in relation to spirit affliction. (Extra thanks to Geoffrey Samuel for his help in understanding the complex nature of this term [email communication, March 2024]).

8. See, for example, Gotsang Repa's 1512 *The Life of the Madman of Tsang* (rgod tshang ras pa sna tshogs rang grol. 1969 [1512]. *gtsang nyon he ru ka phyogs thams cad las rnam par rgyal ba'i rnam thar rdo rje theg pa'i gsal byed nyi ma'i snying po*. Published as *The Life of the Saint of Gtsang*.
9. Lodro described himself using the Indian term 'yogi' rather than Tibetan terms *ngakpa* or *hön*.
10. In addition, DiValerio references another two Tibetan terms used to refer to such figures: *druptop nyönpa* (mad *siddha*) and *neljor nyönpa* (mad yogin), *druptop nyönpa* being used most often to refer to the 'more famous and exalted figures', with '[l]esser-known figures' viewed as 'mad yogins' or 'mad lamas' (2015: 2–3).
11. Interestingly, I came across another description of a practitioner doing this – in that instance, a *lhawa* (spirit-medium) in Rebkong, described by Snying bo rgyal and Rino (2008: ix).
12. 'Aged butter' or pig fat is usually used for this.
13. The patient's constitutional 'type' according to Tibetan medicine classification based on the three aspects of wind, bile and phlegm is also important here.
14. In fact, this differentiation between 'traditional' and biomedical medicine as best for chronic and acute conditions respectively has been described in many communities (Hepburn 1988: 69).
15. This case will be examined in more detail in Chapter 4.
16. Multiple historical and contemporary factors have impacted on Tibetans' views of both Tibetan medicine and biomedicine, and the ways in which such biomedical tests were being used in contemporary Amdo and elsewhere to apparently 'rule out' certain causative factors. See Deane (2024) for some examination of this.
17. Roasted barley flour – a staple of the Tibetan diet, also used extensively in religious contexts, for example in making offering cakes such as *tsa tsa*, and *lü* ('effigies', 'scapegoats').

Chapter 2

Heart, Mind or Wind?

Tibetan Medical Conceptions of Mind, Mental Health and *Nyoné*

> *First you have* nying lung *[heart wind], and then you have your* sok lung *[life-sustaining wind], and then maybe you will become* nyoné.
>
> —Dr Dechen (39, Xining)

In Chapter 1, we saw some of the ways in which doctors, religious practitioners and lay Tibetans in Amdo discussed *nyoné*, its causes, symptoms and treatments in relation to the intertwining concepts of *nying* (heart), *sem* (mind) and *lung* (wind). Evident here was a common focus on sadness or life difficulties in the causation of *nyoné* – as Tsering (27, Xining) told me: 'It is usually because something *happened*, and that causes sadness, or depression . . . Something *happened* and then that can cause you *nyonpa*'. As we heard from Tibetan medicine doctors in Amdo, key here is the role of wind. In this chapter, we will explore Tibetan medical understandings of wind and its relationships with 'heart' and 'mind' in the context of mental health – and particularly the condition of *nyoné*. Through an exploration of Tibetan medical textual descriptions alongside examination of previous research in this arena, we will build up a clear picture of how these concepts are understood by Tibetan medicine doctors and lay people across diverse Tibetan communities, in advance of examining 'religious' notions of wind and its role in Tibetan Tantric practices in Chapter 3.

In the previous chapter, we saw much focus on the notion of *nying né* (heart illness) in lay narratives of *nyoné*. Key to such perspectives is the Tibetan understanding of *sem* – 'mind' – associated with the heart, as opposed to the brain.[1] As a result, the term *nying né* may refer to either problems of the physical organ of the heart (similar to a biomedical diagnosis of 'heart disease', for instance) or conditions related to the mind and/or emotions. In contrast to these numerous mentions of *nying*, only a handful of lay interviewees discussed the role of *lung* here. Some remembered discussions about *lung* among parents or grandparents in previous decades, but interviewees mostly told me that it was not something that they themselves were very familiar with. Interestingly, this focus on 'heart illness', rather than 'wind illness', in discussions on mental health and *nyoné* in Amdo contrasts significantly with my previous research in Darjeeling (Deane 2018, 2019b). There, both lay Tibetans and Tibetan medicine doctors I spoke to frequently brought up the notion of *lung*, and descriptions of *lung* and *sok lung* were central to many lay narratives of mental health and illness – particularly in relation to difficult life circumstances, stresses and traumas. There, I frequently heard descriptions of 'high wind', 'wind problems' and 'wind illness' (in both English and Tibetan) to describe illnesses related to the mind, or simply everyday instances of worry or anxiety. A number of other researchers too have discussed the centrality of this concept in narratives of mental illness in some Tibetan communities. For example, Jacobson explored in some detail *lung* illnesses in his own, earlier research in Darjeeling (2000, 2002, 2007; see also Gutschow 1997 and Millard 2007 for work in other regions), and Adams (1998) and Janes (1995, 1999b) have examined the 'politicization' of *lung* diagnoses in Lhasa.[2]

As we saw in Chapter 1, many discussions on *nyoné* (and mental illness more broadly) in Amdo were focused on afflicted individuals' experiences of diverse difficult or distressing life events and circumstances. Examples included bereavements (especially multiple or particularly traumatic bereavements), significant loss of property such as the theft of a family's yak herd, forced marriage and/or marital abuse, or pressures related to schoolwork or exams. This reflects the findings of researchers working in other Tibetan communities too. For example, in Lhasa – alongside the politicization of *lung* illnesses – Janes described everyday 'family troubles' such as drinking problems, unemployment and arguments within the family as causes of *lung né* of various kinds (1999b: 398). Similarly, working in Zangskar in the 1990s, Gutschow described a case of lung-related 'insanity' resulting from the theft of a man's entire earnings (1997: 191–95). Thus, despite some differences in terminology, a little exploration suggests that lay interviewees and Tibetan medicine doctors in Amdo are in fact referencing similar processes through which some kind of suffering might lead to *nyoné*, where the interconnections between heart, wind and mind are key. In this chapter, we will explore these interrelating concepts in Tibetan medical perspectives, the ways in which they may be involved in the causation and development of *nyoné*, and what this means for treatment. We will start, then, with an examination of Tibetan medical perspectives on *lung*, alongside the multitudinous *tsa* (channels) in which it is understood to flow within the body, *khorlo* (chakras) and *tiklé* (drops) – which together make up what is often referred to in the English-language literature as the 'subtle-body' or Vajra-body system of Tibetan medical theory and practice. Firstly, we will explore medical textual descriptions of *lung*, before examining the ways in which this concept intertwines with notions of 'heart' and 'mind', and their relevance to the causation and treatment of *nyoné*.

Lung: Notions of 'Wind' in Tibetan Medicine

> [A]ccording to Tibetan medical theory, the intrinsic, natural functioning of the mind depends on the balance of pranic [lung] currents. (Epstein and Topgay 1982: 71)

As I described in the Introduction, there has been a certain amount of research already on Tibetan understandings of the role of *lung* in mental health and illness (cf. Deane 2018, 2019b; Epstein and Topgay 1982; Gutschow 1997; Jacobson 2000, 2002, 2007; Janes 1995, 1999b). The close relationship between *lung* and the mind is key here, with the mind and wind traditionally described as being like a rider and their horse: the horse (wind/*lung*) needs the rider (mind/*sem*) for direction; but equally, the rider (mind/*sem*) needs the horse (wind/*lung*) for energy/movement: they work together, the mind said to be 'inseparably linked' to the body through the wind (Rapgay 1984: 50). Any disturbance in the mind will therefore affect the wind and its flow within the mind and body; likewise, any disturbance to the wind will affect the mind. Thus, whilst all three of the *nyépa* (energies) are understood to be linked to various mind-body organs, functions and processes, it is the *lung* that is most commonly implicated in any kind of mind and mental functioning and dysfunctioning – and it is therefore key to our understanding of *nyoné*.

These concepts of mind and body and their connection through *lung* are also key in Tibetan Tantra, as we will explore in Chapter 3. There, mind-body practices designed to manipulate the wind within the body in order to affect the mind and consciousness are key to Tibetan Buddhist and Bon ideas about enlightenment and how to achieve it. Furthermore, it is the 'subtle' (Tib. *trawa*) nature of wind that is also understood to allow spirits and deities to possess individuals, potentially causing illness this way (a topic we will explore in Part II). Thus, this notion of wind is fundamental not only to Tibetan conceptions of mind-body structure and (dys)functioning but also to an individual's relationship to the wider world. In her key 2010 paper on *lung*, Yoeli-Tlalim described the 'culturally defined' nature of our understandings of bodily structure and functioning, and 'the ways in which and purposes whereby these can be manipulated'. Here, culturally specific religious concepts and sociopolitical structures can come into play (2010: 319), as we see clearly in Tibetan notions of *lung*: part of a Tibetan 'ethno-psychology'[3] whereby culturally determined concepts of the person and of the ways in which *lung* is integral to mind and body help to – as Kirmayer, Adeponle and Dzokoto assert – 'locate the individual in society, and underlie ascriptions of causality and agency in health and illness' (2018: 24).

Of course, the notion of bodily 'wind' is not limited to Tibetan traditions – Yoeli-Tlalim references Kuriyama's (1995) work on concepts of *pneuma*/wind/*qi* across diverse European and Asian traditions, arguing that such perspectives 'reflect and define notions of the self' as well as perceptions of the body, making them 'central to any investigation of what defines health and illness' (Yoeli-Tlalim 2010: 319). Indeed, Low and Hsu describe how the notion of 'wind' is 'recruited across cultures as a way of thinking about a host of phenomena that define fundamental aspects of the physical and spiritual world', arguing that 'ideas of wind persistently overlap with notions of spirit, divinity, breath, smell, and shadow' (2007: S2). The Tibetan concept of *lung* is a perfect example of this: bringing together medical and religious notions of mind and body into (sometimes uneasy and even contradictory) coexistence, and tracing its origins back to early Indian religious and medical traditions, *lung* is integral to Tibetan explanations of mind-body structure and functioning.[4]

Clearly reflecting the Indian Ayurvedic concept of *vāta*, we find description of *lung*'s characteristics, functions and dysfunctions in Tibetan medical texts such as the *Gyüshi*. Here, it is one of the three *nyépa* (Skt. *doṣa*; fault, energy) of *lung* (Skt. *vāta*), *tripa* (Skt. *pitta*) and *béken* (Skt. *kapha*) – usually translated into English as 'wind', 'bile' and 'phlegm' respectively. However, with the Tibetan term *lung* being *also* a translation of the Indian Tantric concept of *prāṇa* (breath, life-force), we find the concept of *lung* presented in 'two distinct but closely related ways' in the Indo-Tibetan medical and Tantric traditions (Marek and Oliphant 2017: 418). For example, Garrett and Adams note that the circulatory system that is portrayed in early Tibetan medical literature is 'roughly based on the classical Indian Āyurvedic tradition', but this structure is 'significantly different' from the circulatory system described in Indian Tantric texts, on which Tibetan Tantric descriptions are based (2008: 86–87).

In addition, Tibetan medical traditions also link *lung* to specific Buddhist notions of attachment, with the three *nyépa* said to derive from the Buddhist 'three poisons' (Tib. *duk sum*) – desire/attachment (Tib. *dö chak*), hatred/anger

(Tib. *zhé dang*) and delusion (Tib. *ti muk*) – which ultimately all stem from ignorance (*ma rig pa*) (*Gyüshi II* 2015: 35). We thus have one Tibetan term taking in two separate – if related – Indian medical and Tantric concepts. As Samuel argues, these processes of assimilation and adaptation in Tibet of Indian medical and Tantric notions of 'wind' mean that Tibetan *lung* is not identical to either Ayurvedic *vāta* or Tantric *prāṇa*. Instead, it 'encompasses elements from both' and also has 'an additional layer of meaning' as a result of its connection to the Buddhist concept of attachment or desire (2019: 773). However, despite this conflation into a singular term '*lung*' in the Tibetan language, differences remain between the Tibetan medical and religious traditions in relation to its structure and functioning in the body – as we shall explore below and, in more detail, in the next chapter.

Moreover, when we explore the Tibetan and Indian textual material, it is not simply that there are clear differences *between* the medical and Tantric traditions; in fact, there is also some diversity *within* these two traditions, with winds, channels and chakras described differently across the multiple Indian and Tibetan medical and Tantric traditions. As a result, while many attempts have been made to 'match up' medical and religious Indo-Tibetan notions of this 'subtle' body over the centuries, we might argue that such endeavours are rather tricky given the significant diversities across the texts overall. Indeed, as Garrett and Adams conclude, 'descriptions of the body in South Asian literature are so numerous and so complex that few differences are fully reconciled' (2008: 87), and it is of course from this 'South Asian literature' that so many of the Tibetan textual traditions derive. However, all is not lost. In fact, notions of 'wind'/'breath' in these two divergent Indian traditions originate from the same ancient Indian Vedic sources (something we will explore in more detail in Chapter 3). Over time, these traditions diverged and evolved, leading to significant differences between medical and Tantric narratives, each tradition maintaining 'its own doctrine of bodily winds' (Zysk 2007: S113). While there have been historical and contemporary attempts to bring these diverse approaches back together, this remains rather problematic. This was evident during my time in Amdo, where conversations with Tibetan medical and Tantric specialists demonstrated diverse perspectives on, for example, whether differing descriptions in the medical and religious traditions are in fact referring to the same thing. And it was clear that for those specialists with knowledge and skill across the spheres of *both* medicine and Tantra, this endeavour was no less complicated.

In this chapter, we will focus on Tibetan medical perspectives on *lung*, and the channels in which the various wind currents are said to flow throughout the body. *Lung*, *tripa* and *béken* are understood to be composed of the five elements of earth, air, water, fire and space, with *lung* said to be predominantly composed of air and space,[5] its characteristics rough, light, cold, motile, compact and subtle (Rabgay 1985: 48). Within this tripartite system, *lung* is predominant due to its fundamental role in mind-body functioning as well as its relationship with the other two *nyépa*. For example, Rapgay describes a 'constant interaction of opposing factors or polarities' of 'hot' *tripa* and 'cold' *béken*, mediated by *lung* (1984: 49). Understood to reside predominantly in the lower part of the body (while also pervading the whole mind-body), *lung* is particularly related to the skin, bone, tissues, joints, pelvic region and large intestine. Moreover, there are three types of *lung* – gross, subtle and very subtle – and it is the 'very subtle' wind that passes from one life to the next: the 'completion and fruition of virtuous and non-virtuous karma [action] which determine birth and death' in Dharmic perspective (Rabgay 1985: 48).

Despite the numerous connections between the Tibetan medical tradition and Buddhism, the relationship between 'medicine' and 'religion' is complex. Adams argues that historically – particularly between the seventeenth and early twentieth centuries – medicine was part of 'an entirely Buddhist educational system', in a context where Tibetan culture was also 'predominantly a Buddhist culture'. Here, boundaries between 'religion' and any other aspects of the culture were 'more often than not, never clearly made' (2001: 555). With this in mind, some scholars have described a 'Buddhicization' of the Tibetan medical tradition (Gerke 2013; J. Gyatso 2004). Indeed, it seems that such descriptions of the so-called 'Buddhist' basis of Tibetan medicine can be overstated. What *is* clear, however, is that the concept of *lung* does indeed span the spheres of religion and medicine, and is fundamental to Tibetan conceptions of mind-body, health and illness in both medical and Tantric contexts, with broad implications for practice across Buddhist and Bon traditions. Key too is the related notion of *tsa* – the channels within which *lung* is understood to flow, and which are also integral to Tantric and medical practice.

Tsa *(Channels)*

The Tibetan 'subtle body' comprises *lung* (wind), *tsa* (channels), *khorlo* (energy centres/chakras) and *tiklé* (drops). This system can be seen depicted in Tibetan medical paintings dating back to those commissioned by Desi Sangye Gyatso in the seventeenth century (see, for example, copies of such paintings published in works by Baker and Shrestha 1997; and Williamson, Young and Shrestha 2009). Within this system, wind is understood to be transported through thousands of channels running throughout the body. These channels intersect at a number of chakras – particularly down the centre of the body, where side channels to the left and right of a central channel are understood to converge at key points down its length from the crown of the head to the genitals. The Tibetan *tsa* are equivalent to the channels in the Indian systems known in Sanskrit variously as '*nāḍī-, sirā-/śirā-, srotas-* or *dhamanī-*' (Garrett and Adams 2008: 88), and are understood to transport not only wind but other substances too, including bodily fluids such as blood, water, nutrients and waste products (Gerke 2013: 83).[6] Due to their various functions in transporting these diverse substances, these channels have been translated variously into English as 'veins', 'arteries' and 'nerves'. Indeed, both Tibetan and non-Tibetan medical practitioners and authors often use such English terms despite the reality that the Tibetan '*tsa*' is in fact 'not directly equivalent to any of these' (Garrett and Adams 2008: 88). Moreover, while a number of different categories of channels are described in the *Gyüshi* – for example, the *tsa kar* ('white channels') and *tsa nak* ('black channels'), translated in much contemporary literature as 'nerves' and 'blood vessels' respectively (see Men-Tsee-Khang 2008: 62) – there has been 'considerable debate' in the commentarial texts over 'what these categories actually refer to' (J. Gyatso 2015: 87–88). And, similarly to in the Ayurvedic tradition, there is also much debate in Tibetan medical texts over the exact pathways of these hundreds of channels within the body (Garrett and Adams 2008: 90; see also J. Gyatso 2004: 87–88).[7] Furthermore, despite many descriptions of so-called 'circulatory' systems here, the *tsa* are in fact predominantly understood to be 'open-ended ducts or fine networks' (Gerke 2013: 88). Part of this complexity is no doubt a result of the development of notions of *tsa* across different historical periods, influenced by multiple – and unrelated – medical and philosophical systems (Ibid.: 89).

These numerous channels are classified in the *Gyüshi*. For example, Chapter 4 of the *Explanatory Tantra* describes how the channels may be classified functionally, with four types: channels of formation (Tib. *chakpé tsa*),[8] channels of existence (Tib. *sipé tsa*), connecting channels (Tib. *drelwé tsa*) and vitality/life channels (Tib. *tsé tsa*) (*Gyüshi II* 2015: 23). Descriptions of the 'life channels', for example, list three types: one that circulates throughout the head and body, one that moves in association with the breath and one that wanders within the body like the *la* (life-force) (Ibid.: 24). It is through this network of channels – within which wind, blood and other substances are understood to flow – that the external and internal parts of the body are connected (Ibid.).

Five Tibetan Wind Currents and Their Indian Background

Key in the *Gyüshi* are descriptions of the five 'principal' wind currents, each of which may be subject to increase, decrease and/or disturbance – potentially leading to disorder in the mind and/or body as per the location(s) and functions of that particular wind:

- **Life-sustaining wind** (Tib. *sok [dzin] lung*): located in the centre of the body/at the crown of the head; enables respiration and swallowing; related to the senses (and said to have gross, subtle and very subtle aspects)[9]
- **Ascending wind** (Tib. *gyen gyu lung*): localized in the chest, also circulating in the throat region; produces the voice
- **Pervasive wind** (Tib. *khyap jé lung*): localized in the region of the heart, but pervading the body; facilitates movement in the extremities; responsible for the circulation of the blood and lymph in the body
- **Fire-accompanying wind** (Tib. *mé nyam lung*): localized around the navel; supports digestion and is responsible for bowel movement
- **Descending wind** (Tib. *tur sel lung*): localized in the bladder, large intestine and reproductive organs; involved in menstruation, childbirth and expulsion of urine and faeces

It is clear that these five *lung* currents originate in classical Ayurveda, where Zysk describes five breaths (Skt. *prāṇa*) that 'regulate and promote various internal functions' (1995: 38):

- **Front breath** (Skt. *prāṇa*): located in the mouth; ensures respiration and swallowing
- **Upward moving breath** (Skt. *udāna*): produces speech
- **Diffused breath** (Skt. *vyāna*): circulates in the limbs, motivating their movement
- **Concentrated breath** (Skt. *samāna*): promotes digestion
- **Downward-moving breath** (Skt. *apāna*): ensures excretion and childbirth

However, Zysk notes the differences between various Indian medical compilers' respective discussions of these winds, which he asserts, 'reveal a plurality of sources' on this topic. Thus we find, for example, that texts compiled by Ayurvedic doctor Caraka (*c.*200 BCE–200 CE) 'incorporated both medical and non-medical data' related to wind, in contrast to those by Suśruta (*c.*100–400 CE), which included only teachings that were specifically medical (Zysk 1995: 51–52).[10] Here we have a clue to the origins of Indian notions of 'wind', which date back *prior* to the medical traditions, to the mind-body practices of Indian ascetics whose practices, including breath control, 'gradually gave rise to a standardized list of the five *prāṇás*', including the anatomical locations and physiological functions of each (Zysk 1995: 45). Following these early practices, we find the notion of 'wind' and its relationship to the mind and body diverging into separate Indian medical and Tantric traditions, as Zysk describes:

> Continuing the development of previous doctrines of wind and breath, the classical medical tradition, as preserved in the *Caraka* and *Suśruta Saṃhitās*, established a specifically medical pneumatology . . . It codified the physiology of *prāṇá* and the five breaths and the diseases arising from abnormalities in the physiology of each breath. In quite a different direction, a pneumatology developed around ascetic techniques and the importance of breath in the attainment of higher states of consciousness. These doctrines find their codification in the texts of Yoga. As both the medical and Yogic traditions derive their doctrines of wind and breath from the ascetic Upaniṣadic thinkers, some overlapping can be expected. (1995: 52)[11]

Thus, in the Tibetan medical system, which derives its notions of *lung* from these early Indian conceptions of wind/breath, we find a delineation into the five key *lung* currents described above – each understood to be located in a different area of the body, associated with a different element and related to different functions of the mind-body.

These five *lung* currents in the Tibetan medical system have been described in more detail elsewhere (Yoeli-Tlalim 2010; see also Deane 2019b), and so I will not give too much elucidation here. More important in this context is to note the significance of one particular wind current – the *sok (dzin) lung* – in relation to *nyoné*. In my previous research in Darjeeling, I encountered a focus on the *sok tsa* (life-sustaining channel) and the *sok (dzin) lung* (life-sustaining wind) in many discussions on mental illness, including *nyoné* (Deane 2018). However, there is dispute over the identification of this channel in relation to the other, physical, channels and their functions, which Garrett and Adams note 'was, and still is, hotly contested among medical and religious scholars' (2008: 91–92). In addition, Tibetan medicine doctors and scholars – both ethnically Tibetan and non-Tibetan – have made various equivalences between the Tibetan *tsa* and biomedical anatomical concepts. For example, Dorjee, Jones and Moore assert that 'some of these channels are part of the nervous system' (2005: 164); and Clifford, that the *sok tsa* is linked by some to the vagus nerve (Clifford 1984: 133). Interestingly, the *sok tsa* is in fact translated into English in two different ways in the Men-Tsee-Khang's (Tibetan Medical & Astro Institute's) 2008 English translation of the *Gyüshi*, as Gerke points out (2013: 87) – translated in the section on embryology as 'central life channel' (Men-Tsee-Khang 2008: 51), in contrast to its translation as 'aorta' (Ibid.: 61) in this same translation's fourth chapter, on anatomy.[12]

Given these diversities, such 'matching' endeavours between Tibetan medicine and biomedical anatomy remain problematic – not least due to the fact that *Gyüshi* descriptions include both physical and immaterial channels (Samuel 2019: 780). These discussions over the specifics of channels – and the *sok tsa* in particular – will become even more important when we explore Tantric notions of the 'central channel', and whether they can be equated with the *sok tsa*, in the next chapter. But first, let us explore the ways in which *lung* may become disrupted, and the implications of this for mind and mental health.

Disordered *Lung*: Causes and Symptoms

While disruption in any of the three *nyépa* may lead to psychological and/or physiological symptoms, it is wind's close relationship with the mind that means it is often implicated in cases of mental ill-health, including *nyoné*. As we saw in the previous chapter, this was not always evident from some of my discussions in Amdo, where many narratives instead focused on '*nying*' (heart). However, it is certainly evident in the Tibetan medical texts and in Tibetan doctors' explanations of these kinds of conditions. For example, we find sixty-three main types of wind illness described in the *Gyüshi*, classified under two main groups: general (forty-eight types) and specific (fifteen types), with diverse psychological and physiological symptoms. Furthermore, there are specific causes, symptoms and treatments related to the five key wind currents mentioned above, depending not only on the particular wind current affected, but the *manner* in which it is affected – whether it is increased/in excess, decreased/in deficiency or 'disturbed'.[13]

For example, in general, an *increase* in wind will result in symptoms including the body becoming thin and darker in complexion, a preference for warmth/heat, shivering, constipation, talkativeness, dizziness, a loss of strength, drowsiness and impairment in the senses (*Gyüshi II* 2015: 39–40). In contrast, a *decrease* in wind will likely manifest a loss of energy, lack of talking, unclear memory (*Gyüshi II* 2015: 40), 'confusion in perception' and/or lethargy (Drungtso 2004: 224), among other symptoms. A *disturbance* in the wind may lead to an agitated mind; restlessness; dizziness; buzzing in the ears; feeling cold; a dry, rough, red tongue; and a bitter taste in the mouth (*Gyüshi II* 2015: 41). In addition, Rabgay describes a large number of 'general' wind symptoms including restlessness, delirium, vertigo, tinnitus, chill, insomnia, yawning, anger, pain in *lung* 'focal points', dry heaving and distended abdomen – with symptoms often worse during the night, at dawn and post-digestion (1985: 53–54) – as well as 'specific' symptoms such as 'fright', 'restlessness' and/or talkativeness resulting from disorder of the pervasive wind; and 'general malaise', fatigue and deafness being potential symptoms of ascending wind (Ibid.: 60–61).

In terms of causation, as with the other *nyépa*, factors that can disrupt the regular functioning of wind in the body can be summarized under four categories: i) diet, ii) behaviours, iii) seasonal changes and iv) harmful spirits (Drungtso 2004: 210). Thus, for example, the rainy season is viewed as a common time for wind disorders to manifest (*Gyüshi II* 2015: 37), with the ingestion of bitter foods, prolonged fasting, lack of sleep, forcible retention of urine and/or faeces, 'excessive' sexual intercourse, prolonged crying and grief all considered conditions (Tib. *kyen*) that can contribute to its manifestation (*Gyüshi II* 2015: 37). Similarly, Rabgay describes factors such as vomiting, exposure to cold, talkativeness and malnutrition (1985: 49–50), but particularly pertinent here – as we saw in the previous chapter – are the psychological factors and mental activities described in the texts and by doctors, such as 'excessive joy or sadness' and 'depression' (Epstein and Topgay 1982: 74), 'immense grief' and 'mental activity' (Drungtso 2004: 210). Indeed, Adams argues that '[f]eelings of anger and frustration are *as important* as the cold foods one has eaten, the changing climate, and political oppression' in understanding *lung* disorders (1998: 83).

Notable here – particularly if we focus on some of the more 'psychological' factors described – is the clear overlap between *causes* and *symptoms* of various wind disorders. These demonstrate a kind of circular relationship between mind and wind, whereby disturbance in any of the wind currents is understood to lead to certain kinds of mental or emotional disturbance, and any kind of mental or emotional disturbance is similarly understood to lead to a disturbance in the flow of *lung* (Epstein and Topgay 1982: 73). Thus, Epstein and Topgay describe a form of *nyoné* 'primarily characterized by depression' – '[o]ften precipitated by separation from possessions or family' (Ibid.: 77). They describe how individuals suffering from this form of *nyoné* may become aggressive or delirious, with a loss of control over their body, speech or mind, often suffering from insomnia and/or speaking senselessly (Ibid.: 81). Indeed, in the previous chapter, we saw an example of this in Samdrup's narrative about his neighbour who became *nyoné* after the theft of his yak herd, with his description of the man 'going around everywhere, talking nonsense . . . and hitting people'. This is evident in others' ethnographic research too, with previous researchers describing narratives of wind illness linked to 'stress', 'worry' and loss (Jacobson 2002, 2007; Janes 1999b; Prost 2006 – see also Deane 2018, 2019b). Indeed, if we accept the Tibetan notion that a healthy, well-functioning mind depends on the undisturbed flow of *lung* throughout the body (Epstein and Topgay, 1982: 71), then it is logical that any disturbance to the *lung* will have an effect on that individual's mental health. Similarly, with the wind so closely related to the mind, its functioning and the senses, it is not surprising to hear that any strong emotions or mental activity, such as worry, will affect the functioning of the *lung*.

Disruption in one or more of a person's wind currents is understood to occur through various steps, usually beginning as a minor problem and escalating over time, as Rapgay describes:

> Initial disorders are said to arise from disturbances in the flow of rLung through its natural channels or pathways. Repeated aggravation, however, leads to an increase of rLung beyond its normal range, but still confined to its natural channels . . . With continued disturbance and aggravation, rLung increases beyond a critical point, whereupon, it overflows its natural channels and disrupts the other two pathophysiological factors [*tripa* and *béken*] and the bodily processes dependent on them. In a similar way, if one of the other pathophysiological factors is disturbed and aggravated, it will also overflow and affect the circulation of rLung. (1984: 50)

The fundamental role of wind in the mind-body becomes clear through such descriptions, with any disruption to its natural functioning likely to lead to a diverse range of physiological and/or psychological symptoms depending on the particular *lung* current(s) involved and the type of disruption occurring.[14]

Finally, as I noted above, pertinent to many discussions on *nyoné* is the particular wind current known as the *sok (dzin) lung* (life-sustaining wind) and its associated channel, the *sok tsa* (life-sustaining channel). Indeed, referencing some biomedical diagnoses, Epstein and Topgay assert that in terms of 'mental disorders', it is this current which is the most relevant (1982: 72):

> Most common anxieties, minor depressions, and uncontrollable surfacings of emotion are attributed to primary disturbance and aggravation of the balance of the *sok lung* . . . When the life-bearing current is more seriously affected, i.e. through invasion of its channels by other increased currents, symptoms of violent or hysterical behaviour may appear. If severely affected, psychosis may result. (1982: 74)

These kinds of causes are described in the commentarial texts too, such as in Sanggye Gyatso's chapter on 'The Healing of Life-Wind Illness' in his seventeenth-century *Extended Commentary on the Instructional Tantra of the Four Tantras* (Tib. *men ngag yon tan rgyud kyi lhan thabs zug rngu'i tsha gdung sel ba'i katpū ra dus min 'chi zhags gcod pa'i ral gri*), which lists grief, worry, lack of sleep and anxiety amongst others, with symptoms of *sok lung* disturbance including 'distress, panic, obscure dreams . . . wavering awareness, confusion' (Chui 2019: 88–89). Similarly, at the Qinghai Province Tibetan Medicine Hospital in twenty-first-century Xining, Dr Tangun (50), described 'general causes' of *nyoné* such as 'problems in the family; for example, if your father and mother, or another relative dies in an accident'. Because of that, he explained, 'you will become *nyoné* – because your *sok lung* becomes disturbed'. Indeed, the role of the *sok lung* current in the causation of *nyoné* was discussed by a few Tibetan medicine doctors in Amdo – particularly in relation to its location in the centre of the body, and its consequent proximity and relationship to the *nying*. In the previous chapter, I recounted Dr Dechen's description of *sok lung né* as 'a state between *nying lung* and *nyoné*': 'First you have *nying lung*, and then you have you *sok lung*, and then maybe you will become *nyoné*'. Through such descriptions, we start to see how the heart, mind and wind are interconnected, and how these connections may be implicated in the causation of *nyoné*, as we shall explore in more detail next.

Heart, Wind, Mind: Understanding the Connections

A connection between mind and heart is emphasized by Tibetan medicine doctor and author Phuntsok Wangmo's description of various causes of 'mental diseases': 'weakness of the physical heart; strong, unrelenting sadness, or the experience of a sudden event resulting in intense sadness' as well as 'poor diet' and 'provocations' [i.e. spirits] – all of which, he tells us, can lead to 'seven types of depression' (2015: 155). Similarly, Epstein and Topgay reference both the *Gyüshi* and the renowned Tibetan physician Dr Yeshe Donden when they describe 'predisposing causes' of *nyoné* including depression, 'mental discomfort', 'mental exertion' and a 'weak heart' (1982: 76). Here, the *nying* is important both as a physical organ and also as the seat of the mind, implicated in the emotions. So how can we understand the link between *lung* – particularly the *sok lung* – and *nying*, and the mechanisms by which, as Dr Dechen (39) explained, *nying né* may lead to *sok lung né* and, ultimately, to *nyoné*?

As I mentioned in Chapter 1, Tibetan descriptions of *nying né* – literally, 'heart illness' – can mean that a person is suffering from some kind of problem with their heart – for example, in the sense of the biomedical understanding of 'heart disease' or any other condition related to the heart organ and its functioning – or that someone is experiencing some kind of emotional state or activity, such as sadness, worry or anxiety. As Dr Nyima (38, Rebkong/Xining) explained, '*Nying* is a huge category . . . a big concept – it's also related to the mind, and emotions'. Moreover, we have seen how disruptions in the different wind currents may be both a cause and result of various psychological states and/or activities, and this is in part due to the relationship between heart and wind. One factor here is simply the very *location* of some of the wind currents in the body, as described in the *Second Tantra* of the *Gyüshi*:

> One of the channels (which is thick and only few inches long) goes along the middle (of the body by the heart), and thus the vital channel [*sok tsa*] is formed

> . . . Five hundred channels surround the channel of existence at the heart (i.e. the vital channel [*sok tsa*]), and it is this channel that brings about mental clarity. (Dhondhen and Kelsang [trans.] 1983: 39–40)

In Amdo, Dr Nyima explained clearly in a mixture of English and Tibetan:

> *Nying* is one of the locations of *lung*, so that means that when someone gets *lung né*, it's very likely that it will be harmful for their heart; and also when patients get *nying né*, that means that the *lung* will also become disordered. So because of that, *nying né* and *lung né* have some common symptoms, and when we are treating these, we also have some common medicines. Therefore at some level, these illnesses are very similar.

In addition, as the different *lung* currents are connected, a disturbance in any one of the other *lung* currents may also affect the *sok tsa* and *sok lung* specifically – nudging it out of its place and into the area of the heart, as Clifford explains: '[S]udden extreme anger carried by the "pervasive wind" swells the currents travelling in the life vein [*sok tsa*], pressuring the most subtle life-wind [*sok lung*] out of place and into the heart; it is this disturbance that causes consciousness to become distorted' (1984: 133).

Thus, we have the medical notion of '*nying lung (né)*' – wind in the heart (illness)/heart-wind illness – where one or more wind current(s) is out of its usual place, specifically entering the area of the heart and thus leading to *lung né* symptoms such as palpitations, 'heart swings' and a 'rapid, fluttering heart beat' (Janes 1999b: 394). Rabgay describes symptoms of *nying lung né* including 'mental disturbances' and 'frequent sighing' (1985: 58); Clifford describes 'high blood pressure and other cardiovascular diseases' (1984: 133); and Dorjee and Richards list the symptoms of '[i]nsanity from *wind* disease in the heart' described in Chapter 34 of the *Third Tantra*: 'headache; forgetfulness; insanity; irritability for no reason; talking without meaning or purpose even when not spoken to and not responding when addressed; the patient may become hysterical and sigh a great deal when he hears unpleasant things; shortness of breath; insomnia; an empty feeling in the heart' (Dorjee and Richards 1985: 22).

In Amdo, Dr Nyima (38) explained this as a process of escalation – particularly where treatment for early signs of *nying lung* are not sought, or are unsuccessful: 'It's most likely that when the disease is not heavy [severe], it's called "*nying lung*" or something like this, and then when it becomes heavy [severe], it's called "*sok lung*"'. In Xining, Tibetan medicine doctor and professor Dr Pema (40) described to me that a case of *nying lung né* might become worse and thus upset the function of the *sok tsa*. This, he explained, can create disorder of the *sok lung* – therefore a disturbance in the *sok lung* could be caused by either a *nying lung* disturbance escalating, or directly from some disturbance to the *sok tsa*/*sok lung*. In Chabcha, yogi Lodro (42) told me that *sok lung* is 'an illness where a person's heart is affected by the wind. This results, he said, in various symptoms: 'for example, the person mumbles or speaks nonsense, or becomes *nyoné*'.

In addition, in Amdo I heard explanations focused on the notion of 'controlling' one's mind or emotions, as a way of preventing this kind of escalation, with those unable to do so at greater risk of such conditions. For example, in Rebkong, Bonpo lama Tsering (57) asserted: 'If you cannot control your *nying*, then you cannot control your *sem* . . . This can cause you to have *nying lung*'. Janes also reported similar explanations from Tibetan medicine doctors he interviewed in Lhasa, some of whom described people who are 'narrow minded' or unable to 'control the mind properly' as being 'most likely' to develop *lung né* (1999b: 400). In Amdo, there was often a specifically religious aspect to these assertions, whereby Buddhism or Bon was described as providing Tibetans with a way of managing difficult life events and experiences, and thus apparently preventing a person from becoming affected in this way. For example, in Xining, Lhakpa (38) told me: 'From my perspective, we have Buddhism – we have a religion to rely on – so sadness, depression, or something like that, doesn't really cause us [Tibetans] much *nyoné* . . . For those who are sad or depressed, we can rely on our faith'.

Similarly, in Rebkong, Gelugpa Geshe Dhondup (50) asserted that *nyoné* was less common among Tibetans than among other ethnic groups in the area because of Tibetan Buddhist understandings of karma. However, he was confident that other religious traditions too might also offer some prevention:

> *Nyoné* can be caused by factors inside the person himself – for example, if your mind is out of control, it is not well balanced . . . As for the prevalence of *nyoné*, I can't say how common it is, but generally it's more common among Chinese or Hui Muslims than Tibetan people, because Tibetan people – because of religion – they have some explanation. For example, if I have hardship in this life, then I think maybe this is karma from my previous life: I did something bad, so this is why [I have hardship now]. So this kind of explanation helps Tibetans to find an explanation for why they are having this kind of hardship and to find balance. But for other people, like Chinese people, they don't have these kinds of explanations, so they can't find any other explanations, so the situation gets worse and worse – that's the kind of reason why they get *nyoné* – why it's more common among Chinese than Tibetans. And between Chinese and Hui Muslims, it's more common in Chinese people [because Hui people have religious beliefs].

For Geshe Dhondup, then, Muslim traditions and beliefs are *also* understood to have some benefit in terms of constructing meaning and associated coping mechanisms for adherents – but not to the extent that Buddhist ones are thought to. Indeed, such explanations highlight the role that Tibetan Buddhist/Bon concepts and practices can play in people's everyday engagements with life's ups and downs, with some interviewees describing the importance of 'keeping the mind calm' in maintaining a healthy mind and preventing problems such as 'unhappy mind' or *nyoné*.[15] Here, lay Tibetans as well as religious specialists may discuss Dharmic concepts quite generally, or reference particular practices, as offering some kind of 'protection'. This topic has been explored in more depth in Tibetan refugee communities in Dharamsala: for example, Prost quotes an elderly Tibetan woman there explaining that '*Chos* [Dharma/religion] helps me with this [*lung* disorder], it stops me from becoming too agitated' (2006: 121); and Hussain and Bhushan describe Tibetan research participants reporting that Buddhism provides them with understanding and also a 'method to overcome difficulties of the life and maintain peace of mind', based on the essential Buddhist tenets about the inevitability of suffering and its causation in attachment (2011: 581). Similarly, Lewis describes lay Tibetan exiles' use of Buddhist *lo jong* ('mind training') practices, which 'centre on using both compassion and emptiness to train the mind in combatting distress', (2018: 348–49). This 'active' process, she argues, helps people to create what she terms a 'spacious mind', or 'broad thinking' (Tib. *sem pa chen po*) (Lewis 2013, 2018).

Of course, it is difficult to assess to what extent such perspectives and practices have an impact on an individual level, and help members of diverse Tibetan communities to manage difficult life circumstances, but such explanations quite clearly fit into these Tibetan understandings of 'heart illness' and its relationship to emotions and mental activities. Further, they help us to piece together a picture of how these three concepts – heart, wind and mind – are connected, and thus how they may be involved in the causation of *nyoné*. As we have heard, with particular emotional states leading to disruption in the regular flow of wind through the body, wind may become displaced in the area of the heart, causing *nying lung [né]* – 'heart-wind disorder'. Left untreated, the *sok tsa* and *sok lung* may become affected, potentially leading to *sok lung [né]*. This then has the potential to result in symptoms including *nyoné*: with the *sok lung* being so closely related to the senses, an afflicted individual may find one or more of their senses disrupted or unclear, and may experience hallucinations and/or delusions among a host of other potential symptoms. Indeed, as Prost notes, 'severe *lung* disorders both stem from, and give rise to, serious distortions in perception' (2006: 120).

For many lay Tibetans, attempting to make sense of the complex relationships between these three factors can, perhaps unsurprisingly, be quite tricky, and I encountered quite a variety of explanations – and a fair amount of uncertainty – among lay interviewees in Amdo. For example, when I asked Lodri (68, Haixi/Xining) what might cause *nyoné*, he responded: 'I'm just guessing, but maybe most of the people who are *nyönpa* – it's maybe because their heart is not good, and then their wind [becomes disordered], and they have an uneasy mind [Tib. *sem kham ma dewa*]. Mostly now, if people go to see doctors, they say this is *nying lung*'. In contrast, Khandro (22, Trika/Xining), did not refer to *lung* at all when I asked about *nyoné* and other illnesses related to the mind, instead using a combination of English and Tibetan terms for 'heart illness', as we saw in the previous chapter: 'I think *sem né* and *nying né* are the same . . . *sem né* is heart disease; *nying né* is also heart disease . . . Because *sem* and *nying* in Tibetan are the same – the heart'. When I asked her specifically whether such things are related to *lung*, she responded: 'I think that *lung* and heart disease are different. Older people say that *lung* is just a disease – it's not related to *nyoné* or *nying né* . . . Maybe [with *lung né*] your body is missing something – missing something that you need'.

Sonam (27, Rebkong) linked *lung né* to a lack of energy in the body, telling me that '*lung né* is different from *sems né* . . . We say that if you don't eat meat for a long time, then in your body there is not much energy. This is called *lung né*'.[16] In contrast, Buddhist Studies student Migmar (30, Golok/Xining) understood the notion of *lung* being 'out of place', but linked it to the brain (Tib. *lépa*), telling me that someone may become *nyoné* if '*lung* goes in the *wrong* direction – maybe it goes to your brain – and then *that* causes *nyoné*'.

However, Wangtso (34, Rebkong/Xining) also described some symptoms of *sok lung* similar to those we have already heard about *nyoné*, including a reluctance to speak and an afflicted individual 'doing crazy things – dramatic things . . . destroying things . . . throwing things at people'. In contrast, others told me that they had never heard of *sok lung*, or, as Yeshe (80) responded, '*Sok lung*? I don't know this . . . Usually we go to the [Tibetan medicine] doctor – they know about these things'. Her granddaughter too, in her mid-thirties, asserted, 'I don't know what *sok lung* is – we [lay people] don't know about this', and Wangchuk (31, Golok/Xining) told me that while he knew that *sok lung* is 'described in books', he himself did not know about it.

In addition, some interviewees related *sok lung* specifically to anger (Tib. *lung lang* – literally, 'rising wind'), as well as excessive 'thinking' or studying, as we heard in the previous chapter. This echoes a description from Craig in Mustang, where one man explained to her how his 'thinking a lot' led to an unhappy 'heart-mind' and his illness of disturbed *la* and *nyoné*. As a result, he experienced headaches, a 'blood pressure problem', nervousness and sensitivity to light (2012: 140). In Amdo, Dawa (30, Trika/Xining) told me, '*Sok lung* can really increase if you've been studying a lot, and then people get angry really easily . . . get into fights really easily'. He suggested that 'this is something that's quite common, so I think it's something quite separate from *nyoné*. And Wangtso (34, Rebkong/Xining), suggested that *sok lung* was 'not a kind of sickness – it's a kind of anger . . . *Sok lung* is kind of a term to describe someone expressing anger, so I don't think this is a kind of *nyoné*. In contrast, she described a 'a real *nyonpa*' she had seen in a neighbouring village as a child: 'That person was really a *nyonpa* . . . he would try to harm other people – harm children . . . He was very violent – very aggressive . . . Sometimes he was very quiet, sometimes he got kind of mad, and then he could be very violent. He was about twenty years old then. He was born like that'.

At the Qinghai Province Tibetan Medicine Hospital in Xining, Dr Chaksham (40, Trika/Xining) told me that some of his older Tibetan patients had some knowledge of *lung* and its related conditions: 'maybe not the detail, but if you tell them they have a *lung* illness, they have *some* understanding'. In contrast, he said that in his experience many younger Tibetans don't know about these things at all, and he attributed this to younger generations of Tibetans often having less knowledge of Tibetan culture and/or language in general than their older relatives.[17] As I described earlier, this contrasts sharply with the situation in Darjeeling, where many of the lay Tibetans I spoke to were very familiar with the notion of *lung*, commonly using it to describe not only illnesses but also everyday emotional states such as sadness or anxiety – sometimes referred to simply as 'high wind' (Tib. *lung topo*) (Deane 2018: 139). Here, then, a person's wind was understood to have been affected by a stressful or frightening situation, even though they were not described as suffering from an 'illness' as such.

What are we to make of these differences in narrative between Darjeeling and Amdo? I think there are a number of factors at play here. Firstly, as several Tibetan medicine doctors in Amdo suggested, more comprehensive knowledge of Tibetan medical concepts of mind and body amongst lay Tibetans has perhaps declined over time. Indeed, working in Rebkong, Nianggajia and Fjeld heard from one Tibetan medicine doctor that none of his Tibetan or Chinese-speaking patients understand the 'complicated medical concepts and technical terms', and that clinical encounters usually did not include 'intricate medical theory to explain the conditions' (2017: 65). In Xining, Dr Nyima also told me that he thought people's experiences and knowledge of biomedicine had impacted on their engagement with Tibetan medicine, asserting:

> Because of western medicine, now many [lay] people have a *little* bit of knowledge of western medicine, and *less* knowledge of Tibetan medicine . . . When *I* was a child, I heard about *lung* and *lung né* a lot – mostly from elderly people; they would say, 'Oh, I have *lung né*, and I need to get some treatment . . . [or I should] eat some soup . . . eat meat, or drink some milk'[18] – something like

> that. But nowadays, it's really rare – older people talk of *lung* and *lung né*, but *younger* people – if I tell them it's a *lung* problem, they are not so familiar with this concept.

Of course, the influence of biomedicine and related Western concepts of science and scientific knowledge come not only through Chinese-language schooling using Western scientific, anatomical concepts but also in people's experiences of medicine. As Dr Chaksham (40) explained, patients have become quite used to getting scans and tests from doctors, advancing certain ways of viewing the mind and body, health and illness. This is turn affects how doctors themselves describe the body and illness to patients: some of them told me that they rarely spoke of *lung*, *tripa* or *béken* in any detail with patients, as patients were unlikely to have much knowledge of these concepts.[19] Moreover, the use of scans and other biomedical tests is not limited to *biomedical* hospitals but is also common at state-affiliated Tibetan medicine hospitals such as the one in Xining, where doctors commonly use such equipment alongside traditional diagnostic methods such as pulse analysis and questioning of the patient. I would argue that in this context, patients become more and more used to receiving test results and scans on paper and film, and the organs and body parts which can be *seen*, pointed at, scanned and measured by doctors – and described with evidence of good or poor functioning in terms of numerical values and graphs – perhaps become more tangible than the rather ephemeral notion of *lung* – which indeed, is understood to be only really 'felt' and experienced by advanced-level Tantric practitioners. Thus, perhaps 'medicine' increasingly becomes about the physical body (including the brain), its structure and functioning as evidenced by what can be seen through such equipment. *Lung*, of course, cannot be seen in the body – and neither can these notions of 'mind' be seen, scanned or tested in this way. In contrast, I would suggest that the heart may be a more tangible entity for non-specialists to relate to health and illness.[20]

Treating *Lung*-Related *Nyoné*

According to the Tibetan medical texts, determining causation in any case of illness can be done through various means including pulse diagnosis, urinalysis and/or questioning of the patient. However, in Amdo many lay interviewees predominantly spoke of *mo* (divination) for illnesses like *nyoné*, discussing the consultation of a *mopa* (diviner) either to determine causation and/or to get advice on which medical and/or religious practitioner(s) to consult. In cases where *lung* disruption has been determined, in the earliest stages diet and behavioural specifics are key (Rabgay 1985: 63–64). The

Gyüshi, for example, lists foods for *lung né* more broadly including mustard oil, molasses, garlic, onion and horse meat, with bone soups also serving as medicine (*Gyüshi I* 2015: 12), and Epstein and Topgay also describe the benefits of a high protein intake (particularly from meat), hot milk and cooked dough made from grains (1982: 79).[21]

Behavioural guidelines for *lung né* describe a suitable environment, suggesting that patients stay in a 'warm, not too light or bright environment' with a comfortable and warm bed, wear warm clothing and stay around 'congenial, amiable friends' and 'pleasant friendly speech' (Epstein and Topgay 1982: 79). In the second or 'moderate' stage of *lung né*, dietary and behavioural treatments should be used alongside medication, and in the third or 'advanced' stages of *lung né*, stronger treatments should be prescribed (Rabgay 1985: 65–68). For lay interviewees in Amdo too, a person understood to be suffering from *nyoné* caused by sadness or some other emotional difficulties was said to be best suited to being in a calm environment, surrounded and looked after by caring family or community members. In addition, where *lung né* is thought to be related to spirit affliction, the *Gyüshi* stipulates the importance of consulting a ritual specialist (see Chapter 5 for more on this).

As we saw in the previous chapter, at the Qinghai Province Tibetan Medicine Hospital in Xining, Dr Dechen described medicines and external therapies for those with *nyoné* caused by *lung* disorders, classified into 'soft' techniques (including herbal compress) and 'hard' techniques (including the use of *telwa*/*telpa* – metal instruments used to apply extreme heat to particular points on the body [see Figure 1.1). The *Gyüshi* describes the use of medicinal butters for *nying lung né*, which may be taken orally, applied externally and/or used in the form of a suppository (Dorjee and Richards 1985: 23); and in the sections focused on treatment in the *Subsequent Tantra*, we find description of treatments including poultices to treat *nyo bok* – 'madness' or 'delirium' (*Gyüshi IV* 2015: 633). However, despite the availability of such medical treatments at the Tibetan Medicine Hospital in Xining, as we heard in Chapter 1, doctors working in the Department for Wind Illnesses and Impurities in Xining often struggled to manage and treat patients with *nyoné* – particularly when they were first admitted. Such narratives can highlight the contrast between the 'schematic' approach often found in historical medical texts and the 'fragmented and messy picture' of medical reality, which Gutschow has described in her research in Zangskar (1997: 189). Indeed, in Xining, Dr Dechen acknowledged the limitations of the *Gyüshi* texts particularly, explaining that she had found it hard to correlate the Tibetan medical knowledge based on the *Gyüshi* with the patients 'because the patients were out of control'. We have already heard how biomedical sedatives were utilized as a way to 'calm' these patients, but, overall, biomedicine was described by many of the Tibetan medicine doctors I spoke to as limited in its utility for such illnesses. Dr Dechen, for example, told me, 'The effectiveness of the two different medicines is different – Tibetan medical methods are more applicable [for treating the patient] . . . the Chinese [bio]medicine is only [treating the] surface level [of illness]', and this was a view I heard often in Amdo. However, for others, biomedicine had potential to treat severe cases, as Dr Tenpa (36) (who also worked at the Qinghai Province Tibetan Medicine Hospital) suggested, 'If it is a really serious case of *nyoné*, there are these foreign treatments'. Indeed, he told me that at the hospital it was possible to prescribe Diazepam (a type of benzodiazepine medication, usually used to treat anxiety), Chlorpromozine (an anti-psychotic medication) and Promethazine (sedative) when necessary.

In terms of Tibetan medicines, there are a variety of formulae described in the medical texts for the treatment of different forms of *lung né*, *nying né* and *nyoné*. For example, Rapgay lists a number of medicinal compounds for the treatment of *sok lung né*, which he explains were specified by the chief pharmacist at the Tibetan Medical Center Pharmacy in Upper Dharamsala in India. A key ingredient here is eaglewood (Tib. *a gar*), with several medicinal compounds having this as their principal ingredient. 'Eaglewood-15', for example, contains eaglewood, white sandalwood, red sandalwood, nutmeg and saffron, among its fifteen ingredients, while 'Eaglewood-35' includes eaglewood, clove, cardamom, garlic and pomegranate amongst its thirty-five ingredients (1985: 53). Chui translates Sanggye Gyatso's medicine recipe for *sok lung né*, which is 'particularly recommended for insanity', and includes ingredients such as 'four types of myrobalan', sweet flag, clove, snow lotus, black salt, aconite and the urine from an eight-year old boy (Chui 2019: 90).[22] In Amdo, Dr Nyima also mentioned the use of 'Mutig 70' – a *rinchen rilbu* ('precious pill')[23] used to treat wind disorders as well as other conditions. Containing seventy ingredients including pearl, purified mercury (Tib. *tsotel*), bonnet bellflower and saffron, it is described by the Men-Tsee-Khang for use in treating 'lung(loong) disorder of the heart and life channel' and 'insanity' among other conditions (Men-Tsee-Khang).[24]

In Chapter 1, we heard a little about the biomedical Number Three (psychiatric) Hospital in Xining. However, many of my interviewees in Amdo clearly asserted that such a medical environment was unlikely to be helpful for this kind of illness – whether it was caused by *nying né* or spirit affliction. As I mentioned there, the emphasis on the importance of a 'calm' environment in the recovery of such patients likely contributes to this perspective; regardless of any perceived efficacy of the treatments offered there, several interviewees explained to me that such an environment – surrounded by other patients with *nyoné* – would most likely make a patient feel worse, potentially exacerbating their condition.[25] As Dr Pema (40) told me:

> If a patient with *nyoné* comes here [the Tibetan Medicine Hospital], there might be some treatment you could give them according to the severity of their illness. Over there [at the Number Three Hospital], they might be put in restraints and treated roughly, and given injections. This could affect their stress level, mental state and the chances of recovery – for less serious cases, this could make things worse. If someone comes here [Tibetan Medicine Hospital] and has their illness treated, it won't be as stressful. There will be many types of different patients around, and they will be treated somewhat normally, helping them to feel at ease . . . I think the environment here is good . . . If you use a lot of western medicine, the strength of the patient will decrease and their overall health will deteriorate.

Indeed, for the majority of Tibetans I spoke to, it made little sense to them to take such a patient out of their family/community environment and into a strange – and potentially stressful – hospital environment if at all possible. As Lhakpa (38, Golok/Xining) explained, she felt that even people *without nyoné* would probably be negatively affected by being in such an environment, 'surrounded by people with *nyonpa*', so it would most likely affect a person with *nyoné* even more significantly. Her friend Migmar (30, Golok/Xining) agreed, telling me that 'Maybe seventy percent or eighty percent of people will be affected [by this situation] – even if they are not *nyonpa* – because if you are surrounded by those people [with *nyoné*], it will become worse'. Similarly, Yeshe (80) told me, 'If you go to the *nyonpa* hospital, then you will become *more nyonpa* – because of the environment'.

Finally, there was also a particular discourse around the ways in which doctors from these different medical traditions practise and engage with patients. Working in Lhasa, Adams described Tibetan patients' preference for Tibetan medicine doctors over biomedical doctors – explained by the focus placed on doctor–patient interactions in the Tibetan medical tradition, where 'attending to the "thoughts of the patient" is considered an essential component of physical cure' (2001: 558). Indeed, the *Gyüshi* describes 'compassion' as one of the six prerequisites of a good doctor, with the importance of possessing the Buddhist concept of *bodhicitta* (Tib. *jang chup sem*, mind of enlightenment) delineated clearly in the text (*Gyüshi II* 2015: 95). In addition, shared cultural references, understandings and language will probably impact on patients' and their families' treatment choices.[26] Even without knowledge of the complexities of *lung*, *tripa* or *béken*, or the mechanisms by which they may be involved in a case of illness, these pan-Tibetan understandings of 'heart' and 'mind', and the ways in which difficult circumstances or experiences are seen to have the potential to lead to *nyoné*, will allow Tibetan patients to communicate effectively with Tibetan medicine doctors and religious specialists.

*

From these explorations of textual and ethnographic material, we can start to make sense of the complex ways in which mind, heart and wind are interconnected in Tibetan medical perspectives, and therefore how disturbances in one or more of these various factors may be implicated in the causation of *nyoné*. Key, of course, are the various *lung* currents, disruptions within which may lead, or at least contribute to, the development of *nyoné* – particularly in cases where *lung* is understood to have become disturbed in the area of the heart, or where the *sok lung* has become disrupted, affecting the senses. Thus, with the Tibetan understanding of the mind as residing in the heart and the location of several key wind currents also around the heart area, certain mental states and activities are understood to impact negatively on the flow of *lung*, and disordered *lung* may also lead to certain negative mental states. Tibetan medical treatments for *nyoné* are therefore often focused on treating some form of *lung né*, with many medical formulae and external therapies aimed at 'stabilizing' a patient's *lung*. And yet, as we saw in Chapter 1, it was in fact the *heart* and 'heart illness' that were the focus of many discussions on *nyoné* in Amdo – particularly among lay interviewees. Indeed, while there are clear narratives of these various facets of causation amongst Tibetan medicine doctors – reflecting Tibetan textual explanations – there is significant diversity in how lay Tibetans understand and discuss these different concepts within different Tibetan communities in both the PRC and in exile. What is evident is how clearly the relationship is understood between difficult and/or negative experiences and mental states and *nyoné* – as evidenced by multiple narratives in Chapter 1.

With much of the Tibetan understanding of *lung* coming directly from Indian notions of *prāṇa* and *vāta*, we can trace these concepts of 'wind' back to early Indian texts. But we see clear evidence of specific Tibetan ideas here too – for example in the tying of the three *nyépa* with the 'three poisons', and in Buddhist/Bon notions of attachment and their link to *lung* particularly. However, despite these clear conceptions of *lung* and its relationship to heart and mind in relation to illness, there remains debate over the specifics of the 'subtle-body' system, as we have seen. This is evident, for example, in debates over the location and even existence of some of the described channels in the body. This becomes even more pertinent when we turn to explore Tibetan *Tantric* notions of *lung* and *tsa*, where we encounter channels that may or may not be the same as those described in the medical texts, and which may or may not be seen to have a physical existence. Again, the purported connections between wind and mind are key here – the basis of many Buddhist and Bon practices – and it is to this subject that we turn next, in Chapter 3.

Notes

1. Consequently, it is common to see people point at their heart when saying things like 'In my *mind*, I really think . . .'.
2. In addition, researchers have equated certain *lung* conditions with biomedical psychiatric categories including generalized anxiety disorder (Jacobson 2002, 2007) and schizophrenia (Millard 2007).
3. Kirmayer, Adeponle and Dzokoto describe such 'ethnopsychologies' or 'indigenous psychologies' as being 'rooted in particular cultural ontologies – assumptions about what the world is made up of, the sources and kinds of agency, and available modes of explanation and understanding of human action experience' (2018: 22).
4. Furthermore, the politicization of *lung* conditions in both exile and Chinese-controlled Tibet – as explored, for example, by Adams (1998), Jacobson (2002), Janes (1999b) and Prost (2006) – also demonstrates its relationship to particular sociopolitical factors, as mentioned by Yoeli-Tlalim, above. Here, it has become a way to express suffering, dissatisfaction and other emotions related to the contemporary political situation and related difficulties for many Tibetans. In Amdo, Bassini found that some *nying né* patients 'related their illnesses to experiences of historical vicissitudes', referencing 'issues such as the suffering that resulted from abuse and forced labour during the Cultural Revolution, land disputes, the loss of family members, and extreme poverty' (2013a: 239). In contrast, this was not something I encountered during my own research there, where interviewees certainly discussed sociopolitical factors including, occasionally, those related to life under Communist Party rule with me, but in more direct ways. Perhaps this is at least in part related to the passage of time, and the passing away of so many of those with direct experience of this time period by the time I was in the area in 2018.
5. In comparison, *béken* is understood to be composed of water and earth, and *tripa* of fire.
6. Gerke notes that the first documented mention of the *tsa* in a Tibetan medical context is to be found in eighth- to tenth-century Tibetan medical texts found in Dunhuang, although here the reference predominantly regards the practice of bloodletting (2013: 83–84).
7. For example, Garrett and Adams assert that '[t]he precise enumeration of various types of channels and their functions' is a 'contested topic', with debates among Indian medical scholars 'common' (2008: 87).
8. The three 'channels of formation' are in turn linked to the three *nyépa*, with each of these channels extending to a particular area of the body: one upwards to the brain and associated with the upper part of the body and *béken*, one extending to the middle part of the body and associated with *tripa*, and one extending downwards to the genitals and associated with the lower part of the body and *lung* (*Gyüshi II* 2015: 23).
9. Branching off from this around the heart centre are said to be four channels 'radiating out in each of the four cardinal directions', with the channel in front (i.e. east) relating to 'the consciousness and the five senses' (Millard 2007: 266). Thus, as Millard explains, 'sensory data that is gathered by the brain is rendered intelligible by the heart centre' – illustrating why disturbances here may lead to sensory disturbances.
10. Additionally, Zysk describes two later Ayurvedic medical texts dated from *c.*seventh–eighth centuries CE, which were key in the development of the 'classical āyurvedic doctrine of the five bodily breaths' (2007: S110). These two texts are said to have been authored by Vāgbhaṭa and Vṛddhavāgbhaṭa ('The Elder Vāgbhaṭa') – although, as Zysk explains, it is not clear whether these are in fact one and the same person, with the two texts being very similar to each other (2007: S110–11).

11. These early Indian practices related to wind will be explored in more detail in Chapter 3.
12. In addition, J. Gyatso notes that one issue with this 'central channel' is that it is described in the *Four Tantras* as 'singular in the embryonic stage and double in the mature connecting channel stage', where these differing states are described as 'black' and 'white' (2015: 216–17).
13. This is one of the factors that contribute to the difficulties of attempting to 'match up' these Tibetan concepts and diagnostic categories with biomedical ones, as some have tried, with boundaries between different categories being frequently drawn quite differently in the different systems. For example, Epstein and Topgay note that a biomedical case of 'clinical depression' 'could represent imbalance of at least four of the five major pranic currents' (1982: 78), and *sok lung né* has been equated with a number of different biomedical diagnoses by previous researchers. Millard, for example, found that Western patients diagnosed by the resident (Tibetan) Tibetan medicine doctor at a Tibetan medicine clinic in Edinburgh (UK) as having *sok lung* had been diagnosed by their biomedical psychiatrists with 'schizophrenia' and 'bipolar disorder' (2007: 257–59). Other researchers have equated certain cases of *sok lung* with post-traumatic stress disorder (PTSD) in exiled Tibetans (Benedict, Mancini and Grodin 2009).
14. Some of these understandings of wind/breath and its disruption in the mind-body can be traced back to the early Indian medical texts – for example, to Caraka's description of 'unexcited, excited and normal wind' (Zysk 1995: 50). In addition, as Zysk explains, texts compiled by both Caraka (*c.*200 BCE–200 CE) and Suśruta (*c.*100–400 CE) both describe:

    > two channels which transport *prāṇá* throughout the body: the *prāṇá*-conveying vessels (*prāṇávahasrotas*) which originate in the heart, and the large vessels (*mahāsrotas*) which also carry nutritive fluid (*rasa*). Injury to them due to emaciation, suppression of the natural urges, roughness, physical exercise, hunger and other harsh factors, causes one to cry out with curses, double over, have shallow or frequent loud and painful respiration, become bewildered, dizzy, tremble or die. (1995: 49)

15. This was a notion I also heard discussed frequently in Darjeeling (Deane 2018, 2019b).
16. This perhaps relates to Tibetan medical theory, wherein different foods are described as beneficial for different *nyépa* and different facets of health.
17. There are probably many contributing factors here. Dr Chaksham, for example, mentioned Chinese schooling as one of the factors contributing to this situation, whereby many Tibetan students – often away at Chinese-language boarding schools from a young age – learn through the mediums of Chinese language and Western science.
18. All foods known to be good for *lung* disorders, as delineated in the *Gyüshi*.
19. Indeed, Dr Chaksham told me that of the three *nyépa*, bile (Tib. *tripa*) was the one that lay people were usually most familiar with due to its connection with gallstones, which were not uncommon in the Tibetan population. However, he explained, their knowledge of this *nyépa* generally did not extend beyond this physical condition with which it was associated.
20. There is much more to be said here – particularly about the 'biomedicalization' of 'Tibetan medicine' driven by state reforms, as well as broader cultural changes both within and around Tibetan medical and healing traditions in the PRC and in exile. Unfortunately, there is not the space here to explore this in depth, but other researchers provide clear examinations of the situation in diverse ethnically Tibetan contexts, such as Adams (2001, 2002), Adams and Li (2008), Craig (2012), Janes (1995, 1999a, 2001, 2002) and Schrempf (2011). See also Deane (2024) for more discussion of this situation in Amdo.

21. Such dietary guidelines also reflect those described in the early Indian medical texts; Zysk describes, for example, texts by Caraka which assert that 'unwholesome' foods could 'damage' *prāṇa*, whilst 'wholesome' foods can 'promote' it, with 'milk, soups, meat juices and certain elixirs' in particular understood to increase and maintain *prāṇa* (1995: 48).
22. See Chui (2019) for a discussion on some of the 'secret medicines' – ingredients described in medical commentaries such as Sanggye Gyatso's, including 'the heart of a man that has been killed by knife' and 'the flesh of a bastard child', and how we might understand these substances – some of which are explicitly listed as treatments for *sok lung* illness – and the description of soup made from human flesh (Tib. *sha chen*) as a treatment for *lung* conditions in the *Yutok Nyingtig* text.
23. These ritually empowered pills usually contain precious stones, such as turquoise, amber, coral and/or pearl (Gerke 2019) alongside mercury sulphide ash. See Czaja (2015) and Gerke (2019) for more on these compounds.
24. https://mentseekhang.org/precious-pills/ [retrieved April 2024].
25. One example of this came from Dolma (22), who described her 50-year-old neighbour who had become *nyoné* after having been married and widowed twice, leaving her 'very sad'. Dolma had helped the neighbour's adult children, who did not speak Chinese, to take her to the Number Three Hospital. However, she explained that on arrival the patient's family had concluded that 'there were too many other *nyoné* patients there', and so felt that this was not a good environment for her, taking her home and consulting lamas instead.
26. Indeed, for some Tibetans in Amdo (particularly in more rural areas) not fluent in Chinese, language difficulties can be a major factor here, with a majority of biomedical doctors in the area being Han Chinese.

Chapter 3

WIND, MIND AND *NYONÉ* IN TIBETAN TANTRA

> *If a practitioner controls the* sok lung *[life-sustaining wind] effectively, then he won't become* nyonpa, *but if he can't control it well, he may become broken* – nyonpa.
> —Lama Wangyal (62, Rebkong)

In the previous chapter, we examined the concept of 'wind' in Tibetan medical contexts, exploring the ways in which the medical notion of *lung* is related to the mind, heart and mental health, and may therefore be implicated in the manifestation of *nyoné* in Tibetan medical perspectives. We will now turn to the role of *lung* in the sphere of Tibetan Tantra,[1] and the ways in which wind can be related to *nyoné* in Tibetan religious perspectives. While Tantra's Indian roots demonstrate the early connections made between breath and ritual practice, here the concept of *lung* has taken on additional layers of meaning as a result of its particular role in Tibetan Tantric theory and practice (Samuel 2019: 773).

Again, the relationship between wind and mind/consciousness is key here, with practices designed to manipulate the *lung* and the other components of the 'subtle body' in order to alter the mind-body in the pursuit of enlightenment. As the Kadampa scholar G.K. Gyatso (1931–2022) tells us, 'All pure Dharma practitioners know how important it is to control the mind, but we cannot really control our mind without controlling our winds' (1994: 147). These kinds of practices focused on the winds and channels (Tib. *tsa*) are integral to Hindu, Buddhist and Bon Tantric traditions. However, it is only within the Buddhist and Bon traditions that a connection is made between the *tiklé* ('drops') that are understood to be carried through the body by the winds, and the notion of *bodhicitta* – the 'mind of enlightenment' – which is so important in Buddhist Mahayana and Vajrayana, and Bon traditions. It is through these kinds of *tsa lung* (channel-wind) practices[2] that the practitioner ultimately aims to direct the *lung* currents – containing the drops – into the central channel, where they will dissolve, thereby 'curtailing' the activity of the mind and leading to enlightenment (Marek and Oliphant 2017: 418–19).

Across multiple Indian and Tibetan Tantric traditions, the manipulation of wind currents through the channels and chakras within the subtle-body system[3] is key to the pursuit of realization. And in Tibetan Buddhist and Bon traditions, Tantric practices span a diverse range of individual and group activities, from rituals performed in worship to peaceful deities, to practices including transgressive, antinomian and/or sexual activities (Samuel 2013c: 36). While such practices may look strange or even 'heterodox' to outsiders, and may sometimes appear to be focused on 'worldly' objectives, it is important to remember that they are always aimed, ultimately, towards the goal of enlightenment. From Tibetan perspectives, Tantric practice is the key way to attain realization – an 'advanced path for elite practitioners' (Ibid.) – superior, for example, to the approaches of the Mahayana and Theravada Buddhist traditions. Viewed as a more rapid path to enlightenment, Tantra is understood to be powerful and effective and, consequently, also difficult and risky – a kind of 'high-stakes, high-reward' approach. Indeed, as we saw in Chapter 1, such practices are viewed by both practitioners and non-practitioners as complex, effective and potentially dangerous activities that are suitable only for experienced practitioners, and are to be conducted only under the close guidance of one's teacher.[4] Indeed, potential problems and how to manage them are described at some length in Tantric texts.[5]

As we saw in Chapter 1, a common narrative of *nyoné* in Amdo was that of 'madness' caused by 'incorrect practice': stories of Tantric practices conducted too quickly, too soon, beyond the guidance of a teacher and/or simply performed incorrectly, leading to a practitioner becoming *nyoné*, either for a short period of time, or for many years – potentially, the rest of their life. In addition, we have already encountered the figure of the *lama nyonpa* in Chapter 1 – the lama who apparently *appears* 'mad' but is in fact said to be enlightened. As Ardussi and Epstein note, this 'mad saint' is 'a figure of some importance in Tibetan popular religious literature' (1978: 331), and this was evident in Amdo, where everyone I spoke to about it was well aware of the concept even if they had never met such a figure themselves. At first glance, the strange and often transgressive behaviour of these *lama nyonpa* may seem to run counter to much of what we know about Buddhism, but again here we find echoes of Indian traditions in the stories of 'mad' Indian Tantric practitioners (see Morinis 1985). Some exploration here of historical and contemporary narratives about such practitioners will help us to understand how Tibetan mind-body concepts might explain this notion of 'madness' too.

In this chapter, then, we will first explore the notion of *lung* and its related concepts within the broader Tantric 'subtle-body' system in Tibetan Buddhist and Bon traditions, examining practices focused on the manipulation of *lung* within the body to understand why and how these are understood to, ultimately, bring about a practitioner's enlightenment. Through this exploration, we will be able to make sense of those narratives from Amdo about practitioners who apparently conducted such practices 'incorrectly' and became *nyoné*.

Moreover, as I briefly explained in Chapter 2, one of the complexities of *lung* is the fact that this Tibetan concept derives from not one but *two* Indian concepts and terms – *vāta* in the Indian Ayurvedic medical system, and *prāṇa* in the Indian Tantric system – both understood to flow through channels (Tib. *tsa*; Skt. *nāḍī*) throughout the body. This situation has led to much debate, and some confusion, amongst Tibetan scholars and practitioners over the centuries, as we shall see – and this was no less evident in Amdo. Over the course of this chapter, we will start to build up a picture of the ways in which Tibetan 'religious' and 'medical' perspectives on 'wind' converge and diverge – something that was especially clear in discussions with Amdo-wa who were specialists of both traditions. We will turn our attention to the early Indian origins of this concept in order to understand its key relationship to the mind and enlightenment, and its twin roles in the medical and religious traditions. As we then explore what happens when things 'go wrong' in Tantric practice, and what should be done when and if they do, it will become clear how such practices can be linked to *nyoné*, as we heard about in Chapter 1. Finally, as we turn to the notion of the *lama nyonpa*, we find a further way in which to understand the concept of 'madness' in Tibetan religious contexts as we explore these complex connections between mind and *nyoné*.

Wind and the Subtle-Body System in Tibetan Tantra

> [T]he 'energies' or 'wind-energies' . . . are at the root of both samsara and nirvana. It is by way of the energies that one goes either to liberation and full enlightenment or to the lower realms of existence. (Dhargyey 1985: 105)

The notion of a mind-body system of winds and channels is as significant in the Tibetan Tantric traditions as in the medical traditions – not least because, in addition to its role in the functions of the physical body, *lung* is sometimes described as the 'foundation' for 'mental and sense consciousnesses' (Epstein and Topgay 1982: 72). Thus, Tantric texts contain detailed descriptions of the relationship between *lung* and mind/consciousness across diverse mental states – for example, during dreaming and waking, at the time of death and at the moment of attaining enlightenment. It is these 'interdependent relations' of wind and mind that enable an 'inconceivable number' of Tantric techniques, as fourteenth-century teacher, the Third Karmapa, Rangjung Dorjé (1284–1339) explained. Manipulation of *lung*, he told us, can be 'a means to alleviate maladies' across several domains: 'negative states of mind, localized spirits within the subtle body, and negative forces within the world' (Duckworth 2017: 414).[6] Indeed, such techniques of manipulation have the potential to 'restructure' the self and the emotions (Samuel 1989: 203), through practices which manipulate both breath and 'inner winds'. Thus, Lipman tells us: '[Y]oga works gradually on harmonizing the relationship between body, energy, and mind. Through movements and asanas [postures], one controls breathing and thus motility; through control of motility, one can control the mind; through controlling the mind, one can in turn influence motility' (2010: 78).

Tantric concepts of bodily channels and ways of working with them came to Tibet from India alongside Buddhist knowledge – particularly through the *Kālacakra Tantra* text during the eleventh century (Gerke 2013: 85). Encompassing the second stage of a set of practices within the Mahayoga and Anuttarayoga Indian Buddhist Tantras (Samuel 1989: 200), complex descriptions of the subtle body and practices aimed at its manipulation – such as the 'internal' *tsa lung* (channel-wind) practices, and 'external' *trül khor* (magical movement)[7] practices involving physical exercises (Samuel 2013c: 37–38) – contrast with the first-stage practices, which focus on so-called 'deity yoga' based on the visualization and evocation of particular Tantric deities.[8]

As I have already briefly mentioned, the Tibetan Tantric concept of *lung* originates in the Indian Tantric notion of *prāṇa*. Often translated into English as 'breath' or 'life-force', *prāṇa* in fact refers to a 'variety of subtle inner "flows" within the body' (Samuel 2019: 773),[9] and has a rather complex relationship with the breath. For example, Guarisco examines the Tantric system laid out by thirteenth-century Drukpa Kagyu Buddhist scholar Gyalwa Yangönpa Gyaltsen Pal (hereafter, 'Yangönpa') (1213–58) in his text *Secret Explanation of the Vajra Body* (Tib. *rdo rje lus kyi sbas bshad*), which Guarisco has translated and annotated. Here, Guarisco describes *lung* and breath as flowing 'in synchrony' with each other – closely related but not the same (Guarisco in Yangönpa 2015: 67).[10] As in Tibetan medical traditions, in Tibetan Tantric traditions, the channels through which these winds are understood to flow intersect at various chakras (Tib. *khorlo*; 'energy centres'). Whilst numerous such intersections are described, in Tantric practice there is a focus on a small number understood to be situated down the centre of the body through the head and torso. This is because, among the thousands of channels said to run throughout the body, integral to Tantric practice are the central channel (Tib. *wuma*; Skt. *avadhūti*) running from the crown of the head to the genitals, and the channels directly to the right and left of this – the *kyangma* (Skt. *lalanā*) and *roma* (Skt. *rasanā*)[11] – which intersect with the central channel at various chakras. In *Secret Explanation of the Vajra Body*, Yangönpa described the central channel – 'the chief of the five energy-winds' – thus: 'straight like the trunk of a plantain tree; slender like a lotus stem; luminous like a sesame oil lamp; and red like the lacquer tree's flower' (Yangönpa 2015: 281, 47).

Across the various Tibetan Tantric traditions, there is a diversity of perspectives on some of the specifics of these channels and their functioning as well the number and location of chakras, with four or five commonly described in the Buddhist Tantras – a system probably dating to the eighth century (Samuel 2013c: 40).[12] Similarly, there is variation in the number of 'principal' winds described, with one eighteenth-century commentary on the *Kālacakra Tantra*, for example, describing 'ten main winds: life-sustaining wind, downwardly expelling wind, coexisting wind, upwardly moving wind, pervading wind, *nāga* wind, turtle wind, lizard wind, *devadatta* wind, and *dhanaṃjaya* wind' (Dorjé, trans. by Kilty 2009: 147), in comparison to the 'five' winds of the *Guhyasamāja Tantra*. Indeed, Samuel describes 'disagreements about the exact form of the channels and disagreements concerning whether the distribution of the channels differs in men and women' (2019: 780). Moreover, as Samuel notes, there are also disputes over the material existence of *lung* and *tsa* – particularly at the 'coarse level of ordinary perception' (Ibid.). While for some scholars, a lack of physical evidence was a concern – J. Gyatso describes, for example, Yangönpa's conclusion in *Secret Explanation of the Vajra Body* that if the central channel lacked material existence, this 'would disqualify the viability of the Buddha's tantric teachings' (2015: 206) – for others, it is their apparent connection to mind that is paramount. For example, Guarisco describes debates among scholars about whether the central channel has material existence or, rather, is 'real' by virtue of the 'concrete effects' it can have on mind and body through practice (Guarisco in Yangönpa 2015: 49).

With multiple traditions evolving through different teaching lineages, perhaps it is not surprising to encounter such diversities across the different texts. And we might suggest – as some Tibetan scholars have – that any concerns over discrepancies between traditions and over the physical existence (or not) of these structures, or attempts to 'map' Tantric descriptions onto structures within the physical body such as the spinal cord (as some scholars and researchers have attempted to do),[13] are quite unnecessary. As Samuel argues, unlike in the medical traditions, the *material existence* of the chakras and channels is not a 'central issue' for many Tantric practitioners (2013c: 41). Rather, the focus here is on their *utility* – i.e. how one might *use* these 'maps' of the subtle body in meditative practice. Thus, Garrett describes how sixteenth-century medical commentator Lodrö Gyelpo argued that the three channels do not exist in the body – citing 'an unidentified Vajrayana scholar' in his assertion that 'the tantric presentation of three channels is a trope developed to enhance contemplative practice' (2008: 65). From such perspectives, the utility of these 'channels' is not based on any kind of material existence that can be *seen* or *found* in the body through some kind of 'testing' – indeed, they do not need to 'exist' in the way we might think of biomedical concepts of the body 'existing' for them to be of use to practitioners. Instead, there can be a 'functionality' of a central channel, even without any 'provable' material existence. Similarly, Samuel (2008: 283) cites Silburn's assertion on earlier Indian traditions that the chakras are 'by no means physiological and static centers of the gross body': instead, they can be understood as 'centers of power belonging to the subtle body, centres that the yogin alone . . . can locate with as much accuracy as if they belonged to the body' (Silburn 1988: 25–26). Thus, Samuel explains that from a Tibetan Tantric perspective, the 'co-existence of apparently irreconcilable descriptions' of these subtle-body structures is not necessarily problematic, as each description is 'valid in its own context' (1989: 201) – the channels and chakras are 'ways that we can experience the world through our body' (Lipman 2010: 80). It is not that these diverse Tantric texts are contradicting each other but, with each practice having its own specific aim, 'different channels and chakras are put into function to achieve those aims' (Norbu 1986: 124). In this way, diverse descriptions of the subtle body can even be explained as being appropriate for different practitioners (Samuel 1989: 201), referencing the key Mahayana Buddhist concept of 'skilful means', which helpfully explains the diversity – and value – of a range of texts and practices both across and within Buddhist traditions.

Moreover, while there is significant diversity across different traditions' teachings on the various channels and chakras, the Tantric texts do in fact share a number of key elements – in particular, a predominant focus on the 'central channel' and the manipulation of wind currents into and through it. Such practices are based on the notion that realization can occur through the 'stilling' of the *lung* within the central channel. For example, in the fifteenth-century commentarial text on the *Kālacakra Tantra*, *Ornament of Stainless Light: An Exposition of the Kālacakra Tantra* (Tib. *phyi nang gzhan gsum gsal bar byed pa dri med 'od kyi rgyan*), Khedrup Norsang Gyatso explains that, in the completion stage of practice, '[t]hese winds are stopped from flowing in the left and right channels and brought into the dhūtī [central channel]' (K.N. Gyatso, trans. by Kilty 2004: 475–76).

In some traditions, the process of bringing the various *lung* currents into the central channel, and raising them up through the chakras, is conceptualized in terms of awakening and raising *Caṇḍālī* (Tib. *tumo*), a female Tantric deity (Samuel 1993: 239–40).[14] Often referred to as 'inner heat' practices, due to a practitioner's raising of his/her body temperature, these may even be conducted while sitting outside in the snow. Sometimes, the *roma* channel (Skt. *rasanā*) is associated with 'method', and the *kyangma* channel (Skt. *lalanā*) with wisdom/knowledge (Guarisco in Yangönpa 2015: 52), emphasizing the key Buddhist notion of enlightenment through the union of wisdom and means.

These practices, focused on the manipulation of *lung* inside the mind-body complex, are a result of what Dalton describes as an 'internalization of ritual performance', wherein these kinds of 'internal yogas' contrast with earlier '"external" methods of worship' (2004: 2). Dalton describes three periods in the development of Tantric ritual, whereby the practitioner's attention was focused progressively inwards: 'first from the external altar to himself, then to his physical anatomy and embodied experience, and finally to the subtleties of his internal physiological processes' (Ibid.: 3), during which concepts of the 'subtle body' and its various facets emerged over time (Ibid.: 27).[15] Thus, Gray quotes Indian scholar Abhayakaragupta's categorization of 'five types of disciples', distinguished by the nature of their practice, whereby the 'greatest of the great' (highest) level of practitioner works entirely through his/her own body (Gray 2007: 69–70). Through such practices, a 'Tantric logic of correspondence' can link body, mind and universe – enabling the practitioner to mediate between mind, body and the external world (Duckworth 2017: 413). Here, 'the five elements in the outer world have a symbiotic relationship with five elements that make up the human constitution', with 'a series of fivefold correspondences where the five elements are related to the five mental poisons, the five *skandhas*,[16] the five solid organs, the five orifices, the five seasons, the five transcendental wisdoms, the five cosmic Buddhas, and so on' (Millard 2005 and 2006: 18).

With the body now the basis for meditation practice and the subtle-body system of winds, channels, chakras and drops serving as 'a guide to operating simultaneously with both "body" and '"mind"' (Samuel 1989: 201), these connections – between *lung* and mind, and between *lung* and breath – are taken full advantage of in Tantric practice. Thus, Dalton is clear in emphasizing that this 'interiorization' of ritual (a process that started across various Indian traditions during the eighth and ninth centuries)[17] should not be viewed as a 'psychologization': it is not simply a case of the practitioner 'imagining' his/her body in various new ways; instead, he explains, 'the ritual space' moved from the external shrine to the interior of the practitioner's body (2004: 26). Thus, by the end of the tenth century, 'a new ritual discourse of the bodily interior was in place', whereby '[t]he tantric subject had become the site for the entire ritual performance; the body's interior provided the devotee, the altar, the oblations, and the buddha to be worshipped' (Ibid.: 2). This 'internalization' of practice and de-emphasizing of the mandala as a literal map of sacred sites also had an added advantage: through a 'mapping' of sacred places onto the practitioner's body, these places become 'transportable' (DiValerio 2015: 71) – removing the need for physical pilgrimage to geographical sites that may have been difficult or even impossible to access at different times in history. Instead, the practitioner was now able to engage with such places from any geographical location. Thus, in Gray's 'Introduction' to his translation of the eighth-century Indian Buddhist *Cakrasaṃvara Tantra*, he describes a 'body mandala':

> [T]he mandala is mapped onto the practitioner's body, which is transformed into a 'network of dakinis' (*dakinijala*).[18] Here the mandala serves as what Tambiah has termed an 'indexical symbol,' capable of shifting between multiple levels of referentiality. The tradition presupposes that the mandala, along with the deities who inhabit it, pervades the cosmos at its various levels, including the microcosmic level of the body. (Gray 2007: 56)

In this way, the body can also be linked to the cosmos – 'two aspects of embodied temporality' (Wallace 2009: 289). For example, in the *Kālacakra Tantra*, we are told that in the cosmos 'time' is characterized by the 'movement of the sun through the twelve houses of the external zodiac'. At the individual level, time is measured by 'the number of inhalations and exhalations that take place in the course of a day and night when the vital energies (*prāṇa*) circulate through the twelve subtle channels (*nāḍı*) in the navel cakra, or in the internal zodiac' (Ibid.).[19] Thus, Wallace explains, 'Just as planets take hold and govern certain zodiacal houses as their respective fields in the celestial sphere, they also preside over the elements carried by the vital energies that circulate through the left and right sides of the body' (Ibid.: 292), and we sometimes find the *kyangma* channel associated with the 'lunar wind/energy' and the *roma* associated with the 'solar wind/energy', or vice versa (Guarisco in Yangönpa 2015: 52–53).

Bodhicitta *and Red and White Drops*

Samuel has described a 'considerable overlap' between the various Hindu and Buddhist traditions, with Tantras passed down through a series of Indian teachers known as *siddhas* – some of whom occur in both Buddhist and Hindu Tantric lineages during the seventh to eleventh centuries (Samuel 1989: 201).[20] What was new in the Buddhist context, in contrast to the Hindu traditions, was the connection made between this subtle-body system and the concept of *bodhicitta* (Tib. *jang chup sem*). Often translated as 'buddha mind' or 'mind of enlightenment', *bodhicitta* is a defining feature of Mahayana and Vajrayana Buddhism, with its focus on the desire to attain enlightenment *for the benefit of all sentient beings*. In the Vajrayana and also Bon traditions, *bodhicitta* is connected to the subtle-body system specifically through the notion of the drops that are understood to be carried through the channels by the wind. Here, *bodhicitta* can be viewed not only as a 'state of mind' but also as a 'quasi-material substance' (Ibid.: 199) – one that can be manipulated via Tantric mind-body practices focused on the Vajra body. Indeed, the 'arousing' of *bodhicitta* became an integral part of practice in all Tibetan schools of Buddhism and Bon – with *bodhicitta* 'vows' being an essential preliminary to Tantric practice, and meditations to develop *bodhicitta* important in all Tibetan traditions (Ibid.: 205).

In the Tantric texts, we encounter two kinds of *bodhicitta*: 'red *bodhicitta*', connected to female sexual fluid; and 'white *bodhicitta*', connected to male sexual fluid. In addition, these two substances are also associated with the fundamental Mahayana Buddhist aspects of wisdom and means/compassion respectively. Whilst '[i]n general', Khedrup Norsang Gyatso tells us, the red and white drops are understood to be 'found in every part of the body',[21] the white drop is 'primarily situated in the cakra of great bliss in the crown of the head' and the red drop is 'primarily to be found in the cakras of the secret place and the navel' (K.N. Gyatso, trans. by Kilty 2004: 183). Moreover, Cozort explains that the origin of these drops is the 'indestructible drop' understood to reside in the heart. The size of a large mustard seed, this is said to comprise a 'white top and red bottom' but is, in fact, really *two* 'indestructible drops': the '"eternal" indestructible drop, which is the very subtle wind and mind' and the 'lifetime indestructible drop, which is a subtle material object and is destroyed at the end of a person's lifetime'. The former is understood to be located inside the latter (Cozort 1986: 72).

Thus, achieving 'mastery of the essence-drop' through subtle-body practices, as Samuel explains, involves 'freeing up' the 'knots' (i.e. chakras) in the channels, and 'accumulating the *tiklé* (which supports or constitutes *bodhicitta*) in the central channel' (2019: 781). In order to do this, practitioners must first become familiar with the channels through 'visualization', and then by 'using the mind to direct the vital breath currents' along the channels, as Chaoul explains:

> In this way, one allows the vital breath currents to circulate through the channels more evenly in terms of the rhythm of inhalation and exhalation and seeks a greater balance in terms of the quantity and strength of the breath through the different channels . . . With powerful exhalations and nurturing inhalations, the practitioner clears away the obstacles that are the poisons that impede the flow of the vital breath currents. (Chaoul 2007: 134)

Additionally, this notion of the 'red drop' and 'white drop' associated with male/female energies and compassion/wisdom also gave rise to ritualized Tantric sexual practices focused on sexual union between a male and a female practitioner. Here, there is a focus on the male/female 'polarities', and the process of 'arousing' *bodhicitta* is also connected to sexual arousal and orgasm (Samuel 1989: 199–200).[22]

Karmic Wind vs Wisdom Wind

In Tantric practices aimed at directing the wind (containing the drops) into the central channel, a key distinction is made between what is known as *lé lung* ('karmic wind') and *yéshé lung* ('wisdom wind'). Karmic wind is understood to drive rebirth within samsara,[23] passing from life to life, and is described as flowing through the *roma* and *kyangma*, which run either side of the central channel.[24] It is often linked to, or equated with, the breath (as is evident in Norbu's description of 'inhaling' karmic wind, below). In contrast, the wisdom wind is understood to flow through the central channel, and is associated with enlightenment. Thus, Guarisco describes karmic wind as 'inseparable from thought' and 'associated with emotions' – its movement 'essentially discursive thought, conception, and judgement' (Guarisco in Yangönpa 2015: 72–74) – whereas wisdom wind 'represents the mind's [true] nature . . . characterized by bliss, clarity, and non-thought' (Ibid.: 74).

In Amdo, former Gelugpa monk Tsetan (38, Rebkong) explained this succinctly to me: 'In Tantric teachings, there are two different kinds of *tsa*: the *tsa wuma*, and the *tsa roma* and *tsa kyangma* – one is about truth, and the other is *namtok*. So these two are in parallel'. The aim for the Tibetan Buddhist/Bon Tantric practitioner is thus to transform the 'karmic wind' into 'wisdom wind' in order to attain realization. Namkhai Norbu explains:

> There are many types of prana, and they support the many types of dualistic mind; as long as the prana circulates in the many and various channels, these dualistic minds persist. But when the prana is brought into the central channel, its essential nature – tiklé, or kundalini – is activated and enters the channels. Dualistic mind is then overcome, and realization achieved. The vital energy will not normally enter the central channel except at the time of death or during sleep. Only practice will otherwise cause it to do so. (Norbu 1986: 124)

The upper tips of the *kyangma* and *roma* side channels – through which the 'ordinary' breath/karmic wind is understood to travel – are said to connect at the nostrils, either side of the central channel. Similarly, the lower tips of these two channels are understood to sit alongside the central channel at its base. Ordinarily, the winds travelling through these two side channels do not enter the central channel; the challenge for a Tantric practitioner is to 'cause the ends of the right and left channels to touch the central channel', allowing *lung* to enter the central channel during practice (Garrett and Adams 2008: 92–93). For example, in Norbu's recent commentary on the Dzogchen Buddhist text, *Union of the Sun and Moon Yantra* (Tib. *trül khor nyi zla kha sbyor*), he describes how the practitioner should direct wind through the channels:

> Inhale the karmic air directly, slowly and deeply through the Roma and Kyangma channels; then direct it pushing it down and apply a light closed hold[25] so as to capture it in the central channel. Stretching your chest so as not to push out the abdomen and vigorously drawing your sides in, tense your body thoroughly, applying a contracted hold. In that moment, imagine that the force of the HŪṂ, visualized at the navel in the central channel, instantaneously absorbs all the karmic air, just as a magnet draws iron filings.
>
> Then relaxing your nostrils, lips, and teeth, softly sound a long HŪṂ so that its vibration resonates deeply throughout the body. At the same time imagine that all traces of 'outer' karmic vision, such as material objects and of 'inner' karmic vision, such as your body of flesh and blood, together with all illnesses, provocations of energy and disturbances, are purified in their own condition and all phenomena of the universe manifest in a dimension of uninterrupted clarity in the form of infinite HŪṂs of different sizes, like dust specks we see in rays of sunlight. Train in all this with diligence.
>
> Thus, after having inhaled the karmic air through the solar and lunar paths, by holding it closed and applying a contraction, the karmic air is captured within the central channel; then intoning the sound HŪṂ, the whole universe is purified in the dimension of the HŪṂ. Mastering these phases of expansion and reabsorption, all the karmic *prāṇas* will completely enter into the central channel and all the illusory visions produced by dualism will manifest as primordial wisdom. (Norbu 2008: 192–93)

Wind is said to enter the central channel 'naturally' at several points during one's lifetime: birth, death, during sexual intercourse and when wind 'flows in a balanced way' (Guarisco in Yangönpa 2015: 76). However, for those of us untrained in manipulating *lung* through practice, such occasions pass by unnoticed and 'largely wasted'. In contrast, for Tantric adepts, trained in *tsa lung* practices, such moments 'afford the opportunity to recognize the wisdom wind' (Ibid.: 76). At death, for example, the coarse and subtle bodies separate (Cozort 1986: 97), and all the various *lung* currents are understood to 'dissolve' into the 'very subtle life-sustaining current' (Epstein and Topgay 1982: 72), which itself then dissolves – along with the consciousness – converging into the indestructible drop at the heart (Drungtso 2004: 103). Without intervention, the consciousness will then move through the intermediate state between death and rebirth known as the *bardo*, to rebirth manifesting as another sentient being. An advanced Tantric practitioner, however, is able to harness this process to, ultimately, 'transform the very subtle life-sustaining prana into the basis of the "metaphoric clear light" and "illusory body" – and subsequent freedom from rebirth' (Epstein and Topgay 1982: 72)[26] – i.e. to escape samsara for nirvana – to achieve enlightenment. Indeed, Tantric practitioners may spend considerable time familiarizing themselves with this process of dying during their practice, in preparation for the time when death eventually occurs.

It is clear, then, that much Tibetan Tantric practice is focused on the *lung* and its manipulation in order to affect change within the mind-body complex. Specifically, much focus is on the 'relocation' of *lung* into the central channel – often described as a process of 'converting' karmic wind into wisdom wind through its direction from the side channels into the central channel. However, we can take this one step further – according to Buddhist notions of non-duality (Tib. *nyimé*), the karmic wind and wisdom wind can, in fact, be seen to be *one and the same*: these two 'opposing' winds are simply the same thing, approached from different perspectives – from an unenlightened versus an enlightened mind – as Guarisco quotes from the late Dilgo Khyentse Rinpoche: '[T]he wisdom wind and the karmic wind are the same thing. If this wind is brought under control, it engenders wisdom; if it is not controlled, it gives rise to the ordinary mind, together with its poisons' (Dilgo Khyentse Rinpoche, cited by Guarisco in Yangönpa 2015: 78). Thus, Guarisco concludes that the central channel 'symbolizes the nondual reality; a reality beyond concrete or not concrete; internal or external; and all other ways in which the mind may conceive things to exist' (Guarisco in Yangönpa 2015: 49). From this perspective, we can see why questions of the 'material existence' or 'exact location' of the various channels, winds and chakras may be said to be rather irrelevant; ultimately, all these things are merely tools to enable a Tantric practitioner to access his/her innate buddha-nature – a state of realization beyond ordinary conception.

I include these various details in order to paint a picture of how complex – and perhaps *intense* – these *tsa lung* practices might be for those who undertake them. When we read of the complex physical and cognitive exertions that these high-level practices involve – in light of our understandings of *lung* from the previous chapter – perhaps we can start to imagine why and how problems may result from their incorrect undertaking. Moreover, while the focus of these kinds of Tantric practices is clearly on the manipulation of the various facets of the subtle body for the purposes of, ultimately, attaining enlightenment, due to *lung*'s dual role in Tibetan Tantra and medicine, some such *tsa lung* practices are also understood to be able to treat *lung* disorders – as well as disorders of the other *nyépa* too. Thus, Chaoul tells us:

> With the help of movements that guide the mind and vital breath currents into different areas, the channels-breaths practices bring the possibility of healing or, in other words: harmonising body, energy, and mind, or the body-energy-mind system. This is a goal of yogic practices and also a model of good health that is in line with the concept of health and well-being in Tibetan medicine. (2007: 135)

For example, in his biography of Yangönpa, Chen Ngawa Rinchen Den describes how the Buddhist scholar was able to prevent illness spreading through his body via his manipulation and 'blocking' of *lung* (Chen Ngawa Rinchen Den, cited by Guarisco in Yangönpa 2015: 154).

Moreover, knowledge of body structure and functioning, and understandings of the maintenance and restoration of health, are key to Buddhist practice in a very practical sense, with health described as 'an individual's finest possession' in early Buddhist writing (Yoeli-Tlalim 2010: 320). Lusthaus describes how Asaṅga, author of the key *Yogācāra-bhūmi* text, for example, 'draws on the medical understanding of his day to understand how the mind and body work, and what implications that holds for Buddhist practice . . . Health is necessary for a productive life conducive to advancing on the Path' (2017: 50). Indeed, a practitioner who is not burdened by poor health or pain is of course more easily able to focus on their practice – but Tantric Buddhism developed this notion further, with four aims discussed in texts: 'prevention of illness, cure of illness, securing longevity and attaining spiritual liberation'. Thus, the Tantric Buddhist practitioner learns to control *lung* not only to, ultimately, achieve spiritual realization but also – in the meantime – to maintain health, thus allowing him/her more time and ability to practise (Yoeli-Tlalim 2010: 320).

Indian Roots and Tibetan Notions of the 'Central Channel'

In both Indian and Tibetan Tantric traditions, the ultimate aim of these kinds of practices focused on the manipulation of bodily winds is to become 'liberated' – a being 'beyond the bounds of karmic conditioning' (Samuel 1989: 203).[27] We saw in the previous chapter how much of the *Gyüshi* understanding of the body originates in Ayurvedic descriptions of the body, with the doctrine of five bodily winds traced back to the Indian classical period. Here, I would like to explore early Indian concepts of wind and breath in a little more detail, to give greater context to Tibetan Tantric practices that work with this 'energetic' body.

The concept of a network of subtle channels in the body can be traced back 'at least as far' as the *Bṛhadāraṇyaka Upaniṣad* text (*c.*700 BCE), with breath control delineated alongside mantra repetition in the *Jaiminīya*

Upaniṣad Brāhmaṇa, *c.*800 – 600 BCE (Mallinson and Singleton 2017: xii–xix). Samuel describes early discussion of 'subtle-body' concepts in the *Taittiriya Upaniṣad*, dating from the fourth or fifth century BCE, where five bodies or 'selves' – each one 'shaped like a human being and pervading the one before' – are said to include the physical body ('formed by food') and a 'body or self made of vital breath (*prāṇa*)', and there is also discussion of a 'central channel' (2013c: 33).[28] Moreover, Mallinson notes that a 'connection between the mind and breath' was taught 'as early as the *Chāndogya Upaniṣad* (6.8.2)', with the *Amṛtasiddhi* being 'the first text to teach that mind, breath and *bindu* [drops] are connected, a notion found in many subsequent *haṭhayoga* texts' (Mallinson 2020: 415).

However, Indian notions of bodily 'wind' date back much further than this: Mallinson and Singleton describe how the concept of *prāṇa* as 'life-breath' is found 'from the beginning of India's literary record', included in Vedic sacrificial practices (2017: 128), and Zysk describes a 'relatively unbroken development' of the notion of bodily winds that can be 'traced from earliest times to the centuries around the beginning of the common era' (1993: 211). He traces a process by which understandings of breath/wind originate in the practices of ascetics, diverge into separate but related perspectives in Indian medical and religious traditions, and finally start to converge again during the sixteenth century (Zysk 2007: S113).[29] This process includes the 'development of a doctrine of bodily winds and respiration' among early Indian ascetics, who practised meditation and 'ecstatic techniques' aimed towards achieving long life and immortality – within which, the control and arresting of respiration (Skt. *prāṇāyāma*) was key (Zysk 1993: 202–3). Such practices could be both preliminary, conducted in order to 'purify the channels', and/or advanced, aimed towards acquiring supernatural abilities and/or liberation (Mallinson and Singleton 2017: 130–31). Zysk names the *Ṛgveda* and *Atharvaveda* (*c.*1500 – 1000 BCE) as the key texts for 'tracing an early evolution of vital breath' in India (1995: 35), telling us how 'breath was equated with, contained in, and associated with all micro/macro cosmic elements which produced and maintained life' (Ibid.: 37). A later split from the *Upaniṣadic* tradition led to the development of a separate 'medical physiology' focused on *prāṇa* and the bodily winds in India, with its own specialized treatises (Zysk 1993: 206).

Thus, we have the 'twin origins' of 'wind'/'breath' concepts in Indian medical and religious practice from which the Tibetan medical and Tantric traditions draw, and which were then developed further by Tibetan scholars and practitioners. Perhaps unsurprisingly, this has led to a certain amount of discussion – and no little confusion – with multiple similarities and diversities evident between the Tibetan Tantric and medical notions of 'wind' and its related channels. A much-debated topic, for example, has been the 'central channel' key to these two Tibetan traditions. With their shared origins in the practices of ancient Indian ascetics, might we assume that the 'central channel' of the Tantric system (Tib. *tsa wuma*) and the 'central channel' of the medical system (Tib. *sok tsa*, life-sustaining channel) are one and the same – simply one concept with two different names? Given our focus on the *sok tsa* and *sok lung* in the previous chapter's discussion on mind and mental health, this might be a rather pertinent question for us. Well, it's complicated. Focusing on the central channel and the channels to its left and right, a number of religious and medical scholars – including Lodro Gyalpo (1509–79), Desi Sangye Gyatso (1653–1703/5) and twentieth-century scholar Tsultrim Gyaltsen – do indeed view these three channels in the *Gyüshi* as the three channels of Tantric tradition (Garrett and Adams 2008: 89).[30] Similarly, Adams quotes a contemporary Tibetan medicine doctor in Lhasa asserting that the channels described in Tantric and medical texts are 'ultimately the same' – it is only the ways in which practitioners *utilize* them that are different: the doctor using his/her knowledge in the diagnosis and treatment of illness, and the Tantric practitioner using this knowledge to attain enlightenment (2001: 547).

However, other scholars disagree, and Garrett and Adams have described a 'centuries-old controversy in Tibetan literature': how the Buddhist Tantric textual descriptions of this system might be 'reconciled' with those in the Tibetan medical texts (2008: 87).[31] Here, for example, the existence of the *sok tsa* in relation to the other channels is 'hotly contested' amongst both medical and religious scholars (2008: 91–92), and Guarisco references Yönten Gyamtso's argument that the Tantric *tsa wuma* 'is neither the life channel (Tib. *sok tsa*) nor the spinal cord' (Tib. *gyungpa*) – for these, he says, are 'coarse channels' (Guarisco in Yangönpa 2015: 50). Equally, G.K. Gyatso describes the position of the central channel *in front of* the *sok tsa*: 'Immediately in front of the spine there is the life channel [Tib. *sok tsa*], which is quite thick; and in front of this is the central channel [Tib. *wuma*]' (1994: 125). In fact, the absence of physical structures related to the Tantric central channel and its two side channels was noted by Buddhist scholars in the thirteenth century (J. Gyatso 2004: 88), and an equivalence between the two traditions' 'three channels' was only explicitly made in the fifteenth century – by a medical writer who, J. Gyatso explains, 'casually remarked' that the vitality/life channels (Tib. *tsé tsa*) of the medical system followed the path of the Tantric *roma* and *kyangma* – running down the body either side of the *wuma* (Ibid.). There followed, she tells us, a 'sustained effort to locate this tantric system within the medical system of channels' described in the *Gyüshi*, whereby some scholars made efforts to distinguish between 'outer' and 'inner' versions of various channels, allowing a distinction between the 'medical body' – that of an ordinary (unenlightened) human being – and the body of a Tantric practitioner or *enlightened* human being (Ibid.).[32]

In Amdo, discussions on this topic were varied and complex too. *Ngakpa* and Tibetan medicine doctor Aku Wangchuk (72, Rebkong) explained that the *tsa wuma* materially exists only in the first few weeks of life, asserting:

> Some people say that it [the *tsa wuma*] is still there later in life and it's invisible . . . but this is not true . . . The *tsa wuma* is there at the beginning of life, and the basis of consciousness [Tib. *kün zhi nam pa shé pa*] is located inside this. Then slowly, it will disappear, but when we meditate, we can still focus on it – we can meditate [on it], but from our body we can't find it.

Tibetan medicine doctor Dr Nyima (38, Rebkong/Xining), who had also spent some time studying Tantric concepts of mind-body with a Nyingma *ngakpa*, told me definitively that these two channels are the same. The problem, he explained, was that '[a]ctually [Tibetan medicine] doctors don't know about the *tsa wuma* and this kind of thing – they don't even know what is mind! Even fewer people know what is *sok lung* . . . So that's why if you ask more people, you will get very varied answers'. Moreover, a further complication in attempting to 'unite' Tibetan Tantric and medical accounts of subtle anatomy is the aforementioned 'diversity' we find in the South Asian literature from which the Tibetan concepts are derived (Garrett and Adams 2008: 87). It is clear that there exists a multiplicity of textual descriptions of the body – not only historically but also among recent and contemporary practitioners and scholars too.

When Things Go Wrong: Practice-Related Wind Illnesses

In Chapter 1, we heard several Amdo narratives of *nyoné* apparently caused by 'incorrect' religious practice – from Rinchen's narrative about a 'monk who became crazy because he read a Buddhist text' to a young monk's description of an elderly lama with *nyoné* in Rebkong. Perhaps this should not be surprising: if we follow the premise that, conducted correctly, *tsa lung* and *trül khor* practices have the potential to radically alter the mind-body complex of the practitioner, ultimately leading to their enlightenment, then it should also follow that conducted *incorrectly*, such practices might result in some unintended – potentially negative – effects on the mind and body.[33] Indeed, Gutschow refers to the possibility of 'Tantric overload' as a cause of 'wind disorders and insanity' (1997: 185), and Rapgay notes that a 'special understanding of the pitfalls of meditation practice is included in Tibetan conceptions of mental illness' (1985: 52), explaining that this can occur, for example, if *lung* becomes 'stuck' or out of place.

In Amdo and beyond, such explanations are often focused particularly on the *sok lung* and *sok tsa*. We have already seen how the *sok lung* may be involved in *nyoné* and other mental illnesses from a Tibetan medical perspective, and 'disturbance' of the *sok tsa* is described by Epstein and Topgay as a 'hazard of meditation practice' that may affect both beginners and advanced practitioners. This is, they assert, a condition well understood by Tibetan doctors and Tantric practitioners, who are 'well versed in the predisposing causes, symptoms, and treatments of this disorder' (1982: 74–75). For example, Garrett cites twelfth-century Sakya scholar Drakpa Gyeltsen's description of the *sok lung* as 'generally responsible for the integrated relationship between mind and body', and his assertion that disturbance in it may lead to 'insanity or death' (Garrett 2008: 65–66). Similarly, Yönten Gyamtso specifies that symptoms of *lung* entering the *sok tsa* may include 'madness and unconsciousness' (Gyamtso in Lingpa 2013: 407, n. 261), and Henning references Jonang scholar Tāranātha's (1575–1634) commentary on the *Kālacakra Tantra*, wherein symptoms including 'lack of consciousness, craziness, and ultimately death' are described as potential consequences of 'damage' to the *sok lung* (Henning 2009: 244). In Amdo, as we read in the quote at the beginning of this chapter, Gelugpa lama Wangyal (62, Rebkong) explained how if a practitioner controls their *sok lung* effectively, then they should not suffer from *nyoné*. However, if they are unable to 'control it well', 'the *sok lung* can become uncomfortable [Tib. *mi dewa*] . . . [and] the heart becomes affected by *lung* – the *lung* goes into the heart'. This, he explained, may lead to *nyoné*.

Similarly, Dr Pema (40, Xining) told me, 'In Buddhist practice, meditation is very complicated – if you don't do the very correct way, it causes so many mind problems – there are many possible side effects, for example the *sok lung* may become blocked – [we call this] *sok lung* or *nyoné*'. For yogi Lodro (42), in Chabcha (see Figure 3.1), the state of a practitioner's mind-body was key here. When I asked him about possible negative effects from conducting *tsa lung* practices, he told me: 'The *lung* can become disturbed – especially if your body is weak, and the mind is uneasy/uncomfortable [Tib. *sem kham ma dewa*], and then you try to do practices. Then your *sok tsa* or your *lung* may become disturbed, and your *lung* becomes out of control'.

Such descriptions also lend weight to the argument that the 'central channels' of Tibetan Tantra and medicine – the *tsa wuma* and *sok tsa*, respectively – are not one and the same. For example, Guarisco describes Yangönpa's assertion that negative effects such as 'insanity or seizures' may occur when *lung* currents and mind enter the *sok tsa* but *not* when they enter the *tsa wuma*, whereupon only 'positive qualities' will arise (Guarisco in Yangönpa 2015: 46, 234). However, it is not only the *sok tsa*/*sok lung* that may be implicated here: Marek and Oliphant describe, for example, 'health

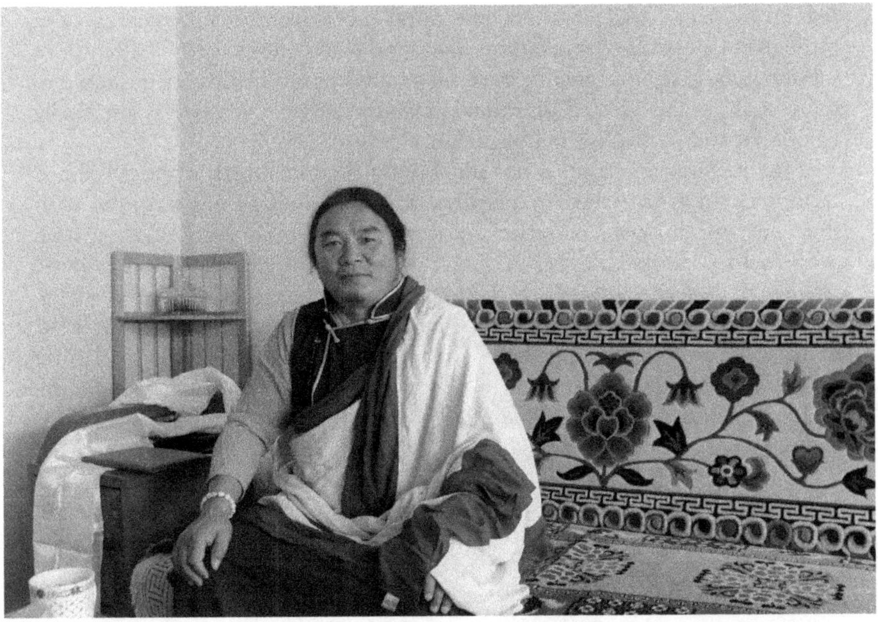

Figure 3.1. Yogi Lodro at his home in Chabcha, 2018. © Susannah Deane.

problems' and specific mental states that may arise if *lung* becomes 'isolated and immobilized' in a number of specific channels, or becomes 'imbalanced, traveling, or trapped in incorrect channels' (2017: 418–19).

Again, we encounter narratives of power and risk inherent in Tantric practice, with intense sensations expected during the course of practice but dire consequences warned for those who do not practise correctly. For example, Khendrup Norsang Gyatso's fifteenth-century commentary on the *Kālacakra Tantra*, *The Ornament of Stainless Light: An Exposition of the Kālacakra Tantra*, describes how '[m]editation on the winds held together should continue until the head begins to hurt, until the yogi sees his body encircled by light, or until the heart starts to jump'. However, he explains, '[i]f meditation continues after these signs appear, there is a danger of death' (K.N. Gyatso, trans. by Kilty 2004: 502). Indeed, this reflects the *Kālacakra Tantra*'s own caution that '[i]f one continues to practice the *prāṇāyāma* after those symptoms occur, the *prāṇā* congeals in the navel-*cakra*, or if unrestrained, it causes death by violently splitting the *uṣṇīṣa*[34] and leaving the body' (Wallace 2001: 52).

Epstein and Topgay discuss a form of *sok lung* disorder that is 'a complication of improper meditation practice', and is, they assert, 'more likely to arise in meditators who are improperly instructed in methods designed to concentrate the mind':

> A kind of manic state in which the mind races. Instead of becoming calm through the practice of meditation, the mind reacts to the forceful attempt to subdue it and becomes unable to settle on any object. It jumps from topic to topic, making the affected individual anxious, restless, and often dramatically emotional and insensitive to the guidance of teachers . . .
>
> If the meditation object is not suitable for the individual, if the developed concentration is tarnished by negative states of mind or not balanced with sufficient mindfulness, or especially if the mind is not concentrated with proper effortlessness, sok-*lung* may develop . . . If strain develops in the mind's attempt to concentrate itself on the object of meditation, if rather than being gently guided into one-pointedness the mind is forced into submission, if the mind squeezes and tightens in its attempt at concentration, then the mind is said to 'rise up' in its attempt to find the object. As the mind rises up, the pranic current on which it is mounted rises with it, producing the symptoms and signs of sok-*lung*. (1982: 74–75)

There is a hint here – in Epstein and Topgay's mention of 'negative states of mind' – of the concept of *namtok*. Usually translated as 'conceptual thoughts/awareness' in classical Tibetan and Buddhist and Bon literature, as I mentioned in Chapter 1, in colloquial Tibetan it is often translated into English as 'suspicion' or 'doubt'. Discussions on this topic in Amdo emphasized the necessity of a good foundation in Buddhist knowledge for practitioners embarking on such high-level Tantric practices. Indeed, in that chapter, for example, we heard Tamdrin (26, Rebkong) describe the difficulties of understanding the key Buddhist concept of 'emptiness' (Tib. *tongpa nyi*[35]), relating it to his uncle's *nyoné*, and telling me that if a practitioner cannot understand well the Buddhist concepts discussed in the texts, 'maybe they will get *namtok*', and perhaps 'become *nyoné*'. To avoid this, he asserted, 'we have to go slowly, step by step, towards the buddha [enlightenment]'.

Similarly, *ngakpa* and Tibetan medicine doctor Aku Wangchuk (72, Rebkong) asserted:

> When you practise [Tantra], if you have *namtok*, things will definitely go wrong. You need to totally eliminate *namtok*, but to do that, you have to understand *a lot*. For example, you need to understand the Buddhist concept of non-self. But if you can eliminate *namtok*, then you will have no problem [with such practices].

Linked to this, some Amdo-wa emphasized the importance of practitioners' 'faith' (Tib. *dépa*) in their practice, such as former Gelugpa monk Tsetan (38, Rebkong), who told me, 'You must have faith in Buddha's teachings . . . His knowledge is also mysterious – you cannot know everything, but you must still have the faith'. Ardussi and Epstein discuss this in reference to what they term '*chos-smyo*' – 'Dharma madness' – which they say may 'befall the practitioner who exhibits self-doubt' (1978: 330). However, they also link this to spirit affliction, asserting that '[a]ny scruple or hesitation (*rnam-rtog*) shown by an unthoroughly trained meditator leaves him open for demonic attack' (1978: 330–31).

These kinds of causative factors, where *lung* becomes trapped or 'out of place', or a practitioner suffers due to *namtok* or a lack of faith, were sometimes described by Tantric practitioners and Tibetan doctors in Amdo as 'inside causes'. As Epstein and Topgay suggested above, in Amdo such instances were often blamed on 'improper' or 'incomplete' instruction, or students not following teachings correctly – perhaps due to their own eagerness or arrogance in their engagement with high-level practices. For example, in Rebkong, Geshe Dhondup (50) asserted that such cases 'usually result from incorrect practices, with the practitioners not having the proper guidance or teachings from teachers'. Indeed, in Vajrayana, the relationship between student and teacher is key, as Chaoul explains:

> Although instructions are provided in the text, it is not advised to practise them just on the basis of reading a text. Instead, one should receive oral explanations from an authorised teacher, giving one the key to open the door to one's experiences. Most practitioners would not even look at such a text without having an appropriate introduction to it by a lama or master. (2007: 135)

These narratives of *nyoné* related to 'incorrect' practice emphasize again the risks inherent in high-level Tantric practice. In Amdo, I often heard descriptions of Tantric students' mistakes or 'arrogance' in going 'too quickly' into advanced practices, or apparently not listening to their teachers. Some of the religious specialists I spoke to in Amdo were keen to assure me that these kinds of cases are uncommon in monasteries, where experienced practitioners are protected by their prior knowledge and practice of Buddhism, and they are studying with experienced and knowledgeable teachers. In Rebkong, for example, Gelugpa Geshe Dhondup (45) described practice-related *nyoné* as very uncommon in the monastery, asserting that 'because of religious teachings and practices, practitioners find a way to keep themselves calm, and to control everything, so these kinds of causes [of *nyoné*] from inside yourself are really, really rare'. Similarly, Bon lama Tsering (57) suggested that only 'one out of every one hundred' practitioners suffer from such *lung* problems during their practice. It was not too frequent, he explained, because 'usually when people go on retreat, they have initiation and guidance – otherwise they usually would not go'. In his introduction and translation of Tenzin Gyatso, H.H. Dalai Lama's commentary on the *Kālacakra Tantra*, Hopkins explains what this kind of 'initiation' involves:

> Initiation means to cleanse and purify defilements; to authorize students to hear about and cultivate the tantric paths and to achieve special feats; to empower the attainment of beneficial qualities; to set potencies for attaining levels of the path and the fruits of those paths; to sprinkle water; to pour potencies and cast seeds into the mental continuum of the initiate; to convey a new style of behavior and its attendant releases from distorted states; and to cause initiates to be endowed with a blissful mind . . . [A]ll of these activities are central to the initiations of the Kalachakra system. (Hopkins in Tenzin Gyatso 1985: 67–68)

In reality, of course, it is difficult to gauge how frequently practitioners suffer from any such problems during practice, and to what degree, but interviews in Amdo suggest that in fact many people view this as rather more common than the geshe suggested. For example, Aku Wangchuk (72, Rebkong) told me that 'this happens a lot' – most of these afflicted practitioners, he said, had done 'something wrong [in their practice]'. Certainly, the number of interviewees in Amdo who described such cases would support the Aku's perspective that these complications are not uncommon. Of course, these kinds of problems will not be experienced by all meditators, and indeed if one is doing one's practice correctly such things should not happen at all – but it is clear, both from my interviews in Amdo and descriptions in the Buddhist and Bon texts, that this is a well-known risk when conducting complex Tantric practices working with the *lung* in this way. As we heard Aku Wangchuk assert in Chapter 1, a Tantric teacher would usually warn students of these kinds of potential problems, and the complexities involved in 'integrating' and 'controlling' the channels, winds and drops, where mistakes in practice can lead to *nyoné.*

Of course, any *non*-specialists who choose to engage with Tantric texts or practices might be expected to be even more susceptible to these kinds of problems – due their lack of knowledge and/or experience. In Rebkong, Ngawang (42) described how his lay brother – who, he said, loved reading all kinds of books – had become *nyoné* after he had 'read about sacred mantras and Tantras': 'Finally he suffered from some strange illness . . . He became *very* dangerous – like, driving the wrong way on the road . . . confused'. Ngawang described how two lamas had been called to perform rituals to help his brother, reporting that these had successfully treated him and he was now well.

Finally, we might remember from Chapter 2 that according to Tibetan medicine, 'mental exertion' has been named as a causative factor for *nyoné.* This too, is often traced to *lung* disturbance, with 'mental strain of any kind' described as a potential cause of *sok lung* disturbance (Epstein and Topgay 1982: 74), and 'too much worry or meaningless conversation' listed as a causative or contributory factor in wind disorders in the *Gyüshi* (*Gyüshi II*

2015: 37) – a perspective also evident in both lay people's and doctors' narratives in Amdo. Indeed, we heard in the previous two chapters how 'too much thinking' and/or 'too much study' may sometimes lead to *lung* problems and/or *nyoné* – and this is something that I also encountered in my previous research in Darjeeling (Deane 2019b). Researchers working in other Tibetan communities have discussed this too; in Dharamsala, for example, Lewis described the propensity for *lung* disorders amongst monks and nuns studying for philosophy exams (2013: 321). Indeed, high-level philosophical or Tantric study is nothing if not intensive, in terms of the amount of time and mental activity that it requires from students. Thus, in Amdo, former Gelugpa monk Tsetan (38) asserted that the 'most common cause' of *nyoné* in practitioners is that 'the person keeps practising a lot – not relaxing or participating in any other activities'. Similarly, Gelugpa lama Wangyal (62) explained, 'Some people do meditation every day – if they stay alone and study, then they may get *sok lung* [*né*], and then they may become *nyoné*'. Indeed, several researchers have described how *sok lung* disorder is viewed by many Tibetans as a common condition among monks (see Prost 2006: 125) – perhaps even '*most commonly* identified in monks as the product of intellectual overexertion' (Benedict, Mancini and Grodin 2009: 489). Prost has described the condition of '*lung tsha po*, or literally "hot strong wind"', which leads some monks to become 'hot-tempered, nervous and irritable' due to their 'constant preoccupation with abstract considerations' (Ibid.). Thus, in a very pragmatic sense too, conducting religious study and/or complex practices alone can be a risky business – best approached very carefully and under the guidance of an experienced teacher if one wants to maintain one's health and sanity.

Treating Practice-Related *Lung Né* and *Nyoné*

In the previous chapter, we explored the treatment of *nyoné* related to wind illness and heart illness within the Tibetan medical traditions, which predominantly focus on medicinal formulas and external therapies. We heard too that when dealing with *lung né*, it is often said to be best – and indeed, most effective – to treat such conditions in the early stages. In relation to practice-related *lung né*, then, the student–teacher relationship is key: Epstein and Topgay tell us, for example, that a 'sensitive teacher' will be able to recognize this kind of practice-caused *lung* condition at an early stage, by 'engaging in slow, quiet conversation with the individual and observing the way his or her mind and speech jump from subject to subject'. Further indications of this kind of problem can be ascertained, they suggest, through observation of a practitioner's appearance and behaviour, such as his/her 'pallor', 'appearance of the eyes', restlessness and/or 'reluctance to answer questions'. Physical symptoms, such as aching in the back, neck and shoulders may also be present (1982: 75). However, in these cases, Epstein and Topgay assert that 'medical' treatment is not always necessary – instead, they describe how a change in meditation practice, or 'careful instruction on the method of meditation', perhaps alongside general dietary and behavioural advice for wind disorders, may be enough to treat 'less advanced cases' of *sok lung* disorder (Ibid.). Similarly, when I discussed this with Geshe Dhondup (45) in Rebkong, he emphasized the importance of *tsa lung* practices (under guidance from a teacher) in treating *nyoné* caused by such 'inside causes'. Indeed, we find such practices well described in Tibetan Tantric texts alongside medical treatments. For example, Marek and Oliphant have translated excerpts from *Oral Instructions on the Methods for Correcting the Defects of the Isolated Wind*,[36] wherein four therapeutic approaches are described for each listed *lung* disorder: a bodily technique, object of visualization, medicinal substance and a blessing (2017: 419–22). For example, for the so-called 'defect of crazy wind':

> First, the cause: It arises from earlier experiences of intense suffering, and of the seventy-two channels that exist at the heart, either the forty-second becomes stuck or the thirtieth rises up.
>
> The four methods of eliminating defects [are as follows]: First, the technique of the body is, having assumed the *vajra* posture, put the two fists inside of the *vajra* posture and lift the crossed legs into the sky. For the object of visualization, contemplate that light rays emanate from a white drop the size of a small lentil amulet at the center of the Dharma Chakra touching the channels. For the substance, together with the cross-legged *vajra* posture, splash the body with waves of cold water. The blessing resembles the earlier [blessing]. (Marek and Oliphant 2017: 420–21)

In Amdo, *ngakpa* and Tibetan medicine doctor Aku Wangchuk (72) told me that practitioners with practice-related wind disorders can 'rarely' treat themselves – instead, he asserted, usually they will consult a doctor, and may also change their practice. And when I asked former monk Tsetan (38) about this, he explained:

> For these kinds of practices, first you need to manipulate the *lung*, and at the end of the practice, there is a way to release it within the body . . . And if you do not do the practices correctly, then you will get problems . . . I'm not sure how you treat this kind of *nyoné* or other problems from practice, but usually it depends on the person himself . . . Maybe he has to rest for a few days . . . after a few days or a few weeks perhaps he will recover . . . I think *probably* moxibustion and acupuncture can help, and also bloodletting and herbal poultice – these could help, but I'm not really sure.

At the Qinghai Province Tibetan Medicine Hospital in Xining, Dr Dechen (39) described having successfully treated a nun who had become *nyoné* this way, with Tibetan medicine. Dechen explained that while initially this nun had been 'very abnormal', 'physically unwell' and 'spitting' at the nurses, over time the patient had become 'better and better – even greeting the nurses' and eventually able to leave the hospital.

Despite these various routes for treatment of practice-induced *nyoné* related to *lung* – described in the texts, and also discussed by contemporary practitioners – those I spoke to in Amdo were very much divided over how successful they thought any such 'medical' treatments for this kind of *lung né* were likely to be. Indeed, a number of people told me clearly that they viewed such treatments – or even *any* treatment – as of little or no use for such cases. For others, as we have seen, remedy was possible through further practices, as is described in some of the commentarial texts.

Madness as Enlightenment: Realization or Performance?

And finally, what of the figure of the *lama nyonpa* – the 'crazy lama' or 'mad yogin' whom we first met in Chapter 1? Should we conclude, as I was told in Amdo, that this is a practitioner who may well *appear* to be *nyoné* but is, in fact, an enlightened Buddhist master – one who has conducted their Tantric mind-body practices so successfully that they have now transcended duality to become fully realized? And if so, how might one tell the enlightened *lama nyonpa* from the *lama* who has, unfortunately, simply become *nyonpa*?

As we have already seen, the *lama nyonpa* or *tokdenpa* is a well-known figure in Tibetan society, with lay people as well as religious specialists describing the activities of famous historical and more recent or contemporary practitioners. For example, some Amdo interviewees discussed the renowned eleventh-century Buddhist yogi Milarepa,[37] as well as other historical figures such as Tsangnyon Heruka (the 'Madman of Tsang' [also known as Sangyé Gyeltsen], 1452–1507). Indeed, most of the people I spoke to in Amdo talked more readily of historical examples such as these than of any recent or contemporary figures. However, Nyingma yogi Lodro (42, Chabcha) was emphatic that there were still many of these types of practitioners in contemporary Tibet – in fact, he reported, he had so far met three such figures.[38] And, while the majority of the *lama nyonpa* that we read about in the Tibetan traditions are male, DiValerio discusses a few female examples too, such as Sönam Peldren (1328?–72?), who was said to perform miracles. With her biography focusing often on 'the theme of religious "madness"', she is said to have 'acquired a cult following after her death' (2015: 225).

Ardussi and Epstein describe the 'tricksterlike' figure of the *lama nyonpa* as '[o]ne of the most fascinating characters that runs through the oral and literary traditions of Tibet' (1978: 327). The reported behaviour of these practitioners ranges from the bizarre to the shocking: in Chapter 1, for example, we heard of a *ngakpa/hön* apparently (temporarily) removing his intestines, having cut open his own torso; and one biography of Tsangnyon Heruka describes him eating the rotting brains of some slain men that he came across during his travels (also encouraging others to eat spoonfuls of the maggot-infested flesh and brains too) (Smith 2001: 68). Ardussi and Epstein describe this figure as 'a sociopath' who engages in the kinds of behaviour that Tibetans 'purport to disdain': 'drinking to excess, fornicating, thieving, defying authority, playing magical tricks' (1978: 327). In fact, they describe six 'principal attributes of the saintly madman', which include a 'generalized rejection of customary behavior which society-at-large, and the monastic establishment in particular, regard as appropriate for a religious man', an 'inclination towards bizarre modes of dress', 'disregard for the niceties of interpersonal behavior, particularly with regard to social status' and a 'professed disdain for scholasticism', alongside the 'use of popular poetical forms, mime, songs, [and] epic tales' in their teaching, and '[t]he use of obscenity and vulgar parlance' (Ibid.: 332–34).

My experiences in Amdo echoed other scholars' assertions that Tibetans often speak of these figures with 'great fondness' (DiValerio 2015: 6). Indeed, explanations for their strange (and often transgressive) behaviour tend to focus on the narrative that they are 'really' enlightened figures (Ardussi and Epstein 1978: 327) – unbound by the usual conceptualizations of the ordinary (i.e. *un*enlightened) mind. Samuel notes that some of these unusual practitioners even became well known for curing illnesses (1993: 304) – and this was the case in Amdo too, where some such practitioners were reported to have various abilities to heal themselves and/or others. For example, Shukho (32, Golok) told me about a living rinpoche she had heard about who spontaneously produced medicine pills from his body. People with all kinds of illness would visit him, she said, because these pills would cure any illness. Contemporary practitioner and author Nida Chenagtsang describes too the various ways in which practitioners can use such magical powers in healing others, such as in mending broken bones or cases of poisoning (Joffe 2019: 114–15).

A link is often made between these Tibetan practitioners and the Indian *siddhas* of the eighth to twelfth centuries. These practitioners developed a number of new rituals and 'entirely new sets of rules incumbent on those following the vows that sometimes required them to act as insane as others certainly believed them to be' (Davidson 2002: 338). However, as DiValerio and others have pointed out, the 'complex and multidimensional' relationship between the Indian *siddhas* and Tibetan *lama nyonpa* was no simple 'copying' from India to Tibet (2015: 93) – rather, influences encompassed a number of Buddhist and non-Buddhist South Asian religious movements (Ibid.: 75); these probably included Theravādin Buddhist societies in Thailand and Sri Lanka (Samuel 1993: 308), and Hindu traditions in India (Ardussi and Epstein 1978: 337). Indeed, Ardussi and Epstein describe this figure as 'a complex assemblage of multiple historical movements and scholastic traditions' (Ibid.: 327), arguing that this particular 'pattern of madness' was indigenous to Tibet (Ibid.: 337).

How, then, can we understand this particular concept of *nyoné*, and how might we relate it to the kinds of 'madness' that we have encountered so far? For example, if we were to witness someone exhibiting the kinds of strange behaviours described here, we might assume him/her to be experiencing 'normal' *nyoné* – i.e. 'madness' caused by any one of the factors we have explored so far (for example, *nying né*, *lung né* or perhaps some form of spirit affliction, which we will examine in Part II). We would probably conclude that the person was suffering from an 'illness' (Tib. *né*) requiring some form(s) of treatment. Indeed, the reported behaviours of some of these *lama nyonpa* do match some of the commonly described symptoms of the illness of *nyoné* that we saw in Chapters 1 and 2, such as eating non-food items or taking off one's clothes in public. As Wangchuk (31, Golok/Xining) said, 'The behaviour of the *tokdenpa* is *like* a *nyonpa*, but actually he is not *nyonpa*, right?' Similarly, Ardussi and Epstein assert that this figure of the *lama nyonpa* 'shares a number of behavioral characteristics' with those who have *nyoné* related to disordered *lung*: 'He is sociopathic, extroverted, aggressive, argumentative, and engages in debate, singing, dancing, and so on' (1978: 334).

Perhaps unsurprisingly, then, there have often been discussions and disputes over the status of some historical figures, with disagreements over whether they might be *lama nyonpa* or simply *nyonpa*. For example, DiValerio describes madness as 'a recurring theme' in the biography of Shuksep Jetsün, whose 'strange' behaviour led to questions over whether she was a *siddha* or simply *nyoné* (2015: 225–26), and Norbu has described meeting a 'very strange' practitioner, whose behaviour was 'as unfathomable to the intellect as Milarepa's' and who 'suddenly seemed to go crazy' (1986: 103). While initially, Norbu reports that people referred to this man as 'The Lunatic', they later began to speak of him as 'a realized being, a saint' (Ibid.: 104). Similarly, Pitkin describes the figure of Amgön Rinpoche (1853–1945), a hermit at Drikung Til in central Tibet, whose 'disregard for clothing, money, food, and his own appearance; his tendency to speak bluntly to everyone, even the powerful nobility' – displayed alongside great yogic powers – led some to think him 'crazy' (2016: 99).

However, some differences between these different forms of *nyoné* are also apparent – not least the fact that, as Ardussi and Epstein assert, the *lama nyonpa* 'seems to be in full possession of his mental faculties' (1978: 331–32). Indeed, when I asked Wangchuk (31, Golok/Xining) how we (as non-experts) might determine the situation if we saw such a person in the street or elsewhere, he suggested this too, saying, 'I think if you meet that kind of [*lama*] *nyonpa*, and you *ask* him some questions, he will talk to you correctly – about Buddhism . . . He will give you the correct answer'. Moreover, a further difference between the 'ordinary' *nyonpa* and the *lama nyonpa/tokdenpa* is demonstrated in the texts by descriptions of the apparently 'miraculous' activities of the latter – such as Milarepa passing his hand through a rock, and levitating (Chang 1977: 385–86). Similarly, Norbu has described how his uncle developed 'remarkable powers' (including communicating with animals) over several years in retreat, leading people to refer to him as a *tokdenpa* (Norbu 1986: 68). And DiValerio describes popular stories about the aforementioned Amgön Rinpoche, who was apparently 'renowned for his miraculous powers, including the ability to transform himself into a young monk, or to travel in an instant to Lhasa to buy dumplings' (2015: 226). In Amdo, Rinchen (26, Rebkong/Xining) told me (in a mix of English and Tibetan):

> Some lamas do magic – *drub tak* [miracles] – if they are enlightened, they can do these things . . . But there are many levels, right? I don't know the level, but if they reach some level they can do some of this kind of magic . . . Enlightenment is the final level, but before you reach the final level – even if you are not [yet] enlightened, you can do some of those crazy activities – do magic . . . These kinds of magical powers are *high* level. First you must do many, many practices, then one by one by one, you can get to that high level.

In fact, the kinds of 'transgressive' behaviours of these practitioners mentioned above – such as eating human flesh, or showing disdain for Buddhist texts – are also said to indicate the high level of attainment they are understood to have reached as a result of their Buddhist practice, having transcended beyond a dualistic mind that categorizes everything as 'good' versus 'bad', 'pure' versus 'impure', etc., as DiValerio explains:

> [A] highly realized Buddhist master lives without such discursive categories mediating and distorting his experience of reality. When viewed from this perspective, the Madman of Tsang's adorning himself in human remains indicates that he has transcended the unenlightened distinction between repulsive and nonrepulsive . . . This state is sometimes explained as the yogin's having transcended 'worldly concerns'. (2015: 7)

Indeed, a *lama nyonpa* is able to engage in supposedly 'polluting' behaviours *because* 'they have the appearance or form (but not the reality) of being polluting' (Ardussi and Epstein 1978: 335). In Amdo, yogi Lodro (42) explained how such a practitioner might experience apparently 'good' and 'bad' foods in the same way: 'In the case of a *lama nyonpa*, for example, if someone offers him some plates of food, and one is good, and one is bad, he can taste the same flavour in both . . . In this case, this person knows everything – he knows that everything is false [i.e. empty of inherent existence]'.

To illustrate this point further, the yogi discussed his own teacher – a '*lama tokden*', who had passed away in 2009 – describing how his behaviour had demonstrated his transcendence of duality: 'For example, if you gave him a container full of *very* hot water, he would instead say that that water was cold; or if you showed him a container of cold water, he would say it was hot'.

From a Tantric perspective then, the *lama nyonpa*'s strange behaviour indicates an *enlightened* mind. As Larsson describes in the case of Tsangnyon Heruka, while some observers thought him to be mad, '[t]he reason for his unusual behaviour was not ordinary madness, however, but rather his mastery of the *rtsa lung* practices' (2011: 436). Having transcended ordinary conceptual thoughts to achieve non-duality, his/her 'insane' behaviour is not actually insane at all; in fact, it simply demonstrates the practitioner's understanding of the true nature of reality according to the Dharma – the ultimate *sanity*, if you will. It is the rest of us, *un*enlightened, stuck in samsara, who are the 'mad' ones – our 'normal' behaviour an indication of our limited understanding of true reality. After all, from a Tantric Buddhist perspective, such 'dualities' of 'good'/'bad', 'purity'/'impurity' are nothing more than 'a product of our own unrealized nature' (Ardussi and Epstein 1978: 337). We return again to the concept of *namtok*, as DiValerio explains:

> This 'madness' is often said to result from the fact that these individuals have abandoned all *namtok* . . . *Namtok* are preconceptions, which are, from the Buddhist perspective, *mis*conceptions. These conceptual thoughts act like lenses, distorting our vision of the world around us. Only those who are free of such thoughts can experience reality directly. (2015: 7)

Having abandoned all *namtok* then, the *lama nyonpa* has only 'pure vision' – behaving in an 'eccentric' way because he/she has 'an abundance of "realization"' (DiValerio 2015: 7). Thus, DiValerio tells us, for example, of Urgyenpa Sengé (1229/30–1309), who he says was often referred to as a 'madman'. On his arrival in Ngari, Urgyenpa Sengé apparently ascertained that 'the lady of the house' was wondering to herself if he was 'a madman or a *siddha*'. In response, he asked her, '"Am I the crazy one, or is it you?"' (Ibid.: 224–25).

Moreover, once a practitioner is understood to have attained realization and transcended duality, their incredible feats and ability to perform 'miraculous' activities can be understood in this context, as Norbu explains:

> One has gone beyond all limits, and in that state such activity becomes natural rather than really miraculous at all. Miracles are usually thought of as actions someone might perform in relation to seemingly external objects, changing them in some way. But, as the division of reality into internal and external is an illusion, when that illusion is overcome it is possible to go beyond all usual limits, as the great yogi Milarepa did, when he sheltered from a hailstorm by actually getting inside a yak's horn that was lying on the ground, even though it's said that the yak's horn didn't get any bigger, and Milarepa didn't get any smaller. (1986: 156)

In fact, such behaviours may be not simply an *expression* of the practitioner's attainment of non-duality but also a *method* for attaining it. As Ardussi and Epstein explain, the practitioner's transgressive behaviour may here be seen as a part of 'a deliberate process' through which he/she aims to understand the key concept of non-duality (1978: 335) – a way of training him/herself 'to overcome conceptual distinctions and realize emptiness' (DiValerio 2015: 8).

However, in his comprehensive exploration of this topic, DiValerio argues that such figures were, in fact, neither 'mad' nor 'realized'. Instead, he asserts that these *lama nyonpa* were engaging in a form of 'Tantric fundamentalism' – taking a *literal* approach to particular parts of Tantric texts, rather than the more common *figurative* interpretations (2015: 14). Thus, their behaviour, he tells us, was 'neither spontaneous nor nonsensical' – rather than some kind of 'wild eccentricity' resulting from the transcendence of worldly concerns, this was instead the 'upholding [of] a well-defined set of spiritual commitments in a purposeful and ordered, if uncommon, manner' (Ibid.: 75). In fact, DiValerio relates much of this to a specific Tantric Buddhist practice known as the 'Practice of the Observance' (Tib. *tülzhuk*), which is described in a number of Indian texts as 'a time-delimited period of wandering homelessness during which an advanced meditator takes on new dress, practices, and attitudes toward the world' (Ibid.: 41–42). He notes that there are chapters dedicated to this practice in Tantras including the *Hevajra*, *Cakrasaṃvara* and *Guhyasamāja* (Ibid.), where some of the texts instruct the practitioner to 'behave like "a madman"' (Ibid.: 42). While there is much diversity in detail across the texts, we do find some common descriptions of *where* this practice should be performed – including in charnel grounds, or under an isolated tree (Ibid.) – with the prescribed practices including 'wandering, consuming impure substances, drinking alcohol, eating whatever one finds, singing and dancing, behaving fearlessly, like a lion, or without concern for what others might think, like a child' (Ibid.).

DiValerio argues that this understanding of the *lama nyonpa*'s activities has been lost over time: with knowledge of the Practice of the Observance having faded, the myth of the highly realized 'crazy lama' has come to predominate. Moreover, one more recent figure has been key in forming our perception of this: DiValerio describes how Chögyam Trungpa (1939–87), through coining the term 'crazy wisdom', was able to create 'specific circumstances ensuring that his behavior would be interpreted in this manner' (2015: 238). Here, his frequent drunkenness, and eccentric and even abusive behaviour, was justified by both himself and many of his followers as the result of his 'enlightened' state:

> Trungpa variously described 'crazy wisdom' as 'the action of truth,' or as 'controlling psychic energies.' He described crazy wisdom as 'very timid or cowardly,' but also as 'what characterizes a saint in the Buddhist tradition.' Trungpa said the 'essence' of crazy wisdom is 'hopelessness.' At the same time, Trungpa talked about crazy wisdom as the totality of the good qualities manifested by the eight forms of Padmasambhava.[39] Trungpa also asserted crazy wisdom to be a pedagogical mode, a sort of skillful means or *upāya.* (2015: 239)[40]

In this way, DiValerio argues, Trungpa played a key role in 'bringing about this state of affairs in which Western commentators so readily employ the notion of "holy madness" in making sense of Tibet's (and India's) past' (2015: 237).

And yet, I think it important to consider *why* this understanding of the *lama nyonpa* as *tokdenpa* has proved so popular – not least because, as Samuel asserts, it can be rather tricky to ascertain 'what is literal and what is metaphorical' in the Tantric texts (1993: 415). Indeed, he points out, there may be several, equally valid, layers of interpretation of Tantric concepts and practices – as we have already seen, for example, in the concept of *bodhicitta*/drops. Both material and immaterial, *bodhicitta*/drops can be simultaneously understood as i) an altruistic motivation to attain enlightenment for all sentient beings, ii) a 'drop' transported through the body by the wind and/or iii) the seminal fluid of the practitioner – in fact, it may be all of these things at once for a practitioner. Thus, we have a situation where practices may well have originally been interpreted literally, becoming symbolic over time . . . likewise, they may have been initially intended to be interpreted symbolically, only later *mis*interpreted as literal practices (Samuel 1993: 418) – the picture, unfortunately, is rather unclear. Add to this the fact that, as we saw above, Tantric techniques of *lung* manipulation are understood to have the potential to 'restructure' the self (Samuel 1989: 203), as well as allowing a practitioner to mediate between mind, body and the cosmos through a 'Tantric logic of correspondence' (Duckworth 2017: 413), and it should not be surprising to hear that such practitioners are understood to be able to perform the kinds of miraculous and horrifying feats we have heard about here. Moreover, as we shall explore in Part II, so-called 'deity yoga' practices are understood to give a practitioner access to the 'power' of an enlightened deity – a *bodhisattva* who has transcended the 'worldly' confines of samsara – through their practice, thus allowing all manner or 'miraculous' activities.

From a Tibetan Buddhist/Bon point of view, of course, the ultimate aim of all of this is enlightenment – manipulating the mind-body through *tsa lung* and other practices to transcend duality, to go beyond samsara to nirvana. Any 'ordinary' magical powers (Tib. *tünmong ngödrup*) are nothing more than a 'by-product' of conducting these practices correctly (Samuel 1993: 423) – enabled by the control a practitioner has gained over mind, body and space.[41] In this context, 'madness' – signifying a practitioner's transcendence of duality – is in fact the 'proof of his success': unaffected by dualistic notions of hot/cold, edible/inedible, purity/impurity, etc., the practitioner becomes 'living proof of the Mahāyāna thesis that the liberated man is outside the laws of karma' (Ardussi and Epstein 1978: 335). Equally, from a Tantric perspective, it is quite logical to claim that engaging in such activities is one method by which a practitioner may achieve realization – *training* the practitioner to overcome dualistic notions of 'purity'/'impurity', etc. through ingesting 'impure' substances, dishonouring normally revered Tantric texts and/or even harming other beings.

*

It is evident from our discussion here, and in the previous chapters, that the relationship between wind, mind, heart and *nyoné* in Tibetan medical and Tantric traditions is rather complex. It is clear that while the Tibetan notion of *lung* has its roots in Indian Ayurvedic and Tantric notions of *vāta* and *prāṇa*, *lung* also has its own meanings in Tibetan Tantric and medical theory and practice. Here, its role in transporting the drops – and the drops' relationship with *bodhicitta* – mean that its manipulation through complex and lengthy mind-body practices are key to attaining realization in the Buddhist and Bon traditions. These 'high-risk, high-reward' practices are suitable only for advanced practitioners, and only under the guidance of a teacher. A foundational knowledge and understanding of Dharmic principles are integral to conducting such practices successfully, as is engagement with the requisite preliminary practices following initiation. As we heard in Amdo, and as we read in the historical Buddhist and Bon texts, the risks arising from incorrect practice can be significant, and religious or medical interventions may or may not remedy the situation.

I have attempted here to make sense of this complicated picture, exploring Tantric notions of *lung* alongside the other facets of the subtle-body system and their relationship to the mind and consciousness, examining their manipulation in Tantric practice and the ways in which such practices can be understood to lead to realization but also to disorders of the mind such as *nyoné*. As we have seen, in this context, 'madness' can be seen to result from both *successful* and *unsuccessful* practice. It may be a consequence of a practitioner's failure to control the *lung*, leading to sensory distortions and/or perhaps succumbing to *namtok* while engaging in these high-level practices. Equally, 'madness' might be an indication of a practitioner's realization – now impervious to dualistic notions of 'purity'/'impurity', etc. – or simply his/her attempts to get there, through the enactment of the principle of non-duality. Next, in Part II, we will explore the role of spirits and deities in Tibetan medicine and religion, seeing that they too can be linked to both the illness of *nyoné* and to realization. The key role of *lung* will again be evident – this time in its ability to connect spirits' immaterial bodies to the subtle aspects of human bodies, and humans' ability to transform themselves into enlightened Tantric deities.

Notes

1. As Samuel notes, while there is much debate over definitions of exactly what constitutes 'Tantra' (Tib. *gyud*, 'thread') in Indian contexts, its definition in Tibetan contexts, in contrast, is 'quite uncontroversial'. Here, it is 'regarded as a highly elevated and spiritually profound tradition' (2013c: 36), and the corpuses of Tibetan Tantric texts, known as the *Kangyur* in both Buddhist and Bon traditions, are understood by Buddhists to have been taught by the Buddha in his Tantric aspect of Vajradhara, and understood by Bonpos to have been taught by Tonpa Shenrab.
2. In Tibetan contexts, Chaoul asserts that these 'magical movement' practices are most prevalent in the Kagyu, Nyingma and Bon traditions (2007: 140); such practices related to manipulation in the body can also be found in multiple Indian traditions including Saivite and Jain practices (Samuel 2008: 289, 332–33).
3. Referred to in Buddhist and Bon texts as the 'illusory body' (Tib. *gyu lü*).
4. This was something I had encountered in my previous research in Darjeeling too, where many discussions on the topic often focused on the notion of overly enthusiastic Westerners supposedly 'jumping too quickly' into Buddhist practices, leading to *nyoné* (Deane 2018: 152–53). Indeed, there is a growing body of research on the 'complications' of meditation practice amongst Western practitioners, with depersonalization and 'derealization experiences' described predominantly by novice students (Epstein and Lieff 1981: 138 – see also Lindahl 2017; Lindahl et al. 2017; Lindahl et al. 2023; VanderKooi 1997; and Helderman 2024).
5. This notion of potential dangers linked to wind practices is not exclusive to Tibetan Tantric traditions. Greene, working on Chinese Buddhist traditions, for example, describes how 'meditation on the breath . . . can, if performed incorrectly, disturb the body's "winds" and lead to death' (2017: 373). Similarly, Epstein and Lieff note the

research done in the area of Transcendental Meditation – with practitioners experiencing panic attacks and/or anxiety, amongst other symptoms (1981: 138; see also Lazarus 1976).

6. Here, Duckworth (2017) is translating Rangjung Dorjé's *Key to the Essential Points of Wind and Mind.*
7. The Sanskrit term 'yantra yoga', or simply 'yoga', is sometimes used by Tibetan authors writing in English. These two varieties of practice are also sometimes combined, and referred to as *tsa lung trül khor* – 'magical movement [of/with] channels-breaths' (Chaoul 2007: 133).
8. These practices, related to *yidam* deities, will be explored in in Part II.
9. In this context, there is also an equivalence with the Chinese notion of *qi* (as opposed to *feng* – which may also refer to external wind) (Chaoul 2007: 133).
10. This is evidenced, for example, by such notions as the 'subtle' *lung* apparently remaining after breath has ceased at death (Guarisco in Yangönpa 2015: 67).
11. In some traditions, the *roma* is described as being red and the *kyangma* white; in others, this is reversed. (The *wuma* central channel is often depicted as blue in colour.) And while in some traditions the *kyangma* and *roma* are deemed to be on opposing sides in women and men, in others there is no difference according to gender (Guarisco in Yangönpa 2015: 53).
12. In addition, there is also diversity across the different Tantric traditions over the structure of the chakras – for example, in the *Guhyasamāja* system the crown chakra is understood to have thirty-two petals, whereas in the *Kālachakra* system it has only four (Cozort 1986: 119–20).
13. Indeed, this is another debate that dates back centuries, as Guarisco notes (Guarisco in Yangönpa 2015: 50–51).
14. As Samuel notes, this deity corresponds to Kuṇḍalinī – the Hindu Tantric female serpent deity (1993: 240).
15. See Dalton (2004) generally for a detailed exploration of the development of such practices in Tantra.
16. This refers to the five material and mental factors that give rise to craving and clinging (form, feeling, perception, mental formations and consciousness).
17. See Flood for a descriptive example of this in the form of the Pāñcarātra tradition, for example (2006: 113–17).
18. Tib. *khandroma.* This term is used to refer female deities and, in the Tibetan traditions, may also refer to human female practitioners who have reached a certain level of spiritual attainment.
19. Moreover, Wallace points out that the 'celestial sphere' too is understood to be 'of the nature of wind, which is nondifferentiated from the wind of vital energies that supports a human body'. These two types of wind, as she explains, 'support their respective spheres by holding and transmitting the elements of earth, water, fire, wind, space, and gnosis' (2009: 289).
20. Several scholars have also noted the possibility of Chinese Taoist influences on the development of these kinds of mind-body practices in India – see, for example, Samuel (1989, 2013c) and White (1996).
21. Cozort, for example, describes how the drops 'coat the inside of the channels "like frost"' (1986: 72).
22. There is much more to say on the Tantric sexual practices, but unfortunately not the space to explore this here; I suggest work by Dalton (2004) and Samuel (1989, 2008) for more on this.

23. In Buddhist understanding, samsara refers to the endless cycle of death and rebirth experienced by all sentient beings, only escapable through enlightenment.
24. Moreover, according to the *Kālacakra Tantra*, the 'collective karma' of sentient beings is said to produce karmic winds that 'mold and dissolve the cosmos by amassing and disintegrating the atomic particles that constitute the cosmos' (Wallace 2001: 57) – again, linking the micro- and macrocosm.
25. This term (Tib. *kyilwa* – 'to retain') refers to a way of holding the breath, concentrating it in the lower part of the lungs (Norbu 2008: 387, n. 93).
26. In addition, for such advanced practitioners, it is also possible to 'direct' their *lung* in terms of a further rebirth within samsara, should they wish to.
27. Of course, understandings of 'liberation' differ between Hindu and Buddhist traditions; in the Buddhist and Bon traditions, we find the notion of nirvana as 'extinction'.
28. Interestingly, as Samuel notes, in these early Indian understandings, these various 'bodies' were viewed as *obstacles* to liberation (here, understood to be union with Brahman). In contrast, the later Hindu and Buddhist Tantric traditions viewed them instead as tools that could be utilized through yogic practices *towards* realization (2013c: 34).
29. In addition, as Zysk (2001) notes, 'medical' and 'religious' approaches have become connected once again more recently in the sphere of what he has termed 'New Age Āyurveda'.
30. Lodro Gyalpo, for example, draws equivalences between the white and black 'existence channels' of Tibetan medicine and the Tantric *kyangma* and *roma* channels respectively (Garrett and Adams 2008: 90).
31. There are some political dimensions to this debate too, in relation to the aforementioned process of 'Buddhicization' in the Tibetan medicine tradition, and Gerke references J. Gyatso's 2004 work on Buddhist state control over medical institutions here, arguing that the 'reworking' of Indian Tantric ideas into Tibetan medical texts should be understood in the context of a 'Buddhist hegemony' in Tibet in the seventeenth century (Gerke 2013: 94). Unfortunately, there is not the space to examine this topic in more detail here; I would suggest looking at work by Gerke (2013) and J. Gyatso (2004, 2015) for comprehensive explorations of this.
32. J. Gyatso includes an interesting discussion of the various ways in which some scholars have attempted to both find and 'match up' (or even connect) the descriptions of the three channels across these two traditions (2004: 87–89).
33. As others have noted, this notion of practice-related illness/madness is not solely a Tibetan concept but is found in other Tantric and Buddhist traditions too. Mallinson and Singleton, for example, describe tenth-century Śaiva scholar and practitioner Nārāyaṇakaṇṭha's warning that 'excessive practice' of prāṇāyāma may lead to laboured breathing, abdominal swelling, epilepsy and insanity (2017: 128); and Ahn describes psychological and physical symptoms of 'maladies of meditation' including depression, hallucinations, cold feet and ringing in the ears in East Asian Buddhist traditions (2017: 390–91; see also Pierce Salguero's forthcoming volume, *Meditation Sickness: A Sourcebook on the Dangers of Buddhist Practice*).
34. This refers to the protuberance at the crown of the head, frequently depicted on the historical Buddha, and understood to be the thirty-second of the thirty-two 'marks of the Buddha'.
35. The key Mahayana and Vajrayana Buddhist assertion that all phenomena are empty of intrinsic existence.
36. Tib. *rlung dben pa'i skyon bcos thabs kyi man ngag*. Authored by the Indian teacher Virūpa, and translated into Tibetan in the twelfth century, this particular text belongs to a corpus of commentaries focused on the *Cakrasaṃvara Tantra* (Marek and Oliphant 2017: 419).

37. In fact, DiValerio notes that Milarepa is not commonly referred to as a 'holy madman' in the same way as the Madmen of Ü and Tsang or Drukpa Künlé; however, '[t]he mythology of Milarepa has had a major impact on the way Tibetans today think about the holy madman phenomenon' (2015: 169).
38. In comparison, he said that he had seen 'more than thirty' people suffering from the illness of *nyoné* in his lifetime so far. Similarly, DiValerio reported a 'wide range of responses' from contemporary Tibetan religious specialists when asked about this: 'One lama stated that "holy madmen" are difficult to find, but as long as there is good meditative practice in the world, they will exist somewhere. One lama said that they surely do exist, but that they are very rare; they were easier to find in old Tibet' (2015: 9).
39. Tib. *guru tsen gyé*; these are the eight principal forms assumed by Padmasambhava at different points in his life.
40. It is important to note too the ways in which Trungpa's use of this term has been deployed to justify abuse within not only his organization, Shambala, but also within other Tibetan Buddhist organizations. For example, allegations of sexual abuse against Sogyal Rinpoche (1947–2019) – founder and former spiritual director of Rigpa, an international Tibetan Buddhist organization – have specifically described how he used the concept of 'crazy wisdom' to justify his behaviour in response to allegations of sexual abuse (https://www.lionsroar.com/wp-content/uploads/2017/07/Letter-to-Sogyal-Lakar-14-06-2017-.pdf, retrieved 1 May 2023; see also Gayley 2018: 179), and Gardener (2021) has asserted that '[m]uch of Trungpa's iconoclastic behavior – including his alcoholism, cruelty to animals, and sexual misconduct – was categorized by his community as "crazy wisdom"'. Gardner described how the '"crazy wisdom" label has been used by some in the Vajradhatu community to enable and perpetuate abuse, and to justify harm' (Ibid.); Langenberg has also described how Chögyam Trungpa used this concept to 'encourage a sexually liberal environment in which devotion to a charismatic guru, Tibetan Vajrayana philosophy, and the North American sexual revolution converged' – in this environment, Trungpa and several other teachers in his lineage 'are all alleged to have perpetrated sexual abuse in the Shambhala community' (2024: 105).
41. Indeed, the notion that the mind has 'great transformative power over matter' can be traced back to early Indian history, where Harvey describes a 'standard list of meditation-based "psychic powers"' in the Pali *suttas* (1993: 37).

Part II

SPIRIT

Chapter 4

Madness-Causing Spirits, Tantric Deities and 'Impurities' in Contemporary Amdo

> *I know of a woman with* nyoné. *She went to herd her animals, and then she slept on the mountain, and then after she came back she was* nyonpa . . . *It was a very powerful place – because of the mountain deity there.*
>
> —Nyima (31, Golok)

In Part I, we explored the role of *lung* and its role in mind-body structure and functioning. It became evident how wind – and its connections to mind and heart – is integral to Tibetan understandings of *nyoné*, in both medical and Tantric contexts. In this second part of the book, we will turn to look at the role of spirits and deities in the causation of *nyoné*. Here, in both everyday activities and Tantric practices, human–non-human interactions have the potential for both benefit and harm. Moreover, as we shall see, *lung* is again important here – the 'subtle' (Tib. *trawa*) nature of the body being key both to spirit afflictions and to Buddhist and Bon practices involving Tantric deities.

Moreover, we will encounter a different kind of practitioner here too, the *lhawa* – 'spirit-medium' – who becomes possessed by a deity in order to perform ritual healing activities. While I only met a few of these practitioners during my time in Amdo, their engagements with spirits and deities also form an essential part of a hierarchical structure of human–deity relations, where differential levels of spiritual 'power' between enlightened and unenlightened beings is key to understanding everyday life in many Tibetan communities. And, as we shall see in Chapter 6, a *lhawa*'s journey often begins with a period of 'madness' before their recognition as a spirit-medium.

In discussions about *nyoné* in Amdo, narratives of *dön né* – spirit affliction/illness – were common. While I encountered differing views over whether the most common cause of *nyoné* was heart illness or spirit illness, almost everyone I spoke to mentioned a case of spirit or deity affliction within either their family or their community. In Tibetan communities, spirit illness is another concept that spans the intertwining spheres of medicine and religion. For example, while 'madness-causing spirits' (Tib. *nyo jé gyi dön*) are described in Chapter 78 of the *Gyüshi* medical text's *Third Tantra* alongside other illness-causing spirits, in Amdo treatment for such conditions was most often described as the purview of ritual specialists rather than medical practitioners. Moreover, the notions of *tsa* and *lung* – so important in the functioning of mind-body, as we saw in Part I – are key here too, with spirits understood to be able to 'invade' an individual's mind-body through the subtle *lung*. In addition, many Amdo interviewees discussed notions of impurity/pollution. Commonly referred to by the term *drip*[1] in many Tibetan communities, in Amdo the term *mi tsangwa* – literally, 'unclean' – was more common among those I spoke to. Its relationship to *dön* appeared rather complex: understood in diverse ways by different people, as we shall see here.

In Amdo, local spirits and deities were often discussed under the general umbrella term '*dön*'. They were understood to vary in their ability to affect humans, as *ngakpa* and Tibetan medicine doctor Aku Wangchuk (72, Rebkong) explained: 'Just like us human beings – some people are very strong, some people are very weak – *dön* are the same: some *dön* are strong; some weak'. For example, low-level water spirits known as *lu* were described by interviewees as predominantly causing minor diseases, such as skin rashes, in people, but more powerful spirits and deities such as mountain deities or 'family gods' were implicated in more severe illnesses – including *nyoné* – and even death. These kinds of spirits and deities are generally understood by lay Tibetans and religious specialists to be *un*enlightened beings (Tib. *jiktenpé lha*); as likely to harm as to help humans, they should be dealt with cautiously. However, I also heard descriptions of *nyoné* related to enlightened Tantric deities, in the context of high-level 'deity yoga' (Tib. *lhé neljor*) practices that focus on *yidam* (tutelary deities). In this chapter, then, we will explore some of the often quite diverse narratives of spirit- and deity-related *nyoné* that I encountered in Amdo, alongside these related concepts of *drip* and *mi tsangwa*. Their place within the overlapping spheres of medicine and religion will start to become clear.

Spirit Affliction and Madness in Amdo

In Xining, Tibetan medicine professor Dr Pema (40) described *dön* as 'something outside your body – some *outside* force . . . some sentient beings who hurt you, take over or control your consciousness'. And among my interviewees in Amdo – medical and religious specialists as well as lay people – spirit illness/affliction (Tib. *dön né*) was described as a common cause of *nyoné* by many. For example, at the Qinghai Province Tibetan Medicine Hospital, Dr Tangun (50) told me that 'most' cases of *nyoné* are caused by *dön*, although he – like the other Tibetan medicine doctors I spoke to – reported seeing few cases himself. In fact, I was told that the founders of the Tibetan Medicine Hospital's Department for Wind Illnesses and Impurities had initially considered naming the department a *Dön Né* Department, but Dr Dechen (39) explained that there had been several concerns about this, including a worry that the notion of spirits or spirit illness 'may not be locally or culturally acceptable'.[2] She also explained how the founders had been aware that there was sometimes some stigma attached to *nyoné* and/or *dön né*, describing how some patients suffering from *nyoné* might feel embarrassed, preferring to say that they had some kind of other illness instead, and they might feel 'uncomfortable' going to a 'department for *dön*'.[3] Thus, the department's name (Lung Né Drip Tsen Khak – 'Department for Wind Illnesses and Impurities') – referring only to *lung* and *drip*, and leaving out reference to *dön* or *nyoné* – was chosen. In fact, the majority of Tibetan medicine doctors I spoke to in Amdo rarely saw patients with any kind of spirit illness anyway, with people frequently consulting religious specialists instead. It was almost exclusively those doctors who were also ritual specialists who described treating such patients. The various reasons for this will become clear as we explore the topic over the course of this chapter.

We might first want to consider the different kinds of spirits understood to make up the Tibetan pantheon, and which of these may be implicated in the causation of *nyoné*. In Rebkong, *ngakpa* Penpa (53) described 'uncountable' numbers of *dön* – 'many, many different ones' – with the 'most common' being the *gyalpo*.[4] In Xining, Tibetan medicine practitioner and Buddhist *ngakpa* Dr Sonam (69) described '360 kinds of *dön*', spanning 'three different levels', or realms: the upper realm, middle realm and lower realm. Tibetan medicine professor Dr Pema (40) explained that it is 'very hard to say' how many of the multiple *dön* that exist might cause *nyoné*, and Dr Rinchen (55) agreed, describing the 'many, many kinds of *dön* that can cause *nyoné*' and noting the two different systems of classification in Tibetan medicine, which describe either eighteen or fifteen kinds of *dön* involved in illness.

Within these discussions, I found that there was often a focus on entities known as *gyalpo* (also sometimes referred to as *gyal dön*) in Amdo narratives.

In Rebkong, for example, *ngakpa* Tsephal (55) told me that those afflicted by *gyalpo* 'often' become *nyoné*, and in Xining, Dr Rinchen (55) asserted, 'The *main dön* who causes madness is the *gyal dön* – this is the most common cause of madness'. However, I encountered differences of opinion about exactly *how* these *gyalpo* might affect humans – for example, while Dr Rinchen claimed that such spirits exclusively *possess* people (rather than causing harm from a distance, as some spirits/deities are understood to do), others disagreed, and in fact I heard multiple narratives of non-possession affliction involving *gyalpo* in Amdo. In addition, mountain deities such as *zhidak* were often mentioned too, with several people describing the dangers of inadvertently walking through their path or unknowingly sleeping in their territory when walking or herding in the mountains. In Rebkong, Gelugpa Geshe Dhondup (50) told me that problems related to such deities were 'quite common' among Tibetans who sleep on the mountain – as he explained: 'We don't always know where the path of one of these spirits is, and if you bump into them, then they will not necessarily harm you, but they *may*. This is quite common in Tibetan places – if you lie down in the spirit's way, and it bumps into you, then some parts of your body may become disabled'. Similarly, Dhondup (25, Labrang/Xining), told me that it was possible to became *nyoné* 'if you went up on the mountain for herding, and you fell asleep there'.[5]

In addition, in discussions of *nyoné* in Amdo, a number of people raised the topic of *shindré*. Sometimes used interchangeably with the term *dön* to refer to low-level spirits in general, this word is also often used to describe what we would term a 'ghost' in English – in other words, the 'spirit' of a person who has passed away. In Rebkong, Gelug lama Wangyal (62) explained that this can occur when someone dies, and their consciousness (Tib. *namshé*) enters the *bardo* (the intermediate state between death and rebirth) but becomes 'stuck' there. This situation was often explained in relation to a person having some kind of 'unfinished business' (for example, debts owed or grudges held) or 'attachment' to people or belongings – leading to their inability or unwillingness to pass successfully through the usual death-and-rebirth process. Samdrup (27, Ngawa/Xining), for example, told me that he thought this was 'common':

> When we die – when our breath stops – at that time, if a person has hatred or anger towards someone, or if he has unfinished things, or he is reluctant to leave this life, then maybe he doesn't want to go – then maybe he becomes a *shindré*, and comes back. When people die, you go through the *bardo*. And after this, you take another life. So if you don't want to take another life, then you become a *shindré*.

It became clear during my time in Amdo that while some people had quite particular ideas about the different spirits and the ways in which each might affect mind and/or body, there was a notable diversity across such explanations. In addition, others I spoke to discussed spirit afflictions in more general terms, telling me that they were less familiar with spirits overall. For example, Wangtso (34, Rebkong/Xining) asserted: 'If *we* [lay people] are talking about *dön*, *dré* and things like that, we don't know much about the differences [between them] . . . The lamas – *they* will know what's what!' However, I did encounter a general consensus about such entities' (in)visibility, with a majority of those I spoke to telling me that these kinds of spirits cannot be seen by ordinary people. For example, Nyingyal (33, Golok/Xining) told me that 'normal people' cannot see *dön* but that *some* Buddhist practitioners who 'have reached [a] really high level' of practice can see them. His classmate Migmar (30, Golok/Xining) agreed, telling me that while *zhidak* are invisible to humans, they can see each other. Similarly, Dr Chaksham (40, Trika/Xining) described how invisible entities exist, unseen, around us:

> There are some different kinds of beings that we cannot see – many different kinds of *dön* in the three realms: for example, in here – just in *this* building – there are three realms: human, animal and spirit. So right now, the other beings are seeing us, and listening to us – we cannot see them, but these kinds of beings can disturb others, for example, causing someone to become *nyoné*.

The doctor likened this to a mobile-phone signal – invisible but clearly evidenced by its functionality, telling me, 'We cannot see it [phone signal] – we cannot *prove* that it exists, but something powerful is there: because of that we can contact each other and send messages – there is something just subtle here'. Thus, the evidence for spirits and deities can be seen through their interventions in humans' lives rather than through any visibility of the entity itself – for example, a person (or even animal) becoming sick or otherwise afflicted in some way, which can be traced back to a particular spirit or deity. Much like the *lung* described in the previous chapters, it is understood that we do not need to *see* it to know that it is there – the fact that it 'exists' is evidenced by some sickness or dysfunction in the mind-body.

I spoke to *ngakpa* and doctor Aku Wangchuk (72) at length about these topics over lunch near his home in Rebkong one day. He laughed as he told me: 'If you want someone to show you a terrifying *dön*, it's not possible . . . If you want to *see* some [*dön*] – like in the movies – there are no *dön* like that . . . Humans' eyes cannot see *dön* – definitely not – and so the only way to know [they are there] is from the behaviour [of the patient]'. However, he continued, there is in fact a small group of people who *can* see spirits: as Nyingyal had also told me, Aku Wangchuk too asserted that some religious practitioners who have reached high levels of Tantric practice, and have attained certain yogic accomplishments (Tib. *ngödrup*; Skt. *siddhi*), have this ability. As he explained: 'If you say that you can *never* see *dön*, that is also not the right answer . . . If you are [a] Buddhist [practitioner], and you meditate, you can reach different levels [of attainment]: first level . . . second level . . . third . . . fourth . . . If you get to the first level, then maybe you can see *dön*'.[6] In Chabcha, yogi Lodro (42) agreed, telling me, 'There are *many* things which are invisible to ordinary humans, but once you become realized, or you have knowledge, then it is possible to see them – [entities such as] *dön*, *lha*, etc.'

With the majority of people said to be unable to see spirits and deities, then, it is often initially through the display of particular symptoms that a spirit/deity affliction is suspected, with a more definitive diagnosis often made later through procedures such as divination (see below). However, the symptoms of spirit and deity afflictions described in Amdo were quite diverse – with one particular spirit often described as affecting different people in different ways, and entities viewed as 'very common' by some interviewees but seemingly completely unknown to others.

Some narratives of possession described a spirit 'taking over' the mind (Tib. *sem*) or consciousness (Tib. *namshé*) of the afflicted individual, as Buddhist Studies student Migmar (30, Golok/Xining), described: 'When a *dön* or *lha* attacks you, the *namshé* will be controlled by something else – [something] that is not part of you. Therefore at that time, in your body there are two *namshé*, and *your namshé* is weaker than the *namshé* of the *dön* or *lha*. So then it will cause problems'. In Rebkong, Bon lama Tsering (57) explained how a spirit might 'steal your memory, or steal your voice'. When a spirit steals your memory, he explained, then you will no longer be thinking or acting according to your own will – instead, you will behave differently 'because you have no memory [of your own] whatsoever, of yourself or your family'. Similarly, if such an entity steals your voice, 'then perhaps you go on the street and meet a stranger, and say all kinds of nonsense, and others can't understand what you're talking about'. Sometimes, he added, an afflicted person may also be verbally aggressive towards others with no apparent reason. With their behaviour inexplicable to observers, such people, he explained, 'are called "*nyönpa*"'. Nyingma lama Namgyal (32, Chabcha) also described how a spirit affliction can affect the consciousness: 'There are many different symptoms [of *dön né*], but mostly, a lot of patients have problems with their memory, and this affects their *sem*, because their *sem* is not calm – it is conflicted, as if there is an inner fighting going on, causing the mind to go astray'.

In fact, interviewees described different ways in which spirit affliction may affect the various senses. At the Qinhai Province Tibetan Medicine Hospital in Xining, Dr Chaksham (40) told me that some of those afflicted by *dön* might 'see strange colours or something' – 'The doctor cannot see [this], but just the *nyönpa* can see it'. This, he explained, is due to 'the mix' of the spirit's and the person's consciousness, leading the afflicted individual to see and say 'many different things'. Similarly, Dr Dechen (39, Rebkong/Xining) described how patients suffering from *nyoné* caused by *dön* 'can often see and hear things that normal people cannot see and hear'.

In cases of *dré* – 'ghost' – possession, I was told that the cause was usually obvious from the symptoms, with an afflicted individual often talking in someone else's voice – perhaps talking about that person's (unfinished) personal business. For example, several Amdo-wa described afflicted individuals suddenly speaking in the voice of a relative or neighbour who had recently passed away, clearly indicating the possession. Among them, Khandro (22) related a case from her home town in Tsolho: 'I'll tell you a real story that happened in my village. There was an old man, and he got some illness and then died. His family had a little son – aged nine or ten – and then after that old man died, the little boy spoke with the old man's voice . . . The villagers said it's a *dön*'. Similarly, Migmar (30, Golok/Xining) described the case of a 'greedy' man in his home town who had passed away:

> He didn't want to leave behind his belongings – he was attached to them – and so he became a *dré* . . . But he had lent a lot of money to other people, so a lot of the people who had borrowed money from him just kept it secret after he passed away – they didn't mention that they needed to pay it back to his family or anything . . . A girl nearby became *nyoné*, but actually he had possessed her, so then the girl's way of talking, and her behaviour – everything was like that man . . . Then that girl mentioned all the people's names who owed him money. So in this case, there were two *namshé* inside that girl.

As we hear, in many cases of suspected spirit affliction the cause was seen to be evident from the symptoms; here, for example, many people in the community recognized that the deceased man was speaking through the young girl. In such cases, an afflicted individual might initially be labelled '*nyoné*' before this kind of possession is ascertained instead. This was thus a little different from the kind of *nyoné* caused by spirits described above, where some kind of low-level local spirit or deity (rather than the spirit of a recently deceased person) was understood to be involved.

How common is *nyoné* caused by spirits understood to be? Of course, it is hard to ascertain this in any real terms, but narratives of *dön né* of various kinds were quite common among those I spoke to in Amdo – and all of my interviewees discussed *dön* and *lha* as potential causative factors of *nyoné*. Some narratives of spirit and deity afflictions also referenced key Tibetan notions of 'strength' or 'spiritual power' (Tib. *wang tang*), which we will explore in some detail in the following chapters. For example, former Buddhist monk Tsetan (38, Rebkong) explained that it was 'more common' for lay people to be affected by spirits than it was for religious specialists 'because for the monks or religious people, they conduct a lot of Buddhist

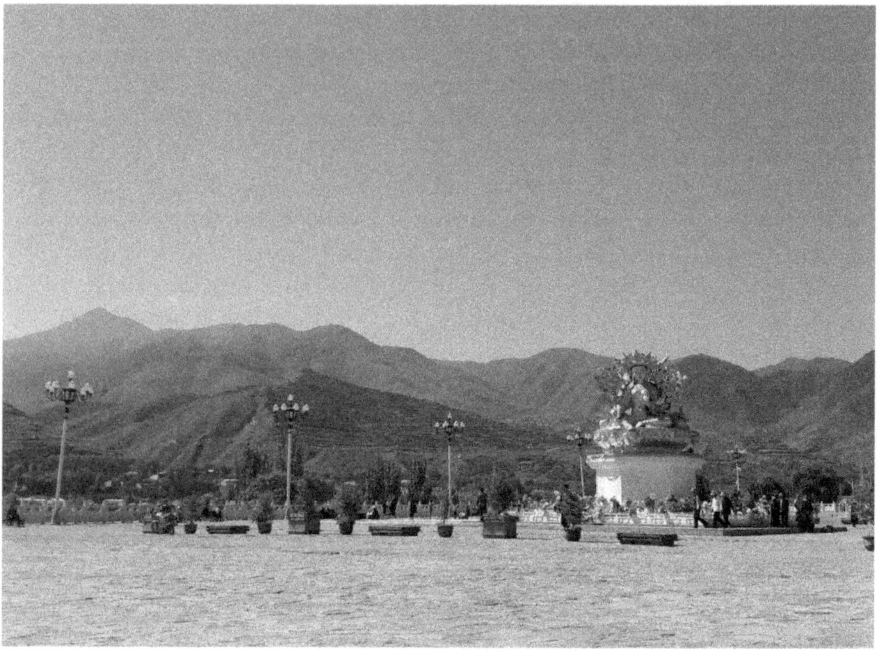

Figure 4.1. Tibetans doing *kora* outside Rongwo Monastery, 2018. © Susannah Deane.

practice' – and it is through these practices that they will have more of this spiritual power. Following this line of reasoning, he added that among lay people, those 'who often practise religious activities' (such as reciting prayers, doing *kora* [e.g. see Figure 4.1] or receiving blessings from lamas) are 'less likely to be affected by spirits'.[7] However, at his monastery in Rebkong, Geshe Dhondup (50) took a different view, telling me that among the monks in the monastery, 'the most common cause of *nyoné* is via the causes from outside, such as spirits – this is the same as for lay people'. He concluded, 'it's not very common but it happens'.

Mi Tsangwa: Impurity and Illness in Amdo

Notable in Amdo were discussions on '*mi tsangwa*', referring to notions of impurity or pollution linked to a number of afflictions including, in some cases, *nyoné*. Sometimes *mi tsangwa* was equated with *drip*, a concept I was more familiar with from my previous research in Darjeeling (Deane 2014b), where people described becoming affected by *drip* from dead bodies (for example, at a cremation ground or a butcher's shop) or wearing someone else's clothes after they had died. For example, Khandro (22, Tsolho/Xining) described how an elderly man in her home town had become *nyoné* as a result of touching an old human skull that he had picked up at a graveyard. She referred to both '*mi tsangwa*' and '*drip*' in her explanation, telling me that neither medicine nor Buddhist rituals performed by lamas had been able to treat her neighbour successfully.

At other times, this concept was explained quite differently, with some descriptions focusing on *mi tsangwa* being 'carried' on objects (such as a bowl, cup or scarf) taken from one house to another, and related to notions of *dön* and/or *lha*. In Rebkong, Norbu (30), for example, told me, in a mix of English and Tibetan, '*Mi tsangwa* is a kind of *dön* – it is one of the *dön*' – i.e. it is a kind of spirit. In addition, *mi tsangwa* was also discussed in cases of *nyoné* (and other conditions) attributed to problematic relationships between two families' differing connections to deities – a kind of 'clash' between different families' traditions. And sometimes *mi tsangwa* was referred to quite generally in lay narratives of *nyoné*, where my questions about specifics led to respondents reflecting that they were not really clear on how or why it occurred. The complex and overlapping nature of these diverse understandings is well illustrated by the following explanation from Lhakpa (38, Golok/Xining), when I asked her about *mi tsangwa*:

> In *our* hometown, if we wear another person's jacket and get some sickness – we say it's *dön* . . . But then if we ask the lama to check out what the problem is, then he will say [it is] 'clothes *drip*' – *drip* from clothes. That is the way the lama will say it, but we [lay people] just say *dön tang zik* ['got *dön*'] . . . He [a doctor we are also talking with] says *dön* is some bad things – it harms your body or something – it attacks you . . . [But] *drip* also attacks you, right?

Similarly, Gabzang (27, Golok/Xining), an English teacher who had helped me with some translation, talked about '*dön*' when I asked him about *mi tsangwa*: 'Maybe *mi tsangwa* is like a spirit . . . It can move [around] . . . but usually *dön* is when we get something from someone else – for example, a cup or something – then you can see that *thing*, but we can't see the thing that is *harming* that person. So we can't see it, but it is moving around'. In Rebkong, former monk Tsetan (38) explained some of these 'misunderstandings' among lay people, from his point of view:

> It is a little bit of a misunderstanding, because people say it's *mi tsangwa* but actually it's caused by *dön* or *dré* or a family deity. So, for example, if a family has faith in a certain deity, and another person takes something from this family,[8] then the family deity may be upset or angry, and so it [the deity] goes to the other family to harm them . . . This kind of *nyoné* or illness sometimes comes as very bad dreams – all caused by that particular deity . . . Usually a lama needs to do a divination to find out the cause. If the lama determines

> that there is some kind of object [involved], he will tell the family the colour or shape of it, and then the family need to find that object and throw it away.

Samdrup (27, Ngawa/Xining) told me that a relative of his had been affected by this, demonstrating his perspective on two slightly different meanings of the word '*dön*':

> Around 2003, one of my uncles had *nyoné* . . . The *ngakpa* said to my uncle, 'A woman gave you something, and then you took that thing, which caused this *nyoné* . . . We call this '*dön tang zik*' ['got *dön*'] . . . It's not *that dön* [i.e. a spirit, as was discussed above] – it's a verb, not a noun . . . it's the same word, but here it means a verb – [for example,] *dön tang zik . . . dön song zik* ['got *dön*'] . . . It means something more like *drip* . . . We say that this family are not good, because they are not good people . . . They are Buddhist, but they are *mi tsangwa* . . . This family is very bad, and so we can't take anything – [for example,] any food – from them. They are *mi tsangwa*.

Having encountered such a variety of descriptions, I asked two Tibetan medicine doctors about this. Dr Chaksham (40, Trika/Xining) explained in a mix of English and Tibetan: '*Dön* and *drip* are a little bit different. *Drip* is like pollution – not clean . . . [But for example,] *lu dön* is *naga* [water spirits] . . . *Naga* is not pollution – it's not human, but it's a *sem can* – a living being . . . *Drip* is not a living being. That's my understanding'. In contrast, Dr Nyima (38, Rebkong/Xining) – also fluent in English – explained *mi tsangwa* simply as a term for the *process* by which a spirit (*dön*) may travel with an object, causing harm to the person who has taken it away from its usual home: '*Mi tsangwa* is *dön* – a *dön* has come with the bowl, cup or other object [from someone's house] because it thinks it belongs to him'. Nyima also took me to meet one of his teachers, *ngakpa* and doctor Aku Wangchuk (72), who gave a similar explanation:

> Usually *drip* is *dön* . . . When you say '*drip*', this is a particular way of harming the body – by *dön* . . . So *drip* is a part of *dön* . . . Many people say that when you say '*drip*', it's some particular kinds of symptoms – for example, the person cannot see, cannot hear, or your tongue not working – you can't speak, or can't speak very well. All these kinds of things are called *drip* . . . it's a particular way to harm the body by *dön*, so in that case, the cause should still be regarded as *dön*.

It was evident from these discussions that there is significant diversity in how the notion of *mi tsangwa* is understood by different people, with some definitively equating it with spirit entities and others seeing it as a separate mechanism/process by which someone might become harmed in various ways. And for many people – as is often the case – such understandings had been inherited from older relatives or other members of the community, and it was perhaps only upon being asked to explain them in more detail by an outsider that they reflected that they were not entirely sure what was meant by it.[9] Moreover, my guess is that there are probably some significant regional differences here, but further research focused on larger numbers of people from diverse geographical areas would be needed to draw any clear conclusions on this.

And finally, some of my interviewees also drew links between *mi tsangwa* and astrology, the elements and the four directions. For example, I met Dr Samphel (72), a retired Tibetan medicine practitioner from Haixi, while he was visiting family in Xining. Similarly to others' explanations about *mi tsangwa*, he also asserted that bringing something from 'outside' the family/ house into your house 'may cause someone from the family to become *nyoné*'. However, he also related this to the 'time of day' and the '*kar ma*' (stars/astrology).[10] He used the example of 'a picture of a lama' – something which is usually 'auspicious'. However, he asserted, 'If it was brought inside the house at the wrong time, that object changes to being a *negative* thing for you'. This 'timing', he explained, was related to 'the person, the [astrological] time, and the direction': in certain configurations, these can have negative consequences – 'then harms can happen'. Other interviewees too described the possible consequences of such confluences – including, but not limited to, *nyoné*. For example, Gabzang (27, Golok/Xining) described several reasons that someone could get *nöpa* [harm] from an object:

> Maybe they took that thing at the wrong time, according to the five elements . . . or maybe it is related to the protective deity [Tib. *sung ma*] which that person [who gave you the object] or their family is worshiping – if that deity is very strong. It won't *necessarily* cause you *nyoné* – maybe you will just get sick, or maybe your family will get sick, or maybe you will have some kind of accident or something like that.

As we can see, key to some of these discussions about *drip* and *mi tsangwa* is the issue of people's differing 'connections' (Tib. *drelwa*) to different deities, potentially leading to problems – including cases of *nyoné*. This was evident, for example, in Tsetan's explanation (above) of a person from one family giving an object to someone from another family/household, thereby inadvertently upsetting a family deity (Tib. *khyim lha*) in the process. Rinchen (26, Rebkong/Xining) also brought up the notion of problems arising from simply wearing clothes from another person – again, linking it to different personal or family gods via the notion of *drip*: 'If your *lü lha* [personal deity] or *khyim lha* [family deity] is different from mine, and I wear your clothes or your hat, *then* I will get *nyoné*, or get some sickness . . . [This is] related to *drip*'.

This was also discussed in relation to romantic relationships, where one person had a connection to a deity unfamiliar to their partner or there was a 'clash' between their different family gods, potentially leading to problems. Rinchen told me, 'For example, if we were partners, but your family god and my family god were different, and then we got married, if we had a baby – that child would be *nyoné*'. Similarly, Dolma (22, Rebkong/Xining) described the importance of *tenpa* (trust/dependency) in relation to different deities, telling me, 'For example, if you want to marry someone, and they rely on different gods, maybe you'll have problems – for example, become *nyoné*'.

In fact, not long after hearing this explanation from Rinchen about the potential problems within romantic relationships, I encountered a corresponding narrative from someone I knew quite well. Norbu (30, Rebkong) had acted as a translator for me when we had been to interview a Rebkong *ngakpa*. Meeting again over coffee in town a few weeks later, he told me that after we had been discussing *nyoné* at length – both in the interview and during our more informal chats about my research – he had suddenly thought about what had occurred in his own family several years previously, and he thought I might be interested to hear about it. Thus, he described his father's period of *nyoné* and subsequent recovery:

> My father suffered something like *nyoné* three years ago . . . His behaviour was *really* strange . . . Suddenly, he was not a normal man . . . He had strong reactions – he damaged things, destroyed windows, and beat a person, saying strange things . . . He was out of control. I was asking him, 'What are you talking about?', but he said, 'I don't know what I am talking about'.
>
> We went to see a doctor – a Chinese [biomedical] doctor – they did body checks; scans of the body, and of the brain, but the doctor said he couldn't find anything . . . Then we just consulted a lama, and he said that maybe my father was possessed by something – but he said, 'There is something wrong, but I can't cure it' . . . At Rongwo monastery, and at another place . . . every place we went – many places . . . Finally, we invited a Nyingma *ngakpa* to our house, and he said, 'I can treat him'. He brought a dog's head and buried it in the ground at the house, and he chanted scriptures for three days, and my father gradually became okay . . . And I thought, Wow, what was this? There was a suspicion – because my girlfriend [at that time] believed [in] *gyalpo*, and the lama who did the divination had said he *thought* that my father was affected by *gyalpo*. And I thought about this for a *long* time . . . This is why I broke up with my girlfriend . . . Because that lama said my father was affected by *gyalpo*, I suspected this for a long time . . . I asked her [my girlfriend] 'What do you believe?' She said, 'I believe [in] *gyalpo*'. Wow – then I realized, OK this is the problem . . . And then I broke up [with her] immediately, and I went back to my hometown, and after we broke up, my father became a normal man immediately – *that* year, my father *really* returned to normal – he recovered

> from that . . . In that girlfriend's village [in the Kham area], they really believe [in] *gyalpo* . . . And [because she was] connected to me – it affected my father.

Here it was Norbu's connection to his girlfriend – whose family had a relationship with a particular *gyalpo* deity (which Norbu and his family had no connection to) – that was understood to have led to his father's *nyoné*. This causative factor had been ascertained through divination, and then apparently evidenced by the fact that Norbu's father had only recovered fully once that 'connection' between the families had been broken by the ending of the relationship. Due to this kind of potential problem, Norbu explained, when a couple plans to marry, there is in fact a Tibetan custom: 'We ask [each other] what we believe at first, and then we decide whether we can marry or not'. If the couple discover that they 'believe [in] different gods', or if one half of the couple has a connection to 'a kind of dangerous god', then, he said, they cannot marry. Subsequently, he told me, when he had initially met his next girlfriend (by this point, his wife), he had asked her 'What do you believe [in]?', discovering that – thankfully – 'we believe [in] the same – the same god'.

I heard this kind of explanation several times during my time in Amdo, and it was often linked to a couple who hailed from different geographical areas.[11] However, I also met several couples in just this situation who mentioned no such issues. Indeed, when I discussed *drip*/*mi tsangwa* with a Tibetan friend and some of her colleagues from Golok, they too brought up the notion of *drip* caused by two people from different areas embarking on a romantic relationship or marrying . . . However, with one married couple present hailing from two places very far apart – and so 'for sure our families are worshipping different protective deities [Tib. *sung ma*]' – this prompted a discussion about why, then, they had not encountered any problems. The friends concluded that perhaps if a couple stay together a longer time, then finally it's 'okay' – wondering aloud whether maybe, over time, the protective deity might 'get used to' the situation.

Lung and *Dön*: Afflicting Humans through Subtle Energy

In Part I, we explored the notion of *lung* and the other facets of the 'subtle body' at some length. Now, examining the role of spirits in human health and illness, we again find it relevant – the 'subtle' nature of both *lung* and *dön* being key to spirits' ability to affect humans. In Xining, Dr Nyima (38) explained to me that while *dön* are understood to be 'living beings' like humans, *unlike* humans they do not have a gross/material body – only a subtle body, a '*lung* body'. It is because of this subtle nature, he said, that a spirit is able to 'easily' connect to the *lung* within a human's body – particularly the *sok lung* – and thus take over control of his/her mind-body. The afflicted individual may then be aware that his/her behaviour is bad or strange, but will be unable to control him/herself; or, perhaps the person cannot understand what he/she is doing, with the *dön* now 'controlling the mind through the *lung*'. Dr Nyima likened *dön* to an army of soldiers, and *lung* to their weapons: the *dön*, he explained, 'use *lung*' to control the afflicted human.

With this in mind, Dr Nyima stressed to me that in order to understand *nyoné* and *dön né*, people need to have some knowledge of Tibetan Buddhism: 'For most doctors, *dön* is the most difficult part – because it's related to Buddhism . . . and also not only the *basic* Buddhist concepts. So in order to understand *dön né*, you have to understand *küntak* [conceptual phenomena]'.[12] Keen to provide a more comprehensive explanation, Dr Nyima took me to interview Aku Wangchuk (72), a *ngakpa* and Tibetan medicine doctor, under whom he had studied about such topics. Aku Wangchuk explained:

> First, the *dön* will kind of catch or locate the subtle *lung* [Tib. *lung trawa*] . . . and then it controls the consciousness a little – maybe [the person experiences] hearing problems, or can see some different things – see strangely, or hear strangely . . . Then slowly, slowly the *dön* can control the whole body and all *lung*, and the base consciousness (Tib. *kün zhi nam pa shé pa*). Then [the person becomes] totally *nyönpa*.

In fact, *lung* is not the only energy that can be related to *dön*; *tripa* and *béken* may be involved in spirit affliction too – depending on the type of spirit involved. Here, we find the notion of three 'levels' of spirits, briefly mentioned at the beginning of this chapter. Dr Nyima (38) explained: 'We usually say "upper", "middle" and "lower" *dön*. This is related to the location of *dön* – to their location in the universe,[13] and also in relation to your body – *lung*, *tripa*, and *béken*'. Aku Wangchuk explained this for us in more detail, asserting that a comprehensive understanding of the *nyépa* was necessary if I was to research spirit illness as, according to Tibetan medical theory, there is a connection between the three *nyépa* and the three types of *dön*:

> Some *dön* can connect with the *lung*, or *tripa*, or *béken*, and so because of these three different *nyépa*, we have *teng* [upper] *dön*, *bar* [middle] *dön* and *ok* [lower] *dön* – three different [types of] *dön*. If a sickness involves *dön*, then these three *nyépa* are connected to *teng dön*, *bar dön* and *ok dön* . . . Without *lung*, *tripa*, or *béken*, *dön* cannot harm the body – they use *lung*, *tripa* or *béken* to harm the person – these can be the tools or 'weapon' of the *teng dön*, *bar dön* and *ok dön* . . .
>
> Usually we say that there are three hundred and sixty *dön*, but not all of these cause *nyoné* – *mainly*, we would say it's *teng dön* which cause *lung*

> disorder, and then cause *nyoné*. However, sometimes *bar dön* or *ok dön* can also cause *nyoné*, so it depends – you cannot say how many kinds or, [for example,] only this one particular *dön* can cause *nyoné*.
>
> When we talk of *teng dön*, *bar dön* and *ok dön*, and these are the outside of the body, these are upper, middle and lower [*dön*]. But the inside of the body is different – in relation to the location of the three *nyépa*, usually we say that *béken* is in the upper part [of the body], and *lung* is in the lower part, and *tripa* is in the middle. But that is in a normal body, when you are *healthy*. But when there is disorder, it is disrupted, and so it is different, and that means that usually, if *teng dön* causes a *lung* disorder, for example, then it is harmful for the head and brain, and *tsa* [channels]. The *tsa* control the body, and that's why [they] can affect the whole body, or [only] part of the body, and lead to different symptoms.

I asked Aku Wangchuk if it is possible for *dön* to affect any one of the five main *lung* described in Chapter 2. Indeed, he explained – '*dön* use all five types of *lung*', depending on the particular kind of spirit involved: 'Just like us [humans] – some people like to eat meat, some people like to eat vegetables, right? So it depends – *dön* can use all five *lung*, but it depends on what *dön* it is, and what it can connect to'.

Upsetting the Gods: Working with Spirits and Deities in Tantric Practice

In the narratives described so far, all of the spirits and deities involved in the causation of *nyoné* and other illnesses are 'worldly' deities – i.e. *un*enlightened gods (Tib. *jiktenpé lha*).[14] This means that they are subject to 'worldly' emotions in the same way that humans are – with the potential to become upset, angry or offended by any human behaviour affecting them, whether intentional or not. Hence, we hear stories of people becoming ill after inadvertently 'bumping into' a mountain god that they could not see on the mountain path, or after chopping down a tree in which an unseen deity was residing. At the other end of the Tibetan pantheon are the Buddhist and Bon Tantric deities – *enlightened* gods who are not subject to such worldly emotions, but who may have both peaceful and wrathful aspects. It is these kinds of deities, known as *yidam* – tutelary deities – with whom Buddhist and Bon Tantric practitioners work in so-called 'deity yoga' practices. These practices form the 'generation stage' (Tib. *kyé rim*) of the high level *Anuttarayoga Tantras* in the New (Sarma) Tantra traditions (i.e. the Gelug, Kagyu and Sakya traditions); the *Mahāyoga Tantras* in the Old (Nyingma) Tantra traditions; and the eighth of the Nine Vehicles of Bon, during which a practitioner works towards evoking an enlightened Tantric deity within him/herself.

Such deities are understood to be very powerful – they are enlightened, after all – and, therefore, much like the *tsa lung* practices discussed in the previous chapter, these are understood to be complex, high-level practices, with initiation from a teacher being imperative and a potential for severe consequences if performed incorrectly. In Amdo, some of my interviewees spoke about these practices in relation to *nyoné*, again describing problems caused by Tantric practices 'gone wrong' – in this case, in relation to engaging with spirits and deities through practice. For example, Rinchen (26, Rebkong/Xining) told me, in a mix of English and Tibetan: 'If a lama gives his student permission to read a text about the high level *ngak* [mantra/incantations], and then he reads this but he does some *ngak* incorrectly, then the *yidam* will get angry . . . then maybe he [the student] will become crazy'. Former Buddhist monk Tsetan (38) explained in a little more detail:

> With practices involving the *yidam*, problems can be caused by incomplete practice. For example, if you forget some steps in the practice, or if you [mistakenly] add something new, the *yidam* may become angry . . . Also for this kind of practice, the practitioner needs to be ready to do the practice . . . It's true, the *yidam* may become angry and harm the practitioner [if something is conducted incorrectly]. So these kinds of rituals must be done step by step; if you miss a step . . . if you misuse or misplace the steps, then the *yidam* may become angry. But at the end of the ritual, there is always a section of the text asking for forgiveness, so at the end of the ritual, you must read the text asking for his forgiveness.

Again, then, we hear about the importance of a good foundational knowledge and skill for conducting these higher-level Tantric practices, just as was described in Chapters 1 and 3 in relation to the *tsa lung* practices. But why might an enlightened Tantric deity harm a practitioner? Not subject to worldly emotions, should he/she, in fact, feel anger or desire retribution for any wrongs committed? We return, therefore, to the concept of *namtok*, and the potential for the practitioner's own mind to create problems – particularly in relation to some of the intense sensations and experiences understood to occur during practice. For example, Buddhist Studies student Migmar (30, Golok/Xining) discussed how a practitioner might find some of the intense sensations during practices 'confusing' if they were not properly prepared: 'The *yidam* is enlightened, and so for example, if someone is practising Yamāntaka[15] meditation . . . maybe all kinds of images of this buddha will arise – maybe, maybe not. If the practitioner gets confused by this, then this can cause a problem'. Moreover, Migmar continued, if a practitioner experiences difficulty with certain parts of such practice – for example, struggling to connect the visualized deity to their own buddha-nature, then the wisdom and compassion cannot connect together – and then 'that might cause *nyönpa*, or cause the practitioner to become abnormal or something'. Further, any arrogance or pride in a practitioner's abilities as he/she works with a deity may cause problems, as he described: 'There are some practitioners who are arrogant, and they say "I am the same as Yamāntaka!", or they don't go to consult their teacher for help – those practitioners' condition will get worse'. We see again, then, the importance of conducting these high-level Tantric practices very carefully – for example, being adequately prepared for any unusual or intense experiences that may arise during practice, and not becoming arrogant in one's own Tantric abilities.

Chöd

And finally, we will briefly explore the well-known practice of *chöd*, during which Tantric practitioners work with *un*enlightened spirits and deities. Here, we are told that careful management of the non-human entities involved is key to successful and safe practice – and in Amdo, problems with this were also described as a potential cause of *nyoné*. This practice involves the practitioner visualizing the dismemberment of their body and the invitation of spirits to feast upon it. Buddhist Studies student Migmar (30, Golok/Xining) speculated how this practice might also cause problems for the practitioner, with the assertion that, again, it is the practitioner's own fears that can be key here. This was well illustrated by our experience as we sat discussing spirits and deities with some of his friends over tea. At one point, as one of the group told us a story about a *dré* one of the curtains in the window next to us moved, startling one of the group especially. Shortly after, Migmar explained how this kind of experience could impact on a practitioner conducting *chöd*:

> When someone is performing *chöd* practice, if it goes wrong, and they become scared by something, then they may become *nyonpa*. It's like that curtain – when we were talking about *dré*, and the curtain moved, you were afraid. It's like this – while you are conducting *chöd* practice, if *dön* or *dré* are near you, and you are saying, 'I am offering my body to those beings', if you get scared by something, then maybe you will be *really* scared, and this may cause problems.

In Amdo, I heard often that Tantric practices that involve *intentional* engagements with both enlightened and unenlightened spirits and deities have the potential to lead to problems, including *nyoné*. For some, the explanation lay in the motivations and behaviours of those non-human entities involved; for others, any problems clearly lay in the mind of the practitioner. We will explore these phenomena in more detail in Chapter 6, where we will again find the notion of *namtok* relevant, alongside key concepts of 'spiritual power' – as we mentioned above.

Diagnosis and Treatment for Spirit and Deity Afflictions

We have seen above that particular symptoms (for example, a very sudden change in a person's behaviour) were often taken as a clear indication of *dön* involvement – but equally, I heard several narratives of people consulting a variety of practitioners before getting a diagnosis and/or treatment of spirit affliction. Dr Dechen (39) described some examples from her experience working in the hospital:

> One case was a Tibetan patient who could speak Chinese fluently, but according to their relatives, they had never spoken Chinese before – so it's obvious that it is caused by a *dön* . . . With symptoms such as hearing or seeing things that are not there, it can be hard to tell, but for those patients who speak in a different way, it's generally clear that they are affected by a *dön*.

Aku Wangchuk (72, Rebkong), suggested that a variety of Tibetan medical diagnostic tools could be used in combination in cases of suspected *don né*: 'Mainly you can definitely read the pulse, and also the behaviour of the patient, and also questioning [the patient] . . . You use all of these diagnostic methods together – then it should be clear'.[16] However, several doctors discussed the difficulties of diagnosing these kinds of illnesses in reality, and, as I mentioned above, the majority of Tibetan medicine doctors I interviewed in Amdo described rarely – if ever – actually seeing such patients.

Moreover, as we heard in some of these Amdo narratives, several of the people I spoke to described utilizing biomedical testing for some cases of *nyoné*. Here, a lack of positive results was often taken as indicative of *dön* involvement – a process of elimination through testing, which leaves *dön* (or perhaps *mi tsangwa*) as the only possible explanation. As Nyingyal (33, Golok/Xining) explained: 'If a case of *nyoné* is caused by *dön*, and you go to the hospital for tests, you can't see anything from those kinds of machines. But if it's caused by *disease*, then there is a result from those kinds of tests – for example, maybe *this* is wrong, or *that* is wrong'.

This multifaceted process of meaning-making in the face of illness probably reflects longstanding notions of spirit afflictions more broadly, wherein diagnosis often comes through *absence* – absence of any other clear explanation, where often a patient has worked through multiple other potential explanatory frameworks and treatment modalities, and yet remains unwell. This, of course, is something we also see in relation to a whole variety of illnesses. For example, Norbang (21, Golok/Xining) described the case of a relative of his who had been ill with unidentified pains down one side of his torso with no apparent cause: 'First we took him to the Chinese [biomedical] hospital, and they checked him out, but everything was ok – all the tests were clear. So we thought maybe it was something like *mi tsangwa*, and so we went to see a *lhawa* [spirit-medium]'.[17]

Buddhist and Bon ritual specialists, of course, diagnose conditions quite differently, with some in Amdo describing diagnosis of *dön né* and *nyoné* through divination (Tib. *mo*) or astrology (Tib. *tsi*). Gelugpa lama Wangyal (62), for example, asserted that 'usually' a lama is able to successfully ascertain the cause of an individual's *nyoné* through divination, and Aku Wangchuk told me that once you have ascertained a *dön né*, 'if you want to know what kind of *dön* it is, then you can use divination'.

In terms of the treatment of *nyoné* caused by spirits, those I spoke to in Amdo generally described medical treatments as likely unhelpful for treating these kinds of cases. Several interviewees were surprised when I asked about their thoughts on treatments available at the various Amdo hospitals for *nyoné*, telling me that medical treatments (either biomedical or Tibetan medicine) are irrelevant for this kind of illness. As Dawa (30, Trika/Xining) said, 'If it's the kind of *nyoné* that relates to your *sem kham* [psychology] or being affected by a *dré*, *dön*, or *nyen* [type of spirit/mountain deity], then what can be done for you at the hospital?'. However, he conceded, 'If you have something related to your brain – if you have *this* type of *nyoné* – then it probably makes sense to go to the hospital'. Responses from other lay interviewees were similar. For example, Wangtso (34, Xining/Rebkong) told me, 'If someone is affected by those kinds of spirits, it's better to consult a lama or *ngakpa* – normally there is no medicine for such things', and Khandro (22, Tsolho/Xining) agreed: 'When someone gets some *drip*, or gets some *dön*, I think it's better to see a lama, because lamas have many methods to deal with these . . . But I think illness is a little bit different . . . For instance, stomach ache – then it's better to see the doctor'.[18]

Amdo doctors I spoke to also stressed the importance of ritual interventions here – used either alone, or in conjunction with medicines and/or external therapies – often explaining that they themselves were not so familiar with this aspect of treatment. For example, when I asked Dr Chaksham (40, Trika/Xining) about the treatment of *dön*-related *nyoné*, he answered:

> This is a little bit complicated to answer. Why? Because in the *Gyüshi* you know there are a *few ngak* [mantra/incantations], and some diseases are [related to] *dön*. [But] in the *Buddhist* texts there is a lot about that . . . The monks have good explanations . . . They tell us to do the *ngak*: *ngak* first, and then medicine. If you do the medicine first, it's not going to help the disease. So first you need to do the *ngak* to control the *dön* – or remove the *dön* from the body. *Then* you give the medicine as well – to cure it.

Similarly, Dr Rinchen (55, Xining) told me that *nyoné* related to *dön* 'cannot be treated only with medicines – medicines alone cannot deal with those kinds of problems . . . The real cause of madness is just *dön*, right? So we should go to a lama, and [they will] do ritual'. However, with a variety of practitioners performing diverse ritual treatments for such conditions, Dr Nyima (38, Rebkong/Xining) stressed to me the importance of consulting a trusted practitioner. In Xining, with few Buddhist, and no Bon, monasteries and temples – and therefore few ritual specialists residing there much of the time – this often meant consulting a lama or *ngakpa* in a patient's home town, as Dr Nyima explained:

> If it's really *dön né*, then ritual healing is definitely more powerful and has more benefits . . . Some doctors send patients to receive ritual healing . . . Usually people will go back to their hometown [for this] – that is easier and convenient for them . . . they can find some *ngakpa* or some very specialist monks . . . Usually, people decide by themselves [which ritual specialist to consult], because it's related to religion. So if the person is Nyingmapa, they will go to a Nyingma practitioner or, if they are Gelugpa, then they maybe will go to a Gelugpa one – it depends . . . [Also] it depends on how skilful the particular lama, *lhawa* or *ngakpa* is.

Dr Nyima noted the often pragmatic nature of health-seeking behaviour, describing many patients' concurrent consultation of both ritual and medical practitioners. However, he also suggested that there might be some other factors at play in patients' and their families' choice of treatment(s) – related to the potential stigma of such conditions, which he said may be viewed as 'kind of embarrassing'. This, he explained, might prevent afflicted individuals from visiting a doctor or hospital, which are rather 'public' places. In contrast, he asserted, 'if you go to a [religious] practitioner, you can go quietly', and potentially keep the person's spirit affliction less known within the wider community.

Perhaps unsurprisingly, religious specialists I spoke also emphasized the importance of ritual intervention for cases *dön né*. In Xining, doctor and *ngakpa* Dr Sonam (69) argued that there was, in fact, usually no way to cure *dön* afflictions through medicine – 'only by ritual'. He related a 'proverb from medicine': 'Illness needs to be cured by medicine, *dön né* needs to be cured by rituals'. Similarly, in Rebkong, Nyingma Geshe Dhondup (50) explained that for spirit-related *nyoné* (or indeed, other spirit-related conditions), particular rituals were necessary to 'expel the *dön*', noting the significant number of diverse rituals appropriate for dealing with the different categories of spirits. As Bon lama Tsering (57) explained:

> It's not the case that these cases can all be treated by one kind of ritual, because you have to know the specific cause. For example, if it is a *gyalpo* that has caused *nyoné* – for this kind of thing, we make *torma* [offerings made of

> roasted barley flour] or ritual, or things like that . . . If it is a different kind of *dön*, then it will need a different ritual. The way to know this is to ask the [afflicted] person's birthdate, and when this *nyoné* started. And *then*, the practitioner can do an astrological calculation or divination, and through this, they will know what kind of ritual this person needs.

Similarly, Aku Wangchuk (72) stressed the importance of accurate diagnosis in determining appropriate treatment, potentially including both ritual and medical interventions:

> First, the doctor should diagnose if it's *nyoné* or not . . . and if it is *nyoné*, if it's [related to] *dön* or not. Then, if it's *dön né*, you need to know what kind of *dön* it is . . . [For example,] if it's *teng dön*, then you use the treatment for *teng dön* – you can use some medicine, and also some ritual . . . But if it's *ok dön* and you use the treatment for *teng dön né* – no matter what you use – then it will be of no use. So you have to clearly know what kind of *dön* it is.

For conditions thought to be caused by *mi tsangwa* related to a particular object or activity, it is similarly important to determine the cause – and lay interviewees recounted having consulted religious specialists here too. Thus Gabzang (27, Golok/Xining) told me: 'First you need to find out what was the *thing* that caused you *dön* . . . So you go to see a lama, and you ask the lama to help, and the lama will tell you which object it was'. He added that while in some places people will consult *lhawa* with these questions, in his village there were no such practitioners and people there generally consulted Buddhist lamas. He explained: 'The lama will find out which object it is by doing a divination or astrological calculation, and then he will say something like, "Recently you took something of . . . colour, and the shape of . . . – you brought that into the house"'. Thus, the problematic object is clearly identified and can then be dealt with.

If a ritual is required for dealing with *dön né* or *mi tsangwa*, it might be done at a local monastery or at a *ngakpa*'s home or temple. Wangtso (34, Rebkong/Xining) told me that in the past, people would invite the monks to their own house to conduct such rituals. However, she explained that sometimes a lama or *ngakpa* will tell you that it is necessary for a particular mantra to be recited for a certain month, and, in this case, 'you need to have many monks' to complete this on your behalf. Nowadays, she said, 'more and more people ask the monastery to do that', but it does not necessarily need to be performed at your local monastery – instead, people might choose a larger monastery in a different area where there is a larger monastic population, for example. Furthermore, she explained, some monasteries will specialize in certain kinds of ritual. And these days, arranging this kind of intervention can be 'very convenient' – you can simply 'make a phone call to arrange it', rather than travelling to the monastery or having monks stay in your home.

However, Gelugpa Geshe Dhondup (50) told me that 'usually' it was preferable to do these kinds of rituals in the patient's home if possible. He described the different ways in which practitioners might approach the treatment of *dön* afflictions:

> There are two different ways to expel spirits. One is in a fierce way, and the other is persuading or convincing [the spirit to leave]. Mostly, practitioners use the fierce method to expel spirits, but sometimes it's possible to convince them [to leave]. So for monks, they don't really do the fierce methods – usually that is done by Bon [practitioners] or *ngakpas*;[19] they have complete methods to expel the spirits. So it's not common to consult monks – this is usually done by *ngakpas*.

Gelugpa lama Wangyal (62, Rebkong) explained one of these methods of 'persuasion', describing how various 'offering cakes' may be offered to the afflicting spirit – 'to try to get this *dön* away from this person quickly'. For this reason, it was best, he explained, for the afflicted individual to be in attendance at the ritual. Different *dön*, he said, have different 'appetites', and so a ritual specialist will 'provide whatever each *dön* wants to eat, and offer the *torma*, and then ask them to cause no further harm to the person'. Moreover, Dr Sonam (69, Rebkong/Xining) explained how some rituals are based around tempting (or forcing) the *dön* away from the afflicted individual, and into an effigy (Tib. *lü*):

> For some *dön* rituals, we need to make some human-like effigy – maybe [out of] roasted barley flour, or sometimes wood . . . We put some clothes [on it] so that it looks like a human. We make something like that, and then we need to perform the ritual, and let the *dön* possess that specific effigy . . . Then we defeat this *dön*, and let this [spirit's] consciousness [Tib. *namshé*] reincarnate in another realm. After the ritual is performed, we need to cut the effigy into pieces – cut the legs, cut the hands, cut the head – and then bury it in the ground somewhere . . . But you need to point these to the opposite direction – for example, if your home is *here* [he pointed one direction], it should be pointing away [in the opposite direction].

Dr Sonam said that during this kind of ritual, ideally, the patient should also be instructed to recite something – but in reality, this can be difficult. The afflicted person – with his/her consciousness at that time overtaken by the possessing *dön* – may become angry, and/or attempt to escape if he/she discovers that the family plan to conduct such a ritual, and so the family may need to 'keep it secret' in advance of its commencement.

In cases of *mi tsangwa/dön* associated with a given object from another household, it was usually said that the object would need to be disposed of once it had been identified by a lama or *ngakpa*, as Gabzang (27, Golok/Xining) told me:

> You need to throw that object out . . . What you will need to do depends on the power of that *dön* – there is something following that object, right? – and it depends on the power of that. If it's strong, you might need a high-level lama to manage this, but if it's just medium strength, maybe you can just ask some monks to chant. And if it's really not too strong, maybe you just can just throw it away yourself – just find out what it is and throw it away . . . Maybe you can offer that object to the lama, or maybe the lama will tell you to take it somewhere, and put it in a certain direction – the lama will tell you 'north', or 'south', or whatever – he will tell you the direction [you should place it in].

In addition, while above we saw *chöd* practice described as a causative factor for some cases of *nyoné*, in Amdo it was also discussed as a potential treatment. For example, Dr Sonam (69) described the recitation of the *chöd* text as a useful practice for treating *nyoné* caused by *dön* possession. Similarly, Dragya (75, Golok) told me that when a person has 'harm' (*nöpa*) from *dré*, '[y]ou have to ask the *ngakpa* to perform *chöd*' before administering any medicine: 'If this works to make the *dré* leave, *then* the medicine will work'.

It can be difficult and/or dangerous to deal with certain kinds of spirits and deities, depending both on their 'strength' and on the knowledge and skills of the practitioner – and also on the type of spirit/deity and how 'powerful' it is in comparison with the afflicted individual. As Aku Wangchuk (72) explained, if the *dön* is very powerful and the afflicted individual is very weak, then it may take a long time. However, if the opposite is the case – where the *dön* is weak but the afflicted individual is strong – then it will likely be 'easy' to successfully treat them.[20] Bon lama Tsering (57) explained that Tantric *hön* practitioners were particularly good at these kinds of rituals, due to their advanced levels of practice. However, he added that, even for this kind of specialist, '[i]f the practitioner doesn't have a really special ability in doing this kind of ritual – if he is not skilled enough – it can sometimes hurt the *hön* himself'. In Xining, Dr Rinchen (55) discussed *gyalpo* spirits in terms of their differing 'strength':

> Not all of the *gyal dön* are so powerful . . . Just like people – some people are really powerful, and some are not powerful. In the same way, some *gyal dön* are really powerful, and can make you *nyoné* – really, they can do this – they are really strong. This kind of *nyoné* is really hard to deal with . . . the *gyal dön* is powerful – if he makes you *nyoné*, he will *seriously* make you *nyoné*, and it is hard to deal with that *nyoné* . . . Sometimes a *gyal dön* will just cause some harm – just disturb us just a little – we can deal with that kind of *nyoné* easily.

Thus, the expected efficacy of this kind of ritual was described as depending on a number of factors, including the type of practitioner and their knowledge, skill and 'power'; and the type of spirit/deity involved.

*

As we can see, then, in Amdo, spirits and deities were often at the forefront of discussions about *nyoné* with Tibetan religious and medical specialists as well as lay Tibetans. This reflects what we find in the Tibetan medical and religious traditions, where spirits and their ability to cause illnesses are described in both Tibetan medical and Tantric texts. There was some notable diversity across explanations about the types of entities involved in illness causation – with some, for example, focusing on *gyalpo* as a common cause of *nyoné*, and others unaware of this category of spirit/deity altogether. Similarly, understandings of *mi tsangwa*, and the ways in which this might (or might not) be related to *dön*, were varied. Nonetheless, spirit narratives in general were common amongst those I spoke to, and a majority of interviewees discussed spirits and deities in quite concrete terms – as entities that may be 'bumped into' on a mountain path, and perhaps even seen directly by some religious specialists. It was notable, however, that none of the doctors I interviewed in Amdo spoke much of medical treatments for spirit affliction, and few recalled having seen such patients. Indeed, it was predominantly those doctors who were also Tantric specialists who described treating patients with these kinds of afflictions. In the next two chapters we will explore Tibetan medical and Tantric approaches to this topic in more detail, and we will see how these Amdo narratives sit alongside those from other Tibetan communities, as they have been examined through ethnographic research in different geographical regions, as well as to what extent these reflect what we find in Tibetan medical and Tantric texts. We will be able to build up a complex picture of the different ways in which non-human entities can be understood in medical and Tantric perspectives, and how these play out in connection to *nyoné* for lay people and Tantric practitioners.

Notes

1. Which is related, as Lichter and Epstein explain, both etymologically and semantically to the Buddhist concept of *drip* – 'defilement' – 'cognitive . . . and emotional . . . obscurations upon the path toward enlightenment' (1983: 246).
2. It wasn't entirely clear to me what Dr Dechen was referring to here, but I think one issue in particular is relevant, which will be discussed further below: the fact that 'religious practice' is not allowed in state hospitals, and references to anything deemed 'religious' or 'superstitious' are very sensitive in the current political climate. Additionally, it may be

related to the fact that this hospital served people from both Tibetan and non-Tibetan communities, treating a number of patients from local Han Chinese and diverse Muslim communities, with different beliefs and traditions relating to notions of spirit affliction. However, it was also notable that several Tibetan *ngakpas* reported seeing a significant number of non-Tibetan patients from these communities for rituals related to spirit affliction.

3. Similarly, Tidwell has described a reticence to diagnose *dön* in a patient's notes at this hospital during her own time as a medical resident there, with *dön* 'not an openly recognized category in public hospitals'. Here, she explains, an official diagnosis of *nying lung* serves a 'dual purpose': 'circumventing a taboo diagnosis of schizophrenia or *dön* and indicating a broader category related to heart *lüng*, which covers anxiety and depression' (Tidwell, Nianggajia and Fjeld 2022: 806). During my time in Amdo, it was hard to determine to what extent stigma avoidance played a role. While there is most likely some stigma attached to certain types of illness and/or causation, those I spoke to about this topic talked to me quite openly about this – including sometimes in relation to their close relatives. However, my position as an outsider, and non-medical professional, probably impacted on this, and so it was difficult for me to get any real sense of this stigma avoidance.
4. Often translated as 'king spirit', these entities are sometimes referred to as 'spirits' (Tib. *dön*), and sometimes 'deities' (Tib. *lha*).
5. Working in the region some years earlier, Bassini also encountered similar narratives, with some Tibetans she spoke to linking their *nying né* to having inadvertently offended a local deity by sleeping in the mountains. This, they explained, had drawn 'pollution' onto them, which then manifested itself as illness (2013a: 239).
6. Such abilities gained over the course of practice are understood to include levitation – as we heard about in Chapter 1 – clairvoyance and the ability to access memories of past lives.
7. In fact, there may be multiple reasons why one person is more susceptible to spirit attack than another, from notions of 'spiritual power' to concepts of karma and 'luck' (see Chapter 5 for more on this).
8. It was clear from the multiple explanations I heard that this was not usually about the *stealing* of objects—indeed, whenever I queried this, I was told that the afflicted person had been *given* an object to 'take' away in the form of a gift or loan. The resulting *mi tsangwa* was therefore not linked to any kind of 'moral' notions of taking an object without permission but instead, as Tsetan explains here, to the notion of anger or displeasure from a family deity at something from 'their' house being removed.
9. This situation is most likely exacerbated by Tibet's recent history, whereby many practices designated 'religious' or 'superstitious' during the Cultural Revolution were banned and many traditions were lost, with community members prevented from passing on knowledge and practices to younger generations (see Adams, Schrempf and Craig 2011 and Hofer 2018 for more on this).
10. We might remember the discussion in the previous chapter on the relationship between the individual body and the cosmos, and the importance of 'time', defined through the movement of the *lung* through the body as well as the sun through the twelve zodiacs – as Wallace explains, '[e]ach of the twelve houses of the external zodiac is said to be of the nature of one of the six elements, which determines its dominant characteristics' (2009: 289).
11. There is perhaps something to be explored here on local perceptions about Tibetans from different regions – which may have diverse customs, and markedly different dialects, as

was the case for Norbu and his girlfriend at that time. Indeed, in her exploration of food and illness in Amdo, Bassini asserts that within Tibetan families, 'experiencing well-being also means to live harmoniously and in ordered coexistence with other members of the family', where being ill 'is not merely an individual experience that can be fully investigated within a patient-healer framework; rather, the experience of illness for Tibetans includes and is heavily shaped by the structures of power at work within the family and beyond' (2013b: 458, 454). However, how much any of this influenced Norbu's and his family's understandings of his father's illness is impossible for me to know, and I therefore simply report the case of *nyoné* as it was described to me rather than presuming to attribute any other meanings to Norbu's narrative.

12. This difficulty is perhaps best described as the misconception of the true nature of phenomena, caused by the unenlightened mind.
13. Spirits of the upper regions or planets, spirits of the intermediate regions and spirits of the lower regions/worlds.
14. See Nebesky-Wojkowitz (1993) for a good classification of these.
15. Dorjé Jikjé in Tibetan, this *yidam* was referred to by his Sanskrit name, Yamāntaka, by my Buddhist Studies student interlocutor.
16. The *Gyüshi* also contains comprehensive instructions on diagnosing different types of spirit affliction through urine analysis; see Chapter 5 for more on this.
17. I asked whether there had been a particular reason to consult a *lhawa* rather than a lama, or any other kind of practitioner, and Norbang explained simply that his family had heard that this particular *lhawa* in the area could treat this kind of *mi tsangwa*.
18. We see here an interesting demarcation between conditions seen to be related to specific physical structures within the body (for example, here related to the 'brain' or 'stomach') and those with what might be seen to be a more ephemeral nature – related here to spirits and deities, but also to the mind or 'psychology' more broadly. This, I think, ties into the increasing ways in which 'testable' phenomena are seen to be the purview of medicine – a perspective encouraged by the increasing use of biomedical diagnostic equipment in Tibetan medicine hospitals as well biomedical ones (see Deane 2024 for an examination into this topic).
19. It is interesting that the Geshe links such 'fierce' practices to the Bon tradition, when in most instances they are conducted similarly by both Nyingma and Bon *ngakpas*, but not by the non-*ngakpa* practitioners of either of those traditions (who do not specialize in such rituals). I would suggest that this is linked to longstanding ideas (and misunderstandings) about the Bon tradition in many Buddhist communities, which I occasionally heard expressed by Buddhists in Amdo.
20. Here, of course, we are not talking about *physical* strength but referring to various concepts about spiritual power (Tib. *wang tang*), which will be explored in the following chapters.

Chapter 5

Spirits, Deities and 'Pollution' in Everyday Life and Illness

> *[I]n the pathogenesis of madness, the interference of harmful spirits is said to act as a 'condition' for its development. This condition acts as a helping agent, the immediate external factor that precipitates the changes in consciousness but which cannot act without the predisposing causes. Thus, the cause and condition act together to disrupt the* pranic *[wind] currents that support the mind.*
>
> —Lobsang Rabgay, 'Lung Diseases and Their Treatment'

In the previous chapter, we saw that many discussions about *nyoné* in Amdo focused on spirits (Tib. *dön*), deities (Tib. *lha*) and/or various notions of impurity/pollution (Tib. *mi tsangwa, drip*). In fact, in Tibetan perspectives, spirits and deities may be involved not only in the causation of mental health and illness but also in many different kinds of illness including skin rashes (usually attributed to *lu [dön]*), and conditions likened to epilepsy (Tib. *za yi dön*). Indeed, as we saw in Chapter 4, for many of the Tibetans I spoke to in Amdo, spirits and deities were an everyday reality: a diverse array of unseen forces understood to inhabit the Tibetan environment, which should be dealt with carefully and correctly. Discussed by both young Tibetans in Xining city and their older relatives in more rural areas, they form part of the 'embedded ecology' of Tibetan life (Samuel 2007: 221), whereby Tibetans have a 'direct and intimate' relationship with these kinds of entities (Samuel 1993: 191).

Narratives about spirit-related illness are, of course, not unique to these particular Amdo communities but illustrate perspectives described within multiple ethnically Tibetan communities across Tibet, India, Nepal, Bhutan and beyond.[1] Tibetan notions of the environment – and the non-human entities understood to reside within it – encompass both Buddhist and pre-Buddhist elements. Any discussion of Tibetan spirits and deities can therefore take in a variety of entities including enlightened Buddhist or Bon deities; local mountain gods; gods of the village, home or family; and 'low-level' local spirits. As we will see here, it is evident that, as Samuel asserted in the 1990s, these kinds of deities remain central to what have often been termed 'folk religious' practices in many contemporary Tibetan communities (1993: 177). While these kinds of unenlightened deities are not able to help humans achieve their soteriological goals, they are highly relevant in everyday life – and are implicated in the health of the community not only in terms of its human members but also in the health of livestock and the health of the environment (crops, rivers, lakes, etc.). Subject to worldly emotions, such local deities may be both 'easily offended and readily appeased' (Calkowski 1985: 70). It is therefore important to keep such spirits and deities 'on side' – propitiating them with offerings (most commonly juniper-smoke offerings) regularly, and showing due care to the environment in which they are understood to reside.

In this chapter, we will explore in more detail Tibetan classifications of spirits and deities, the various ways in which they are understood to cause harms through possession and non-possession afflictions, and the related notions of 'impurity' (Tib. *mi tsangwa, drip*) that we saw in Chapter 4. Here, we will see how these kinds of spirit afflictions (Tib. *dön né*) are related to notions of 'spiritual power' (Tib. *wang tang*), and how they may be treated through both medical and religious means.

Spirits and Deities of the Tibetan Pantheon

In the Tibetan pantheon, we find a mix of Buddhist deities and pre-existing Tibetan spirits and deities – some of which were co-opted into Buddhism after its establishment in Tibet. We find a similar narrative in the Bon tradition too. However, a 'Buddhicization' of Tibetan history has made it difficult to tease out the exact history or background to some of these deities, whose status may have changed over the centuries (for example, from originally being an 'opponent' of Buddhism, to becoming a 'protector' of the Dharma). In addition, there is some diversity in how particular entities are 'classified' – as we have seen in the case of *gyalpo* – as well as some notable geographical differences in perspective.

We can find a variety of local spirits mentioned in the early Indian Buddhist and medical texts too. Samuel points out, for example, that a diversity of gods and spirits are described 'on the same level and in much the same terms as the other, human characters' in the Buddhist (and also Jaina) Sutras (2008: 140–41). And in the Ayurvedic *Caraka Saṃhitā* text, it is asserted that 'madness' can be caused by 'an influx of super human powers (demons) brought on by "hostile, inharmonious, vitiated or impure attacks' (Clifford 1984: 171). What is different in the Tibetan context is the way in which these entities were incorporated into Buddhist and Bon practice. Key in Buddhism is the narrative of the 'taming' of Tibet by Indian Tantric master Padmasambhava (also known as Guru Rinpoche; see Figure 5.1). Tibetan Buddhist sources explain how he arrived from India in the eighth century at the invitation of King Trisong Detsen, successfully converting large sectors of the Tibetan population to Buddhism and founding the first Buddhist monastery (at Samye, south of Lhasa) as well as the Tibetan Buddhist tradition that came to be known as the Nyingma ('Old') school. But Padmasambhava also converted the very landscape, subjugating local spirits and deities as he travelled across Tibet. Such was his superior power, some of these entities were even enlisted as 'protectors' (Tib. *sung ma*) of Buddhism – vowing to protect the Dharma. As worldly deities (Tib. *jiktenpé lha*), these kinds of gods remain unenlightened. However, thus 'converted', they now answer to Tibetan Buddhist specialists, who can compel them to behave in certain ways.

As a result of this process of 'Buddhicization', Buddhist specialists such as lamas and *ngakpa*s became indispensable to lay Tibetans, capable of overpowering and subjugating troublesome local spirits and deities in order to prevent them from causing problems. Key here is the notion of 'spiritual power' (Tib. *wang tang*) – the understanding that *Buddhist* power is stronger than all other forms of (non-Buddhist *un*enlightened) power. A similar narrative can be found within the Bon tradition, describing the figure of Tonpa Shenrab – the founder of the Bon tradition, said by Bonpos to date much earlier than the historical Buddha – and his 'conversion' of Tibet many centuries prior to this.[2]

Thus, while many Tibetan notions of spirits and deities – and the ways in which they may be implicated in humans' everyday lives, health and illness – pre-date the arrival of Buddhism into Tibet, they have become fully incorporated into Tibetan Buddhist and Bon worldviews. Indeed, the existence of these unenlightened spirits and deities seemingly confirms the need for the superior power of Buddhism or Bon to manage them, and rituals to deal with spirit/deity afflictions may be conducted by Buddhist or Bon lamas and *ngakpa*s both inside and outside of the monastery.[3]

We find both spirits and spirit-affliction treatments described in key Tibetan medical texts. In the *Gyüshi*, for example, *dön* are mentioned as one of the four 'conditions' (Tib. *lam zhis*, *kyen*) of illness: season, spirits, diet and lifestyle/behaviour[4] (Men-Tsee-Khang 2008: 22, 97, 104). Spirits are

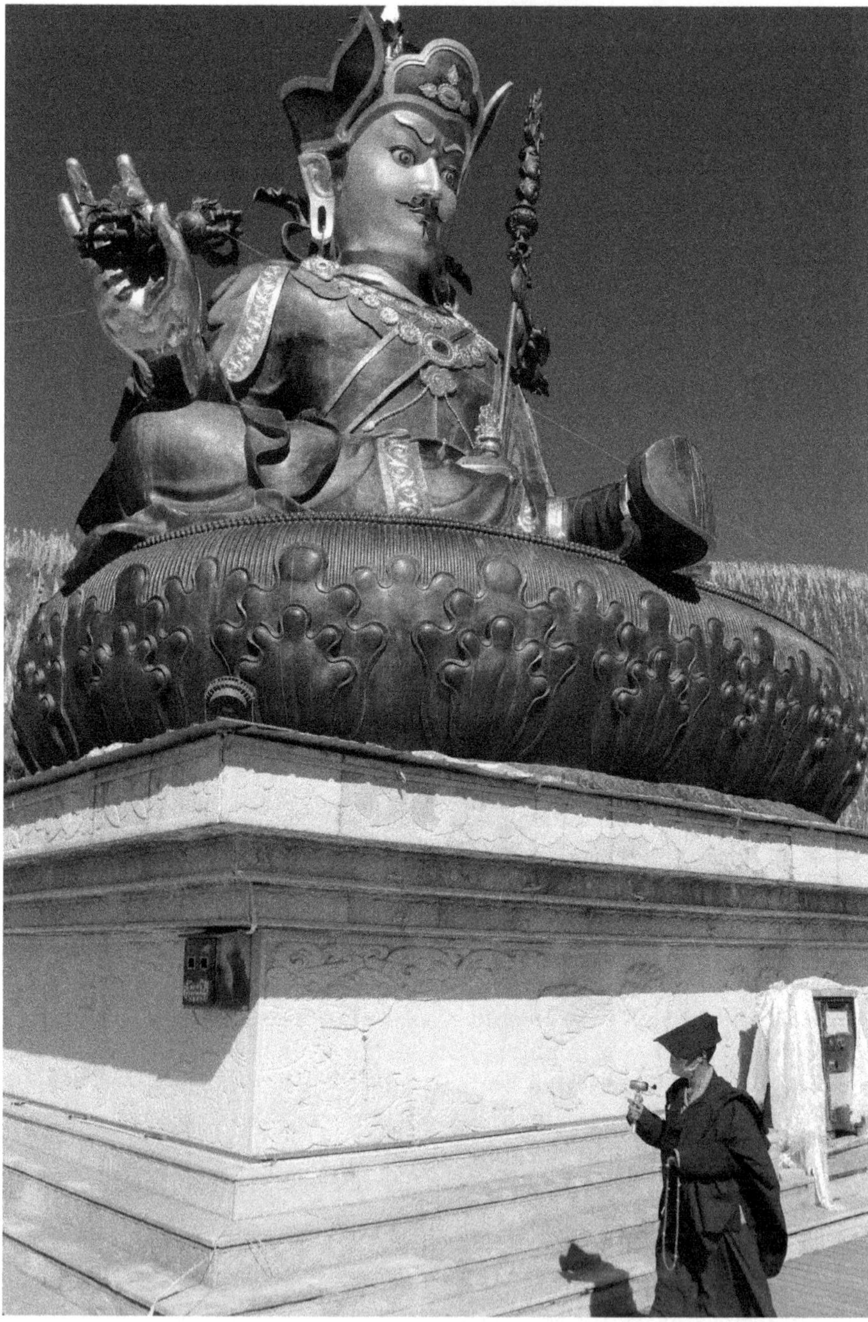

Figure 5.1. Guru Rinpoche statue, sTag lung Monastery, Golok, 2019. © Susannah Deane.

discussed in several places in the text: in the *Oral Instruction Tantra*, in the section on illness-causing spirits in Chapters 77–81 (and Chapters 83–87 in the *Bumshi*) and also under 'children's diseases' in Chapters 72 and 73; and in the chapters on pulse and urine analysis in the *Subsequent Tantra*. Here, we are told, for example, that an 'unstable' *la* pulse indicates spirit affliction (*Gyüshi IV* 2015: 562). They are also mentioned in the context of poison (Tib. *duk*), where poison from elemental spirits (Tib. *jung pö dön*) is described alongside other forms of poison including those from meat and snake venom in Chapter 12 of the *Explanatory Tantra* (*Gyüshi II* 2015: 45).

I think it important to note that while some interpretations (particularly from outside traditions such as certain schools of Western psychology) describe these kinds of non-human entities as abstract or symbolic,[5] as we saw in Chapter 4 this was rarely the case for those I spoke to in Amdo. Here, *dön* were predominantly described as distinct entities with the ability to cause harms including illness, misfortune and even death for those who get on the wrong side of them. This reflects others' findings too – for example, working in Dhortapan, Nepal, Millard discussed the 'everyday reality' of spirits, with the health of both the individual and the community being dependent on 'maintaining a harmonious relationship with these beings' (2007: 261). Here, he describes discussion of 'harmful spirits' (Tib. *nöpa*) as common among both Tibetans and Nepalis in the area, noting that this causative factor was invoked particularly in cases of mental illness (Ibid.: 259).[6] And in Zangskar, Gutschow discusses cases of *nyoné* seen to be related to spirits, where both doctors and lay people 'accept the provisional reality of demons' (1997: 186).

In some Tibetan medical writing too, Tibetan medicine doctors speak in these terms. Yeshe Donden, for example, asserts that '[e]ven though spirits cannot be seen, they definitely do exist and bring harm' (1986: 102). Indeed, this was the way that the doctors I spoke to in Amdo discussed spirits too. However, a few interviewees did express doubts over their material existence. In Xining, for example, Khandro (22) told me: 'Many people say there are no spirits in the world, but some people said they that they really saw these. It's very hard to say – although the science says that there are no spirits in the world, in our real life, some people said that they have encountered something'.

Moreover, in Tibetan religious understanding, there may be multiple ways of interpreting or viewing these types of entities – including the less material. Thus, Clifford argues that at one level, *dön* may be seen as 'embodied forms we give to our negative projections . . . which are then projected outward and turned against ourselves' (1984: 151–52).[7] In Amdo, Nyingma lama Namgyal (32, Chabcha) told me, '*Dön* is not something that can come from outside, but from *sem kham* [psychology] – the state of mind of that person . . . No such thing[s] as *dön* exist'. And in a biography of renowned Tibetan yogi Milarepa, we read of him being troubled by demons before declaring, 'I have already fully realized that all beings and all phenomena are of one's own mind . . . how foolish I am to try to dispel these manifestations physically!' (Chang 1977: 5–6). It was through 'overcoming' these entities, we are told, that Milarepa experienced 'great spiritual growth' (Ibid.: 12–13).

In addition, the experience of seeing spirits can even be viewed as a *symptom* of the kind of disturbances in the senses caused by the wind illnesses that we explored in Part I, where we saw hallucinations and delusions described as a consequence of *lung né*, for example. As contemporary Tibetan medicine doctor and author Thubten Phuntsok asserts, 'Even if objectively something does not exist, the person can see it and thinks that it is a ghost', when in fact 'these visions are caused by wind or blood circulating in the wrong way in the physical body' (2015: 72). And finally, a further layer of explanation describes how an afflicted person's hallucinations might in fact be the result of the possessing spirit's ability to see other beings, as Tidwell described in the case of a *nyoné* patient in Xining (in Tidwell, Nianggajia and Fjeld 2022: 805). We will explore these perspectives in more detail below. First, however, let us take a look at the different types of non-human entities that may be held responsible for *nyoné* and other illnesses.

Classification: Medical and Religious

Much as we might like to find a definitive classification of Tibetan spirits and deities, as we saw in the previous chapter, descriptions of the wide variety of non-human entities that encompass the Tibetan pantheon are varied. This is the case not only in local understandings but also within both Tibetan and non-Tibetan texts and scholarly works, where we find multiple descriptions of entities ranging from powerful protective deities down to local spirits residing in water courses, trees and mountaintops.[8] These entities are frequently categorized into different groups: one common categorization is into 'Eight Classes' (Tib. *lha sin dé gyé*), which is common in Nyingma Buddhist texts (Samuel 1993: 161).[9] In addition, in the previous chapter we heard how spirits can be classified into those of the upper, middle and lower realms[10] – with Tibetan medicine practitioner and *ngakpa* Dr Sonam (69, Rebkong/Xining) describing '360 kinds of *dön*' and Dr Rinchen (55, Xining) noting the two different systems of classification in Tibetan medicine, which describe eighteen or fifteen kinds of *dön* involved in illness. Further, Clifford notes that in the Buddhist texts, *dön* come under the broader umbrella of *gek* – 'obstacle/hindrance' – 84,000 of which are described in the Buddhist Sutras, where 1,080 are *dön* described as causing 'faults of mind' (1984: 154).

Within this pantheon, the Tibetan term '*lha*' is used to refer to three quite distinct types of gods: i) local worldly (unenlightened) deities, ii) 'gods of the Buddhist or Bon heavens' (who are also unenlightened, and therefore exist within samsara), and iii) enlightened Tantric gods (Samuel 1993: 165). Moreover, within the first of these, the differentiation between 'local gods' and what are usually referred to as 'spirits' is not clear cut, with some entities, such as *gyalpo*, sometimes described as *lha* and at other times as *dön*, or sometimes even as powerful ghosts – often said to be the ghosts of lamas who were greedy and irascible (Lichter and Epstein 1983: 249).[11] As we might expect, such classifications are not necessarily a primary concern for lay Tibetans, whose main worry is rather about the potential harm posed by these entities. For example, local deities – if so inclined – can protect individuals, families or even whole communities against harm from local spirits . . . or may instead 'unleash' local spirits on 'someone with whom they are displeased' (Samuel 1993: 189). We might conclude, as Samuel argues, that any 'pantheon' of Tibetan spirits and deities should be viewed 'less a rigid hierarchy than a series of intermeshing patron-client relationships' (Ibid.: 191), with some geographical differences in perspective evident too, as we have seen in Amdo.

In the *Gyüshi* medical text, we encounter spirits predominantly described in the *Oral Instruction Tantra*, with five categories delineated:

- Chapter 77: Elemental Spirits (Tib. *jung pö dön*)
- Chapter 78: Spirits That Cause Madness (Tib. *nyo jé gyi dön*)
- Chapter 79: Spirits That Cause Forgetfulness (Tib. *jé jé kyi dön*)
- Chapter 80: Planetary Spirits That Cause Strokes or Partial Paralysis (Tib. *za yi dön*)
- Chapter 81: Serpent Spirits (Tib. *lu dön*) (*Gyüshi III* 2015: 381–98)[12]

These five classes of spirit are described in some detail in English-language publications by a number of Tibetan medicine practitioners and scholars. For example, contemporary Tibetan medicine doctor and teacher Pasang Y. Arya discusses 'Tibetan medical psychiatry' on his 'Tibetan Medicine Education Center' website. Here, he references these five categories in describing the 'five major mild and aggressive mental disorders' that are related to possession by these classes of spirits.[13]

Every chapter on nosology in the *Oral Instruction Tantra* follows the same structure: cause, secondary cause, types, diagnosis and treatment. Thus, we find *dön* described in Chapter 78 as a 'secondary cause', acting alongside fearfulness/weak heart (Tib. *nying top zhen*), suffering/distress (Tib. *nya ngen*), excessive worry (Tib. *sem lé ché*), unhappy mind (Tib. *yi mi dé*) and/or unwholesome/unsuitable diet (Tib. *zé jö mi trö*) (*Gyüshi III* 2015: 383). Here, as Rapgay explains, spirits act as a 'condition' or 'helping agent' for the development of *nyoné* – an 'immediate external factor that precipitates the changes in consciousness but which cannot act without the predisposing causes' (1985: 48). The *dön* are understood to 'distort the senses through the interaction of the emotions and humors (nyes pas)' (Vargas 2009: 371). As such, there are seven types of *nyoné* described here: (i–iv) *nyoné* arising primarily from *lung*, *tripa* or *béken*, or a combination of all three; (v) *nyoné* arising primarily from a 'distressed mind'; (vi) *nyoné* arising primarily from poison (Tib. *duk*); and, finally, (vii) *nyoné* arising solely from *dön* (*Gyüshi III* 2015: 383–84). The symptoms that an afflicted person experiences will depend on the primary cause; for example, where *lung* is a primary cause of *nyoné*, flesh 'diminishes', the afflicted individual foams at the mouth, and talks and cries excessively. Their eyes will become red and cloudy, and their condition will worsen after eating (Ibid.). In contrast, symptoms of spirit-related *nyoné* arising primarily from *tripa* include anger and violence, with the afflicted individual having a preference for the cold, emitting yellow tears, and seeing 'fire and stars' in front of their eyes. For cases of *nyoné* where the cause is solely *dön*, the afflicted person behaves 'harmfully' (Tib. *nöd*) (Ibid.: 384). In addition, while Chapter 78 explicitly describes 'spirits that cause madness', spirits designated in some of the other chapters may also be implicated in cases of *nyoné*. For example, Clifford describes how the eighteen 'elemental spirits' of Chapter 77 may 'cause a sudden type of insanity' that she characterizes as 'splits in consciousness' (1984: 176–79).

Interestingly, these spirits actually take up proportionally little space in the *Gyüshi* text (Samuel 2001b: 262), and Tibetan medicine doctors' familiarity with these sections of the text will depend very much on their specific medical training and experience, as I found myself during my time in both Darjeeling and Amdo.[14] Moreover, the spirits described in Chapters 77–79 directly reflect what is found in the Ayurvedic *Aṣṭāṇgahṛidayasaṃhīta* text, from which much of the *Gyüshi* derives (Emmerick 1987), but in fact, as Samuel has noted, some of these appear to have little resonance with how contemporary Tibetans think about illness – with some chapters, for example, reflecting 'Indian rather than Tibetan understandings' of spirit-caused illness (2007: 214).

Moreover, as we have already seen, there are some notable differences in the ways in which various spirits are discussed in different Tibetan communities. In Chapter 4, for example, I reported how one *ngakpa* in Amdo described *gyalpo* as the 'most common' spirits involved in the causation of *nyoné*, and Clifford quotes twentieth-century Nyingma Buddhist scholar Mipham Rinpoche saying the same thing (1984: 158). Other Amdo-wa told me that they had never heard of this entity, and emphasized other deities and their role in *nyoné* instead. In Rebkong, Nyingma *ngakpa* Tsephal (55) told me that those afflicted by *gyalpo* 'often' become *nyoné*, but he also spoke of people afflicted by *sadak* (earth spirits), who he said, 'often behave out of control and become *nyoné*'. In contrast, Tibetan medicine doctor Lobsang

Rapgay asserts that of the various beings that inhabit Tibetan cosmology (humans, animals, gods, jealous gods, hell beings and hungry ghosts), it is the hungry ghosts (Tib. *yidak*) who are primarily involved in the causation of *nyoné* (1985: 51). Moreover, there are a variety of ways in which the different spirits and deities may disturb a person or cause them harm – some examples of which we saw in Chapter 4, and which we will take a look at now.

Possession and Non-Possession Spirit Afflictions

It is important to note that spirits and deities may harm humans either intentionally or unintentionally. For example, a local deity may *intentionally* cause harm to individuals it feels have wronged it (for example, if humans have ceased their usual offerings to the deity or polluted its environment). On another occasion, a deity may *inadvertently* harm people with no ill will intended – and this was often described to be the case with non-possession spirit afflictions in Amdo, as we heard in narratives of people 'bumping into' a mountain deity while out in the mountains.

As we saw in the previous chapter, in Amdo possession by a spirit was often said to be identifiable from a person's behaviour – often a sudden change seemingly occurring 'out of nowhere'. Such narratives echo Lobsang Rapgay's description of 'madness primarily due to harmful spirit', where he describes such cases as 'characterized by a sudden change in personality with the individual acquiring the temperament and behaviour patterns of one of the sixty types of harmful spirits' (1985: 51). One example is an afflicted individual apparently speaking in a language previously unknown to them – as we heard in Dr Dechen's (39) description, reported in the previous chapter, of a Tibetan patient who could apparently suddenly speak fluent Chinese, having never spoken it before. In this case, as we saw, it was concluded that it was 'obvious' that the affliction was caused by a *dön*.

Such symptoms can be clearly accounted for if we examine Tibetan understandings of the process of 'possession' – i.e. the method by which a spirit is seen to 'invade' and 'take over' a person's mind-body. As Dr Nyima (38) explained in the previous chapter, it is through the *lung* that a spirit is understood to enter a person's body – often said to be through openings in the third ('ring') fingers on each hand (Millard 2007: 261) – and, again, it is the *sok lung*/*sok tsa* that is often key here. For example, Epstein and Topgay describe how 'psychosis' may result when the *sok tsa* is 'forcefully entered by another energy'. They explain that this is 'usually' a spirit, but is sometimes one of the other *nyépa*, which has become increased. This, they explain, 'disturbs the flow between pranic flow and mind' (1982: 76). For example, Sanggye Gyatso's *Extended Commentary on the Instructional Tantra of the Four*

Tantras names *gyalpo* spirits as one of the causes of *sok lung* disturbance (Chui 2019: 88). Epstein and Topgay thus describe spirits as a 'helping agent' for the development of *nyoné* – the 'immediate external factor that precipitates the change in consciousness but which cannot act without the predisposing causes' (such as 'poor diet', 'a weak heart' and mental exertion', as we heard above) (1982: 76). Similarly, Rapgay explains:

> Invasion by spirit or *nyes-pa* is said to occur through the interior channel, through the current that supports ear consciousness. It is conducted through the anterior channel to the inferior channel, site of the support of mental consciousness. This invasion causes a blockade in the inferior site, occluding or reversing the current of *prana* upon which the mind rests. Thus, control over the functioning of the mind is lost, with loss of memory and hysterical behavior preceding full-fledged psychosis.
>
> Mind, memory, and mental consciousness are thus disturbed. The capacity to sense the pleasant or unpleasant feelings that normally accompany sense awareness is lost. (Rapgay 1985: 49)

Equally, Duckworth translates from the Third Karmapa Rangjung Dorjé's text *Key to the Essential Points of Wind and Mind* to explain how difficulties in the manipulations of wind in the kinds of *tsa lung* practices that we examined in Chapter 3 can also lead to spirit interference:

> If you don't know how to expel Wind when becoming angry, the male spirits will harm you. You will become afflicted by illnesses. Your students will fight, and there will be much discord . . . If you don't know how to expel [Wind] outwardly when prideful, king spirits [Tib. *gyalpo*] will harm you . . . The Demon of the Lord of Death resides in the breath. He stirs at midnight accompanied by brazen spirits. Knowing his signs – anxiety and depression – expel healing Wind outwardly and meditate on your teacher at your heart. (Duckworth 2017: 415–16)

With the afflicted individual's mind-body now host to *two* consciousness (i.e. their own and that of the possessing spirit), he/she 'has not totally lost his mind' but neither 'does the affected person's mind bear its original nature' (Rapgay 1985: 49–50). Thus, as Chaoul explains, 'when there are spirit-provoked obstacles (*gdon*), the vital breath currents cannot flow in the proper way together with the mind, through the channels' (2007: 135).

In addition to this key relationship between spirits and *lung*, as we heard from Aku Wangchuk (72) in Chapter 4, different types of spirits will have a connection to the three different *nyépa*, with the 'spirits of the upper realm' (Tib. *teng dön*) connected particularly to the *béken*, 'spirits of the intermediate/middle realm' (Tib. *bar dön*) connected to the *tripa* and 'spirits of the lower realms' (Tib. *ok dön*) connected to the *lung*. Drungtso explains that spirits such as *kordak* (a low-level spirit) and *gyalpo* are 'mostly responsible for *lung* problems' (2004: 213) in contrast to the *mamo* which are more related to *tripa*, and the *lu*, *nyen* and *sadak* spirits, which are related to disruption in the *béken* (Ibid.: 216, 220). Indeed, this is evident in the *Gyüshi*'s Chapter 78, which describes diverse symptoms of *dön* affliction depending on which *nyépa*(s) are also involved, as Vargas explains: here, madness-causing spirits are said to 'distort the senses through the interaction of the emotions and humors (*nyes pas*). For example, arising from *lung*, one becomes emaciated. Arising from phlegm, one sleeps a lot' (Vargas 2009: 371).

However, not all spirit afflictions involve possession. In the previous chapter, we heard Norbu's (30, Rebkong) description of his father's period of *nyoné*, which was understood to have been caused by a *gyalpo* spirit. In this case, as we saw, the afflicting spirit was not *possessing* the afflicted individual; rather, it was understood that the spirit was causing some 'harm' from a distance as a result of the family's connection to it (via Norbu's relationship with his girlfriend). Nonetheless, the symptoms of non-possession and possession spirit affliction may be similar, as we saw in this description, which included his father's 'strange' and violent behaviour. Indeed, as we have seen, in Amdo, *gyalpo* were often mentioned in relation to *nyoné*, usually described as causing harm from a distance. Similarly, mountain deities – often referred to as *zhidak* – were also generally discussed in this way, as we saw in the previous chapter, where both lay Tibetans and religious specialists discussed the dangers of inadvertently walking through the path of such an entity, or unknowingly sleeping in its territory when walking or herding in the mountains.

In Golok, teacher Lhakpa (38) and her colleagues discussed a *zhidak* in the local area over dinner, with Lhakpa explaining: 'The *zhidak* there was really powerful, and so if you sleep there, then you can get the *nyo* [madness] . . . Just being awake there is ok, but if you *sleep* there . . .' Her colleague Gabzang (27) interrupted to add:

> It's kind of like you are not respecting the *zhidak* . . . Sleeping [on the mountain], it's kind of disrespectful to the *zhidak* . . . so someone slept there, and then became *nyonpa*. We have heard these kinds of things several times . . . Old people say that you cannot even *rest* there – you have to go around the other side.
>
> And if it's *two* mountains . . . At the top there are two mountains, with a small valley in between them – at the top, between the two peaks . . . People say that if you sleep there, then the *za* [*dön*; planetary spirits] can maybe cause you to become *nyoné*.

And, of course, as we have heard, it was generally understood that lay people cannot see such entities, making it easy for them to inadvertently disturb or harm them.

Pollution: *Mi Tsangwa, Drip* . . . and *Dön*?

In Chapter 4, we also heard several Amdo narratives about '*mi tsangwa*' and '*drip*' – impurity/pollution. While the notion of 'pollution' is often discussed in relation to problems of the eyes, colds, numbness and even death in Tibetan communities (Lichter and Epstein 1983: 242), in Amdo, as we have seen, I also heard it occasionally referenced in the causation of *nyoné*. Lichter and Epstein have described multiple potential sources of *drip* including faeces, urine, unclean food, food taken from an unclean place/container, corpses, childbirth, fights and broken vows (1983: 242), and Tucci describes several kinds of *drip* or *mi tsangwa* including 'eating various impure foods' such as that 'offered by a widow or a murderer' or '[b]urnt foods' as well as pouring 'substances producing evil smells or smoke' onto a hearth, which he explains may 'anger the god of the hearth'; 'lighting fires on mountains'; and 'staying in neighbourhoods where *gnyan* [spirits] live' (1980: 173). My own previous research had found *drip* mentioned in the context of dead bodies or wearing the clothes of someone who had passed away (Deane 2014b).

Samuel notes that pollution can result from '[h]aving caused offense to the gods' (1993: 161), and this was something we heard referenced in the previous chapter, with many of the descriptions of *drip* or *mi tsangwa* focused on objects (bowls, clothes, etc.) given or taken from another's home, apparently causing offence to the family deity. In Amdo, I found *drip* or *mi tsangwa* sometimes discussed as a quite direct cause of illness, as in retired doctor Samphel's (72) assertion that *nyoné* can be caused by 'bringing something from outside [the family/house]' into your home. However, as we saw in the previous chapter, there was also sometimes a rather unclear picture – particularly around the relationship between *mi tsangwa* and *dön*, with some interviewees describing these as 'the same' and others hinting at a rather complex relationship between them. For example, Buddhist *ngakpa* Tsephal (55, Rebkong), described 'eight *drib*' in similar terms to the common classification of eight *dön*, and, as we heard in the previous chapter, Lhakpa (38, Golok/Xining) told us that where her family described affliction by *dön*, this was labelled *drip* by the lamas they consulted. She was unsure of the relationship between these things, and a question about this prompted an interesting discussion between her and her husband, whose family – from a different geographical region – described *drip*/*mi tsangwa* and *dön* and the relationship between them quite differently from her. Tucci has also discussed this overlap in meaning – explaining, for example, how the term *drek* refers to both 'demonic beings' and also 'uncleanliness, filth' (1980: 201).

For some, there is an understanding that *drip* may simply increase one's vulnerability to attack from spirits (Samuel 1993: 161). Tucci explains, for example, that pollution 'obstructs a favourable destiny and renders one receptive to all that is unfavourable' (1980: 173). One way in which this may occur is by causing a person's protective deities to 'abandon' him/her – due to the individual becoming 'polluted and impure'. Spirits can then 'take advantage' of the person's new vulnerability and make their attack (Tucci 1980: 173–75, 201).

In addition, we have already heard about the potential problems that may result from two people from different geographical areas entering into a romantic relationship or marriage. This was sometimes referred to in terms of *drip* or *mi tsangwa*, as well as in terms of connections to local spirits or deities, as in Norbu's narrative of his father's illness. In the previous chapter, we heard one couple – whose families had come from very different geographical regions – conclude that perhaps the longevity of a relationship might eventually negate this. This echoes Lichter and Epstein's explanation that in cases of *drip*, the 'degree of seriousness of a pollutant can be modified over time', and they also suggest that changes in social structure can lead to 'previously unacceptable' marriages becoming more routine (1983: 245). This might be particularly relevant in a city such as Xining, where Tibetans from many different regions come together to study at the university or to find work, for example. And finally, we come back to notions of 'suspicion', or *namtok*. As Lichter and Epstein explain, 'People say that pollution is a matter of what one is used to, so that if something ceases to arouse the suspicion that it will make one sick, then it ceases to make one sick' (Ibid.). Similarly, in Rebkong, former Buddhist monk Tsetan (38) spoke of cases of illness where *mi tsangwa* was determined to have stemmed from a particular object, referring back to the notion of *namtok*:

> The illness is caused by this object, but also it's caused by *namtok* . . . Buddhist practices or Buddhism stops *namtok* . . . Everything good or bad . . . clean or dirty . . . beautiful or ugly – everything comes from *namtok*. So if you free yourself from *namtok*, then you will be ok.

Spiritual Power: Hierarchies of Spirits, Deities and Humans

As is evident here, narratives of spirit illness – including cases of *nyoné* – are common across many Tibetan communities. And as we saw in the previous chapter, remediation is often seen to lie predominantly in rituals conducted by Buddhist or Bon *ngakpa*s and lamas, who are understood to have sufficient 'spiritual power' (Tib. *wang tang*) to deal with these non-human entities. In Tibetan understanding, 'hierarchies' of spiritual power see lay people as less powerful than these kinds of local spirits and deities, allowing them to be harmed by these entities. And if a person's *wang tang* is particularly low, they will be especially vulnerable to attack by spirits.

Differential levels of *wang tang* may result – at least, in part – from activities performed in previous and present lifetimes. Calkowski explains, for example, that spiritual power may be 'obtained through application to Buddhist meditational deities, contagiously acquired through the touch of a high lama, [or] achieved through religious initiations actualised by lamas who themselves possess it' (1993: 32–33). And Tibetan discourses describe a clear hierarchy of power, a concept underscored by the Buddhist narrative of Padmasambhava's 'taming' of Tibet through the superior power of Buddhism, which we saw above – and, equally, in the Bon narrative of Tonpa Shenrab. This Dharmic power is understood to be stronger than all other forms of non-Dharmic spiritual power – thus we hear of Padmasambhava's success in converting local deities to Buddhism. However, while these deities were converted, they remained 'worldly', *unenlightened* entities (Tib. *jiktenpé lha*). As a result, they are understood to be beholden to the same emotions and desires as unenlightened humans and, significantly, they hold more power than lay humans but *less* power than advanced Buddhist/Bon practitioners – who derive their power through their practices evoking enlightened Tantric deities. The result of this is that while lay Tibetans are negotiating with these spirits and deities from a position of inferiority – for example, politely requesting their assistance or asking for them to leave a person alone – in contrast, Tibetan Buddhist/Bon lamas and *ngakpa*s are able to negotiate with even the more powerful deities from a position of superiority – compelling the deities to assist them when necessary, and often ritually inducing them to be helpful and to prevent misfortune.[15]

As a result of this power differential, Buddhist and Bon lamas and *ngakpa*s are less likely to become afflicted by local spirits and deities: as *ngakpa* and doctor Aku Wangchuk (72, Rebkong) explained, 'If a person is really powerful, then it's not easy for them to get *dön né*; if the person is weak, then they can easily get *dön né*'. Instead, these kinds of practitioners possess sufficient power to command and subjugate less-powerful, unenlightened spirits and deities – casting them out, or away from, any human(s) they are afflicting. However, another consequence of this situation is the difficulty of dealing with the 'ghost' (Tib. *dré*) of someone who has previously been a religious practitioner with a high level of Tantric knowledge and skill – and who thus has a great deal of power that they might use for good or ill. Indeed, in Amdo former Gelugpa monk Tsetan (38) gave the example of a Tibetan religious specialist with negative motivations who became a ghost after death, telling me, 'These people are strong – they also know everything'.

Moreover, these differential levels of spiritual power can be key in protecting humans in another way too: through the role of the 'family deity' (Tib. *khyim lha*), and its ability to protect family members from any troublesome lower-level spirits and deities. Aku Wangchuk (72, Rebkong) told me, 'In Tibetan culture, we believe that all families have their own *sung ma* [protector deity]'. This kind of protector deity 'is just like a dog for the property – protecting the family', he explained; 'If the *sung ma* is strong, then a *dön* cannot come [inside]; if it is not strong, then a *dön* can come in'. However, he continued, there can be a 'misunderstanding' of the status of some of these deities, causing the kind of problems we heard about in Chapter 4, around taking objects from another's house: 'Some *sung ma* – because of a misunderstanding or something – could be *dön* [spirits]. So if you take an object from another's house, then *dön* may follow that object. This *can* happen, but not always'.

In addition, these unenlightened protector deities may also cause trouble when they are unhappy with events involving the family. In Golok, for example, Pasang (33) related a tragic story of a relative who moved with his family from Golok to Yushu. After they moved, she told me, several family members had died: the father, mother and one brother. When the surviving child married someone from Yushu, they had two children, both of whom had also died. Pasang described how they had consulted a lama, who told them that their *sung ma* was angry that they had left Golok. On discovering this, the lama communicated with the protective deity, and it was agreed that the family would honour the *sung ma* every year on a particular day. Since then, she told me, there had been no further problems.

In addition to *wang tang*, there are also a number of other factors that may impact on an individual's susceptibility to spirit attack and/or *drip/mi tsangwa*. These include an individual's luck (Tib. *lungta*), merit (Tib. *sonam*) and the strength of their life-force (Tib. *la*).[16] As former monk Tsetan (38, Rebkong) told me, 'People may have higher or lower *lung ta*. If you have more *lung ta*, then it is difficult for the spirits to affect you'. And, of course, there is also always the role of karma (Tib. *lé*), as Gutschow explains: '[I]n an absolute sense, all disease is caused by karma' (1997: 185), and when cases of madness – or any other illness or misfortune – remain unresolved despite multiple treatments – particularly the powerful, ritual treatments of experienced lamas or *ngakpa*s – underlying karmic affects are often referenced. In Amdo, Migmar (30, Golok/Xining) asserted that some diseases are simply not treatable – with some having been caused by a person's previous life/lives. These cases of *nyoné*, he explained, are 'incurable'. The fruits of karma can be increased by virtuous action (Tib. *gewa*), and can 'accumulate' or be 'exhausted' (Lichter and Epstein 1983: 240). This contrasts with a person's 'worldly luck' (Tib. *lung ta*), which is 'synonymous with unpredictable good fortune' and flows 'unilineally from gods to humans' (Calkowski 1993: 32). Luck may be 'high' or 'low', and can be increased by religious activities, but it cannot be accumulated.[17]

Clearly, keeping one's local spirits and deities happy is key to maintaining the health and harmony of a household, village or local area, and this is

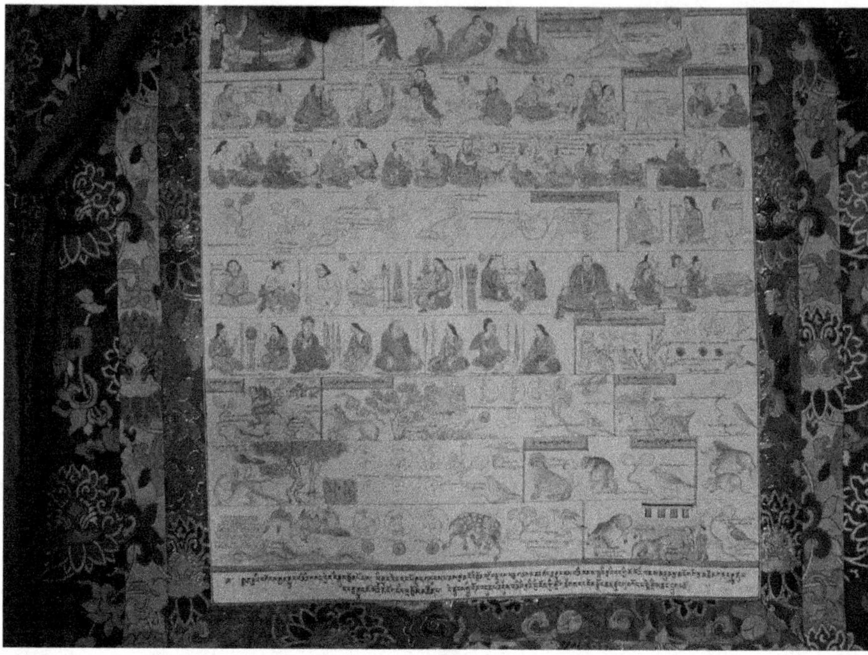

Figure 5.2. Tibetan medical *thangka* depicting pulse examination, Lhasa Mentsikhang, 2010. © Susannah Deane.

done through the making of regular offerings. However, unintentional harm or offence is always possible, and, if one's local or family deities *do* become unhappy, offended or angry – and refuse to be placated through lay people's efforts to right the situation – the superior power of lamas and/or *ngakpa*s is then called upon to deal with the situation, as we shall now explore.

Diagnosis and Treatment of Spirit-Caused *Nyoné*

Diagnosis

As we heard in the previous chapter, Tibetan medicine includes a number of diagnostic techniques for *dön*-related *nyoné*, and a skilled practitioner is understood – at least theoretically – to be able to ascertain a spirit affliction through pulse and/or urine analysis (see Figures 5.2 and 5.3 for pictorial representations of this in the medical *thangka*s). For example, in Chapter 1 of the *Subsequent Tantra*, the *dön* pulse is described as becoming 'irregular', halting and reversing/retracting (*Gyüshi IV* 2015: 561). Indeed, Tidwell describes, in a similar fashion, her own experience of a pulse reading suggesting *gyalpo* affliction in a Qinghai Province Tibetan Medicine Hospital patient (Tidwell, Nianggajia and Fjeld 2022: 804–5). Moreover, the exact *type* of spirit involved can be determined through pulse analysis too: earlier in this *Gyüshi* chapter, for example, we read that the 'appearance' of the *dön* pulse on the wood-element pulse (Tib. *shing tsa*) identifies the involvement of *nyen* and *gyalpo* spirits. In contrast, the appearance of the *dön* pulse on the fire-element pulse (Tib. *mé tsa*) indicates the involvement of *tsen* and *dü* spirits (*Gyüshi IV* 2015: 557).

As far as we can ascertain, pulse and urine analyses do not have an Indian origin: Samuel points out, for example, that while pulse diagnosis does not feature in the classic Ayurveda texts, it in fact forms a 'significant part of both traditional Chinese medicine and the Greek-Islamic system' – both of which we know the Tibetans were acquainted with (Samuel 2007: 218). He characterizes *dön né* as a 'recognisable if somewhat secondary category' in these sections on pulse and urine diagnosis in the *Gyüshi* (Ibid.). Nonetheless, McGrath describes a 'vast and diverse' field of Tibetan-language instructions for channel examination beyond this, including the 'identification of demonic possession' prior to the thirteenth- and fourteenth-century systematization of the *Subsequent Tantra* (2019: 299–300). For example, McGrath notes that Chapter 23 of the *Medicine of the Moon King* text (dating from some time between the eighth and eleventh centuries) 'depicts a diverse landscape of demonic agents' in relation to 'vessel diagnosis' (2017: 503). In his translation of a section of the *Medicine of the Moon King* (Tib. *sman dpyad zla ba'i rgyal po*) text, we find some quite detailed descriptions – including, for example, the assertion that: 'If the Lung and Large Intestine vessels quiver and halt, the affliction derives from spirits of temple grounds . . . If the Lung and Heart vessels quiver and halt, the affliction derives from non-Buddhist extremists disturbing gods and spirits, fornicating in the woods or near a spring, in either a southern or western direction' (Ibid.: 508).

In terms of urinalysis, the influence of various types of spirit may be determined by different forms of 'cream' or foam (Tib. *dri ma*) on the urine, as is described in Chapter 2 of the *Subsequent Tantra* (*Gyüshi IV* 2015: 564). Here, the doctor also looks for sediments or bubbles in the urine in different parts of the urinalysis bowl, using a 'grid' system to indicate the different area(s) of the afflicted person's life in which spirits or deities are active (see Ibid.: fig. 10). This grid divides the bowl into nine sections with vertical and horizontal lines: gods (Tib. *lha*), humans, spirits (Tib. *dön*), house, field, charnel ground/graveyard, self, ancestor and child (Drungtso 2004: 322–33; see also Men-Tsee-Khang 2011: 44–48). For example, *nyen* and *gyalpo* spirits are indicated by bubbles resembling 'fish eyes and [a] stitching like pattern' in the eastern section of the grid; and *tsen* and *mamo* spirits are indicated by a sign in the southern portion (Drungtso 2004: 329–30). Equally, the type

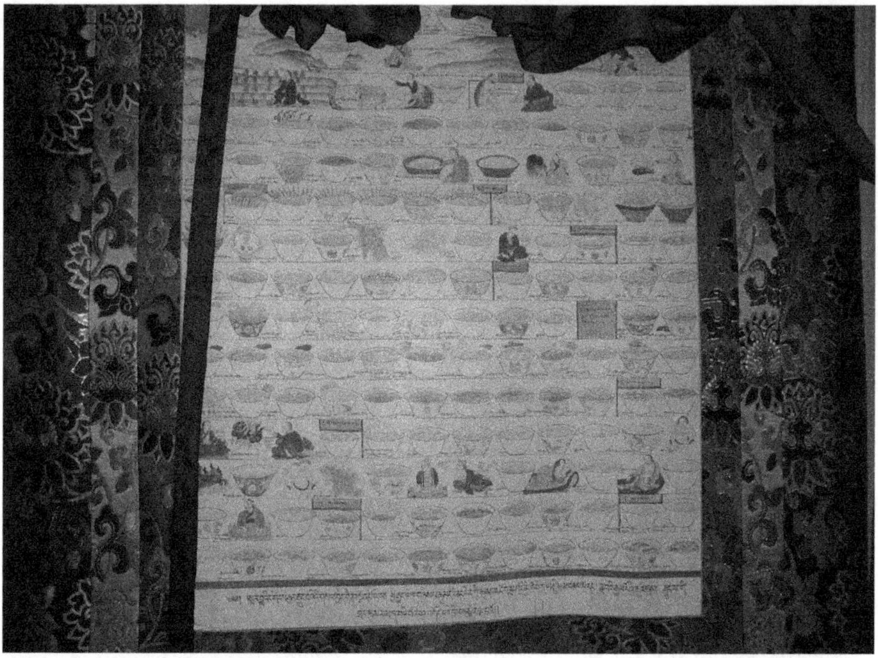

Figure 5.3. Tibetan medical *thangka* depicting urine analysis, Lhasa Mentsikhang, 2010. © Susannah Deane.

of spirit may be ascertained by any patterns in the urine – for example, the 'appearance of a shimmering orb of light in the urine suggests provocation[18] from *rGyal-po*' (Ibid.: 331). If diagnosis is still uncertain following examination of the urine bowl, as described above, a urinalysis divination may be performed. Drungtso describes this method:

> The urine divination is done by the physician holding eight white grains and one brown grain in his hand.[19] Then, he prays to the three jewels of Buddha, Dharma and Sangha and puts one grain in each of the houses while keeping his eyes closed. The physician locates and confirms the harmful spirits as the one on which the brown grain falls. Accordingly he suggests rites and rituals to please the spirits and delivers the patient from harms. (2004: 334–35)

In reality, as we heard in the previous chapter, many Tibetans in Amdo did not in fact seek out an 'medical' diagnostic in the realm of spirit illnesses, and doctors may well not be consulted for such cases at all. Instead, those I spoke to described 'religious' approaches to both diagnosis and treatment – usually focused on the skills of lamas and *ngakpas*. This was something that I had also seen in my previous research in Darjeeling, where I had found that for many Tibetans, religious practitioners such as these were often the first port of call in cases of suspected spirit affliction (Deane 2019a). Within Tibetan communities in Dalhousie too, Samuel reported that spirit afflictions were rarely diagnosed through medical means; instead, here they were predominantly 'self-diagnosed, with confirmation sought from a spirit medium or lama, rather than diagnosed by the doctor', with neither pulse nor urine analysis used at all (2007: 219).

As we heard in Chapter 4, some of my Amdo interviewees described the use of various forms of divination to determine the cause of a person's illness, or perhaps to identify which particular kind of spirit/deity might be involved – as we saw, for example, in Norbu's (30) narrative about his father's illness. I would argue that the use of divination is particularly pertinent in the case of *nyoné*. Here, there is often a suspicion of spirit involvement, but it may not be clear to those involved how or why a spirit is causing trouble for the afflicted person – or even which particular type of entity might be involved. For example, Dhondup (25, Labrang/Xining) told me that even when you are clear that a person's *nyoné* is caused by some kind of spirit affliction, 'clarification' is probably still needed: 'You might need to find out exactly *which* [deity/spirit] they offended . . . Sometimes it's *really* apparent what it was – in that case, you wouldn't need a diviner or astrologer – but maybe you'll do a divination or an astrological calculation if you haven't figured out exactly what it is'. Similarly, Norbu tells us that in the Bon medical tradition, in cases of suspected spirit affliction, 'first of all divination and astrological calculations are performed to determine how the particular class of being has managed to cause the disturbance, what is the present condition, and how to eliminate it' (1995: 133).

I asked Aku Wangchuk (72) whether a divination was always necessary to determine this kind of causation. He explained: 'Mainly you can definitely use the pulse [to diagnose this], and also from the behaviour of the patient, and also questioning [the patient] – so you use all these diagnostic methods together. Then it should be clear'. However, he added, 'If you really don't understand, then maybe use divination'. Of course, with his training in both Buddhism and medicine, this *ngakpa* was able to conduct these different kinds of diagnosis. But in contemporary Amdo, he was in a minority – one of only a couple of practitioners I met who had knowledge and skill in both spheres – and the vast majority of interviewees described consulting separate medical and religious practitioners for these different types of diagnosis.

These kinds of divinatory practices may be performed by lamas, *ngakpa*s, spirit-mediums or perhaps simply a specialist diviner (Tib. *mopa*) or astrologer (Tib. *tsipa*). There are multiple ways to perform divinations, and in Amdo a number of techniques were discussed by different practitioners. Rebkong *ngakpa* Penpa (53), for example, described performing divination using dice, while, in Xining, Tibetan medicine doctor and *ngakpa* Dr Sonam (69) asserted the utility of both divination and astrology (although he explained that he did not conduct these himself). Moreover, McGrath describes in some detail what are known as '*prasenā*' (Tib. *tsé tra drup*) rituals, which may be used for divination: 'a ritual process through which a practitioner may communicate with the divine', which may be done through various means including 'spontaneous visions and voices' (2019: 266). McGrath tells us that there is a particular genre of *prasenā* divination rituals known as '"channel *prasenā* rituals" (*rtsa'i pra sgrub*)', during which a practitioner supplicates 'either sages or goddesses in order to predict the lifespan of a patient, see pathogenic demons with the aid of divine sight, and intuitively sense the appropriate methods for treatment' (Ibid.: 264). The instruments used can include a butter lamp, earth, iron, the sky, a mirror or even one's own thumb (Ibid.: 268).

It was clear in Amdo that divination might be sought at various points during a case of *nyöné* or other affliction: (i) *before* any diagnosis is sought – to determine which practitioner (or even type of practitioner) to consult in the first instance; (ii) *for* diagnosis of the condition and/or of the type of spirit/deity involved; (iii) *after* diagnosis – to ascertain which type of treatment should be sought, or which particular practitioner or even hospital to visit; and (iv) after a diagnosis and following little or no success with treatment(s), with the understanding that further information is needed to treat the person fully. Thus, we heard in the previous chapter how Norbu and his family sought a divination after consulting multiple practitioners including a biomedical doctor and a lama, none of whom were able to offer a clear diagnosis or treatment path for his father's *nyoné*. The pragmatism of so much health-seeking behaviour is again evident in such narratives, where afflicted individuals and/or their families may utilize multiple diagnostic and healing modalities for a single case of illness. We will see more of this in the process of accessing and utilizing treatment(s) in the next section too, as we move on to an exploration of the types of treatments relevant to spirit- or pollution-caused *nyoné*.

Treatment

In Rebkong, *ngakpa* Penpa (53) had told me that while *nyoné* caused by 'normal' (i.e. non-spirit) causes can be treated by medical therapeutics, '[i]f the person is possessed by, or harmed by, *dön*, there is only *ngak* [mantra/ritual]'. Indeed, this is also emphasized in Tibetan medical texts: in the first chapter of the *Subsequent Tantra*, focused on pulse analysis, for example, we are told that ritual specialists might need to conduct offering and exorcism rites (Tib. *dö*, *tré*) in cases of spirit affliction (*Gyüshi IV* 2015: 561). In other sections, such as those on spirit-caused *nyoné* in the *Oral Instruction*

Tantra, the treatments listed include oil massage, medicinal bath, purgatives, bloodletting[20] and medicinal butter[21] (*Gyüshi III* 2015: 385). Where spirit illnesses are particularly related to *lung*, we find descriptions of medicinal compounds with ingredients including molasses, coriander, ginger, nutmeg, human bones and beer; and ingredients for moxibustion including blue-lotus root, saffron crocus and long pepper. For cases solely related to *dön*, the burning of incense comprising the urine, faeces, bile, nails, hair and skin of cat, ram, owl and/or fox is recommended (*Gyüshi III* 2015: 385). And, as I have also noted elsewhere (Deane 2019a: 326), the Men-Tsee-Khang's Museum in Dharamsala has displays of medicinal ingredients including precious stones such as agate, tiger's eye and quartz described for the treatment of various *dön né*.

In addition, depending on their knowledge and training, some medical and ritual practitioners may use a broad range of treatments detailed in other Tibetan medical texts or elsewhere (Clifford 1984: 199–203). Clifford describes, for example, an 'all-purpose psychiatric incense' made by Dodrag Amchi, a lama–doctor in Bodhnath, Nepal, that was understood to be effective for treating 'insanity' and 'emotional instability' – and that included three varieties of frankincense along with nutmeg, juniper and three types of myrobalan, among other ingredients (Ibid.: 201). Equally, in his 1995 work on the Bon tradition, renowned religious teacher Namkhai Norbu describes the use of yak heart to 'eliminate provocations of energy (*gdon*) caused by the Gyelpo' (1995: 145), and Chui has described the 'secret medicines' listed in commentarial texts for the treatment of conditions including those related to *gyalpo* spirits. Here, we find ingredients such as various animal and human hearts, flesh and blood described in, for example, Sanggye Gyatso's *Extended Commentary on the Instructional Tantra of the Four Tantras*. Similarly, Chui also references Pasang Y. Arya's description of the use of the 'heart of parrot killed by knife' to 'protect one against *gyelpo* spirits and speechlessness due to mental disorders' (Chui 2019: 89, fn. 25).[22] Other medicinal compounds specified for *sok lung* attributed to a 'powerful evil spirit, which is hard to eliminate', include the 'secret medicine' known as 'Fierce Wild Garuda' mixed with multiple herbs and other ingredients (Ibid.: 91).

Moreover, as McGrath notes, 'non-empirical' approaches to diagnosis and treatment – such as divination, mantra recitation and spirit exorcisms – 'can be found throughout the texts of the Tibetan medical tradition' (2019: 263). And indeed, as we have already noted, the importance of ritual interventions for spirit afflictions is clearly conveyed in the *Gyüshi*. In Chapter 12 of the *Explanatory Tantra*, for example, we read that *dön né* can be cured by performing ritual (*Gyüshi II* 2015: 47), and a few pages later, in Chapter 13 ('Behavioural Guidelines'), the importance of 'supreme medicine [Tib. *men chok*], precious stones *and secret mantras* [Tib. *sang ngak*]' are again emphasized (*Gyüshi II* 2015: 48 [italics mine]). In the *Oral Instruction Tantra* too, in the chapters on *dön*, we find religious treatments described. For example, in Chapter 77, it is said that illness caused by elemental spirits will be helped by the recitation of mantras and the making of *torma* and grain offerings, amongst other things (*Gyüshi III* 2015: 383). And in Chapter 3 of the *Subsequent Tantra*, ritual interventions, blessings and the accumulation of merit are also suggested where a spirit affliction has been identified (*Gyüshi IV* 2015: 561). However, as J. Gyatso points out, these descriptions of ritual treatments take up only a small portion of the text ('less than 10 pages, scattered through a work of more than 660 pages') (2015: 422–23, n. 95); instead, there is far more detail to be found in the medical commentaries. Chui describes, for example, how the *Extended Commentary* 'employs a collection of ritualistic and peculiar medicines' which are 'seldom found' in the *Gyüshi* in reference to spirit-caused illnesses (2019: 88).

It is perhaps not surprising, then, that many contemporary Tibetan-medicine doctors also discuss the importance of 'religious' treatments for *dön né*: Pema Dorjee, for example, argues that any pharmacological treatment(s) for spirit affliction would 'always be accompanied by specific spiritual practices' (2005: 41), and Yeshe Donden asserts that ritual practices should be conducted *before* any medicines are taken – otherwise, 'no matter how much medicine is given, it cannot be effective'. Here, he describes activities such as 'the conduct of rituals, giving food offerings, having rites of exorcism performed by competent lamas, receiving blessings, making donations to religious persons, gaining merit through giving to the destitute, and so forth' (1986: 103). Indeed, this echoes the findings of others' research – see, for example, Millard's work on spirit and *drip* afflictions in Dhortapan, Nepal (2007: 260). And in my previous research in Darjeeling too, many of the Tibetans I spoke to emphasized the need for ritual interventions for spirit afflictions rather than medical ones (Deane 2018, 2019a). This was also the case in Amdo, as we saw in Chapter 4, where a majority of interviewees described ritual treatments as the best approach for spirit-related conditions, including *nyoné*. The type of ritual intervention conducted for a case of spirit affliction will depend on a number of factors, including the type of spirit/deity thought to be involved, certain factors related to the afflicted individual and also on the practitioner themselves. For example, in Rebkong, we heard Bon lama Tsering (57) describe how ascertaining the appropriate ritual for someone seeking his assistance involves performing an astrological calculation for the afflicted person, alongside a determination of what type of spirit was involved in this particular case. Equally, *ngakpa* and doctor Aku Wangchuk (72, Rebkong) described the importance of first ascertaining whether the afflicting *dön* is from the upper, middle or lower realm, in order to allow him to prescribe the correct ritual intervention.

Moreover, there are a number of different ways to expel a spirit, as we heard in Chapter 4, with multiple rituals of varying length and form described in different traditions. In Xining, Tibetan medicine doctor and *ngakpa* Dr Sonam (69) described 'three versions' of such rituals: 'longest; middle; and shortest', the longest 'probably' lasting a full day. In contrast, *ngakpa* Penpa (53, Rebkong) told me that the longest ritual he knew of for dealing with *dön* took ten days. As we have seen, methods of expulsion include tempting a spirit with offering cakes and casting it away from, or out of, the afflicted individual with force. In Zangskar, for example, Gutschow has described ritual treatment whereby the rinpoche performed a ritual commanding the spirits to leave the man's body and go instead into ritual effigies prepared by his assistants. Following this, the rinpoche blessed the afflicted man, and gave him an amulet to 'ward off' any future spirits from attacking him (1997: 193–95). In such rituals, as we heard described by Dr Sonam in the previous chapter, the afflicting spirit(s) are made to enter the effigy and then destroyed within it: the spirit's body is offered to the Tantric deities represented in the mandala, with its consciousness 'sent to rebirth in the heaven of Guru Rimpoch'e' (Samuel 1993: 265). Similarly, Norbu has described Bon 'ransom' rituals, which involve drawing an afflicting spirit away from the person (or people) it is harming and into an effigy, usually made of barley flour.[23] One such example is the class of *dö* rites, which are aimed at stopping the harm being caused by spirits including *lha*, *lu*, *nyen* and *gyalpo* (Norbu 1995: 77).

In Rebkong, former monk Tsetan (38) explained how the nature of the afflicting spirit can determine how it is dealt with:

> Some spirits should be killed, rather than controlled. This depends on how the spirit acts – for example, if the spirit is really dangerous, it's better to kill it . . . if it is not really dangerous, or not really powerful, then it can be controlled. For example, the *zhidak* [mountain deities] listen to lamas – the lamas can order them to do this, and not do that . . . or to protect this [particular] village or place. These kinds of spirits can be controlled.

In Xining, doctor and *ngakpa* Dr Sonam (69) described how particularly powerful spirits that are difficult to deal with must be brought into a fire to kill them. He described such a ritual being performed close to his village after the patient's family had already tried many methods to rid him of this *dön*, none of which had proven successful. Dr Sonam described how, during this ritual, as the *ngakpa* made the required fire and started to put objects into it to burn, the afflicted man – sitting in the next room – exclaimed, 'It's so hot, I am burning!' Dr Sonam added that recovery following ritual intervention is often 'very fast' – in some cases, he said, a patient's condition is clearly becoming 'better, better, better' even while the ritual is being conducted.

A range of religious texts may be used in these kinds of rituals. For example, Wallace describes 'Tantric medicinal *mantras*' mentioned in the *Kālacakra Tantra* (Tib. *dus kyi 'khor lo rgyud*), including in the sixth section of the 'Chapter on the Individual' (vs. 107–60), where she notes some discussion on 'ritual tantric methods of protecting pregnant women and infants from diseases caused by malevolent spirits' (2001: 24). Lopez has translated a ritual based around the *Heart Sutra* text (1997),[24] which he notes is described as being a cure for a 'wide range of calamities, misfortunes, dangers, and afflictions', including spirit possessions. Here, this Buddhist text is used as a mantra: during the process of the ritual, the Sutra is repeated 252 times, and the offending spirit is tempted away from an afflicted person and into an effigy (Tib. *ngar mi*) or 'ransom' (Tib. *lü*) of him/her, before being 'both cajoled and threatened' to agree to 'release the patron [i.e. host] from their power'. Interestingly, Lopez notes here the combination of elements of 'pre-Buddhist Tibetan religious practice' (particularly the creation and use of a dough effigy) and Buddhist elements (for example, the fact that the work is 'structured like a standard Buddhist *sādhana*' and based on a key Mahayana Buddhist text) (Ibid.: 215–16), highlighting again the multilayered nature of human–spirit relations in Tibetan communities. And in Muses' edited translation of *The Initiation Ritual of the Fierce Guru with Phurba*, we read that this initiation can also be used to treat cases of *sok lung* illness or other 'mental disturbances' – including *nyoné* – caused by *gyalpo* spirits, where no other treatments have worked. It is explained that for an afflicted Tantric practitioner who has been unable to overcome this through other means, the initiation ritual should be practised one thousand times in front of him/her – this will 'definitely' bring about a cure. However, for a lay person similarly afflicted, we read that only 108 or 216 repetitions of the mantra will be necessary to cure them (Muses 1961: 39).

And finally, another form of treatment that spans these overlapping medical and religious spheres, and which may also be utilized in the treatment of *dön né*, is the use of a variety of 'precious pills' (Tib. *rinchen rilbu*), which we also saw briefly in Chapter 2. These compounds contain 'between twenty-five and 160 plants and minerals', alongside 'precious' ingredients such as gold; silver; rubies; diamonds; turquoise; and, famously, *tsotel* – a compound of processed mercury sulphide and other metals and rock components (Gerke and Ploberger 2017: 583). Drungtso describes, for example, the 'precious wish-fulfilling jewel', which is based on a thirteenth-/fourteenth-century formula containing around seventy ingredients and which can be used for the treatment of numerous conditions including fainting, hypertension, impaired sense organs, insanity and 'sudden ailments caused by different spirits' (2004: 481). These pills are usually accompanied by specific instructions for their ingestion (for example, to be taken at a specific time of day, on a particular day) and, as Samuel notes, these types of pills are based on the 'alchemical tradition of Indian *Vajrayāna* medicine' rather than the *Gyüshi* (Samuel 2007: 216, fn. 4).[25]

Moreover, there may also be certain things that patients, and/or their families, can do themselves to improve the situation, or to prevent it reoccurring. For example, in the *Kālacakra Tantra*, we read that 'carrying a precious stone of the color red, which belongs to the class of the substances that predominantly arise from the fire-element, is believed to prevent evil spirits from entering one's body' (Wallace 2001: 50). And Rapgay describes how practices 'designed to ward off further harmful influences' can be beneficial – for example, activities that generate merit (Tib. *sonam*) are understood to be helpful when the accrued merit can 'subdue' negative influences (1985: 51–52). In Amdo, Nyingma lama Namgyal (32, Chabcha) told me that often a lama can recommend some Buddhist texts for the afflicted person to chant daily. And Clifford references Patrul Rinpoche's suggestions, which include 'performing charitable and virtuous activities' and wearing 'blessed protection circles and charms as amulets' (1984: 165) – something also described by Gutschow in the context of Zangskar (1997: 194), above. Similarly, in Rebkong, Rinchen (26) described a combination of treatments for *nyoné* and other illnesses caused by wearing the clothes of someone with a different family god: 'I think the lama can fix it – they can give you a special amulet, and then they do some ritual'. In more complex cases, as we saw in the narrative of Norbu's father's illness, there may be a 'connection' or 'relationship' to an offending spirit or deity that needs to be dealt with. As we saw in that case, not only was a ritual intervention performed to deal with the *gyalpo* but Norbu himself broke off his relationship with his girlfriend – the relationship that was understood to be tying his family to the *gyalpo* causing harm.

With several factors potentially involved in one case of illness, it is not surprising to hear people describe the use of multiple potential treatment modalities across the interrelated spheres of medicine and religion. Again, we see the pragmatism of so much health-seeking behaviour: in cases such as spirit-caused *nyoné*, a patient and/or their family might wish to address not only the particular spirit understood to be causing trouble but also the luck and spiritual power that have contributed to this particular person (rather than their neighbour, for example) becoming afflicted. Moreover, with *lung* or another of the *nyépa* most likely disrupted either as cause or consequence of a spirit affliction, it would make sense to also seek medical treatment(s) to address this aspect of causation.

However, as I have already mentioned, it was notable in Amdo that the vast majority of people I spoke to advised consulting a Buddhist rather than any kind of medical practitioner for cases of *nyoné* understood to be related to *dön* and/or *mi tsangwa* – despite the broad variety of medicinal treatments delineated in the *Gyüshi* and other Tibetan medical texts for *dön né*. This is something described by other researchers too. Samuel notes, for example, that in many Tibetan communities, in reality, spirit afflictions are less often diagnosed by Tibetan medicine doctors, and more often via divination by a religious specialist (2009: 93). I think that there are a number of reasons for this – not least the fact that in Amdo (as I had also experienced in Darjeeling), several Tibetan medicine doctors reported being unfamiliar with the *Gyüshi*'s chapters on spirits, and were rarely consulted for conditions thought to be related to spirit afflictions. In Rebkong, Gelugpa lama Wangyal (62) asserted that 'many Tibetan medicine doctors in contemporary society have a hard time identifying these things' – this kind of diagnosis of *dön né*, he told me, 'can only be done by very skilful and specialized [Tibetan medicine] doctors'.

This lack of familiarity is a result of multiple factors, not least the fact that, as J. Gyatso describes, while the *Gyüshi* describes multiple forces that can contribute to illness, 'including karma, luck, behavior, state of mind, and even demons', in reality, 'it is most concerned with imbalances of the humors in the body and physical injuries', and there are no instructions for the doctor here on 'how to become adept at healing rites or magic' (2015: 393). In Amdo, I met two practitioners who were specialists in both Tibetan medicine and Buddhist ritual, one of whom, Dr Sonam (69), worked at a Tibetan medicine hospital. But these kinds of practitioners were not the norm in contemporary Amdo, and the vast majority of practitioners I interviewed were specialists of *either* medicine or religion. In communities like this in the PRC, changes in medical training over the past few decades have led to increased divisions between the so-called 'medical' and 'religious' spheres, with a majority of contemporary Tibetan medicine practitioners not learning so-called 'religious' aspects of Tibetan medicine. In Lhasa too, Vargas has described a 'reticence' from not only Tibetan medicine doctors but also other hospital staff and professors in the medical college to talk about spirits and spirit illnesses, as a result of the state-sanctioned 'separation' of religion from medicine (2009: 374). And, as Dr Sonam explained, while he was able to conduct ritual treatments for his patients, such rituals are not allowed to be performed by doctors inside the hospital – they are deemed, he said, 'too religious': 'It's against the discipline here. They do it somewhere else – not here – it is not allowed [in the hospital]'.[26] Equally, he was unable to teach his medical students such rituals, which he himself had learnt in the course of his *ngakpa* study. Instead, he told me, for such cases he would prescribe any medicinal treatments and perform any required external therapies (such as moxibustion, which I watched him do for a patient one day) in his hospital clinic, and then later conduct any necessary ritual treatments for the patient in his own home, outside of his hospital working hours.

*

It is clear from these discussions that notions of spirit affliction have a significant part to play in Tibetan understandings of *nyoné*, its causation and treatment – both in Tibetan medical and religious texts, and within Tibetan communities. Also evident is a diversity in perspectives with regard to the different kinds of spirits and deities likely to be involved in cases of *nyoné*, and also their relationship – or not – with *mi tsangwa* or *drip*. As we have seen, afflictions from spirits and deities may or may not involve possession, but, either way, *lung* is again significant here – a spirit or deity's 'subtle' nature enabling it to affect humans. Moreover, the ways in which the causation and treatment of spirit afflictions are explained through concepts of 'spiritual power' illustrate the hierarchical nature of human–deity relationships so key to Tibetans' understanding of the world and their place within it. Here, in both Buddhist and Bon communities, Tantric practitioners have a vital role in mediating between humans and non-human entities, the power they access through their Tantric practices being fundamental to their abilities to subjugate spirits and deities in a way that lay people cannot. Through these ritual services performed for, and within, the local community, the Tantric practitioner thus enacts again and again the narrative of Padmasambhava's 'taming' of Tibet and its landscape – or, in the case of Bon practitioners, a similar narrative of Tonpa Shenrab's 'taming' of Tibet.

As we have seen here, there are often multiple factors at play that influence contemporary Tibetans' health-seeking behaviour around spirit-caused *nyoné*, including limited knowledge about Tibetan medical theory amongst many lay people, and changes in Tibetan medicine doctors' knowledge and practice. In this way, illnesses thought to be related to *dön* and/or *mi tsangwa* may be either taken to a Tantric specialist in the first instance or perhaps diagnosed through a process of elimination via hospital biomedical tests that prove inconclusive. It is clear from these narratives that while there may be diverse perspectives on different types of *dön* and *mi tsangwa* in different communities, the effects of these human–deity relations are keenly felt by many – being fundamental to the ways in which health, illness and healing continue to be understood in many contemporary Tibetan communities, and sometimes even emphasized by the failure of medicine to treat these kinds of illnesses.

Notes

1. There is a vast amount of anthropological research in this area – much of it, as Samuel notes, taking a predominantly functional approach to this topic, exploring notions of spirit attack 'as a way of dealing with situations of structural inferiority and vulnerability'

(2007: 220). And during her own work in Xining as both doctor and researcher, Tidwell references Cassaniti and Luhrmann's more recent 2014 theory of 'cultural kindling', whereby 'spiritual experiences' are 'formed, learned, embodied, interpreted, recognized – kindled – and confirmed through sociocultural looping processes' (Tidwell, Nianggajia and Fjeld 2022: 810). There is unfortunately not the space to explore the various theoretical approaches to spirit afflictions and related experiences here; instead, we shall limit our discussion to Amdo narratives as they were presented to me, in relation to some Tibetan medical and Tantric textual descriptions of these categories and experiences. I hope future research will explore some of these ideas in more depth in this context.

2. See Karmay 1972 for more on this topic. In fact, this narrative of a 'taming' of the landscape by Dharma practitioners could be said to be a 'common motif' in Tibetan communities: Millard describes a Bon narrative in Dhortapan, Nepal, about a more recent Bon lama, Tsultrim Nyima, who was said to have conducted a similar taming of troublesome local spirits when Tibetans first arrived in the area in the 1960s (2005 and 2006: 11).
3. In some Tibetan communities, there may also be spirit-mediums who deal with low-level spirits and deities (something I have also discussed in my previous research focused on Darjeeling [Deane 2018]). However, in Amdo, few of my interviewees mentioned spirit-mediums in our discussions on *nyoné* and its treatment unless I brought them up – usually then explaining that such practitioners were rare in Xining and/or their own home town, although some people had heard of them working in other regions. The Rebkong valley has its own specific tradition of spirit-mediums related to the annual summer Lurol festival. We will explore this topic a little more in the next chapter.
4. These sit alongside the fundamental 'causes' (Tib *gyu*) of *lung*, *tripa* and *béken*.
5. As I have noted elsewhere (Deane 2018: 95), this interpretation is reflective of some of the psychodynamic theories of psychology that focus on the role of the unconscious and which were more prominent in Western psychiatry in the decades prior to the 1980s, at a time of growing interest in and knowledge of Tibetan religion and culture. I think it worth noting the impact of drives to 'secularize' the Tibetan medical tradition here too. Vargas describes, for example, how in the 'increasingly secularized and/or "biomedical" Tibetan environment [such] as the Mentsikhang and the Tibetan Medical College in Lhasa', where medical training is 'focused on being "scientific" and secular in its theoretical and practical content', spirit illnesses are 'mostly described in empirical and psychological terms, often focused on symptomatology'. She adds, 'At the medical college, students are taught that *klu* and *gdon* either do not really exist or are mental projections of some kind', and describes illnesses traditionally attributed to spirit affliction being instead referred to as 'environmental diseases' (Vargas 2009: 373). I discuss this secularization and its impacts on health-seeking behaviour in more detail in Deane (2024).
6. Here, Millard found that, while *all* cases of 'mental illness' were related (at least in part) to *nöpa*, *not all* cases of *nöpa* were related to mental illness – with a majority, instead, being 'physical disorders' (2007: 263).
7. From this perspective, they can be understood as devoid of any intrinsic existence. However, from a Buddhist or Bon philosophical point of view, in fact, we are *all* devoid of intrinsic existence – so this is not a simple solution of spirits being 'unreal' in comparison with 'real' humans.
8. One of the first English-language accounts of Tibetan spirits and deities was Réne de Nebesky-Wojkowitz's *Oracles and Demons of Tibet* (1956; reissued 1993). More recent

research has examined these entities in greater detail (see, for example, Anne-Marie Blondeau 1998).

9. In fact, this list usually includes ten classes of deities: *lu*, *sa dak*, *nyen*, *tsen*, *gyalpo*, *dü*, *ma mo*, *za*, *nö jin* and *lha* (Samuel 1993: 161–63, Cornu 1997: 247–53).
10. Norbu notes that this is a classification also found in the Bon tradition (1995: 143).
11. In addition, *gyalpo* are described by some as particularly dangerous: as a result of their previous lives as religious practitioners, they are understood to hold significant knowledge and power (Calkowski 1985: 107).
12. The corresponding chapters in the *Bumshi* text are Chapters 83–87 of the third volume.
13. https://tibetanmedicine-edu.org/tmm/tm/psychology-and-psychiatry/psychology-and-psychiatry/ [retrieved April 2024]. See also Donden (1997), Drungtso (2004) and Clifford (1984) for English-language discussions on these spirit illnesses.
14. In relation to my findings in Darjeeling, see Deane (2018, 2019a); for more on how a 'secularization' of medical training inside China over the past few decades has impacted on doctors' knowledge and practice, see Adams (2001, 2007), Deane (2024) and Hofer (2018). Add to this the fact that these chapters on spirit illness are not easy to interpret – there is much abbreviation, and the assistance of a knowledgeable scholar/practitioner is usually necessary to make sense of it (Clifford 1984: 173) – and we can understand why many contemporary Tibetan medicine practitioners may profess a lack of familiarity with these sections of the text.
15. I have examined this in more detail elsewhere (Deane 2018, 2019a). See Deane 2019a for a narrative of spirit affliction and the impact of differential levels of 'spiritual power' on the harms caused to the afflicted individual and also her friend in Darjeeling.
16. See Deane 2018 and 2019a for more on this topic.
17. Intention is also relevant here: as Lichter and Epstein explain, while intention is key in matters of *sonam* and karma, it is unimportant in matters related to conditions/secondary causes such as offending or harming any local spirits or deities (1983: 242).
18. 'Provocation' is a fairly common translation of *dön* in some of the contemporary English-language literature on this topic, perhaps indicating a discomfort with some of the more traditional translations such as 'spirits' or 'demons' that we see in older works – particularly, perhaps, when writing for Western audiences. In addition, some contemporary Tibetan medicine doctors have taken an integrative approach to this topic, such as Thubten Phuntsok's description of how the 'eight classes on nonhuman beings get angry and create all kinds of bacteria and viruses', or how 'unclean circumstances' can lead to 'problems with blood and wind circulation', with the potential to lead to 'depression or schizophrenia' (2015: 72).
19. The text does not specify what grains might be used here; perhaps barley, rice, and/or any other grains available to practitioners in different regions.
20. Interestingly, this seems to contradict the assertion in the *Subsequent Tantra* that bloodletting is contraindicated for conditions caused by spirits (*Gyüshi IV* 2015: 621).
21. See Clifford for a list of the ingredients for this substance in English (1984: 186).
22. Here, a link is made between the violence of the death from which some of these substances are obtained and the potency of the resulting medicine (Chui 2019).
23. For a description of a Bon effigy ritual conducted in a Tibetan community in Nepal for a woman thought to be unwell from a spirit attack, see Millard (2005 and 2006: 24–25).
24. The full title of this ritual text is *The Procedure for Repelling Demons Based on the Heart Sutra, The Summation of the Vast, Intermediate, and Condensed Mothers*, and the text is attributed to Kumārabuddha.

25. In fact, Samuel noticed in his own research that people may often be rather relaxed about these specific instructions (Samuel 2007: 216, fn. 4). See Gerke and Ploberger (2017) for a translation of the *Gyüshi*'s chapter on *rinchen rilbu.*
26. As Dr Nyima (38) pointed out, such rituals are usually noisy – including chanting, drums and other instruments, and often involving multiple practitioners – so they could not be 'hidden' in these hospital settings.

Chapter 6

Invoking the Gods

Spirits and Deities in Tantric Practice

[T]hrough the force of our meditating on an imagined Deity body, eventually our continuously residing body, or very subtle wind, will become an actual Deity body.

—Geshe Kelsang Gyatso, *Tantric Grounds and Paths*

In Chapter 4, we heard again about cases of *nyoné* related to Tantric practice – this time in relation to those practices focused on a practitioner's intentional dealings with spirits and deities. For example, we heard former Gelug monk Tsetan (38, Rebkong) describe how *nyoné* can be caused by 'incomplete' deity yoga practice, where a practitioner has forgotten some of the steps in the practice or was not sufficiently prepared to undertake it. In addition, multiple Amdo interviewees described the risks arising from *chöd* practice – during which a practitioner engages with (unenlightened) low-level spirits – citing such factors as a practitioner losing control of these entities, or struggling with 'doubt' or fearfulness during practice.

In this final chapter, we will explore what exactly practitioners are doing in these Buddhist and Bon deity yoga and *chöd* practices, and for what purpose. This will help us to understand the various ways in which their endeavours might 'go wrong' – potentially leading to *nyoné* or other problems. In deity yoga practices, we are again looking at methods to attain realization through manipulation of the mind-body. In Chapter 3, we saw this described in terms of the Tantric *tsa lung* practices; here, we find this achieved through a practitioner's visualization of him/herself as an enlightened deity – a practice described as the 'essential method' of achieving buddhahood by the renowned fourteenth-century Tibetan Buddhist master Tsongkhapa (Lopez 2000: 525). And, much like the *tsa lung* practices explored in Part I, these deity yoga practices too are understood to be complex and difficult – suitable only for practitioners sufficiently prepared and initiated by their teachers. We will hear again about the problems of *namtok*, and this exploration will also bring us back to the figure of the *lama nyonpa* ('mad lama'), whom we last saw in Chapter 3. Long described in fond terms in Tibetan literature, this practitioner is said to appear mad to ordinary folk – *as a result of his enlightened state*. However, as we shall see here, some scholars have argued that his outlandish appearance and activities can be viewed simply as a mimicing of Tantric deities. Here, questions about non-duality and performance come to the fore again as we try to make sense of extraordinary tales, both historical and contemporary.

And finally, we will briefly examine a class of Tibetan religious practitioners who intentionally seek possession by deities – the *lhawa* (spirit-mediums). The crucial difference here, of course, is that these practitioners are working with *un*enlightened deities, usually in order to perform divinations and/or healing. While only occasionally mentioned in this context in Amdo, such spirit-mediums are well established in many Tibetan communities. Particularly interesting to our discussion here is the initial period of 'madness' that many such practitioners experience prior to their identification as a spirit-medium, as we shall explore below.

Enlightened Gods: Deity Practice in Tibetan Tantra

Tibetan Buddhist and Bon deity yoga practices (Tib. *lhé neljor*) are focused on the evocation of an array of Tantric *yidam (lha)* – 'tutelary deities'. On initial exploration, it may sound as if a practitioner is *taking on possession* by a Tantric deity or perhaps simply *imagining* him/herself as that figure. In fact, again, what we are actually talking about is a *total transformation* of the practitioner, whereby he/she ultimately aims to transform him/herself *into* the chosen enlightened deity through complex, multi-stage, mind-body practices. This is, asserts Germano, the 'imaginative appropriation of a new subjectivity, self-identity, and body-image as a male or female buddha' (1997: 314). Moreover, while these practices are key to Tibetan Buddhist and Bon traditions, Samuel in fact describes a pre-Vajrayana history to this process in Mahayana Buddhist communities, where 'the basic orientation of the practice of Buddha recollection (*buddhāntcsmṛti*)' developed by focusing on summoning buddhas and communicating with them. He describes how practitioners increasingly sought to identify with these figures 'as a mode of obtaining insight' (2008: 259), and we can see the ultimate result of this 'identification' in some of the Tibetan practices that we will explore here.

As with the *tsa lung* practices described in Part I, we are speaking here not only about altering one's 'consciousness' but about the 'mind-body complex as a whole' (Samuel 2010: 40). This is a complex process by which, as J. Gyatso asserts, the 'visualized identity' of a Tantric deity is effected across 'three dimensions of personhood: bodily form, verbal expression, and mental state'. Here, she explains, an understanding that 'a person's identity, experience, and existence are self-created' – and can therefore be wilfully manipulated – allows the possibility of this transformation for a practitioner in possession of the correct training and skill (J. Gyatso 1997: 266). Thus, twentieth-century Nyingma scholar Khetsun Sangpo explains that, as part of this process, practitioners must 'put aside' their ordinary sense of themselves: 'Instead, we think that our body is the body of the enlightened deity associated with our practice' (Klein and Sangpo 1997: 540). Here, the notion of 'divine pride' (Tib. *lhé nga gyallhé nga gyel*) is key, as Harding explains:

> Generally, this means maintaining the deep sense of actually being the deity, pure and perfect in every way. It is not the feeling of dressing up in a costume and mask, assuming another weird form, or superimposing an alien personality on top of the old one. A sense of confidence in being the actual deity counteracts one's sense of ordinariness and frees one from all the limitations usually imposed by our mundane sense of self. (Harding in Kongtrul 1996: 16)

Initiation

Key to deity yoga is a practitioner's initiation or 'empowerment' (Tib. *wang*) into each practice, whereby the student is 'formally introduced and admitted to the *maṇḍala*', and the relevant Tantric text (often both in verse and 'quite condensed') is 'explained in detail' (Samuel 1993: 244–45) by the Tantric teacher. During this process, the student is also initiated into a 'relationship' with the *yidam*: 'Once initiated, practitioners are empowered to accomplish, emulate, and experience themselves as the deity' (Klein and Sangpo 1997: 540).[1] For example, Bentor describes the 'ripening initiation' – so-called because it 'activates the disciples' capacities to engage in the practice':

> In receiving initiation, the disciples gain the first inner experience of the meditation, such as seeing themselves as enlightened beings. When both guru and disciple are worthy, the disciple shares in the meditation of his or her guru. They also share in the meditation of the entire lineage of teachers, who have achieved direct experience in that meditation. (Bentor 2000: 329)

Bentor quotes a twelfth/thirteenth-century text, *The Outline of the Jewel Mound of Instructions* (Tib. *man ngag rin chen spungs pa'i dkar chag*) and its description of 'two essential roles of the initiation: 'cleansing the disciples' impurities and endowing them with efficacy'[2] (2000: 329). Initiations vary in complexity, but key here is the 'guru' – the teacher – who becomes an 'external, identifiable form' of the enlightened deity. Consequently, the student's relationship with their guru is integral to practice: the 'connecting factor between one's own buddha nature and the visualized deity' (Harding in Kongtrul 1996: 12), and the 'covenant' (Tib. *dam tshig*, Skt. *samaya*) between student and teacher must be protected and respected, or it is thought that these practices will not be successful (Ibid.: 11–12).

Yidam *Deities*

Many *yidam* deities are understood to be manifested forms taken by enlightened beings in order to impart teachings to humans. Here, the deity represents the second of the 'three bodies of the Buddha' (Tib. *kyu sum*, Skt. *trikāya*): the heavenly body (Tib. *long chö dzok pé ku*; Skt. *saṃbhogakāya*), key to Mahayana and Vajrayana Buddhist and Bon doctrine. Some of these *yidam* are common across Mahayana traditions while others are specific to Tibetan traditions, including some figures who are based on historical lamas. Some – such as Avalokiteśvara and Tārā – will be well known by lay Tibetans: a focus of devotion, they are often depicted in statues and murals at monasteries, as well as in the form of Tibetan *thangka* paintings and/or statues in Tibetan homes and other buildings. Other deities are relatively unknown to lay people, and are only really the concern of those practitioners who work with them in their Tantric practice (Samuel 1993: 165).

However, these figures are not only heavenly deities residing in celestial realms known as 'pure lands'. They are also understood to correspond to 'real potentialities' both within human beings and in 'the universe as a whole' (Samuel 1993: 164). Here, a *yidam* represents a particular state of 'mind-body configuration', the potential for which exists in all of us. It is thus through practising with a deity that a practitioner is able to 'manifest' this aspect (Samuel 2001a: 80–81). Consequently, while it may be tempting to categorize these entities from a dualistic perspective – are they 'real' deities, or merely symbolic? – this question cannot be answered so simply. The *yidam* can be both a deity within the cosmos *and* a potentiality within any person:[3] if we all have an innate buddha-mind, as is understood in Mahayana and Vajrayana Buddhism and Bon, then theoretically any one of us can access this enlightened potentially through the correct practice. Here, such Tantric deities are both *result* and *method* of these practices: a manifestation of the pure mind of enlightenment, and a route to achieve it. In this way, a Tantric deity's 'existence' can be understood to be a *result* of Tantric practice: as Samuel explains, a Tantric deity such as Avalokiteśvara, for example, 'is brought into existence through the millions of Tibetans who do Avalokiteśvara practices, develop appropriate qualities, and thus, to a certain degree, "become" Avalokiteśvara' (1993: 247).[4]

Nonetheless, in Amdo, lay people often discussed these figures in quite tangible terms – for example, deities who were the recipients of their prayers and offerings, or figures who might protect them. Again, here we see that such entities may be conceptualized in different ways by different people, and perhaps at different times. Indeed, the discussions I had in Amdo illustrated Samuel's assertion that these entities are 'not understood in the same way by all Tibetans, or even all lamas' (1993: 248).

Becoming a Deity: Generation and Completion Stages in Deity Yoga Practice

As mentioned in Chapter 4, deity yoga practices form the 'generation stage' (Tib. *kyé rim*) of the *Anuttarayoga Tantras* in the Sarmapa Buddhist traditions, the *Mahāyoga Tantras* of the Nyingma Buddhist tradition and the eighth of the Nine Vehicles of Bon. However, slightly confusingly for the non-expert, as Cozort explains, *within* deity yoga we can also talk about a 'generation stage' and a 'completion stage'. In the former, the practitioner 'generates a vivid imaginative visualization of one's transformation into a deity'; in the latter, the practitioner 'completes' this transformation by 'actually bringing about a new physical structure, that is, by transforming one into an actual deity, a Buddha' (1986: 27). While this means that these *yidam* practices actually come *before* the *tsa lung* practices we explored in Part I, deity yoga practices are also complex and difficult high-level practices within the traditions.

Evocation instructions for deity yoga practices can vary significantly in length, but will all contain five essential elements: i) refuge and arousing of *bodhicitta*, ii) visualization of the Tantric deity, iii) homage and recitation of that deity's mantra, iv) dissolution into emptiness and v) conclusion and dedication of merit accrued (Samuel 1993: 233–34). In addition, some of these practices may also include 'preparatory purifications' of the practitioner and the environment, and the more complex visualizations will incorporate the multiple deities of the *yidam*'s mandala – all of which must be 'visualized precisely' by the practitioner (Ibid.: 234–36) – and/or 'lengthy discussion of the symbolic significance of all the details mentioned in the description' (Cozort 1986: 81). These are designed to enhance the practitioner's 'divine pride' – i.e. 'the sense that one actually *is* the deity one imagines'. The meditator is often assisted in this task by the use of a *thangka* (Tibetan painting, often on silk or cotton cloth) based on the textual description of the deity in its mandala (Ibid.).

In the generation stage of deity yoga practice, the practitioner must recreate and hold in their mind the extremely detailed depiction of a chosen *yidam* within its buddha realm. The *yidam* (in either peaceful or wrathful form) is usually depicted at the centre, with or without a consort and/or subsidiary deities or other figures. For example, Samuel explains the 'basic structure' of a mandala assembly: '[A] central deity surrounded by four or (especially for the Nyingmapa) eight other deities, who are conceived of as aspects of, or projections from, the central *yidam*. Each deity may have a consort, and there may be several circles of such deities, with attendant figures, adding up to several hundred deities' (1993: 235–36).

As we can imagine, then, recreating and holding this in one's mind is no easy task for a practitioner – Samuel describes the 'considerable' imaginative control required here (1993: 236), referencing Jackson's description in relation to the *Kālacakra Tantra*:

> One is said to have accomplished the generation stage of the Kalacakra when one can visualize the entire *maṇḍala* in a drop the size of a mustard seed at the tip of one's nose, with such clarity that one can see the whites of the eyes of all 722 deities – and can maintain this visualization with uninterrupted one-pointed concentration for four hours. (Jackson 1985: 32)

Following success in this generation stage, in the completion stage of deity yoga practice, the practitioner aims to *become* that deity within its mandala – ultimately, there is 'full union' between practitioner and *yidam*, as Harding explains: 'the guru's mind and the disciple's mind are recognized as identical (*thug.r yid dbyer med*), and all the enlightened attributes of the guru are reclaimed as one's own' (Harding in Kongtrul 1996: 12). In his explanatory text, contemporary scholar G.K. Gyatso (1931–2022) explained that through continued practice:

> we shall gradually perceive that Deity body more and more clearly. The generic image will become more and more transparent until it finally disappears altogether and we attain a yogic direct perceiver of the imagined Deity body. If we then improve this yogic direct perceiver by means of completion stage practices, eventually we shall obtain the actual divine body, the illusory body. (1994: 79)

Thus, for example, when conducting *yidam* practice focused on the deity Heruka, the practitioner's illusory body becomes 'the shape of Heruka' (G.K. Gyatso 1994: 177), and the practitioner not only transforms him/herself into the deity but also transforms his/her very *environment* into the environment of the deity. Bentor explains:

> By means of the generation process, ordinary perception of the world and its contents – all its inhabitants – dissolves away and is replaced with the mandala and the enlightened beings inhabiting it. Through such practice, one conceptualization is replaced with another – though the later conceptualization is somewhat more 'true,' since it is in this form that actual reality appears to enlightened beings. However, the shift from one conceptualization to another demonstrates both the relative nature of each and the workings of the human mind in creating such conceptualizations. The nature of mental construction is more apparent with regard to the mandala than with regard to the external world, and this serves to illuminate the dreamlike nature of ordinary reality, as well. Eventually both conceptualizations will dissolve. (Bentor 2000: 330–31)

Eventually, the practitioner's visualization of themself as 'an enlightened being at the center of a mandala' is 'gathered back . . . and dissolved into emptiness'. Indeed, this 'dissolution' illustrates the true nature of the visualization as 'an empty illusion', which also works to prevent the practitioner developing 'attachment to the reality created through the generation itself' (Bentor 2000: 332).

Perhaps unsurprisingly, when we are talking about this transformation of the mind-body of a practitioner, the subtle-body system is again key. For example, in the *Kālacakra Tantra*, it is explained that the 'limitless karmic winds generate the numerous world-systems of the Buddhafields' in the same way that 'the karmic winds of the *prāṇas* . . . generate the body of a sentient being' (Wallace 2001: 57). What this means for deity yoga practice can be illustrated by a description from Cozort, where we can see similarities with the completion practices that we explored in Chapter 3:

> Within the vivid visualization of oneself as a deity and one's environment as divine, one practices penetrative focusing on important points of the body, causing the currents of energy (winds) that course through the body to enter and dissolve in the central channel and then into the indestructible drop in the center of the heart. Using the very subtle and powerful mind of 'clear light' that dawns as a result of the total dissolution of the winds in the indestructible drop, one realizes emptiness. Rising up in the form of a deity in an illusory body – a body made of wind – and meditating on emptiness with a mind of clear light, one swiftly amasses the collections of wisdom and method, overcomes all of the obstructions to liberation and omniscience, and achieves the final rank of Buddhahood. (Cozort 1986: 65–66)

Lama Nyonpa

In exploring deity yoga practices, we must also return again to the *lama nyonpa*, who we first met in Part I. One aspect of their practice is particularly relevant here: in Chapter 3, we explored the 'Practice of the Observance', during which the practitioner is expected to take on 'new dress, practices, and attitudes toward the world' while wandering homeless for a period of time (DiValerio 2015: 41–42). In his in-depth work on this topic, DiValerio has described how, for some such practitioners, copying the dress of a wrathful Tantric deity was an 'essential' aspect of their practice (Ibid.: 43). Thus, we find descriptions of historical practitioners such as the Madmen of Ü and Tsang, Künga Zangpo and Tsangnyon Heruka respectively, all imitating Heruka[5] in terms of clothing and hairstyle. For example, much of Künga Zangpo's dress followed the iconography of Cakrasaṃvara, apparently including 'wearing a human skin in addition to the tiger pelt prescribed in the tantras' (Ibid.: 48–49, 58). Indeed, DiValerio concludes that Künga Zangpo was going beyond instructions on dress in these texts, 'dressing as best he could like the deity himself' (Ibid.: 58) – he and Tsangnyon Heruka enacting a 'sort of lived deity yoga' through their behaviour (Ibid.: 63). In this way, these famous *lama nyonpa* 'lived as the deity in the present: dressing like him, speaking like him, acting like him' – turning 'long periods of their lives into a very literal form of deity yoga', enacting their union with him both 'bodily and publicly' (Ibid.), and 'citing the tantras' in justification (Ibid.: 67). Indeed, Künga Zangpo was described in one text as 'identical' to the deity Cakrasaṃvara, and Tsangnyon Heruka as 'Great Vajrasattva, in the form of a man' (Ibid.: 64–65). Moreover, some of these renowned *lama nyonpa* were even said to be emanations of particular Tantric deities, such as the fourteenth-century female practitioner Sönam Peldren, who claimed to be an emanation of Vajravāhārī (Ibid.: 225).

Again we see that this figure of the 'mad lama' might be interpreted in a several ways: as an emanation of a specific Tantric deity . . . or simply as a practitioner *performing* the role of the deity through his/her behaviours and dress. And, as we saw in Chapter 3, this 'performance' itself can also have multiple layers: both a way to aid the practitioner in their quest to overcome duality and as a way to teach others the same. And there may be different appraisals of these characters by different observers, with some proclaiming them 'fake'; others viewing them as enlightened, holy madmen; and others still seeing them as suffering from 'madness' in an ordinary sense. For example, DiValerio notes that one biography states that Tsangnyon Heruka's unusual mode of dress led some to mistake him for a demon while others 'wondered if he was a *siddha*' (2015: 66).

Working with Spirits: *Chöd*, Ransom Rites and Subjugation of Spirits and Deities

Chöd

As we have seen in the previous two chapters, a number of Buddhist and Bon Tantric practices necessitate engaging with a variety of spirits and local deities – some of which were discussed in relation to cases of *nyoné* in Amdo. One of these was *chöd* – a well-known practice in both Tibetan Buddhist and Bon traditions.[6] This practice, while sometimes performed in monastic contexts, is particularly associated with non-monastic yogic practitioners (Samuel 1993: 477). Here, the practitioner 'works to overcome attachment and ego-clinging' through the ritual offering of the body (Norbu 1986: 65) – visualizing the cutting up of his/her own body and offering it up to Tantric deities, local gods and spirits.[7]

Practices of self-sacrifice have a precedent in early Buddhism, where the giving up of one's own body was a 'cherished topic' (Orofino 2000: 398).[8] The Tantric traditions approach this concept from a ritualized perspective, where the practitioner dances and chants to the rhythm of a drum and a human-thighbone trumpet, invoking 'all the spirits and gods of the universe' and offering them 'the gift of his body' (Ibid.). In addition, *chöd* practice is often conducted in places understood to be haunted, such as graveyards or charnel grounds, where a practitioner can encounter 'elemental spirits and unseen forces' in order to 'evoke terror and anxiety' (Sheehy 2005: 42–43). Orofino describes the practice:

> The gcod pa [practitioner] visualizes the transference of his consciousness into a ḍākinī, who cuts the head off his physical body and then places the corpse inside the cranium, which stretches to cosmic proportions. The corpse is subsequently transformed in accordance with the wishes of the guests, multiplied infinitely, and offered to them as a gift.[9] Then the offering is divided into various categories: the white offering, in which the yogin visualizes that his body is transformed into ambrosia to be consumed by the higher deities and by the three jewels: the buddhas, devas, and ḍākinīs; the multicoloured offering, in which his body is transformed into all kinds of riches and material goods and offered to the dharmapālas, the protector spirits of the Buddhist law; the red offering, in which the dismembered flesh and blood are multiplied infinitely to appease the demons and fierce spirits; and finally the black offering, in which the officiant visualizes that all the errors and wrongdoings of the world are absorbed into his body, which is then offered as a meal to the demons. These offerings aim to satisfy all spirits, both higher and lower, in order to placate negative impulses and to eliminate definitively the ills of the world. (2000: 405)

While many of those I spoke to in Amdo discussed the non-human entities described here in quite tangible terms in our conversations on *chöd*, ultimately, as Orofino explains, from a Buddhist/Bon perspective, '[t]he foremost demon to be severed is attachment to the ego, and all that flows from it: pride, vanity, arrogance, and presumptuousness' (2000: 398).

This is also clear in DiValerio's description of the so-called 'Secret Practice' that was so central to the Madmen of Ü and Tsang's practice (DiValerio 2105: 50–51), and which is described, for example, in *Instructions for the Secret Practice of Great Glorious Nāropa* (Tib. *dpal na ro pa chen po'i gsang spyod kyi 'khrid*) authored by Tsangnyön Heruka. Here too, the practitioner visualizes the destruction of his/her own body (here, 'being chopped into pieces by the goddess Vajrayoginī') and its offering to various spirits and deities within the six realms of existence. However, as DiValerio explains, there are multiple layers of meaning here – not least in the interpretation of these spirits and deities:

> The next part of the meditation is a test of the practitioner's level of accomplishment. He is to try to tame various spirit-beings present in the area where he is meditating – but according to the text, he is ultimately not taming entities external to himself, but his own delusions and failings, which are externalised and personified as independent entities. The 'demons' referred to throughout the text are in fact conceptual formations (*rtog pa*, here synonymous with *nam tok*). (2015: 51–52)[10]

And, as we heard in Chapter 4, in Amdo (as in my previous research in Darjeeling [Deane 2014a: 454]), *chöd* was described as both cause and treatment for certain forms of *nyoné*. For example, Dr Dechen (39, Xining) told me that if a patient is 'seriously *nyoné*' from a *dön* affliction, their family may ask a Tantric practitioner to chant mantras including those of *chöd* rituals.

Taming Spirits

Another sphere in which Buddhist and Bon specialists engage with unenlightened spirits and deities is through rituals conducted for members of the lay community. In Amdo, as we have heard, when spirit afflictions were suspected in cases of illness or misfortune, afflicted persons and/or their families would commonly consult a Buddhist or Bon practitioner, who could perform the necessary ritual(s). We have seen already how a hierarchical understanding of spiritual 'power' underlies these interactions, with Tantric practitioners understood to have access to the requisite power to subjugate the kinds of unenlightened spirit(s) or deity(-ies) involved. In Amdo, Yogi Lodro (42, Chabcha) explained, 'If someone is realized [Tib. *tokden*] or has knowledge [Tib. *rigpa*], it is easy [for them] to exorcize *dön* or these kinds of problems'.

Indeed, for many Tibetan Tantric practitioners, conducting rituals to subjugate these lower-level spirits and deities can be a significant part of their practice, and Tantric specialists may be called upon to perform a broad range of ritual activities in the community. As Samuel has noted, this was also the case for the Indian Tantric gurus who preceded them, and the types of ritual services performed by today's Tibetan Tantric practitioners can be classified into 'four Indian-derived subdivisions': (i) calming or pacifying, (ii) increasing (wealth, long life, etc.), (iii) empowering and (iv) destroying or overcoming (1993: 246). Nyingma philosopher Jamgön Mipham (1846–1912) describes a similar classification in his commentary *Luminous Essence: A Guide to the Guhyagarbha Tantra* (Tib. *'od gsal snying po*), where examples he gives of 'pacifying activities' include the assuaging of illness, malevolent forces and obstacles; while 'subjugating activities' include 'summoning, . . . binding, suppressing, . . . killing, and expelling' as well as 'terrorizing, such as destroying something or driving someone insane' (Mipham 2009: 131–32). As we heard in Chapter 5, Amdo doctor and *ngakpa* Dr Sonam (69) explained that the chosen method will depend on the practitioner, and he described the process of making and destroying a 'human-like effigy' explaining that recovery can be 'very fast' with such rituals: 'Some patients even get better while I am performing the ritual'.

Another example of this practice is provided by a group of practitioners known as 'hail masters'. With hail understood to be brought by malevolent spirits, it is up to specialist practitioners to prevent it (Klein and Sangpo 1997: 539). The importance of deity yoga is explicit here – it is not simply about 'spiritual power' but about the practitioner's presentation as a terrifying deity: Anne Klein and hail master Khetsun Sangpo explain how these practitioners must 'learn to identify' with a 'fierce' *yidam*: this leads the troublesome spirits to see the hail master *as this deity*, rather than as an ordinary human. This protects the practitioner as, of course, such low-level spirits would not attempt to harm a Tantric deity (Ibid.: 539–40).

However, these engagements with lower-level spirits and deities through *chöd* practice and subjugation rituals performed on behalf of the community can also be a source of problems for practitioners – particularly those, yet again, thought to be insufficiently prepared or skilled to undertake them. As we saw in Chapter 4, some cases of *nyoné* were attributed to practitioner's dealings with these entities – something we will explore in more detail below.

Unenlightened: Madness and Spirit-Mediumship

And finally, in many Tibetan communities, there is also another kind of practitioner who willingly enters into a close relationship with deities to access their power – the spirit-medium, usually referred to in Amdo as *lhawa*.[11] These practitioners work with *un*enlightened deities, usually ritually becoming possessed by a worldly deity in the service of healing and/or divination for the local community. During my time in Amdo, this was something I encountered in a rather limited way, with only a couple of interviewees describing first-hand contact with such practitioners in the context of *nyoné*, and my own encounters limited to interviewing one *lhawa* in Rebkong. However, I am including some discussion of these practitioners here as they form an interesting part of our picture of *nyoné* in Tibetan communities, and I think it is important to consider how this too fits into Tibetan understandings of 'madness'.

Firstly, we should note that Amdo is home to a particular group of *lhawa* who populate the Rebkong valley. These practitioners are renowned for their participation in the annual Lurol festival, where each village hosts a ceremony focused around the ritualized possession of a local deity.[12] While the Rebkong *lhawa* have historically had 'many functions' – including performing healing – in recent times, their primary role has been participation in the Lurol festival (Snying bo rgyal and Rino 2008: 45). This certainly seemed to be the case while I was in the region in 2018 and 2019; while I interviewed one elderly Rebkong *lhawa* who described treating illnesses – particularly those related to spirit afflictions – many lay Tibetans I spoke to in the area told me that such practitioners did not conduct healing any more. Indeed, the vast majority of lay Tibetans I spoke to in Amdo explained that they had not consulted any *lhawa* for treatment of illness, and/or they did not know of any who conducted such practices. A slight difference was notable for a handful of people I spoke to who either lived in or hailed from Golok, several of whom mentioned *lhawa* they knew of who conducted healing rituals there. However, none of them had attended such rituals for the treatment of *nyoné*, and they too usually recommended Buddhist or Bon lamas or *ngakpa*s as best placed to treat such conditions. As such, I will not explore the healing activities of *lhawa* here. More relevant for our discussion in this context is the well-documented role of 'madness' in the transition to *becoming* a spirit-medium. While this is not particularly relevant in the case of these Rebkong *lhawa*, it is something that has been described in relation to spirit-mediums practising across Tibetan and Himalayan regions, as we shall see.

Within Tibetan communities, there are a variety of practitioners who work as spirit-mediums. Best known, perhaps, is the Nechung Oracle, key advisor to the Fourteenth Dalai Lama, and one of a class of practitioners who become possessed by key protector deities of Tibet within the monastic setting.[13] More common are the local spirit-mediums, male or female members of the lay community who usually live and work outside the monastic setting. While these practitioners may initially appear to be entirely independent of Buddhist or Bon institutions, in fact in many areas they have a close relationship to the monastic establishment – either receiving a lama's 'permission' or 'blessing' to practice (Berglie 1976: 93), or working 'under some degree of supervision' from lamas in the area (Samuel 1993: 292).[14] Again, we can see here a clear illustration of Tibetan notions of *wang tang*: with spirit-mediums' spiritual power deriving from unenlightened deities, it is ultimately weaker than that of Tantric practitioners, whose power derives from the enlightened Tantric deities with whom they engage through their practice. Spirit-mediums form an integral part of this hierarchical structure of spiritual power and, in Nepal, Berglie even found spirit-mediums woven into the narrative of Padmasambhava's taming of Tibet. Here, his interviewees claimed that the first spirit-mediums had been invited to Tibet by Padmasambhava in order to cure illnesses that were afflicting Tibetans at that time (1976: 96).[15]

While there is often a hereditary aspect to spirit-mediumship in Tibetan communities (for example, a practitioner having a *lhawa* parent, aunt or uncle), there is frequently also a narrative of initiatory illness. Working in Ladakh, for example, Rösing described how 'madness' frequently played a 'fundamental role' in the beginning stages of a path towards recognition as a spirit-medium (2006, 128–29), with an afflicted individual displaying symptoms such as 'erratic roaming around, various aches and pains, vivid dreams, confused visions and hallucinations, or perhaps indecent or nonsensical behaviour and running away' (2006, 114). Similarly, Berglie (working with Tibetan refugees in Nepal) described initial signs including an afflicted person seeing divine beings, 'demons', 'strange' animals, etc. that no one else sees; and one individual who apparently became 'just like a "madman" (*smyon pa*)' (1976: 88–89). In southwest Tibet, Diemberger related the narrative of woman who fell ill at age 32 – explaining, 'It was as if I had gone insane' – before she was recognized as a spirit-medium (2005: 123); and in Ladakh, Day described how this kind of madness or 'illness' may not be immediately recognized, with novices 'rendered incapable by "fits" and "unsettled minds" for months or years while families and friends search for cures and specialists provide no help at all' (1989: 273). Indeed, Day notes, all four of the spirit-mediums she spoke to in Ladakh 'dwelt upon their loss of control; "fits", "unsettled mind", the experience of "death" and generally "abnormal" behaviour', emphasizing that this 'madness' was key 'above all other factors' here (Ibid.: 277).[16]

How might we understand this initial period of 'madness' so common in *lhawa* narratives? Much like in the unwanted spirit possessions we saw in Chapters 4 and 5, in the case of spirit-mediumship, the possessing deity is understood to enter the practitioner's mind-body through the channels (Tib. *tsa*). Thus, Turpeinen explains how once a deity has chosen its preferred medium, the individual starts to suffer from 'god sickness' (Tib. *lha né*) – 'a sign of the god attempting to enter the medium through the subtle channels (*rtsa*) of the energy body' (2019: 44).[17] Narratives about this period of *nyoné* are therefore often focused on the need to 'purify' and/or 'open' these channels – something usually done by a senior oracle or a lama (Turpeinen 2019: 44). Before such a purification, the person is thought to be vulnerable to attack by other spirits and deities entering the channels – thus causing the kind of symptoms we saw above, and including, as Diemberger describes, '[u]ncontrolled visions, voices, fainting, weakness, and the experience of a death-like state' (2005: 120). And here again, we hear of the importance of the hierarchical structure of spiritual power within Tibetan religious traditions. Indeed, in Ladakh, Day described the 'prominent role' of rinpoche in confirming 'god-inflicted madness' and either 'banning the spirits or referring villagers to senior oracles for training' (1989: 281).

These purification and initiatory rituals are understood to perform two functions: allowing the 'correct' deity unobstructed access and blocking the 'door' to malevolent spirits (Diemberger 2005: 130–33). The latter are prevented from entering the body not only through the 'control' that the practitioner can now exert over his/her own channels but also as a result of a lama's 'authorization' to practice (Ibid.: 137). In addition, in some areas, there may also be some Buddhist elements to spirit-mediums' practice. In his research in 'Upper Tibet' (sTod and Byang thang), for example, Bellezza describes how a majority of spirit-mediums' 'trance ceremonies' were 'prefaced with Buddhist prayers in which refuge is taken and the protection of the Buddhist divinities sought' (2011: 9).[18] Again, the practitioner – who is dealing predominantly with unenlightened deities – is seeking protection and authentication from the higher power of the Tantric deities and their practitioners.

Pride and Doubt: When Practice Goes Wrong

As we saw in Chapter 4, in Amdo a number of my interviewees discussed the risks of practices focused on intentional engagement with spirits and deities, and I heard a range of narratives about how and why practitioners might suffer from *nyoné* as a result of deity yoga or *chöd* practice, for example. Much like in our discussions of practices 'gone wrong' in Chapter 3, people spoke of practitioners improperly prepared for deity yoga practices, and dealing with problems like *namtok*.

We have heard already that Tantric texts can be extremely complex. Indeed, in his examination of the *Cakrasaṃvara Tantra*, for example, Gray notes that the text was *designed* to be inaccessible to those who had not been initiated into the tradition. This inaccessibility, he says, was achieved in several ways, including 'listing the mantras in reverse order' and encrypting them through puzzles that code consonants and vowels by assigning them numerical values (2007: 133). These methods, of course, will increase the risk of misinterpretation and confusion for those not sufficiently experienced or knowledgeable about the practices. In addition, in Part I, we explored the complex manipulations of *lung* involved in many completion-stage practices – and how *lung né* problems (including *nyoné*) may result from errors in these practices. The manipulation of *lung* through the bodily channels is key in deity yoga practices too, and we might therefore not be surprised to hear that errors in this aspect of practice could equally cause problems such as *nyoné* here. And, as we saw in Chapter 4, some Amdo interviewees also spoke of problems arising from practitioners' dealings with different kinds of spirits and deities as part of their Tantric practice. Here, we will explore these various causes of *nyoné*, and the ways in which they might be remedied.

Problems with Deity Yoga

As we saw above, deity yoga practices require considerable skill and an appropriate mindset to be conducted successfully. Contemporary practitioner Khenchen Thrangu Rinpoche (b.1933) explains:

> In the visualization of the form of the deity, or the visualization of the syllables of the mantra, if your mind is too tight, too tense, then the natural clarity of the visualization is diminished; and if your mind is too relaxed, you become distracted. (Khenchen Thrangu Rinpoche's commentary, cited by Harding in Kongtrul 1996: 120)

In Amdo, interviewees spoke of problems in deity yoga resulting from factors including 'confusion' and 'arrogance' during these complex practices. We have heard, for example, about the key notion of 'divine pride' in a practitioner's identification with the chosen Tantric deity. And yet, in Amdo, Buddhist Studies student Migmar (30, Golok/Xining) asserted that one cause of *nyoné* is a practitioner's arrogance or 'pride' in their ability to become an enlightened deity. He described practitioners who are 'arrogant', for example, explaining that they may proclaim that they are 'the same as' the deity. The difference between these two states of mind is key, with a clear distinction between 'confidence in one's own innate buddhahood' ('the psychological key to gaining enlightenment rapidly') and the problems of 'false pride and a sense of entitlement' (Nālandā Translation Committee 1997: 141). Indeed, as we heard above from Bentor, the 'dissolution' of the practitioner's visualization of themself as an enlightened being at the end of the practice is intended to prevent them from developing an 'attachment' to this reality (2000: 332).

In addition, in Chapter 4, we heard Migmar describe how 'confusion' could occur during deity yoga practice, explaining that a practitioner may see 'all kinds of images of this buddha' and, 'if the practitioner gets confused by this, then this can cause a problem'. He continued: 'If someone is practicing [Buddhist deity] Yamāntaka meditation, their appearance may change – maybe their face or body will change to become similar to Yamāntaka's face or body . . . In addition, when they are completing the practice, if the practitioner struggles to understand or complete the practice correctly then that might cause *nyoné* or other problems'.

It becomes clear that a practitioner may experience some quite intense sensations during Tantric practices. These might be internal and/or external: for example, Kohn quotes a lama's description of wind 'kicking up', the sky turning black and the appearance of a rain-less rainbow at a *Kālacakra* initiation conducted by the Dalai Lama (1997: 227), and notes that the text advises practitioners to look out for internal or external signs that the deities have come. One lama whom Kohn interviewed described three categories of internal signs: 'signs of the body, such as shivering; signs of speech, such as spontaneously singing; and mental signs, such as suddenly becoming very happy'. And Lopez translates Tsongkhapa's *The Stages of the Path to Enlightenment* (Tib. *byang chub lam rim chen mo*) text, noting that it includes 'instructions on how to deal with experiences (Tib. *nyams*) that may occur as a result of meditation'. This, he explains, 'refers to the various apparitions, hallucinations, and visions (both visual and auditory) that may occur in the course of meditation'. He emphasizes that it is key for the practitioner to determine 'whether the various supernatural beings that materialize before the meditator are real or not', and Tsongkhapa thus describes some techniques, as Lopez explains: 'If what appears really is a buddha or bodhisattva, one should ask them to bestow magical powers (siddhis). If the meditator is simply overwhelmed by a multitude of apparitions, he or she should shift attention to the first of the apparitions to appear, until it disappears' (Lopez 2000: 528).

Dudjom Rinpoche, Jigdrel Yeshe Dorje (1904–1987) described such 'signs' occurring 'in reality, in experiences, or in dreams' (2011: 271–72). He adds that when a practitioner focuses his/her energy on the practice,

> it is quite common for bad deeds from the past to surface, so that all sorts of unwanted things happen to us: we fall physically ill, feel mentally anguished,

> experience the manifestation of negative forces and obstacle makers, fall victim to hostile people, bandits, and thieves, find ourselves subject to people's criticisms and false accusations, and so on. (Ibid.: 272)

Dorje explains that, given that these are signs that 'we are purifying ourselves', the practitioner should respond by 'don[ning] the great armour of diligence that renders the practice impervious to unpleasant circumstances' (Ibid.).

We can imagine, perhaps, how such sensations and experiences might cause anxiety or confusion in a less-experienced or improperly prepared practitioner. In Amdo, Buddhist Studies student Nyingyal (33, Golok/Xining) spoke of younger, less-experienced monks and *ngakpa*s who 'become *nyonpa*' from conducting their practice incorrectly. This is particularly the case, he asserted, if they are anxious while they are practising: 'Maybe this will cause *nyonpa*'. As Dorje explains, not only can it be 'hard to distinguish' which of these signs are 'genuine', and which are 'obstacles caused by demons', it may also be the case that even the genuine signs can become problematic: 'the moment we attach any importance to them, they will turn into demonic obstacles' (2011: 272).

We thus return to the notion of *namtok*. As we have already discussed, this term refers quite specifically in Buddhist terms to the incorrect understanding of the world that results from our lack of realization – i.e. the misapprehension that things have intrinsic existence, on the basis of which, we (as unenlightened beings) create the ego. However, it is also often used in a broader sense, as we see here. In Chapter 1, we discussed Ardussi and Epstein's description of *namtok* as 'hesitation' or 'scruple' (1978: 330), and in his co-authored dictionary of Modern Tibetan, Goldstein translates this predominantly as 'superstitious beliefs, taboos' (Goldstein et al. 2001: 630). In Amdo too, it was often used in ways that suggested notions of doubt, suspicion or a lack of faith in a practice, leading to confusion or anxiety for a practitioner. Thus, Tamdrin (26, Rebkong) told me (in English) about how his uncle, a monastic practitioner, had apparently become *nyoné* following deity yoga practices: 'He researched the high level deity, but he misunderstood some things . . . He was between trust and suspicion, and he lost his mind'.

We can see here that many of these explanations for practice-related *nyoné* focus not on the activity of the *yidam* themselves but on the practitioner and their state of mind – both in terms of their preparedness and knowledge/understanding of key concepts and what to expect during these practices, and also on their faith in the Dharma as they engage in them. In contrast, when we explore narratives of *nyoné* related to practices involving lower-level spirits and deities – such as in the case of *chöd* practice, or in rituals aimed at subjugating local spirits and deities – much of the discussion in Amdo was on the activities and danger of the entities themselves, as we shall explore next.

Chöd: *Inviting in Spirits*

As we have seen, a number of interviewees in Amdo described *chöd* as a potential cause of madness, and this is something that has been described by other researchers too. Evans-Wentz, for example, asserted that an unsuccessful *chöd* practitioner risks 'an unbalancing of mind and psychic constitution, possibly leading to madness or even death' (1967: 281). In Amdo, this was discussed by both the lay interviewees and the Buddhist and Bon ritual specialists I spoke to. Much like similar discussions on deity yoga, some of these narratives were focused on the importance of correct initiation and preliminary practices. For example, Bon lama Tsering (57) told me:

> *Chöd* can cause you to get *nyoné*, because when you do *chöd*, you need a rinpoche's guidance and permission to practice – proper initiation from your teacher – and you also need to perform preliminary practices [Tib. *ngön dro*] before you can do *chöd*. Without this kind of initiation or permission, if you do it by *yourself*, sometimes it can cause you to become *nyoné*, and even kill you – maybe as a result of the *dön*.

Indeed, a number of Amdo interviewees spoke explicitly about the dangers of spirits and how they might harm a practitioner during this practice. As we have seen above, a key aspect of *chöd* is the practitioner's offering of his/her (visualized) dismembered body to spirits to feast on, as a means to 'overcome attachment and ego-clinging' (Norbu 1986: 65). Moreover, as we have heard, *chöd* is traditionally practised in 'graveyards and charnel grounds at night', as well as 'lonely and desolate places, such as caves and mountain peaks'. Here, Norbu explains, the 'terrifying energy' of these places 'serves to intensify the sensation of the practitioner' (Ibid.: 67). Again, we can imagine that this practice might have the potential to cause fear and/or confusion in a meditator not fully prepared or skilled to undertake it – regardless of whether the 'spirits' involved are external entities or projections of the mind, as explained by Machig Labdron (1055–1149), the founder of this tradition. Orofino translates from a poem attributed to her, *The Great Collection of the Teachings* (Tib. *bka' tshoms chen mo*):

> The root of all demons is one's own mind.
> If one feels attraction and desire
> in the perception of any phenomenon,
> one is captured by the demons.
> When the mind grasps at phenomena
> as if they were external objects
> one becomes contaminated. (2000: 413)

Orofino asserts that good practitioners understand the 'psychological significance of this macabre banquet', whereby the deities (Tib. *lha*) evoked during the *chöd* ritual are 'symbolic images of his [the practitioner's] desires and wishes', while the spirits are 'nothing but projections of the practitioner's mind, embodiments of his disquiet and fear' (Ibid.: 405). Similarly, as we heard in the previous chapter, Amdo lama Namgyal (32, Chabcha) asserted: '*Dön* is not something that can come from outside, but from *sem kham* [the psychology, state of mind] of that person. No such thing[s] as *dön* exist . . . The eternal state of mind has so many conflicts, and has many problems, but there are no *outer dön*'.

And yet, we have seen that these entities may be described in quite tangible terms. In Amdo, for example, *ngakpa* and Tibetan medicine doctor, Aku Wangchuk (72) described how some kind of *dön* or *mi tsangwa* can impact on ritual practice:

> *Mi tsangwa* means 'not clean', so we can use this term generally – for example, 'This cup is not clean' – but also sometimes, *mi tsangwa* can also be *dön.* [For example] when you do some ritual, if there is *dön*, then maybe some bad things will happen, and then you cannot continue your ritual practice. So at the beginning of a ritual, we have a ceremony to send all the *dön* out. First, a kind of offering is performed: [you say] 'I will give you [*dön*] all this, so please go – take your food, take these offerings, and leave. But still, maybe some will remain. Then [the practitioner] will negotiate – more strongly: 'If you don't leave, I will conduct a strong ritual'. Then if some *dön still* stay, then the practitioner will use some very strong ceremony and expel them.

Again, then, we encounter spirits in multiple ways, described at certain times seemingly as 'real' entities with their own motivations, at other times as simply manifestations of a practitioner's mind. Similarly, Orofino describes the ambiguous and multiple meanings of *māra*, from which Tibetan notions of *dü* expand, as both a 'popular god with his own place within the cosmology of early Buddhism' and as 'etymological meaning of "he who causes death," and Mara is thereby associated with everything that is deceptive, transient, or that brings about spiritual death' – concepts then built upon within the *chöd* tradition (2000: 400–1).[19] He notes, however, the difference between the 'tangible demons (*thogs bcas kyi bdud*)' – which 'belong to visible reality' and consist of all the phenomena that, through sensory experience, arouse desire – and 'intangible demons (*thogs med kyi bdud*)', which 'comprise purely mental events' and which 'arise when the categories of good and evil are separated in the mind and one distinguishes between what one wants and what one rejects' (2000: 401).

Perhaps the translation often found in books directed at Western audiences (audiences possibly presumed to be less comfortable with notions of spirit entities) – 'provocations' – is in fact a good one. In Amdo, I encountered narratives that held spirits and deities to be both a cause and a consequence of *namtok*: where doubts about practice and its related sensations and experiences could cause a practitioner to become susceptible to *dön*, so too could an experience with *dön* cause a practitioner to experience *namtok*. As Yangönpa explains, when the various wind channels 'are opened [by concepts and negative actions], [one will] receive a provocation'. He describes the different 'provocations' that will afflict the different channels: 'at the lungs there is the channel of the *tsen*; at the heart, that of the *gyalpo*; at the liver and kidney, that of the *mamo*; at the stomach, that of the *theurang*; and at the small intestine, that of the *lu*' (Yangönpa 2015: 259). Similarly, Norbu describes a 'great variety' of non-human beings that have the capacity to cause disturbances by 'directly influencing the sphere of an individual's energy', referencing the *nyo jé gyi dön* (madness-causing spirits) described in Chapter 78 of the *Third Tantra* (Norbu 1995: 142–43). However, he also translates *dön* as 'to doubt', asserting that a person may be '"provoked" by something that gives rise to doubt' (Ibid.: 143), demonstrating again the multiplicity of spirits beyond a duality of 'real' versus 'unreal' in Tibetan understandings. And ultimately, of course, according to Buddhist and Bon Dharmic perspectives, *everything* is 'devoid of an independent or intrinsic nature', as Lopez explains:

> [E]verything in the universe, from physical forms to the omniscient consciousness of the Buddha, is contingent, depending for its existence on its causes, on its parts, or on a designating consciousness. Nothing exists in and of itself, nothing is able to stand alone. To believe that anything, whether it be a person, a material object, or an idea, exists autonomously, without depending on anything else, is ignorance, and this ignorance is the cause of all suffering in the universe. (2000: 524)

Here, spirits and deities are both as 'real' and 'unreal' as humans, and should be approached as such.

Subjugating Spirits

As we saw in Chapters 4 and 5, a key part of lamas' and *ngakpas*' practice in both Buddhist and Bon traditions is often the performance of rituals for their local communities. These rituals are often directly aimed at managing local spirits and deities – particularly when these are understood to be afflicting lay members of the community through illnesses such as *nyoné* or other kinds of harm. As we have already seen, it is through their Tantric practices – focused on engagements with enlightened Buddhist or Bon deities – that Buddhist and Bon ritual specialists access the higher spiritual power necessary to successfully perform such rituals. This power not only enables a practitioner to subjugate trouble-causing, unenlightened spirits and deities, as we saw in Chapter 5, but also protects the practitioner from being harmed by these less-powerful entities. In Amdo, doctor and *ngakpa* Aku Wangchuk (72) spoke of both *wang tang* (spiritual power), and also *nüpa* (power, ability, potency), as he explained:

> If a person is really powerful, then it's not easy for them to get *dön né*. For example, if I am conducting a *Tamdrin* practice and become really powerful, then I will not easily get *dön*: if the weak *dön* even *see* me – see my breath – then they will disappear, or it may be harmful for them [to come close to me] . . . If you are chanting Tamdrin, then from the body, mind, and speech – from these three levels – you can get power from Tamdrin, get empowered from this, so you can be very, very strong. So for these people, *dön* are really, really easy [to deal with] . . . Some people do [Tantric] retreat for four or five years – even fifteen or twenty years – *these* people are really strong.

This echoes what we heard from hail master Khetsun Sangpo, above, about the necessity of identifying with a 'fierce' *yidam*. As he explained: 'If you can clearly and with an unwavering mind visualize yourself as, for example, Hayagrīva,[20] then worldly deities cannot harm you' (Klein and Sangpo 1997: 541).

*

And finally, in Amdo I heard occasional references to madness and other afflictions caused by protector deities (*sung ma*).[21] These deities occupy a curious place in the Tibetan pantheon. Deriving from both 'Tibetanized Indian divinities' and indigenous Tibetan deities (Bell 2019: 1254), they may be enlightened or unenlightened – and there may even be differing categorizations of particular deities depending on who one asks.[22] Tasked with protecting the Dharma, these figures may display violence against those who seek to destroy it, and they have 'an especially vicious hatred' for those who break the vows they made to 'practice and propagate' Buddhism (Bell 2006: 65).[23] Thus, in Xining, for example, Dr Nyima (38) explained to me that if a practitioner 'breaks the rules' within the higher levels of Buddhist Tantric practice, then a protector deity might 'punish' (Tib. *ché pa tong*) them.

Bell notes that this issue is, for example, particularly obvious in the case of protector deity Tsiu Marpo, whose 'primary task is to attack those who do not uphold the Dharma' (2006: 54). Thus, we read of Tsiu Marpo being instructed to send illnesses including colic and fainting, and to 'order the *teu rang* demons to cause fits of madness' to foes (Nebesky-Wojkowitz 1993: 167). Similarly, as leader of the *gyalpo* class of deities, the protector deity Pehar has been instructed to 'destroy completely those who break the religious vows' (Ibid.: 117). Indeed, Pehar is known for his capricious nature and propensity to cause harm when offended, and his ability to 'bring epidemics, cause insanity and other illness', necessitating certain rituals to pacify him (Lin 2010: 22). In one initiation text, it is even said that Padmasambhava prophesied a future increase in madness (here, using the terms *nyoné* and also *bok*) due to the influence of Pehar, as well as a particular *teurang* spirit (Muses 1961: 31–33).[24]

Treating *Nyoné* Related to Spirit and Deity Practices

As we saw in Part I, for many cases of *nyoné* or other conditions understood to have been precipitated by problems with Tantric practice, the first line of treatment is often the consultation of one's teacher. More knowledgeable and experienced, the Tantric teacher will ideally be able to guide their student – often through particular religious practices. While there may be recourse through medical treatments – for example, where there is seen to be a problem with the flow of *lung* – as we saw in Chapter 3, for conditions understood to be precipitated by practice, much treatment is seen to lie in the Dharma. Thus, Buddhist Studies student Migmar (30, Golok/Xining), who described, above, the problems that can result from a practitioner's pride (Tib. *ngagel*, pride/arrogance) in their practice, told me, 'Some practitioners will seek support from a higher level teacher; then maybe the teacher will calm their mind [Tib. *sem*], and then tell them what to do'. Then, he said, 'maybe they will get better'.

The pre-eminence of 'religious' remediation is perhaps especially evident when discussing *nyoné* in relation to the concept of *namtok*, which, as we have seen, can be key to a practitioner's problems when engaging with spirits and deities. Here, ultimately both prevention and 'cure' are understood to lie in the Dharma, and in a greater understanding of the realities of Tantric practice and the unusual and/or intense experiences a practitioner might have. For example, Tamdrin (26, Rebkong), who told me, above, about his monastic relative who had become *nyoné* – caught 'between trust and suspicion' during deity yoga practice – explained that this relative had recovered to some degree as a result of studying further and increasing his knowledge of the Dharma. As former monk Tsetan (38, Rebkong) told me, 'Buddhist practices stop *namtok* . . . The sense of good or bad . . . clean or dirty . . . beautiful or ugly – all of this results from *namtok*. So if you free yourself from *namtok*, then you will be ok'.

Similarly, when dealing with problems related to *chöd* practice, again we have heard that ultimately the issue is not necessarily the behaviour of spirits or deities as external entities but the practitioner's own (mis)understanding of them from a Dharmic perspective. In addition, as we have already heard above, while *chöd* practice has the potential to lead to *nyoné* for some practitioners, sometimes it was also described as a form of healing. In Amdo, several interviewees mentioned the benefit of a practitioner conducting *chöd* for the benefit of their afflicted patients. For example, Tibetan medicine doctor and *ngakpa* Dr Sonam (69) described the *chöd* ritual as a key practice for treating *dön* affliction, explaining, 'If a patient is possessed by a *dön*, I can recite this *chöd* text to bring the *dön* out – to defeat it or cast it into another realm'. And it has also been described as a ritual with which an individual might successfully treat themselves. In Lhasa, for example, Jacobson described a lay woman conducting *chöd* as a way of – temporarily at least – decreasing her *lung né* symptoms (2000: 508).

In dealing with *sung ma* too, the greater spiritual power of enlightened Tantric deities is key. As Yogi Lodro (42, Chabcha) told me: 'If you venerate a *sung ma*, and then you offend it, then it may be destructive. Then you need a *yidam lha*, [and] you need some kind of *ngak* [mantra, ritual] for that *yidam lha* . . . If you have a *yidam lha* beside you – or *inside* you – then you can easily control the *sung ma*'. On the other hand, of course, with all unenlightened deities empty of intrinsic existence, ultimately, 'conquering' them is really a matter of overcoming one's own dualistic mind to see the truth of the Dharma.

*

This chapter has again highlighted the complexity, power and risk inherent in Tibetan Buddhist and Bon Tantric practices – and also the fundamental role that non-human entities continue to play in both Tibetan ritual and daily life. As we saw in the previous two chapters, for lay people, the 'everyday' reality of spirits and deities can help to explain cases of illness – particularly, perhaps, when other diagnoses and treatments have failed to precipitate healing. Here, ritual treatments performed by Tantric ritual specialists such as spirit-mediums, lamas and *ngakpa* are informed by longstanding Tibetan notions of a hierarchy of 'spiritual power', and the necessity of specialist Buddhist or Bon Tantric practitioners is demonstrated by the everyday problems caused by unenlightened spirits and deities. Here, lay people need Buddhism or Bon to maintain (or restore) the health and wellbeing of the community; so too do Buddhism and Bon need the spirits and deities to justify the ongoing support of the lamas, monasteries and ritual specialists from that lay community.

For Tantric specialists, problems – including *nyoné* – may arise from their own dealings with a variety of spirits and deities as part of their Tantric practice. Dangers of dealing with unenlightened spirits during *chöd* practice, for example, are said to include 'losing control' of the spirits. And yet, as we have seen, these spirits may be interpreted in a number of different ways, and realization means understanding their true nature: the reality that ultimately these entities have no intrinsic existence – and neither do any of us. Here, then, the problem is not the spirit itself but the practitioner's own (mis)understanding of it. Similarly, in deity yoga practices, problems are often said to arise from the practitioner's own mind. Much like the *tsa lung* practices we saw in Chapter 3, *yidam* practices are complex and lengthy, and involve manipulations of the mind-body that may result in strange or unusual sensations and experiences. For the practitioner, these experiences can lead to doubts, fears, suspicions or simply difficulties in fully realizing the true nature of reality according to the Dharma. Lacking faith, the practitioner may 'lose their mind', becoming *nyoné*. Alternatively, they may become arrogant: seeing themself becoming a powerful Tantric deity, they may be overcome with a false pride, attached to this experience. These things, of course, are more likely to happen in those practitioners who have not sufficiently prepared for undertaking these high-level practices: those without the requisite training, skills or knowledge.

And finally, of course, we have the figure of the *lama nyonpa*. Wearing a human skin like a wrathful Tantric deity, and citing the Tantras in justification, perhaps this practitioner has become a realized being as a result of his/her performances of non-duality . . . Perhaps he/she is simply performing – imitating the enlightened deity but not (yet) enlightened him- or herself . . . Or perhaps he/she is simply 'mad', suffering from the illness of *nyoné*, but misrecognized – or misremembered – as an enlightened practitioner.

In all of these practices, we can see the *yidam* as representative of the buddha-nature within all of us; and the low-level spirits as manifestations of our own negative mental states. It is in working to gain this knowledge and understanding of the world that the practitioner can come unstuck: conduct these practices correctly and, ultimately, realization is possible; conduct them incorrectly – without sufficient understanding of, or faith in, the Dharma – and madness may result.

Notes

1. Yoeli-Tlalim notes similarities with Hindu Tantric empowerment rituals (*dīkśā* or *abhiśeka*) here: 'Both the actual practices and the overall symbolism resemble each other' (2009: 416).
2. As Bentor explains: 'First, the vase initiation transforms disciples into vessels suitable for the generation process in which they transform themselves into enlightened beings. Second, the secret initiation renders the disciples suitable vessels for engaging in the practice of the subtle body, composed of cakras, channels (nadis), and winds (pranas)' (2000: 329).
3. For more on the nature of these entities, see Samuel 1993: 247–50.

4. In fact, Samuel argues that these *yidam* could even be said to be 'more' real than the unenlightened spirits and deities residing with us in samsara, since they 'correspond to underlying properties of the universe and human nature rather than to the illusory realm of karmic appearance' (1993: 164).
5. Here, referring to Hevajra or Cakrasaṃvara. DiValerio notes that Tibetans 'most often leave the Sanskrit term *heruka* untranslated'; '[w]hen translated, it is rendered as *trak-tungwa*, "blood-drinker," connoting the absorbent ground in which bodies are buried, showing the deity's deep association with the macabre' (2015: 57).
6. Uniquely, *chöd* is attributed to female Tibetan practitioner Machig Labdron (1055–1149) in the Buddhist tradition – the only female lama to have founded a major teaching lineage.
7. See, for example, a short description of nineteenth-century practitioner Ayu Khandro (b.1839), and her time travelling around Tibet doing *chöd* practice in 'cemeteries and sacred places' (Samuel 1993: 352).
8. In the Jātaka tales of the Buddha's previous lives, for example, we can read narratives such as the Buddha giving up his body to a tiger.
9. See, for example, Evans-Wentz's translation of parts of the text:

   > Then imagine this body, which is the result of thine own karmic propensities,
   > To be a fat, luscious-looking corpse, huge [enough to embrace the Universe],
   > . . . Having one face and two hands and holding a knife and a skull.
   > Think that she severeth the head from the corpse,
   > . . . And cutteth the corpse into bits and flingeth them inside the skull as offerings to the deities. (1967: 311–13)

10. See DiValerio too for some discussion on the similarities and differences between the 'Practice of the Observance' described here and *chöd*, and confusions resulting from this (2015: 53–54).
11. Other terms include *lhapa* and *lha zhuk ken* – and, in other regions, *pawo* (male) and *pamo* (female).
12. For descriptions and analysis of this festival, see Buffetrille (2008), Dpal-ldan-bkra-shis and Stuart (1998), Epstein and Wenbin (1998), Makley (2013), Sihlé (2018), and Snying bo rgyal and Rino (2008).
13. For more on these practitioners, see Samuel (1993: 292).
14. This is not the case everywhere, however: Turpeinen, for example, references Diemberger's (2005) point that spirit-mediums in rural areas of Tibet do not necessarily have these kinds of close connections with 'elite Buddhist religion' – 'presumably due to lack of access to lamas' (Turpeinen 2019: 50). In addition, it should be noted that, much like the *lama nyönpa* and other Tibetan religious practitioners, there may be debates and disagreements over a practitioner's 'authenticity' (Diemberger 2005: 123).
15. However, this runs counter to evidence suggesting a long pre-Buddhist history for these kinds of practitioners in Tibet (see Samuel 1993: 176).
16. See also Gutschow's description of the case of a Tibetan man in Zangskar, whose 'insanity' was initially diagnosed as a wind disorder following the theft of his earnings while working away from home. After limited success in treating his condition with Tibetan medicines and external therapies, it was thought that he was suffering from a *dön né*, and rituals were performed by Buddhist lamas; however, these were also unsuccessful and it was later concluded that he was an oracle, possessed by a powerful protector deity (1997: 191–95). This narrative illustrates not only the shifting nature of diagnosis for conditions that may be difficult to treat successfully (through either medicine or ritual) but also how these conditions overlap in both their expression and explanation.

17. See Berglie (1976, 1982) for description of the complex ways in which particular deities were associated with different channels by those he spoke to in Nepal. In fact, this connection with the channels is key for the Rebkong Lurol *lhawa* too: as one *lhawa* explained to Snying bo rgyal and Rino, '"When I was possessed I felt like I was being attacked by a power. I felt it in my *rtsa*. I believe the deities possess the *lha pa*'s *rtsa*"' (2008: 116).
18. In some contexts, the spirit-medium's consciousness is also said to be 'guarded' by specific Tantric deities during the ritual (Sumegi 2010: 446). Again, we see how these Buddhist and pre-Buddhist conceptions interact and justify each other, each to some extent 'reinforcing' the efficacy of the other, as Bellezza describes (2011: 26).
19. See also Sheehy here, who references the Pali and Sanskrit Buddhist literature on different types of '*māra*' in this context (Tib. *dü*) (2005: 41–42), pointing out that in the *chöd* system there are 'outer'/'externalized' and 'inner'/'internalized' *māra* (Ibid.: 42), and describes an 'anthropomorphization' of the 'positive and negative expressions of duality' (Ibid.: 41) whereby 'seemingly outward and inward experiences are actually a seamless continuity' (Ibid.: 44). See also Orofino for an examination of Indian Buddhist influences on the development of the *chöd* tradition (2000).
20. Skt. Hayagrīva; wrathful manifestation of Avalokiteśvara.
21. Also referred to as *chö kyong* [Skt. *dharmapāla*] – 'Dharma protector'.
22. See, for example, Lin's examination of the diverse ways in which Pehar was described in different Tibetan texts, and his changing role in Tibetan traditions over time (2010).
23. We can reference here the fourteen Tantric vows, which are understood to lead to fourteen root downfalls (Tib. *tsa tung chu zhi*) if broken.
24. Indeed, there are several mentions of Pehar's ability to cause *nyoné*, as well as other maladies, in the descriptions of him in various Tantric texts – see, again, Lin (2010) for some examples of this and a description of his 'instinct to harm living beings' (Ibid.: 22).

Conclusion

Across these past six chapters, we have explored some of the diverse ways in which 'madness' (*nyoné*) may be understood in text and everyday life, in both historic and contemporary Tibetan contexts. We have heard how *nyoné* may be a form of illness – a symptom of disordered *lung* ('wind') or an indication of a spirit affliction, perhaps – or in fact a sign of realization: a person's 'mad' behaviour being apparently a consequence of their ability to see beyond the false dichotomies of samsara (the cycle of rebirth). In these narratives, we have explored how longstanding Tibetan medical and religious conceptions of mind-body structure and functioning converge and diverge to explain these different forms of *nyoné*. And our focus on Amdo has allowed us to see how these ideas play out in some contemporary Tibetan communities in modern China, where people may have access to a broad variety of explanatory frameworks and healing modalities provided by a diverse range of medical and religious practitioners. Key here are enduring Tibetan notions of the self and the wider world, where fundamental concepts such as 'wind' and 'spirits' link the microcosm and macrocosm. Here, health, illness and healing are dependent not only on a person's own actions but perhaps also on those of their family or wider community as well as the greater forces of the world around them, and the unseen entities understood to reside within it. In this context, we can understand how *nyoné* might result, for example, from a family member's relationship to someone with different deity traditions from them, or from a Tantric practitioner's lack of faith in the Dharma as he/she experiences him/herself as an enlightened deity in his/her own pure land, beyond the realm of samsara. Or perhaps, a practitioner summons the spirits, practising *chöd* in a cremation ground, and then panics when they arrive, and he/she misunderstands their nature and believes that he/she cannot control them.

We have seen that amongst lay people in Amdo, *nyoné* was often linked to heart: here, simplified notions of Tibetan medical theory were often employed to explain instances of *nyoné* in relation to emotions and difficult life circumstances. Where Tibetan medicine doctors described complex connections between 'wind' (Tib. *lung*), 'heart' (Tib. *nying*) and 'mind' (Tib. *sem*), reflecting their descriptions in medical texts, many of the lay people I spoke to in Amdo mainly discussed 'heart illness' (Tib. *nying lung [né]*) related to both everyday difficulties (for example, exam stress) and significant tragedies (e.g. multiple bereavements). In addition, it has become clear how discussions on spirit afflictions – and related concepts of impurity/pollution – were frequent among Amdo-wa, with interviewees describing a variety of spirits and deities thought to cause *nyoné* and other conditions. Diversities were evident here too, with differing ideas about how common some of these entities are and how they might interact with humans.

*

In Part I, then, we explored in some depth how the notion of *lung* is key to Tibetan understandings of mind and consciousness, and the ways in which the relationship between *lung* and *nying* can be related to the causation of *nyoné*. Tibetan medicine doctors explained how disruptions to the different *lung* currents can impact on mind-body functioning. Here, the healthy functioning of *lung* through the channels of the body is both cause and consequence of the functioning of the mind and consciousness. Thus, an individual's state of mind and body will both impact on and be affected by the flow of *lung* through the channels. And with the *sok lung* ('life-sustaining wind') located around the area of the heart – the seat of the mind in Tibetan understanding – this *lung* current is particularly associated with the (dys) functioning of the mind. Here, disruptions in its flow can lead to disturbances in the senses, including hallucinations and other symptoms of *nyoné*.

As we saw, this important relationship between *lung* and mind is also key for Tibetan Tantric practices. Here, the deliberate manipulations of wind through the channels within the body are key to the manipulation of the mind and consciousness towards enlightenment in both Buddhist and Bon traditions. In these practices, *lung* works to transport the 'drops' (Tib. *tiklé*) – linked to both physical substances (male and female sexual fluids) and the *bodhicitta* (Tib. *jang chup sem*, 'mind of enlightenment'). Tibetan Tantric texts delineate the many ways in which practitioners can direct the *lung* – carrying the drops – into and through the central channel. Here, there is a clear delineation between the 'karmic wind' of the unenlightened mind, travelling through the side channels, and the 'wisdom wind' of the enlightened mind, which travels through the central channel. And yet, ultimately, we learn that 'transforming' the karmic wind of ordinary consciousness into the wisdom wind of an enlightened mind is actually a matter of realizing that these two are the same – one wind viewed from the standpoint of either the *unenlightened* or *enlightened* mind. Thus, realization is not simply a cognitive process of the consciousness but an embodiment of the true nature of reality beyond false beliefs about duality.

With the flows of wind so intimately tied to the functioning of the mind, it is perhaps unsurprising to hear that incorrectly conducting these kinds of advanced, complex, 'high-risk, high-reward' practices can lead to all manner of problems – including *nyoné*. As we heard in Amdo, this is understood to be more likely to occur in practitioners who are insufficiently prepared for practice – through a lack of foundational knowledge, or perhaps through over-confidence. The former, particularly, we are told, can lead to *namtok*, where a practitioner's lack of knowledge or faith in the Dharma can leave him/her vulnerable to doubts and fears about the intense physical and psychological sensations experienced during practice. As we have seen, this notion of 'meditation sickness' is found not only in Tibetan Buddhist traditions but has also been described and discussed in other Buddhist and meditative traditions too (see, for example, Greene's 2017 work on Chinese Buddhism).

We explored in Chapter 2 how these complex Tibetan notions of *lung* can be traced back to Indian medical and Tantric understandings of 'wind' (Skt. *vāta*) and 'breath'/'life-force' (Skt. *prāna*). It is of course these twin origins in two different (but related) Indian traditions that have led to centuries of discussion and debate amongst Tibetan scholars and practitioners over whether the winds and channels of Tibetan medicine can be reconciled with the winds and channels described in the Tibetan Tantric texts. What this means in terms of illness and treatment is a certain amount of overlap between medical and religious explanatory frameworks and healing modalities. According to Tibetan medical theory, for example, the treatment of *lung* illnesses is often seen to lie in Tibetan medicine: both medical texts and the doctors I spoke to in Amdo described medicinal formulae and external therapies appropriate for treating different kinds of *lung* illnesses. In addition, as with all illnesses, particular dietary and behavioural considerations are recommended: for *lung* conditions, a healing environment should be calm and warm, and foods including meats and warming foods are ideal. This also means that for those practitioners whose *lung né* or *nyoné* has been precipitated by their Tantric practices focused on *lung* manipulation, particular *lung* medications and treatments may help to restore the healthy functioning of *lung*. In such cases, though, there may also be a particular focus on conducting certain mind-body practices that will impact the *lung*, as advised by a more experienced Tantric teacher. As we heard in Chapter 1, however, not all such cases are understood to be treatable – particularly where they have not been treated in the early stages.

In Part II, we explored the role of spirits and deities in the causation of *nyoné*. As was evident in Amdo, longstanding Tibetan understandings about non-human entities inform many narratives about health and illness, with low-level spirits and deities implicated in the causation of many kinds of disease. This was the case both for *un*intentional engagement with local spirits/deities as well as intentional interactions such as during Tantric practice. Here, some spirits were particularly renowned for their propensity to cause madness – *ngakpa* (ritual specialist) Penpa in Rebkong, for example, was one of several Amdo interviewees to talk about a particular class of spirits known as *gyalpo*. In addition, spirits and local deities may also be related to notions of 'impurity' or 'pollution' – although, as we saw, in Amdo there are diverse perspectives on the connections between them.

Trouble-causing spirits are described in both medical and Tantric Tibetan texts, such as the madness-causing spirits described in the *Gyüshi* medical text or the protector deity Pehar – known for his ability to 'bring epidemics, [and] cause insanity and other illness' (Lin 2010: 22). Thus, theoretically, the treatment of illnesses caused by such entities also comes under the purview of both of these traditions and their practitioners. In reality, of course, it seems that in many places it is primarily religious specialists who are consulted in such cases, using ritual methods to expel spirits/deities and stop them from causing harm. Moreover, as we have seen, these kinds of unenlightened spirits and deities can cause problems for Tantric practitioners too – we heard, for example, about how a practitioner conducting *chöd* practice might 'lose control' of the spirits he/she has summoned. But here, as we explored in Chapter 6, the focus is not on a ritual specialist intervening to cast out an afflicting spirit. Instead, the practitioner him/herself has to recognize a spirit's true nature as a manifestation of his/her own unenlightened mind in order to overcome it. Here, we are reminded of the dual status of such entities as both 'real' and 'unreal' – the ultimate phenomenon to be 'conquered' is in fact the practitioner's own mind, rather than any kind of external factor.

In contrast, in Tantric deity-yoga practices, *enlightened* Buddhist and Bon deities are the focus. Here, the practitioner works with an enlightened *yidam* deity – initially visualizing the deity in front of him/herself before eventually evoking it within his/her own mind-body, transforming him/herself *into* that very buddha. Ultimately, a practitioner's ability to do this is key to successful practice; the form of 'pure vision' that they attain through this is understood to be 'truer and more correct than the practitioner's normal perception of reality' (Samuel 1993: 236).

In these engagements with both unenlightened spirits/deities and enlightened Tantric deities, we have seen how *lung* is, again, key. In the case of low-level spirits and deities, pre-Buddhist ideas about spirit affliction are brought into Tantric notions of mind-body in part through the notion of *lung*. As Dr Nyima explained to me in Xining, the spirits and deities only have a '*lung* body' – a subtle, or energetic, body – and it is this that allows them to connect to a human's subtle energy, entering a person's body through 'openings' in the fingers. And in deity yoga too, it is the subtle aspect of the human body – and a Tantric practitioner's control over it – that allows the transformation from human practitioner to enlightened Tantric deity through a reconfiguration of their very state of being. Here again, we see that 'realization' is not a case of cognitive understanding but a *restructuring* of mind-body. These practices are not only key to the attainment of realization but are also the foundation of a practitioner's spiritual power: having attained control over the subtle energies of the mind-body, the everyday norms of time and space no longer apply to them – and thus we heard about Tantric practitioners levitating, removing their own intestines or travelling through space.

In these discussions, enduring Tibetan notions of human–non-human relations were key. Here, a hierarchy of differential levels of 'spiritual power' (Tib. *wang tang*) inform how lay people, spirit-mediums and Tantric practitioners engage with different types of spirits and deities, and highlights the superiority of the Dharma (Buddhist or Bon). In many of these explanations, pre-Buddhist Tibetan notions of humans and their relationship to the world and the cosmos come together with Buddhist and Tantric notions of mind-body originating in India. Thus, where ordinary (unenlightened) humans are understood to hold less spiritual power than (unenlightened) spirits and deities, it is Tantric practitioners' evocation of enlightened deities that enables them to subjugate the less-powerful unenlightened entities. For spirit-mediums – whose power is accessed through their ritual possession of powerful *un*enlightened gods – their spiritual power is not always strong enough to sufficiently control some of these non-human entities. Hence, we hear about the common period of 'madness' that many spirit-mediums experience at the beginning of their mediumship, as spirits and deities are understood to be fighting for control of their mind-body. Hopefully, under the tutelage of a more experienced spirit-medium, the practitioner learns to control (at least to some extent) the entry and exit of this deity to and from their consciousness through the channels, quelling the symptoms of madness. This new spirit-medium is then able to use the power of this mid-level unenlightened deity for the benefit of the community, including through the control of less-powerful local spirits/deities that may be causing illness or other harms. However, ultimately, these practitioners – and their deities – come under the superior power of the Buddhist or Bon lama, who has more spiritual power than both lay humans and all of these unenlightened non-human entities. This superior spiritual power means that Tantric Buddhist and Bon practitioners are often called upon to subjugate spirits or deities thought to be causing a variety of illness and harms, including madness. And it is through these ritualized engagements with spirits and deities that we can see Tantric practitioners enacting again and again the narrative of the 'taming' of Tibet by the Dharma through the actions of Padmasambhava in the Tibetan Buddhist traditions, and Tonpa Shenrab in the Bon tradition.

Within these discussions about 'madness', of course, we also encounter the figure of the *lama nyonpa* – the 'mad yogin'. This practitioner, as we have heard, may initially *appear* to have the illness of *nyoné* but he/she is actually enlightened. In Amdo, interviewees mostly spoke to me about historical *lama nyonpa*, but I occasionally heard about contemporary figures too: some of these were known only through descriptions online or videos shared through WeChat, but a handful were described second or third hand by those I spoke to.

How might we understand these figures in this broad picture of 'madness'? Indeed, we have heard that it is not always easy for a casual observer to determine the *lama nyonpa* from the lama who has *nyonpa*. DiValerio argues that historical figures such as the Madmen of Ü and Tsang were not enlightened or mad. Instead, they were simply performing a form of 'Tantric fundamentalism' – taking a literal approach to some particular parts of Tantric texts, rather than the more common figurative interpretations (2015: 14). Here, he asserts, the lama simply 'performs' madness rather than experiencing it, in contrast to popular narratives. But perhaps this is not important. According to Tantric Buddhist and Bon understanding, it is at least *possible* for this kind of 'madness' to occur: if a practitioner conducts their practices correctly, manipulating the *lung* to manipulate the mind-body, they will be able to comprehend 'non-duality' and see beyond the false dichotomies of samsara; indeed, they can become an enlightened Tantric deity. Seeing everything 'as it truly is', and acting accordingly (Ibid.: 6), the *lama nyonpa* might indeed be found naked in public, eating dirt or engaging in other strange behaviours. While this may appear to be ordinary 'madness', it is in fact the ultimate sanity – seeing everything as it truly is through the enlightened mind. Indeed, Tantric practitioners understand that it is only in recognizing the 'madness' of samsara that one can overcome it: it is thus those who have accomplished realization who are truly sane: their 'madness' demonstrating that they have 'transcended delusory understandings of the spiritual path' (Ibid.: 172).

But while the *lama nyonpa* perhaps 'performs' madness . . . or, indeed, appears 'mad' due to his/her true enlightenment, and the Tantric practitioner aims to attain the ultimate 'sanity' of realization, people's everyday experiences of *nyoné* reference common themes. Here, narratives of ordinary (e.g. trauma, stress, loss) and extraordinary (spirit affliction, impurity) life events are explained through the lens of wind and its relationship to heart and mind, and to humans' connections to the wider world and the cosmos through longstanding Tibetan notions of spirits, deities and hierarchies of spiritual power. Ultimately, in all of these narratives of madness, people are simply searching for answers – often moving between different explanatory frameworks, healing systems, practitioners and practices across the related spheres of 'medicine' and 'religion' in search of meaning, diagnosis and perhaps healing for themselves and their loved ones.

Glossary

Amdo-wa (a mdo pa): person from Amdo
bardo (bar do): intermediate state between death and rebirth
bar dön (bar gdon): spirits of the middle realms
béken (bad kan): phlegm
bodhicitta: see *jang chup sem*
bok ('bog): mad, insane
Bumshi ('bum bzhi): Bon medical text
chakpé tsa (chags pa'i rtsa): channels of formation
ché pa tong (chad pa gtong): punish
Chi mé Gyü (phyi ma'i rgyud: *Subsequent (Fourth) Tantra*
chöd (gcod): cutting-off ritual (Tantric practice founded by Machig Labdrön [1055–1149])
chö kyong (chos skyong): Dharma protector (see also (*sung ma*)
dam tshig (dam tshig): vow, pledge (Skt. *samaya*)
dépa (dad pa): faith
dorjé lü / ku dor jé (rdo rje lus / sku rdo rje): Vajra body
dö (mdos): thread ritual – a type of 'ransom' ritual using a cross made from sticks and coloured threads
dö chak (dod chags): attachment, desire
dön (gdon): spirit
dön né (gdon nad): spirit illness/affliction
drelwa (sbrel ba): connection
drelwé tsa (*'brel ba'i rtsa*): connecting channels
dré ('dre): spirit, ghost (see also *[shin]dré*)
dri ma (spris ma): cream/foam (in relation to urine)
drip (grib): impurity, pollution (also *mi tsang wa* [mi gtsang ba])
druptop (grub thob): *siddha*; accomplished one
duk sum (dug gsum): three poisons
dü (bdud): demon, demonic forces, Māra
dzé (mdze): leprosy
gek (bgegs): obstacle, hindrance
geshe (dge shes): title given to a monk who has completed the course in Buddhist or Bon dialectics
gewa (dge ba): virtuous action
go (mgo): head
guru tsen gyé (gu ru mtshan brgyad): eight forms of Padmasambhava
gyal dön (rgyal gdon): see *gyalpo*

gyalpo (rgyal po): 'king spirit', type of worldly (unenlightened) deity/local god (also *gyal dön*)
gyen gyu lung (gyen rgyu rlung): ascending wind
gyu (rgyu): cause; primary cause
gyud (rgyud): Tantra (lit. 'thread')
gyu lü (sgyu lus): illusory body
gyungpa (rgyungs pa): spinal cord
Gyüshi (rgyud bzhi): Four Tantras, Four Treatises
hormé (hor me): herbal poultice
hön (dpon): Tantric ritual specialist; *ngakpa*
ja men (rgya sman): literally, 'Chinese medicine'; used in Amdo to refer to biomedicine
jang chup sem (byang chub sems): *bodhicitta*, mind of enlightenment
ja tsa men (rgya rtsa sman): Chinese herbal medicine (Traditional Chinese Medicine)
jé jé kyi dön (rbjed byed kyi gdon): spirits that cause forgetfulness
Jikjé ('jigs byed): Vajrabhairava/Yamantaka (a wrathful Tantric deity)
jiktenpé lha ('jig rten pa'i lha): unenlightened deities (also 'jig rten gyi lha)
jung pö (dön) (byung po'i gdon): elemental spirits
Kangyur (bka' 'gyur): *Teachings of the Buddha* (translated into Tibetan from Sanskrit); foundational texts of the Buddhist and Bon traditions
kar ma (skar ma): stars, constellation, specific astrological moment/time
khandroma (mkha' 'gro ma): female deities; also used to refer to high-level female Tantric practitioners (Skt. *ḍākinī*)
khorlo ('khor lo): energy centre, chakra (Skt. *cakra*)
khyap jé lung (khyab byed rlung): pervasive wind
khyim lha (khyim lha): family god
kora (skor ra): circumambulation – usually of sacred sights such as monasteries, or sacred objects
kordak (dkor bdag): a type of low-level spirit
küntak (kun btags): conceptual phenomena
kün zhi nam pa shé pa (kun gzhi rnam pa shes pa): base consciousness
kyangma (rkyang ma): right channel (Skt. *lalanā*)
kyen (rkyen): secondary causes; conditions (see also *lam zhi*)
kyé rim (skyed rim): generation stage (of the high level *Anuttarayoga Tantras* in the New (Sarma) Tantra traditions) and the *Mahāyoa Tantras* in the Old (Nyingma) Tantra traditions
kyilwa (skyil ba): to retain (the breath)
kyu sum (skyu gsum): three bodies of the Buddha (Skt. *trikāya*)
la (bla): subtle life essence, life-force
lama (bla ma): Tibetan Buddhist or Bon Tantric teacher, senior practitioner
lama nyonpa (bla ma smyon pa): 'mad yogin', 'crazy lama'
lam zhis (lam bzhis): conditions (see also *kyen*)
lé (las): action; the law of cause and effect; karma (Skt. *karma*)
lé lung (las rlung): karmic wind
lépa (klad pa): brain
lha (lha): deity, god
lha sin dé gyé (lha srin sde brgyad): eight gods and spirits
lhawa (lha pa): spirit-medium (also *lhapa, lha zhuk ken* [lha bzhugs mkhan])
lhé neljor (lha'i rnal 'byor): deity yoga
lhé nga gyallhé nga gyel (lha'i nga rgyal): divine pride
lo jong (blo sbyong): 'mind training' (practice)

long chö dzok pé ku: (longs spyod rdzog pa'i sku): heavenly body; enjoyment body (Skt. *saṃbhogakāya*)
lu (dön) (klu [gdon]): water spirits (Skt. *naga*)
lung (rlung): wind, energy (related to both Skt. *vāta/vāyu* (wind) and *prāna* (life-force, breath)
lung lang (rlung langs): anger
lung né (rlung nad): wind illness
Lung Né Drip Tsen Khak (rlung nad grib rigs tshan khag): Department for Wind Illnesses and Impurities
lungta (rlung rta): luck, fortune
lung topo (rlung mtho po): high (i.e. increased) lung
lung trawa (rlung phra ba): subtle wind/energy
lung tsha po (rlung tsha po): hot strong wind (condition)
lü (glud): effigy, ritual 'scapegoat'
lü lha (lus lha): personal deity
men (sman): medicine
menba (sman pa): doctor
men chok (sman mchog): supreme medicine
men gyud (sman rgyud): *lineage physicians*
Men ngak Gyü (man ngag rgyud): Oral Instruction (Third) Tantra
mé nyam lung (me mnyam rlung): fire-accompanying wind
mé tsa (me btsa'): moxibustion
mé tsa (me rtsa): fire-element pulse
mi dewa (mi bde ba): uncomfortable
mi tsangwa (mi gtsang ba): impurity, pollution (also *drip* [grib])
mo (mo): divination
mopa (mo pa): diviner
Mutig 70 (mu tig bdun ju): 'Pearl 70' [medical formulation]
namshé (rnam shes): consciousness
namtok (rnam rtog): conceptual thoughts, discursive thoughts, suspicion (Skt. *saṁkalpa*; *vikalpa*)
né (nad): illness, disease
ngagel (nga gnal): pride, arrogance, conceit
ngak (sngags): mantra, ritual
ngar mi (ngar mi): effigy
ngödrup (gnos grub): *siddhi*, yogic accomplishment
ngön dro (sngon 'gro): preliminary practice
nöd (gnod): harm (see also *nöpa*)
nöpa (gnod pa): harm (see also *nöd*)
numjuk (snum byug): massage of the hands and/or feet with melted butter/fat mixed with herbs
nüpa (nus pa): ability, power, potency
nyam (nyams): experience
nyam yig (nyams yig; lit. 'writing from experience'): commentarial texts
nya ngen (mya ngan): suffering/distress
nyen (gnyan): a type of spirit
nyépa (nyes pa): energy, fault (often translated as 'humour/humor') (Skt. *doṣa*)
nyimé (gnyis med): non-duality
nying (snying): heart
nying lung (né) (snying rlung [nad]): heart-wind illness, wind-in-the-heart illness

nying né (snying nad): heart illness
nying top zhen (snying stobs zhan): fearfulness/weak heart
nyo bok (smyo 'bog): madness, delirium
nyo jé gyi dön (smyo byed gyi gdon): 'madness-causing spirits'
nyoné (smyo nad): madness, insanity
nyonpa (smyon pa): madness, mad person
ok dön ('og gdon): spirits of the lower realms
rigpa (rigs pa): knowledge, reasoning
rinchen rilbu (rin chen ril bu): 'precious pill'; usually a medicinal compound including precious gems
roma (ro ma): left channel (Skt. *rasanā*)
sadak (sa bdag): earth spirits
sang ngak (gsang sngags): secret mantra
sem (sems): mind [generally understood to be located in the heart]
sem kham (sems khams): psychology, state of mind
sem kham ma dewa (sems khams ma bde ba): uneasy/uncomfortable mind
sem lé ché (sems las ches): excessive worry
sem né (sems nad): mind illness, illness of the mind
sem pa chen po (sems pa chen po): 'spacious mind', 'broad thinking'
sem trel (sems khral): anxiety, worry
Shé Gyü (bshad rgyud): Explanatory (Second) Tantra
(shin)dré ([shi] 'dre): ghost/spirit
shing tsa (shing rtsa): wood-element pulse
sipé tsa (srid pa'i rtsa): channels of existence
sok (dzin) lung (srog ['dzin] rlung): life-sustaining wind
sok lung men (srog lung sman): life-sustaining wind medicine
sok lung (né) (srog rlung [nad]): life-sustaining wind/life wind illness
sok tsa (srog rtsa): life-sustaining channel
sonam (bsod nams): merit; good karma associated with virtuous activity
sung ma (srung ma): protective deity (see also *chö kyong*)
telpa/telwa (tel pa): medical instruments used to apply heat to specific points on the body
teng dön (steng gdon): spirits of the upper realms
Tengyur (bstan 'gyur): Commentarial texts in the Tibetan Buddhist and Bon traditions
tenpa (brtan pa): trust, dependency
teurang (the'u rang): a type of spirit variously translated as poltergeist, gnome, or *preta*, often said to afflict children
thangka (thang ka): traditional Tibetan Buddhist or Bon painting, usually on cloth; often depicting buddha figures
tiklé (thig le): drops (Skt. *bindu*)
ti muk (gti mug): delusion
tokden (rtogs ldan): realised
tokdenpa (rtogs ldan pa): realised person
tongpa nyi (stong pa nyid): emptiness; the assertion that all phenomena are empty of intrinsic existence (Skt. *śūnyatā*)
torma (tor ma): offerings made of roasted barley flour
trak lung (khrag rlung): blood pressure
trawa (phra ba): subtle
tré (skrad): exorcism ritual
tripa (mkhris pa): bile

trül ('phrul): magic, illusion
trül khor ('phrul 'khor): 'magical movement'
tsa (rtsa): channels
Tsa Gyü (rtsa rgyud): Root (First) Tantra
tsa kar (rtsa dkar): white channels, often translated as nerves or lymphatic vessels
tsa lung (rtsa rlung): channel-wind (practices)
tsa nak (rtsa nag): black channels, often translated as blood vessels
tsa tung chu zhi (rtsa ltung bcu bzhi): fourteen root downfalls; fourteen root transgressions of the Tantric vows/precepts
tsa wuma (rtsa dbu ma): central channel (Skt. *avadhūti*)
tsen (btsan): type of worldly (unenlightened) deity/local god
tsé tra drup (rtsa'i pra sgrub): a type of divination (Skt. *prasenā*)
tsé tsa (tshe'i rtsa): vitality/life channels
tsi (rtsis): astrology
tsipa (rtsis pa): astrologer
Tso ngon Shing chen Bö Men Khang (mtsho sngon zhing chen bod sman khang): Qinghai Province Tibetan Medicine Hospital
tsotel (btso thal): purified mercury compound ['a compound of processed mercury sulphide, eight metals, and eight rock components, which are all processed over several weeks with numerous plants and other ingredients, and eventually burnt to ash' (Gerke and Ploberger 2017: 583)]
tuk (thugs): intentions, emotions, thought, perception [honorific form of *yi*] (Skt. *manas*)
tumo (gtum mo): Tantric 'inner heat' practice (Skt. *Caṇḍālī*),
tur sel lung (thur sel rlung): descending wind
tülzhuk (brtul zhugs): Practice of the Observance
tünmong ngödrup (thun mong dngos grub): 'ordinary' *siddhis*
wang (dbang): empowerment, initiation
wang tang (dbang thang): spiritual power
yéshé lung (ye shes lung): wisdom wind
yi (yid): intentions, emotions, thought, perception (Skt. *manas*) (see also *tuk*)
yidak (yi dags): hungry ghost
yidam (yi dam): Tantric tutelary deity
yi mi dé (yid mi bde): unhappy mind
za yi dön (gza' yi gdon): planetary spirits that cause strokes or partial paralysis
zé jö mi trö (zas sbyod mi 'phrod): unwholesome diet
zhé dang (zhe sdang): hatred, anger
zhidak (gzhi bdag): a kind of spirit or mountain deity

References

Tibetan-Language Sources

rgod tshang ras pa sna tshogs rang grol.1969 [1512]. *gtsang nyon he ru ka phyogs thams cad las rnam par rgyal ba'i rnam thar rdo rje theg pa'i gsal byed nyi ma'i snying po*, published as *The Life of the Saint of Gtsang*. New Delhi: Śata-piṭaka Series, vol. 69. Edited by Lokesh Chandra, with 'preface' by Gene E. Smith. Tibetan Buddhist Resource Center (TBRC) W4CZ1247.

Yutok Yonten Gonpo [gyu thog yon tan mgon po]. 2015. *bdud rtsi snying po yan lag brgyad pa gsang ba man ngag gi rgyud ces bya ba bzhugs so* [*The Tantra of the Oral Instructions of the Eight Limbs of the Essence of the Amrita*]. Beijing: bod ljongs mi dmangs dpe skrun khang.

English-Language Sources

Adams, Vincanne. 1998. 'Suffering the Winds of Lhasa: Politicized Bodies, Human Rights, Cultural Difference, and Humanism in Tibet', *Medical Anthropology Quarterly* 12: 74–102.

———. 2001. 'The Sacred in the Scientific: Ambiguous Practices of Science in Tibetan Medicine', *Cultural Anthropology* 16: 542–75.

———. 2002. 'Establishing Proof: Translating "Science" and the State in Tibetan Medicine', in Margaret Lock and Mark Nichter (eds), *New Horizons in Medical Anthropology: Essays in honour of Charles Leslie*. London: Routledge, pp. 200–20.

———. 2007. 'Integrating Abstraction: Modernising Medicine at Lhasa's Mentsikhang', in Mona Schrempf (ed.), *Soundings in Tibetan Medicine: Anthropological and Historical Anthropological Perspectives. PIATS 2003: Proceedings of the Tenth Seminar of the International Association of Tibetan Studies, Oxford 2003*. Leiden: Brill, pp. 29–43.

Adams, Vincanne, Renchen Dhondup and Phuoc V. Le. 2011. 'A Tibetan Way of Science: Revisioning Biomedicine as Tibetan Practice', in Vincanne Adams, Mona Schrempf and Sienna R. Craig (eds), *Medicine Between Science and Religion: Explorations on Tibetan Grounds*. New York: Berghahn Books, pp. 107–26.

Adams, Vincanne and Fei-Fei Li. 2008. 'Integration or Erasure? Modernizing Medicine at Lhasa's Mentsikhang', in Laurent Pordié (ed.), *Tibetan Medicine in the Contemporary World: Global Politics of Medical Knowledge and Practice*. London: Routledge, pp. 105–31.

Adams, Vincanne, Mona Schrempf and Sienna R. Craig (eds). 2011. *Medicine Between Science and Religion: Explorations on Tibetan Grounds*. New York: Berghahn Books.

Ahn, Juhn. 2017. 'Getting Sick Over Nothing: Hyesim and Hakuin on the Maladies of Meditation', in C. Pierce Salguero (ed.), *Buddhism and Medicine: An Anthology of Premodern Sources*. New York: Columbia University Press, pp. 390–97.

Ardussi, John and Lawrence Epstein. 1978. 'The Saintly Madman in Tibet', in James F. Fisher (ed.), *Himalayan Anthropology: The Indo-Tibetan Interface*. The Hague and Paris: Mouton Publishers, pp. 327–38.

Arya, Pasang Y. 'Psychology and Psychiatry', Tibetan Medicine Education Center website 2023. Retrieved May 2023 from https://tibetanmedicine-edu.org/tmm/tm/psychology-and-psychiatry/psychology-and-psychiatry/.

Baker, Ian A. and Romeo Shrestha. 1997. *The Tibetan Art of Healing*. London, Thames and Hudson.

Bassini, Patrizia. 2013a. 'Harmony or Hierarchy? The Mindful Body and the Sacred Landscape in Tibetan Healing Practices', in Peregrine Horden and Elisabeth Hsu (eds), *The Body in Balance: Humoral Medicines in Practice*. New York: Berghahn Books, pp. 235–55.

———. 2013b. 'The Hierarchy of Food Consumption and Tibetan Experiences of Gastric and Gallbladder Disorders in Amdo', *East Asian Science, Technology and Society: An International Journal* 7(3): 453–66.

Bell, Christopher. 2006. 'Tsui Marpo: The Career of a Tibetan Protector Deity', M.A. dissertation. Florida: Florida State University.

———. 2019. 'Worldly Protector Deities in Tibet', in Jonathan A. Silk, Richard Bowring, Vincent Eltschinger and Michael Radich (eds), *Brill's Encyclopedia of Buddhism, Volume II: Lives*. Leiden: Brill, pp. 1254–66.

Bellezza, John Vincent. 2010. 'Gshen-rab Myi-bo: His Life and Times According to Tibet's Earliest Literary Sources', *Revue d'Etudes Tibétaines* 19: 31–118.

———. 2011. 'The Liturgies and Oracular Utterances of Spirit-mediums of Upper Tibet–An Introduction to their *bSangs* Rituals', *Revue d'Etudes Tibétaines* 20: 5–31.

Benedict, Adriana Lee, Linda Mancini and Michael A. Grodin. 2009. 'Struggling to Meditate: Contextualising Integrated Treatment of Traumatised Tibetan Refugee Monks', *Mental Health, Religion and Culture* 12: 485–99.

Bentor, Yael. 2000. 'The Tibetan Practice of the Mantra Path According to Lce-sgom-pa', in David Gordon White (ed.), *Tantra in Practice*. Princeton, NJ and Oxford: Princeton University Press, pp. 326–46.

Berglie, Per-Arne. 1976. 'Preliminary remarks on some Tibetan "spirit-mediums" in Nepal', *Kailash* 4: 85–108.

———. 1982. 'Spirit-possession in Theory and Practice: Séances with Tibetan Spirit-mediums in Nepal', *Scripta Instituti Donneriani Aboensis* 11: 151–66.

Besch, Nils Florian. 2006. 'Tibetan Medicine Off the Roads: Modernizing the Work of the Amchi in Spiti', Ph.D. dissertation. Heidelberg: Universität Hiedelberg.

Blezer, Henk. 2011. 'Creation of a Myth: The Zhang Zhung Empire of the Bon Po-S: Khyung Lung Dngul Mkhar', in Henk Blezer (ed.), *Emerging Bon: The Formation of Bon Traditions in Tibet at the Turn of the First Millennium AD. PIATS 2006: Tibetan Studies: Proceedings of the Eleventh Seminar of the International Association for Tibetan Studies, Königswinter 2006 and Oxford 2003*. Andiast: International Institute for Tibetan and Buddhist Studies, pp. 117–63.

Blondeau, Anne-Marie. 1998. 'Tibetan Mountain Deities, Their Cults and Representations', in Anne-Marie Blondeau (ed.), *Papers Presented at a Panel of 7th Seminar of the International Association for Tibetan Studies, Graz, 1995*. Vienna: Austrian Academy of Sciences Press.

Buffetrille, Katia. 2008. 'Some Remarks on Mediums: The Case of the *Lha pa* of the Musical Festival (*glu rol*) of Sog ru (A mdo)', *Mongolo-Tibetico Pragensia* 8: 13–66.

Calkowski, Marcia. 1985. 'Power, charisma, and ritual curing in a Tibetan community in India', Ph.D. dissertation. Vancouver: University of British Columbia.

———. 1993. 'Contesting Hierarchy: On Gambling as an Authoritative Resource in Tibetan Refugee Society', *Proceedings of the International Seminar on the Anthropology of Tibet and the Himalaya*. Zurich: Völkerkundemuseum der Universität Zürich, pp. 30–38.

Cassaniti, Julia and Tanya Marie Luhrmann. 2011. 'Encountering the Supernatural: A Phenomenological Account of Mind', *Religion and Society: Advances in Research* 2(1): 37–53.

Cassaniti, Julia L., and Tanya Marie Luhrmann. 2014. 'The Cultural Kindling of Spiritual Experiences', *Current Anthropology* 55(S10): S333–S43.

Chang, Garma C.C. 1977. *The Hundred Thousand Songs of Milarepa, by Tsangnyön Heruka: Volume II*, 2nd edn. Boulder, CO and London: Shambhala.

Chaoul, M.A. 2007. 'Magical Movement (*'phrul 'khor*): Ancient Tibetan Yogic Practices from the Bon Religion and their Migration into Contemporary Medical Settings', *Asian Medicine* 3: 130–55.

Chui, Tony. 2019. '"Secret Medicine" in the Writings of Sanggyé Gyatso: the Encoded Esoteric Material of Therapeutics', in William A. McGrath (ed.), *Knowledge and Context in Tibetan Medicine*. Leiden: Brill, pp. 85–110.

Clark, Barry. 1995. *The Quintessence Tantras of Tibetan Medicine*. Ithaca, NY: Snow Lion Publications.

Clifford, Terry. 1984. *Tibetan Buddhist Medicine and Psychiatry: The Diamond Healing*. Wellingborough: The Aquarian Press.

Cornu, Philipe. 1997. *Tibetan Astrology*. Boston, MA: Shambhala Publications.

Cozort, Daniel. 1986. *Highest Yoga Tantra*. Boston and London: Snow Lion.

Craig, Sienna R. 2012. *Healing Elements: Efficacy and the Social Ecologies of Tibetan Medicine*. Berkeley, CA: University of California Press.

Czaja, Olaf. 2015. 'The Administration of Tibetan Precious Pills: Efficacy in Historical and Ritual Contexts', *Asian Medicine* 10: 36–89.

Dalton, Jacob. 2004. 'The Development of Perfection: The Interiorization of Buddhist Ritual in the Eighth and Ninth Centuries', *Journal of Indian philosophy* 32: 1–30.

Davidson, Ronald M. 2002. *Indian Esoteric Buddhism: Social History of the Tantric Movement*. New York: Columbia University Press.

Day, Sophie. 1989. 'Embodying Spirits: Village Oracles and Possession Rituals in Ladakh, North India', Ph.D. dissertation. London: London School of Economics and Political Science (University of London).

Deane, Susannah. 2014a. 'From Sadness to Madness: Tibetan Perspectives on the Causation and Treatment of Psychiatric Illness', *Religions* 5: 444–58.

———. 2014b. 'There is Power in Belief': Creating Space for Psychiatric Illness and Healing in the Tibetan Context', *SHARE: Studies in History, Archaeology, Religion and Conservation* 1: 40–48.

———. 2018. *Tibetan Medicine, Buddhism, and Psychiatry: Mental Health and Healing in a Tibetan Exile Community*. Durham, NC: Carolina Academic Press.

———. 2019a. 'Madness and the spirits: examining the role of spirits in mental illness in the Tibetan communities of Darjeeling', in William A. McGrath (ed.), *Knowledge and Context in Tibetan Medicine*. Leiden and Boston, MA: Brill, pp. 309–36.

———. 2019b. '*rLung*, Mind, and Mental Health: The Notion of "Wind" in Tibetan Conceptions of Mind and Mental Illness', *Journal of Religion and Health* 58: 708–24.

———. 2024. '"For this kind of thing, the lama is better": Religion, Medicine, and the Treatment of Madness Among Tibetans in Amdo', in C. Pierce Salguero, Kin Cheung and Susannah Deane (eds), *Buddhism and Healing in the Modern World.* Honolulu, HI: University of Hawai'i Press.

des Jardins, J.F. Marc. 2009. 'Bon Institutions in Contemporary Tibetan Territories and the Dynamics of Religious Authority', *East and West. Bon: The Everlasting Religion of Tibet. Tibetan Studies in Honour of Professor David L. Snellgrove* 59(1/4): 233–44.

Dhargyey, Geshe Lharampa Ngawang. 1985. *A Commentary on the Kalacakra Tantra*, Dharamsala, Library of Tibetan Works and Archives.

Dhondhen, Yeshi and Jhampa Kelsang. 1983. 'The Ambrosia Heart Tantra: The Secret Oral Instructions on the Eight Branches of the Science of Tibetan Medicine, Vol. 1', *Tibetan Medicine* 6: 1–93.

Dhondup, Yangdon. 2011a. 'Reb kong: Religion, History and Identity of a Sino-Tibetan borderland town', *Revue d'Etudes Tibétaines* 20: 33–59.

———. 2011b. 'Rig 'dzin Dpal ldan bkra Shis (1688–1743) and the Emergence of a Tantric Community in Reb kong, A mdo (Qinghai)', *Journal of the International Association of Buddhist Studies* 34(1/2): 3–30.

———. 2013. 'Rules and Regulations of the Reb kong Tantric Community', in Yangdon Dhondup, Ulrich Pagel and Geoffrey Samuel (eds), *Monastic and Lay Traditions in North-Eastern Tibet.* Leiden: Brill, pp. 117–40.

Dhondup, Yangdon, Ulrich Pagel and Geoffrey Samuel. (eds). 2013. *Monastic and Lay Traditions in North-Eastern Tibet.* Leiden and Boston, MA: Brill.

Diemberger, Hildegard. 2005. 'Female Oracles in Modern Tibet', in Janet Gyatso and Hanna Havnevik (eds), *Women in Tibet.* London: Hurst & Company, pp. 113–68.

DiValerio, David M. 2015. *The Holy Madmen of Tibet.* New York: Oxford University Press.

Donden, Yeshi. 1986. *Health Through Balance: An Introduction to Tibetan Medicine.* Delhi: Motilal Banarsidass.

Dorje, Dudjom Rinpoche Jigdrel Yeshe. 2011. *A Torch Lighting the Way to Freedom: Complete Instructions on the Preliminary Practices*, trans. Padmakara Translation Group. Boulder, CO: Shambhala Publications.

Dorjee, Pema, with Janet Jones and Terence Moore. 2005. *The Spiritual Medicine of Tibet: Heal Your Spirit, Heal Yourself.* London: Watkins Publishing.

Dorjee, Pema and Elizabeth Richards. 1985. 'Chapters 60–102 of the Four Tantras: Translated by Dr Pema Dorjee with Elizabeth Richards', *Tibetan Medicine* 2: 7–56.

Dpal-ldan-bkra-shis and Kevin Stuart. 1998. 'Perilous Novelties: The A-mdo Tibetan *klu-rol* festival in Gling-Rgyal village', *Anthropos*: 31–53.

Drungtso, Tsering Thakchoe. 2004. *Tibetan Medicine: The Healing Science of Tibet.* Dharamsala, HP: Drungtso Publications.

Duckworth, Douglas. 2017. 'Rangjung Dorjé's "Key to the Essential Points of Wind and Mind"', in C. Pierce Salguero (ed.), *Buddhism and Medicine: An Anthology of Premodern Sources.* New York and Chichester: Columbia University Press, pp. 413–17.

Emmerick, Ronald E. 1977. 'Sources of the rGyud-bzhi', *(Supplement, Deutscher Orientalistentag vom 28. Sept. bis 4. Okt. 1975 in Frieburg i. Br.) Zeitschrift der Deutschen Morgenländischen Gesellschaft (Wiesbaden)* III(2): 1135–42.

———. 1987. 'Epilepsy according to the *rgyud-bzhi*', in Gerrit Jan Meulenbeld and Dominik Wujastyk (eds), *Studies on Indian Medical History: Papers Presented at the International Workshop on the Study of Indian Medicine. Wellcome Institute for the History of Medicine. 2–4 September 1985.* Groningen: Egbert Forsten.

Epstein, Mark D. and Jonathan D. Lieff. 1981. 'Psychiatric Complications of Meditation Practice', *Journal of Transpersonal Psychology* 13: 137–47.

Epstein, Mark D. and Sonam Topgay. 1982. 'Mind and Mental Disorders in Tibetan Medicine', *ReVision: A Journal of Consciousness and Change* 9: 67–79.

Epstein, Lawrence and Peng Wenbin. 1998. 'Ritual, Ethnicity, and Generational Identity', in Melvyn C. Goldstein and Matthew T. Kapstein (eds), *Buddhism in Contemporary Tibet: Religious Revival and Cultural Identity*. Berkeley and Los Angeles, CA: University of California Press, pp. 120–38.

Evans-Wentz, Walter Yeeling. 1967. *Tibetan Yoga and Secret Doctrines*. Oxford: Oxford University Press.

Flood, Gavin. 2006. *The Tantric Body: The Secret Tradition of Hindu Religion*. London and New York: I.B.Tauris.

Ga, Yang. 2010. 'The Sources for the Writing of the *Rgyud bzhi*, Tibetan Medical Classic', Ph.D. dissertation. Cambridge, MA: Harvard University.

———. 2014. 'The Origin of the Four Tantras and an Account of its Author, Yuthog Yonten Gonpo', in Theresia Hofer (ed.), *Bodies in Balance: The Art of Tibetan Medicine*. Seattle, WA and London: Rubin Museum of Art, New York in association with University of Washington Press, pp. 154–77.

Gardener, Alexander. 2021. 'The Eleventh Trungpa, Chogyam Trungpa', *The Treasury of Lives*. Retrieved 21 May 2023 from: https://treasuryoflives.org/biographies/view/The-Eleventh-Trungpa,-Chogyam-Trungpa/11231.

Garrett, Francis. 2008. *Religion, Medicine and the Human Embryo in Tibet*. Abingdon and New York: Routledge.

Garrett, Francis and Vincanne Adams. 2008. 'The Three Channels in Tibetan Medicine, with a Translation of Tsultrim Gyaltsen's "A Clear Explanation of the Principal Structure and Location of the Circulatory Channels as Illustrated in the Medical Paintings"', *Traditional South Asian Medicine* 8: 86–115.

Gayley, Holly. 2018. 'Revisiting the "Secret Consort" (*gsang yum*) in Tibetan Buddhism', *Religions* 9(6): 179.

Gerke, Barbara. 2007. 'Engaging the Subtle Body: Re-approaching *bla* Rituals in the Himalaya', in Mona Schrempf (ed.), *Soundings in Tibetan Medicine: Anthropological and Historical Perspectives. PIATS 2003: Proceedings of the Tenth Seminar of the International Association of Tibetan Studies, Oxford 2003*. Leiden and Boston, MA: Brill, pp. 189–212.

———. 2011. 'Correlating Biomedical and Tibetan Medical Terms in *Amchi* Medical Practice', in Vincanne Adams, Mona Schrempf and Sienna R. Craig (eds), *Medicine Between Science and Religion: Explorations on Tibetan Grounds*. New York and Oxford: Berghahn Books, pp. 127–52.

———. 2012. *Long Lives and Untimely Deaths: Life-span Concepts and Longevity Practices Among Tibetans in the Darjeeling Hills, India*. Leiden: Brill.

———. 2013. 'On the "Subtle Body" and "Circulation" in Tibetan Medicine', in Geoffrey Samuel and Jay Johnston (eds), *Religion and the Subtle Body in Asia and the West: Between Mind and Body*. Abingdon and New York: Routledge, pp. 83–99.

———. 2014. 'The Art of Tibetan Medical Practice', in Theresia Hofer (ed.), *Bodies in Balance: The Art of Tibetan Medicine*. Seattle, WA and London: Rubin Museum of Art, New York in association with University of Washington Press, pp. 16–31.

———. 2019. 'The Buddhist-Medical Interface in Tibet: Black Pill Traditions in Transformation', *Religions* 10: 282.

Gerke, Barbara and Florian Ploberger. 2017. 'Jewels in Medicines: On the Processing and Efficacy of Precious Pills According to the Four Treatises', in C. Pierce Salguero (ed.), *Buddhism and Medicine: An Anthology of Premodern Sources*. New York and Chichester: Columbia University Press, pp. 582–92.

Germano, David. 1994. *Mini-Encyclopedia of Great Perfection Terminology*. Charlottesville, VA: University of Virginia.

———. 1997. 'The Elements, Insanity, and Lettered Subjectivity', in Donald S. Lopez Jr, (ed.), *Religions of Tibet in Practice*. Princeton, NJ: Princeton University Press, pp. 313–34.

Goldstein, Melvyn C., T.N. Shelling, J.T. Surkhang and Pierre Robillard. 2001. *The New Tibetan-English Dictionary of Modern Tibetan*. Berkeley, CA and London: University of California Press.

Gray, David. B. 2007. *The Cakrasamvara Tantra (The Discourse of Śrī Heruka): A Study and Annotated Translation*. New York: American Institute of Buddhist Studies & Columbia University's Center for Buddhist Studies and Tibet House US.

Greene, Eric. 2017. 'Healing Sicknesses Caused by Meditation: "The Enveloping Butter Contemplation" from the Secret Essential Methods for Curing Meditation Sickness', in C. Pierce Salguero (ed.), *Buddhism and Medicine: An Anthology of Premodern Sources*. New York: Columbia University Press, pp. 373–82.

Gutschow, Kim. 1997. 'A Study of "Wind Disorder" or Madness in Zangskar, Northwest India', in Thierry Dodin and Heinz Räther (eds), *Recent Research on Ladakh: Proceedings of the 7th Colloquium of the International Association for Ladakh Studies held in Bonn/Sankt Augustin, 12–15 Juni 1995*. Ulm: Universität Ulm, pp. 177–202.

Gyatso, Geshe Kelsang. 1994. *Tantric Grounds and Paths: How to Enter, Progress on, and Complete the Vajrayana Path*. London: Tharpa Publications.

Gyatso, Janet. 1997. 'An Avalokiteśvara Sādhana', in Donald S. Lopez Jnr. (ed.), *Religions of Tibet in Practice*. Princeton, NJ: Princeton University Press, pp. 266–70.

———. 2004. 'The Authority of Empiricism and the Empiricism of Authority: Medicine and Buddhism in Tibet on the Eve of Modernity', *Comparative Studies of South Asia, Africa and the Middle East* 24: 83–96.

———. 2015. *Being Human in a Buddhist World: An Intellectual History of Medicine in Early Modern Tibet*. New York: Columbia University Press.

Gyatso, Khedrup Norsang. 2004. *Ornament of Stainless Light: An Exposition of the Kālacakra Tantra*, trans. G. Kilty. Boston, MA: Wisdom Publications.

Gyatso, Tenzin, The Fourteenth Dalai Lama, with Jeffrey Hopkins. 1985. *The Kālachakra Tantra: Rite of Initiation For the Stage of Generation: A Commentary on the Text of Kay-drup-ge-lek-bel-sang-bo by Tenzin Gyatso, the Fourteenth Dalai Lama, and the Text Itself*. London: Wisdom Publications.

Harvey, Peter. 1993. 'The Mind-Body Relationship in Pāli Buddhism: A Philosophical Investigation', *Asian Philosophy* 3: 29–41.

Helderman, Ira. 2024. 'Mindful of the Media: Framing "Adverse Meditation Effects" in Popular Media in the United States', in C. Pierce Salguero, Kin Cheung and Susannah Deane (eds), *Buddhism and Healing in the Modern World*. Honolulu, HI: University of Hawai'i Press.

Helman-Ważny, Agnieszka and Charles Ramble (eds). 2023. *Bon and Naxi Manuscripts*. Berlin and Boston, MA: De Gruyter.

Henning, Edward. 2009. 'The Six Vajra-Yogas of Kālacakra', in Edward A. Arnold (ed.), *As Long as Space Endures: Essays on the Kālacakra Tantra in Honor of H. H. the Dalai Lama*. Ithaca, NY: Snow Lion Publications, pp. 237–58.

Hepburn, Sharon J. 1988. 'W. H. R. Rivers Prize Essay (1986): Western Minds, Foreign Bodies', *Medical Anthropology Quarterly* 2: 59–74.

Hofer, Theresia. 2018. *Medicine and Memory in Tibet: Amchi Physicians in an Age of Reform*. Seattle, WA: University of Washington Press.

Huber, Toni. 2020. *Source of Life: Revitalisation Rites and Bon Shamans in Bhutan and the Eastern Himalayas*. Vienna: Austrian Academy of Sciences Press.

Hussain, Dilwar and Braj Bhushan. 2011. 'Cultural Factors Promoting Coping Among Tibetan Refugees: A Qualitative Investigation', *Mental Health, Religion & Culture* 14: 575–87.

Jackson, Roger. 1985. 'The Kalachakra in Context', in Geshe Lhundb Sopa, Roger Jackson and John Newman (eds), *The Wheel of Time: The Kalachakra in Context*. Madison, WI: Deer Park Books, pp. 1–50.

Jacobson, Eric Emil. 2000. 'Situated Knowledge in Classical Tibetan Medicine: Psychiatric Aspects', Ph.D. dissertation. Cambridge, MA: Harvard University.

———. 2002. 'Panic Attack in a Context of Comorbid Anxiety and Depression in a Tibetan Refugee', *Culture, Medicine and Psychiatry* 26: 259–79.

———. 2007. 'Life-Wind Illness in Tibetan Medicine: Depression, Generalised Anxiety, and Panic Attack', in Mona Schrempf (ed.), *Soundings in Tibetan Medicine: Anthropological and Historical Perspectives. PIATS 2003: Proceedings of the Tenth Seminar of the International Association of Tibetan Studies, Oxford 2003*. Leiden and Boston, MA: Brill, pp. 225–46.

Janes, Craig R. 1995. 'The Transformations of Tibetan Medicine', *Medical Anthropology Quarterly* 9: 6–39.

———. 1999a. 'The Health Transition, Global Modernity and the Crisis of Traditional Medicine: The Tibetan Case', *Social Science & Medicine* 48: 1803–20.

———. 1999b. 'Imagined Lives, Suffering, and the Work of Culture: The Embodied Discourses of Conflict in Modern Tibet', *Medical Anthropology Quarterly* 13: 391–412.

———. 2001. 'Tibetan Medicine at the Crossroads: Radical Modernity and the Social Organization of Traditional Medicine in the Tibet Autonomous Region, China', in Linda H. Connor and Geoffrey Samuel (eds), *Healing Powers and Modernity: Traditional Medicine, Shamanism, and Science in Asian Societies*. Westport, CT: Bergin & Garvey, pp. 197–221.

———. 2002. 'Buddhism, Science, and Market: The Globalisation of Tibetan Medicine', *Anthropology & Medicine* 9: 267–89.

Joffe, Ben P. 2019. 'Mantras for Modernity: Nida Chenagtsang's "Mantra Healing Is an Indispensable Branch of Tibetan Traditional Medicine" (2003) and "A Rough Explanation of How Mantras Work" (2015)', in C. Pierce Salguero (ed.), *Buddhism and Medicine: An Anthology of Modern and Contemporary Sources*. New York: Columbia University Press, pp. 108–17.

Karmay, Samten G. 1972. *The Treasury of Good Sayings: A Tibetan History of Bon*. London: Oxford University Press.

———. 1998. 'The Soul and the Turquoise: A Ritual for Recalling the *Bla*', in Samten G. Karmay (ed.), *The Arrow and the Spindle: Studies in History, Myths, Rituals and Beliefs in Tibet*. Kathmandu: Mandala Publications, pp. 310–38.

———. 1998 and 2005. *The Arrow and the Spindle: Studies in History, Myths, Rituals and Beliefs in Tibet Vols I and II*. Kathmandu, Mandala Book Point.

Karmay, Samten Gyaltsen and Jeff Watt (eds). 2007. *Bon: The Magic Word. The Indigenous Religion of Tibet*. New York: Rubin Museum of Art.

Kilty, Gavin. 2009. 'Brief Presentation of Channels, Winds, and Drops According to Kālacakra Tradition by Dorjé, Changkya Rölpa 1717–1786', in Edward A. Arnold (ed.), *As Long as Space Endures: Essays on the Kālacakra Tantra in Honor of H. H. the Dalai Lama*. Ithaca, NY: Snow Lion Publications, pp. 145–50.

Kirmayer, Laurence J., Ademola Adeponle and Vivian Afi Abui Dzokoto. 2018. 'Varieties of Global Psychology: Cultural Diversity and Constructions of the Self', in Suman Fernando and Roy Moodley (eds), *Global Psychologies: Mental Health and the Global South*. London: Palgrave Macmillan, pp. 21–37.

Klein, Anne C. and Khetsun Sangpo. 1997. 'Hail Protection', in Donald S. Lopez Jnr. (ed.), *Religions of Tibet in Practice*. Princeton, NJ: Princeton University Press, pp. 538–47.

Kloos, Stephan. 2010. 'Tibetan Medicine in Exile: The Ethics, Politics and Science of Cultural Survival', Ph.D. dissertation. San Francisco and Berkeley: University of California, San Francisco with University of California, Berkeley.

———. 2016. 'The Recognition of Sowa Rigpa in India', *Medicine Anthropology Theory* 3: 19–49.

Kohn, Richard J. 1997. 'A Rite of Empowerment', in Donald S. Lopez Jnr. (ed.), *Religions of Tibet in Practice*. Princeton, NJ: Princeton University Press, pp. 225–33.

Kongtrul, Jamgön Lodrö Thaye. 1996. *Creation and Completion: Essential Points of Tantric Meditation*, translated, introduced and annotated by Sarah Harding. Boston, MA: Wisdom Publications.

Kuriyama, Shigehisa 1995. 'Pneuma, *Qi*, and the Problematic of Breath', in Yosia Kawakita, Shizu Sakai and Yasuo Otsuka (eds), *The Comparison Between Concepts of Life-Breath in East and West: Proceedings of the 15th International Symposium on the Comparative History of Medicine–East and West, 1995 Susono-shi, Shizuoka, Japan*. Tokyo: Ishiyaku EuroAmerica Shizuoka, pp. 1–31.

Kvaerne, Per. 1995. *The Bon Religion of Tibet: The Iconography of a Living Tradition*. London: Serindia Publications.

———. 2000. 'The Study of Bon in the West: Past, Present, and Future', *Senri Ethnological Reports* 15: 7–20.

Langenberg, Amy Paris. 2024. 'Better (Buddhist) Sex in the USA: Mindfulness, Non-Harm, and Dr. Nida's *Yoga of Bliss*', in C. Pierce Salguero, Kin Cheung and Susannah Deane (eds), *Buddhism and Healing in the Modern World*. Honolulu, HI: University of Hawai'i Press.

Larsson, Stefan. 2011. 'What Do the Childhood and Early Life of gTsang smyon Heruka Tell Us About His *bKa'brgyud* Affiliation?', in Roger Jackson and Matthew T. Kapstein (eds), *Mahāmudrā and the Bka'brgyud Tradition. PIATS 2006: Tibetan Studies: Proceedings of the Eleventh Seminar of the International Association for Tibetan Studies, Königswinter 2006*. Halle (Saale): International Institute of Tibetan and Buddhist Studies/Andiast Schweiz, pp. 425–52.

Lazarus, Arnold A. (1976). 'Psychiatric Problems Precipitated by Transcendental Meditation', *Psychological Reports* 39: 601–2.

Lewis, Sara E. 2013. 'Trauma and the Making of Flexible Minds in the Tibetan Exile Community', *Ethos* 41: 313–36.

———. 2018. 'Resilience, Agency, and Everyday *Lojong* in the Tibetan Diaspora', *Contemporary Buddhism* 19(2): 342–61.

Lichter, David and Lawrence Epstein. 1983. 'Irony in Tibetan Notions of the Good Life', in Charles F. Keyes and E. Valentine Daniel (eds), *Karma: An Anthropological Inquiry*. Berkeley, CA: University of California Press, pp. 223–59.

Lin, Shen-Yu. 2010. 'Pehar: A Historical Survey', *Revue d'Etudes Tibétaines* 3: 5–26.

Lindahl, Jared R. 2017. 'Somatic Energies and Emotional Traumas: A Qualitative Study of Practice-Related Challenges Reported by Vajrayāna Buddhists', *Religions* 8: 1–22.

Lindahl, Jared R., Nathan E. Fisher, David J. Cooper, Rochelle K. Rosen and Willoughby B. Britton. 2017. 'The Varieties of Contemplative Experience: A Mixed-Methods Study of Meditation-Related Challenges in Western Buddhists', *PloS ONE* 12(5): e0176239.

Lindahl, Jared R., Roman Palitsky, David J. Cooper and Willoughby B. Britton. 2023. 'The Roles and Impacts of Worldviews in the Context of Meditation-Related Challenges', *Transcultural Psychiatry* 60(4): 637–50.

Lingpa, Jigme. 2013. *Treasury of Precious Qualities Book Two: Vajrayana and the Great Perfection, with The Quintessence of the Three Paths–A Commentary by Yongten Yeshe Dorje and Kagjur Rinpoche*. Boston, MA and London: Shambhala Publications.

Lipman, Kennard. 2010. *Secret Teachings of Padmasambhava: Essential Instructions on Mastering the Energies of Life*. Boston, MA and London: Shambhala.

Lopez, Donald S. Jnr. 1997. 'Exorcising Demons with a Buddhist Sutra', in Lopez, Donald S. Jnr. (ed.), *Religions of Tibet in Practice*. Princeton, NJ: Princeton University Press, pp. 511–26.

———. 2000. 'A Tantric Meditation on Emptiness', in David Gordon White (ed.), *Tantra in Practice*. Princeton, NJ and Oxford: Princeton University Press, pp. 523–29.

Low, Chris and Elisabeth Hsu. 2007. 'Wind, Life, Health: Anthropological and Historical Perspectives–Introduction', *Journal of the Anthropological Institute* 13: S1–S17.

Lusthaus, Dan. 2017. 'Health and Sickness of Body and Mind: Selections from the *Yogācāra-Bhūmi*', in C. Pierce Salguero (ed.) *Buddhism and Medicine: An Anthology of Premodern Sources*. New York: Columbia University Press, pp. 49–60.

Makley, Charlene. 2013. 'Reb kong's *Klu rol* and the Politics of Presence: Methodological Considerations', in Yangdon Dhondup, Ulrich Pagel and Geoffrey Samuel (eds), *Monastic and Lay Traditions in North-Eastern Tibet*. Leiden: Brill, pp. 187–201.

Mallinson, James. 2020. 'The Amṛtasiddhi: *Haṭhayoga*'s Tantric Buddhist Source Text', in Dominic Goodall, Shaman Hatley, Harunaga Isaacson and Srilata Raman (eds), *Śaivism and the Tantric Traditions*. Leiden: Brill, pp. 409–25.

Mallinson, James and Mark Singleton. 2017. *Roots of Yoga*. London: Penguin Random House.

Marek, Todd P. and Charles Jamyang Oliphant. 2017. 'Treating Disorders of the Subtle Winds in Tibetan Buddhism', in C. Pierce Salguero (ed.), *Buddhism and Medicine: An Anthology of Premodern Sources*. New York and Chichester: Columbia University Press, pp. 418–24.

McGrath, William. A. 2017. 'Vessel Examination in the Medicine of the Moon King', in C. Pierce Salguero (ed.), *Buddhism and Medicine: An Anthology of Premodern Sources*. New York and Chichester: Columbia University Press, pp. 501–13.

———. 2019. 'Tantric Divination and Empirical Diagnosis: a Genealogy of Channel Prasenā Rituals in the Tibetan Medical Tradition', in William A. McGrath (ed.), *Knowledge and Context in Tibetan Medicine*. Leiden: Brill, pp. 261–308.

McKay, Alex. 2007. 'Himalayan Medical Encounters: The Establishment of Biomedicine in Tibet and in Indian Exile', in Mona Schrempf (ed.), *Soundings in Tibetan Medicine: Anthropological and Historical Perspectives. PIATS 2003: Proceedings of the Tenth Seminar of the International Association of Tibetan Studies, Oxford 2003*. Leiden and Boston, MA: Brill, pp. 9–27.

———. 2011. 'Biomedicine in Tibet at the Edge of Modernity', in Vincanne Adams, Mona Schrempf and Sienna R. Craig (eds), *Medicine Between Science and Religion: Explorations on Tibetan Grounds*. New York: Berghahn Books, pp. 33–56.

Men-Tsee-Khang. 2008. *The Basic Tantra and the Explanatory Tantra from the Secret Quintessential Instructions on the Eight Branches of the Ambrosia Essence Tantra*. Dharamsala, HP: Men-Tsee-Khang Publications.

———. 2011. *The Fourth Part Called the Subsequent Tantra from the Secret Quintessential Instructions on the Eight Branches of the Ambrosia Essence Tantra*. Dharamsala, HP: Men-Tsee-Khang Publications.

———. 2017. *The Oral Instruction Tantra from the Secret Quintessential Instructions on the Eight Branches of the Ambrosia Essence Tantra*. Dharamsala, HP: Men-Tsee-Khang Publications.

Men-Tsee-Khang Tibetan Medical & Astro Institute. 'Precious Pills'. Retrieved April 2024 from https://mentseekhang.org/precious-pills/.

Meyer, Fernand. 2003. 'The Golden Century of Tibetan Medicine', in Francoise Pommaret (ed.), *Lhasa in the Seventeenth Century: The Capital of the Dalai Lamas*. Leiden and Boston, MA: Brill, pp. 99–117.

Millard, Colin. 2005 and 2006. '*sMan* and *gLud*: Standard Tibetan Medicine and Ritual Medicine in a Bon Medical School and Clinic in Nepal', *The Tibet Journal* 30: 3–30.

———. 2007. 'Tibetan Medicine and the Classification and Treatment of Mental Illness', in Mona Schrempf (ed.), *Soundings in Tibetan Medicine: Anthropological and Historical Perspectives. PIATS 2003: Proceedings of the Tenth Seminar of the International Association of Tibetan Studies, Oxford 2003*. Leiden and Boston, MA: Brill, pp. 247–82.

———. 2013a. 'Bon Medical Practitioners in Contemporary Tibet: The Continuity of a Tradition', *East Asian Science, Technology and Society* 7: 353–79.

———. 2013b. 'Bon Religion in Reb kong', in Yangdon Dhondup, Ulrich Pagel and Geoffrey Samuel (eds), *Monastic and Lay Traditions in North-Eastern Tibet*. Leiden: Brill, pp. 141–62.

Mipham, Jamgön. 2009. *Luminous Essence: A Guide to the Guhyagarbha Tantra*. Boulder, CO: Snow Lion.

Morinis, Alan. 1985. 'Sanctified Madness: The God-Intoxicated Saints of Bengal', *Social Science & Medicine* 21(2): 211–20.

Muses, Charles Arthur. (ed.). 1961. *Esoteric Teachings Of The Tibetan Tantra*. Denver, CO: The Falcon's Wing Press.

Nālandā Translation Committee. 1997. 'The Life of Tilopa', in Donald S. Lopez Jnr. (ed.), *Religions of Tibet in Practice*. Princeton, NJ: Princeton University Press, pp. 137–56.

Nebesky-Wojkowitz, René de. 1993. *Oracles and Demons of Tibet: The Cult and Iconography of the Tibetan Protective Deities*. Kathmandu: Pilgrims Book House.

Nianggajia, (sNying dKhar rGyal). 2011. 'Local Health Seeking Strategies and the New Cooperative Medical Scheme in Contemporary Phyed Ri Village, Amdo', M.A. dissertation. Oslo: University of Oslo.

———. 2015. 'The White Pill: Perceptions and Experiences of Efficacy of a Popular Tibetan Medicine in Multiethnic Rebgong', *Asian Medicine: Tradition and Modernity* 10: 221–48.

Nianggajia and Heidi Fjeld. 2017. 'In Search of Trust and Efficacy', *Medicine Anthropology Theory* 4(5): 46–72.

Norbu, Chogyal Namkhai. 1981. *The Necklace of Gzi: On the History and Culture of Tibet*. Dharamsala, HP: Information Office of His Holiness the Dalai Lama.

———. 1986. *The Crystal and the Way of Light: Sutra, Tantra and Dzogchen*. London: Penguin.

———. 1995. *Drung, Deu, and Bön: Narrations, Symbolic Languages, and the Bön Traditions in Ancient Tibet*. Dharamsala, HP: Library of Tibetan Works and Archives.

———. 2008. *Yantra Yoga: The Tibetan Yoga of Movement*. Ithaca, NY: Snow Lion Publications.

Orofino, Giacomella. 2000. 'The Great Wisdom Mother and the *gCod* Tradition', in David Gordon White (ed.), *Tantra in Practice*. Princeton, NJ and Oxford: Princeton University Press, pp. 396–416.

———. 2015. 'A Note on Two Theogonic Myths Found in a Bon Magical Ritual', in Hanna Havnevik and Charles Ramble (eds), *From Bhakti to Bon. Festschrift for Per Kvaerne*. Oslo: The Institute for Comparative Research in Human Culture – Novus Press, pp. 381–93.

Phuntsok, Thubten. 2015. 'Introduction to Mental Disorders According to Traditional Tibetan Medicine', in Shang Shung Edizioni (ed.), *First Integrative Medicine Conference:*

Mental Disorders and Dementia: A Dialogue Between Conventional, Homeopathic, Tibetan, and Chinese medicines, 2014 Barcelona, Spain. Arcidosso: Shang Shung Publications, pp. 69–75.

Pitkin, Annabella C. 2016. 'The "Age of Faith" and the "Age of Knowledge": Secularism and Modern Tibetan Accounts of Yogic Power', *Himalaya, the Journal of the Association for Nepal and Himalayan Studies* 36(1): 96–115.

———. 2017. 'Dazzling Displays and Hidden Departures: Bodhisattva Pedagogy as Performance in the Biographies of Two Twentieth Century Tibetan Buddhist Masters', *Religions* 8: 173.

Prost, Audrey. 2006. 'Causation as Strategy: Interpreting Humours Among Tibetan Refugees', *Anthropology & Medicine* 13: 119–30.

Punzi, Valentina. 2021. 'A Minyag Domestic Rite of Paying a Vow', in Diana Lange, Jarmila Ptáčková, Marion Wettstein and Mareike Wulff (eds), *Crossing Boundaries: Tibetan Studies Unlimited.* Prague: Academia Publishing House of The Czech Academy of Sciences, pp. 430–46.

Rabgay (=Rapgay), Lobsang. 1985. 'rLung Diseases and Their Treatment', *Tibetan Medicine* 9: 47–68.

Rapgay (=Rabgay), Lobsang. 1984. 'Mind-Made Health: A Tibetan Perspective', *Tibetan Medicine* 8: 45–55.

Rapgay (=Rabgay), Lobsang. 1985. *Tibetan Medicine: A Holistic Approach to Better Health*, Tibetan Medical Sciences Series. New Delhi: Sona Printers.

Rapport, Nigel. 1997. 'Edifying Anthropology: Culture as Conversation; Representation as Conversation', in Allison James, Jenny Hockey and Andrew Dawson (eds), *After Writing Culture: Epistemology and Praxis in Contemporary Anthropology.* London and New York: Routledge, pp. 177–93.

Rösing, Ina. 2006. *Shamanic Trance and Amnesia: Traditional Healing in Ladakh.* New Delhi: Concept Publishing Company.

Salguero, C. Pierce. (ed.). 2017. *Buddhism and Medicine: An Anthology of Premodern Sources.* New York: Columbia University Press.

———. (ed.). 2019. *Buddhism and Medicine: An Anthology of Modern and Contemporary Sources.* New York: Columbia University Press.

———. (ed.). [forthcoming] *Meditation Sickness: A Sourcebook on the Dangers of Buddhist Practice.* Honolulu, HI: University of Hawai'i Press.

Salguero, C. Pierce, Kin Cheung and Susannah Deane (eds). 2024. *Buddhism and Healing in the Modern World.* Honolulu, HI: University of Hawai'i Press.

Samuel, Geoffrey. 1989. 'The Body in Buddhist and Hindu Tantra: Some Notes', *Religion* 19: 197–210.

———. 1993. *Civilized Shamans: Buddhism in Tibetan Societies.* Washington, DC: Smithsonian Institution Press.

———. 2001a. 'The Effectiveness of Goddesses, or, How Ritual Works', *Anthropological Forum* 11: 73–91.

———. 2001b. 'Tibetan Medicine in Contemporary India: Theory and Practice', in Linda H. Connor and Geoffrey Samuel (eds), *Healing Powers and Modernity: Traditional Medicine, Shamanism, and Science in Asian Studies.* Westport, CT and London: Bergin & Garvey: pp. 247–68.

———. 2006. 'Healing and the Mind-Body Complex: Childbirth and Medical Pluralism in South Asia', in Helle Johannessen and Imre Lazar (eds), *Multiple Medical Realities: Patients and Healers in Biomedical, Alternative and Traditional Medicine.* New York and London: Berghahn Books: pp. 121–35.

———. 2007. 'Spirit Causation and Illness in Tibetan Medicine', in Mona Schrempf (ed.), *Soundings in Tibetan Medicine: Anthropological and Historical Perspectives. PIATS 2003: Proceedings of the Tenth Seminar of the International Association of Tibetan Studies, Oxford 2003*. Oxford: Brill Academic Publishers, pp. 213–24.

———. 2008. *The Origins of Yoga and Tantra: Indic Religions to the Thirteenth Century*. Cambridge: Cambridge University Press.

———. 2009. 'Religion, Health and Suffering Among Contemporary Tibetans', in John R. Hinnells and Roy Porter (eds), *Religion, Health and Suffering*. Abingdon and New York: Routledge, pp. 85–110.

———. 2010. 'Possession and Self-Possession: Towards an Integrated Mind-Body Perspective', in Bettina E. Schmidt and Lucy Huskinson, *Spirit Possession and Trance: New Interdisciplinary Perspectives*. London and New York: Continuum International Publishing Group, pp. 35–52.

———. 2013a. 'Reb kong in the Multiethnic Context of A mdo: Religion, Language, Ethnicity, and Identity', in Yangdon Dhondup, Ulrich Pagel and Geoffrey Samuel (eds), *Monastic and Lay Traditions in North-Eastern Tibet*. Leiden: Brill, pp. 5–20.

———. 2013b. 'Revisiting the Problem of Bon Identity: Bon Priests and Ritual Practitioners in the Himalayas', *Journal of the International Association for Bon Research* 1: 77–97.

———. 2013c. 'The Subtle Body in India and Beyond', in Geoffrey Samuel and Jay Johnston (eds), *Religion and the Subtle Body in Asia and the West: Between Mind and Body*. Abingdon and New York: Routledge, pp. 33–47.

———. 2014. 'Body and Mind in Tibetan Medicine and Tantric Buddhism', in Theresia Hofer (ed.), *Bodies in Balance: The Art of Tibetan Medicine*. Seattle, WA: Rubin Museum of Art in association with University of Washington Press, pp. 32–45.

———. 2019. 'Unbalanced Flows in the Subtle Body: Tibetan Understandings of Psychiatric Illness and How to Deal With It', *Journal of Religion and Health* 58: 770–94.

Saxer, Martin. 2013. *Manufacturing Tibetan Medicine: The Creation of an Industry and the Moral Economy of Tibetanness*. New York: Berghahn Books.

Schrempf, Mona. 2007. 'Bon Lineage Doctors and the Local Transmission of Knowing Medical Practice in Nagchu', in Mona Schrempf (ed), *Soundings in Tibetan Medicine: Anthropological and Historical perspectives. PIATS 2003: Tibetan Studies: Proceedings of the Tenth Seminar of the International Association of Tibetan Studies, Oxford, 2003*. Leiden: Brill, pp. 91–126.

———. 2011. 'Between Mantra and Syringe: Healing and Health-Seeking Behaviour in Contemporary Amdo', in Vincanne Adams, Mona Schrempf and Sienna R. Craig (eds), *Medicine Between Science and Religion: Explorations on Tibetan Grounds*. New York: Berghahn Books, pp. 157–84.

———. 2015. 'Contested Issues of Efficacy and Safety between Transnational Formulation Regimes of Tibetan Medicines in China and Europe', *Asian Medicine* 10(1–2): 273–315.

Sheehy, Michael R. 2005. 'Severing the Source of Fear: Contemplative Dynamics of the Tibetan Buddhist *gCod* Tradition', *Contemporary Buddhism* 6: 37–52.

Sihlé, Nicolas. 2018. 'Assessing and Adapting Rituals That Reproduce a Collectivity: The Large-Scale Rituals of the Repkong Tantrists in Tibet', *Religion and Society* 9(1): 160–75.

Silburn, Lilian. 1988. *Kundalini: The Energy of the Depths*. New York: State University of New York Press.

Silverman, David. 2000. *Doing Qualitative Research: A Practical Handbook*. London: Sage Publications Limited.

Smith, E. Gene. 2001. *Among Tibetan Texts: History and Literature of the Himalayan Plateau*. Somerville, MA: Wisdom Publications.

Snellgrove, David L. 1967. *The Nine Ways of Bon: Excerpts from "gZi-brjid"*. Oxford: Oxford University Press.

Snying bo rgyal and R. Solomon Rino. 2008. *Deity Men: Reb gong Tibetan Trance Mediums in Transition*. Morrisville, NC: Asian Highlands Perspectives.

Soktsang, Lobsang Dhonden and Colin Millard. 2013. 'Diversity in Unity: The Changing Forms of Tibetan Medicine', *East Asian Science, Technology and Society: An International Journal* 7(3): 467–86.

Stoddard, Heather. 2013. 'Rig'dzin Dpal Ldan Bkra Shis (1688–1743): The "1900 Dagger-Wielding, White-Robed, Long-Haired Yogins" (sngag mang phur thog gos dkar lcang lo can stong dang dgu brgya) & the Eight Places of Practice of Reb Kong (reb kong gi sgrub gnas brgyad)', in Yangdon Dhondup, Ulrich Pagel and Geoffrey Samuel (eds), *Monastic and Lay Traditions in North-Eastern Tibet*. Leiden: Brill, pp. 87–115.

Sumegi, Angela. 2010. 'Being the Deity: The Inner Work of Buddhist and Shamanic Ritual', in Axel Michaels (ed.), *Ritual Dynamics and the Science of Ritual, Vol. II*. Wiesbaden: Harrassowitz Verlag, pp. 443–58.

Thar, Tsering. 2000. 'The *bla ma* in the Bon Religion in Amdo and Kham', in Samten G. Karmay and Yasuhiko Nagano (eds), *New Horizons in Bon Studies: Bon Studies 2. (Senri Ethological Reports 15)*. Osaka: National Museum of Ethnology, pp. 417–27.

———. 2003. 'Bonpo Monasteries and Temples in Tibetan Regions in Qinghai, Gansu and Sichuan', in Samten G. Karmay and Yasuhiko Nagano (eds), *A Survey of Bonpo Monasteries and Temples in Tibet and the Himalaya (Senri Ethological Reports 38)*. Osaka: National Museum of Ethnology, Bon Studies 7, pp. 249–668.

———. 2008. 'Bonpo Tantrics in Kokonor Area', *Revue d'études Tibétaines* 15: 533–52.

Tibetan & Himalayan Library online translation tool. Retrieved March 2024 from https://ttt.thlib.org/.

Tidwell, Tawni L., Nianggajia and Heidi E Fjeld. 2022. 'Chasing *Dön* Spirits in Tibetan Medical Encounters: Transcultural Affordances and Embodied Psychiatry in Amdo, Qinghai', *Transcultural Psychiatry* 60(5): 799–818.

Tucci, Giuseppe. 1980. *The Religions of Tibet*, trans. G. Samuel. London and Henley: Routledge & Kegan Paul.

Turpeinen, Katarina. 2019. 'The Soteriological Context of a Tibetan Oracle', *Himalaya, The Journal of the Association for Nepal and Himalayan Studies* 39: 42–52.

VanderKooi, Lois. 1997. 'Buddhist Teachers' Experience with Extreme Mental States in Western Meditators', *The Journal of Transpersonal Psychology* 29: 31–46.

Van Schaik, Sam. 2013. 'The Naming of Tibetan Religion: *Bon* and *Chos* in the Tibetan Imperial Period', *Journal of the International Association for Bon Research* 1: 227–57.

Vargas, Ivette. 2009. 'Demon Diseases and Tibetan Medicine: The Interface Between Religion and Science', in Edward A. Arnold (ed.), *As Long as Space Endures: Essays on the Kālacakra Tantra in Honor of H. H. the Dalai Lama*. Ithaca, NY: Snow Lion Publications, pp. 367–85.

Wallace Vesna. 2001. *The Inner Kalacakratantra: A Buddhist Tantric View of the Individual*. Oxford: Oxford University Press.

———. 2009. 'Medicine and Astrology in the Healing Arts of the *Kālacakratantra*', in Edward A. Arnold (ed.), *As Long as Space Endures: Essays on the Kālacakra Tantra in Honor of H. H. the Dalai Lama*. Ithaca, NY: Snow Lion Publications, pp. 277–300.

———. 2017. 'Selections from a Mongolian Manual of Buddhist Medicine', in C. Pierce Salguero (ed.), *Buddhism and Medicine: An Anthology of Premodern Sources*. New York: Columbia University Press, pp. 363–70.

Wangda, Jurme. 1996. *Health Seeking Behaviours of Tibetan Refugee Community in Dharamsala, India*. M.Sc. dissertation. Kingston, ON: Queen's University.

Wangmo, Phuntsog. 2015. 'The Treatment of Mental Disorders According to Tibetan Medicine', in Shang Shung Edizioni (ed.), *First Integrative Medicine Conference: Mental Disorders and Dementia: A Dialogue between Conventional, Homeopathic, Tibetan, and Chinese Medicines, 2014 Barcelona, Spain*. Arcidosso: Shang Shung Publications, pp. 149–56.

White, David Gordon. 1996. *The Alchemical Body: Siddha Traditions in Medieval India*. Chicago and London: University of Chicago Press.

Williamson, Laila, Serinity Young and Romio Shrestha. (eds). 2009. *Body & Spirit: Tibetan Medical Paintings*. New York and Seattle, WA: American Museum of Natural History, New York in association with University of Washington Press.

World Health Organization. 2018. *ICD-11 International Classification of Diseases 11th Revision*. Geneva: World Health Organization.

Wylie, Turrell. 1959. 'A Standard System of Tibetan Transcription', *Harvard Journal of Asiatic Studies* 22: 261–67.

Yangönpa, Gyalwa. 2015. *Secret Map of the Body: Visions of the Human Energy Structure*, translated from the Tibetan and annotated by Elio Guarisco. Arcidosso: Shang Shung Publications.

Yeh, Emily T. 2006. '"An Open Lhasa Welcomes You": Disciplining the Researcher in Tibet', in Maria Heimer and Stig Thøgersen (eds), *Doing Fieldwork in China*. Copenhagen: NIAS Press, pp. 96–109.

Yoeli-Tlalim, Ronit. 2009. 'The Kālacakra Empowerment as Conducted by Kirti Tsenshab Rinpoche', in Edward A. Arnold (ed.), *As Long as Space Endures: Essays on the Kālacakra Tantra in Honor of H. H. the Dalai Lama*. Ithaca, NY: Snow Lion Publications, pp. 415–48.

———. 2010. 'Tibetan "Wind" and "Wind" Illnesses: Towards a Multicultural Approach to Health and Illness', *Studies in History and Philosophy of Science Part C: Studies in History and Philosophy of Biological and Biomedical Sciences* 41: 318–24.

You, Xuedan and Yasuki Kobayashi. 2009. 'The New Cooperative Medical Scheme in China', *Health Policy* 91(1): 1–9.

Zysk, Kenneth G. 1993. 'The Science of Respiration and the Doctrine of the Bodily Winds in Ancient India', *Journal of the American Oriental Society*, 198–213.

———. 1995. 'Vital Breath (*Prāṇa*) in Ancient Indian Medicine and Religion', in Yosio Kawakita, Shizu Sakai and Yasuo Otsuka (eds), *The Comparison Between Concepts of Life-Breath in East and West: Proceedings of the 15th International Symposium on the Comparative History of Medicine–East and West*. Tokyo: Ishiyaku EuroAmerica Inc., pp. 33–65.

———. 2001. 'New Age Ayurveda or What Happens to Indian Medicine When It Comes to America', *Traditional South Asian Medicine* 6: 10–26.

———. 2007. 'The Bodily Winds in Ancient India Revisited', *Journal of the Royal Anthropological Institute* 13: S105–S115.

Index

www.ingramcontent.com/pod-product-compliance
Lightning Source LLC
Chambersburg PA
CBHW071248180926
51613CB00002B/167

Fluorescence Applications in Biotechnology and Life Sciences

Fluorescence Applications in Biotechnology and Life Sciences

Edited by

Ewa M. Goldys

WILEY-BLACKWELL

A JOHN WILEY & SONS, INC., PUBLICATION

Published by John Wiley & Sons, Inc., Hoboken, New Jersey
Published simultaneously in Canada

Wiley-Blackwell is an imprint of John Wiley & Sons, Inc., formed by the merger of Wiley's global Scientific, Technical, and Medical business with Blackwell Publishing.

Library of Congress Cataloging-in-Publication Data:

Fluorescence applications in biotechnology and life sciences / Ewa M. Goldys (editor).
p. ; cm.
Includes bibliographical references and index.
ISBN 978-0-470-08370-3 (cloth)
1. Fluorimetry. 2. Fluorescent probes. 3. Fluorescence microscopy. I. Goldys, Ewa M.
[DNLM: 1. Flow Cytometry–methods. 2. Fluorescence. 3. Biotechnology–methods. 4. Microscopy, Fluorescence. QY 95 F646 2008]
QP519.9.F58F578 2008
616.07′56–dc22

2008035473

Printed in the United States of America

10 9 8 7 6 5 4 3 2 1

CONTENTS

PREFACE

It is a great pleasure for me to introduce this book on fluorescence applications in biotechnology and life sciences. Fluorescence is one of the oldest and most established analytical techniques. The phenomenon of fluorescence was first observed by Monardes in 1656 in an extract of *Ligirium mephiticiem*, and since then it has been investigated by a succession of leading scientists, including Sir George G. Stokes, Francis Perrin, Alexander Jablonski, Gregorio Weber, and numerous others. It is also intensely used nowadays, underpinning countless technologies, and a keyword search of fluorescence in research databases returns around a million entries. In light of such a remarkable legacy and scope, any new project of this kind needs strong justification. This group of authors embarked upon it with the conviction that we have new messages to convey and a unique perspective which we would like to share with the broader research community.

First, we saw significant trends emerging in the fluorescence discipline which are already apparent in the research community but have not yet made their way into books. We were well aware that the emphasis in the field of fluorescence is progressively moving toward imaging, supported by the deepening fusion of fluorescence spectroscopy and microscopy and new modalities such as time resolution. Fluorescent images contain vast amounts of data which have only recently begun to be utilized. Fortunately, digital imaging technology is ubiquitous these days, and the wider application of software for image processing and, most importantly, analysis has shifted the goalpost for many fluorescence imaging studies. Finally, there is now greater awareness that biological diversity can be quantified through the analysis of cell populations. We believe the authors were able to capture these emerging ideas.

Second, a unique feature of fluorescence is that it is inherently cross-disciplinary, and we continue to witness its further convergence with other fields. It is traditionally associated with chemistry, but at the same time it is physics which moves forward the boundaries of instrumentation and techniques. The area of fluorescent image analysis, which is clearly in the ascendant, is the domain of mathematicians, statisticians, and software developers in equal measure, but the key users and beneficiaries are actually the life sciences, especially biology, medicine, and biotechnology—hence the need to develop a common language and for researchers and students to build the courage to extend beyond their own discipline, the need which we tried to serve as well as we could. This is best done at early stages in a person's career so we have aimed this book at the level of postgraduate students in the expectation that it will also be suitable for a broad class of more senior researchers who need a similar cross-discipline introduction. This book thus aspires to contribute to the restoration of the unity of science and to overcome the increasing specialization of various fields of inquiry. To this aim, we made sure that this book contains contributions from authors representing a variety of traditional disciplines, chemistry, medical sciences, biochemistry, biology, physics, and engineering. Each of them speaks the language of their discipline, but here they have undertaken to communicate as simply as they could.

We attempted to compile an advanced textbook that looks at fundamental concepts and approaches illustrated with key examples of applications of fluorescence in biotechnology and life sciences. This book might serve as a quick introduction to a specific topic, leading to recent results, and also as a valuable reference material. While an effort has been made to cover most of the important topics in the field, this book is not meant to be encyclopedic in nature, and the content was ultimately influenced by the present scientific interest of the contributors and editor. Some of the contributed chapters survey the literature of relevance for a given topic, some discuss and present new research, while others do all of the above. The book is as up-to-date as possible and we expect it will remain relevant and authoritative in several years time. The chapters have been written by active researchers leading in their respective areas. It is important that each author focused on the areas with which they were deeply involved and in most cases currently working hands on in a laboratory. This gave them a unique perspective which they were encouraged to share with the reader. The chapters include suggestions and recommendations which very rarely make their way to research papers and can only be learned in face-to-face contact and by word of mouth. We were very keen to capture this personal experience and I hope we have succeeded.

We now give a brief outline of the chapters. For the benefit of those whose training did not cover the basics of fluorescence we begin with a fairly comprehensive explanation of the key ideas in our first chapter (Chapter 1). It was written by three outstanding researchers and inspiring teachers, Robert Learmonth, Scott Kable, and Ken Ghiggino, who use intuitive models to convey difficult concepts in a simple and imaginative style. It covers issues such as Jablonski–Perrin diagrams used to interpret fluorescence data and the effect of the environment on fluorescent molecules and goes as far as polarization anisotropy, a powerful technique which is somewhat underutilized. The contents of this chapter have been tested on generations of students at three different universities who gave it their overwhelming thumbs up.

The remaining chapters cover more specific aspects of fluorescence in areas of increased research activity, one of which is fluorescence labeling. We felt there is a need for an integrated and compact guide through the maze of different reagents used in fluorescent labeling, especially for live cells. There is a wealth of information available on this subject, for example, in the *Handbook of Fluorescent Probes* available from Invitrogen (http://www.invitrogen.com), but it can be somewhat overwhelming for the uninitiated. Ian Harper, who directs a major microscopy imaging facility at Monash University in Melbourne, prepared a very detailed text (Chapter 2) to help the readers organize this information. Like many other contributors, Ian has current hands-on experience in this field and was able to share his insights and know-how about fluorescence labeling of cells and tissues which can rarely be seen in print.

While the second chapter focuses mostly on chemical dyes, we must not lose sight of one of the breakthrough fluorescence labeling technologies whose implications we are only beginning to see, that is, genetically targeted fluorescent probes. These are covered in Chapter 3, written by Mark Prescott and Anya Salih. Mark made major contributions to the development of new fluorescent proteins which can work not only as fluorescent highlighters of specific cellular proteins but also as much more sophisticated reporters of various cellular processes. Anya has been involved with bioprospecting for fluorescent proteins found, for example, in the corals living in the

Australian Great Barrier Reef. She uncovered that the fluorescent proteins act as a form of sunscreen, dispersing the sun's energy to prevent sunburn in living corals. These fluorescent corals are shown in one of the figures.

The third labeling technology which we believe is gaining momentum involves fluorescent nanoparticles. Among many different nanoparticles currently under investigation we decided to focus only on fluorescent quantum dots (Chapter 4), as they are commercially available and have been commonly used for several years. The author, Krystyna Tomsia, has been growing semiconductor quantum dots in house, and she was able to demystify some of their aspects and properties. Quantum dot technology has its place in life sciences due to their high brightness and photostability of quantum dots, but challenges remain, and the community is yet to master how to use them in some applications, including flow cytometry. In this context the understanding of quantum dot properties such as their extinction coefficient and methods of conjugation is crucial.

Having covered most important areas of fluorescence labeling, the stage is now set for the next step. The cell culture or tissue has been labeled, the parts of cells or proteins of interest have been imaged, and now the investigators are trying to analyze the results. The traditional method is to make a more or less subjective judgment about the image and the process under investigation. While the human brain is a wonderful qualitative analysis tool, the same cannot be said about human memory, and studies involving looking for similarities in a large number of images are very difficult for us to do. At the same time cells are very diverse, and the only way to capture their representative behavior is by studying cell populations. Fortunately, microscopy images nowadays are taken in a digital format, and we have technological support to extract quantitative information from such images. We believe the life sciences community will greatly benefit from improved awareness of such approaches so one such method, scanning cytometry, is described in the next chapter (Chapter 5). One of the authors, Mick Godlewski, used this technology extensively to examine cancer-related processes. The chapter provides a detailed illustration of how quantitative analysis based on a couple of simple parameters can support an in-depth cell biology investigation.

The next chapter (Chapter 6), by Pascal Valotton and colleagues, follows the same theme of how to make the most of the acquired images. They explain what can be done in the situation when two (or more) different fluorophores label the sample, especially when they happen to stain the same region and the spectra show some overlap—as is often the case with many chemical dyes and also with fluorescent proteins. By using a suitable software package for image analysis, the relative contribution of these individual fluorophores can be untangled in a process referred to as unmixing. The authors are mathematicians, so some equations are given and there is also an illustrative example of tablet analysis. One of the unmixing approaches has deep connections to the discipline of statistics. Both this and the preceding chapter clearly indicate that life scientists gain an advantage by use of statistics as it can give them an additional step beyond the intuitively obvious.

Another research frontier which emerged quite clearly when we were working on this book was optical microscopy breaking through the diffraction limit. We saw several new concepts such as 4Pi and STED microscopies as well as structured illumination microscopy being further developed to a point that commercial instrumentation for the first two has become available. However, at the point of submission, this community was not clear which one will become the leading technology, and also the market penetration of 4Pi and STED was limited. Therefore, instead of describing these we decided to focus on correlative microscopy (Chapter 7), which is the current gold standard for investigations of nanoscale structures in life sciences. The name "correlative" refers to correlation between optical, mostly laser scanning and electron, microscopies. The author of this chapter, Marko Nykänen, is an experienced practitioner, with expertise in the very difficult correlative microscopy of tissues. The chapter describes the cornerstone laboratory techniques required in this field.

The chapter on correlative microscopy shifts the emphasis of this book to experimental methods, and we felt we must do justice to the most powerful ones, that is, fluorescence resonance energy transfer (FRET) and fluorescence recovery after photobleaching (FRAP), described in the next two chapters (Chapters 8 and 9). We are fortunate to have among us Andrew Clayton, Senior Fellow at Ludwig Institute for Cancer Research, who has in-depth understanding of FRET, mostly in the context of cell biology, and who is also an outstanding presenter. The chapter concerned with FRET (Chapter 8) thoroughly organizes different approaches used currently in a unique format of step-by-step instructions, and we hope that it will help dispel the mystery surrounding FRET experienced by its first-time users. FRET utilizes the transfer of energy between two fluorophores which is possible only if they are up to several nanometers apart. Due to this distance sensitivity it is sometimes referred to as a molecular ruler. More experienced researchers will benefit from a comprehensive description of the various FRET variants and methods of performing experiments. Much of that is now coded in modern microscopy software, but to use this software effectively, one must be fully aware of what is behind the scenes. The following chapter (Chapter 9) concerned with FRAP, written by Nick Klonis and Leann Tilley, in a sense mirrors the FRET chapter by describing the technique and its various incarnations. However, it goes a step further and shows how FRAP has supported their own studies of the malaria parasites. Both Leann and Nick are leading researchers in the field of malaria, renowned for their willingness to try new technologies as they emerge.

Another group of technology pioneers led by Trevor Smith wrote the next chapter on time-resolved microscopy (Chapter 10). This microscopy modality is steadily gaining prominence thanks to improved availability of commercial systems and the increasing awareness of the community of how to apply the new tools in various studies. However, much is yet to be learned, and this chapter was prepared in order to better inform the reader about the capabilities of time resolution. There is a fair amount of technicalities involved and Trevor and his colleagues have painstakingly gone through all the details of methodologies and intrumentation. Life scientists need to keep abreast of time-resolved microscopy, one of the reasons being that time-resolved FRET is the gold standard in FRET measurements.

The following chapter (Chapter 11), by Jörg Enderlein focuses on one more microscopy technique, namely fluorescence correlation spectroscopy (FCS). FSC can be used, for example, to determine if two proteins labeled with two fluorophores have been able to combine together forming a larger complex. The chapter describes the underlying concepts and gives numerous practical suggestions of how these measurements should be performed. With increasing number of FCS systems available and the fact that FCS, with its ability to detect interacting proteins, does not have a distance limit (as opposed to FRET), the awareness of this technology is increasing. Jörg and his team are technology developers and in this chapter also explain how to use the two-focus approach to obtain more reliable quantitative, not only comparative, values from FCS.

So far the emphasis has been on fluorescence microscopy, a very powerful method but unsuitable to study rare cells or events even in its most sophisticated variants. It turns out that in many areas, for example, in microbiology or stem cell research, we can often expect only one cell of interest per 10^6 or more other cells. In such situations a different technique is needed, namely flow cytometry. The authors of the following chapter (Chapter 12), Russell Connally, Graham Vesey, and Charlotte Morgan have been developing new approaches to flow cytometry and their applications for decades. They have produced for us a summary of the technique fundamentals and their leading applications. We believe that there is a great future ahead for flow cytometry as the cost of instrumentation will come down and it will become more user friendly. Some of this spirit has made its way to the chapter, especially in the discussion of new light sources.

All the contributing authors were asked to write about fluorescence applications to relate their text to the subject of this book, and they have done so while describing their techniques or methods, but several focused on applications alone, and we have grouped these chapters together. The first such chapter (Chapter 13), about fluorescence in medical imaging, was written by Morry Silberstein. Morry is a leading expert in this and related fields, and his chapter brings this medical perspective to fluorescence. Due to limited light penetration depth, only some health conditions benefit from fluorescence diagnostics, and it is important to be aware which ones do. The next chapter on fluorescence in diagnostic medicine (Chapter 14) explores more detailed applications in the areas of clinical diagnostics, including biochemistry, pathology, cancer diagnostics, and genetics.

Another medically relevant technology, bioassays use fluorescence among other reporting schemes. One of the the authors of the following chapter (Chapter 15), Eva Matveeva, has many years experience in bioassay development in the industry and academia and has spent a recent period developing fluorescence assays. This chapter is especially well set out for teaching/learning purposes, and the readers will appreciate the especially clear presentation of the material. Coauthors Zygmunt and Ignacy Gryczynski have pioneered the technology of metal enhancement, which significantly increases the detection limit of fluorophores.

Further the book makes a detour from medicine back to cell biology. In a very detailed chapter (Chapter 16) Katharina Gaus explains how fluorescence can support the studies of membrane organization. Cellular membranes are an amazingly complex biological system which play a major role in the functioning of cells. Some of the best known objects identified within membranes are lipid rafts, which were discovered some time ago and continue to be the subject of intense investigation. Cellular membranes present challenges as many processes occur in the nanoscale—hence the need for advanced techniques, biological, chemical, as well as physical. The last chapter (Chapter 17), by Ron Clarke, continues the analysis of a selected component of cellular membranes, namely ion pumps, not to be confused with better known ion channels. Ion pumps are also difficult objects to study, as they require specially developed voltage-sensitive dyes, which have been the emphasis of the chapter.

As indicated earlier, the book is designed to assist in cross-disciplinary dialogue at both postgraduate and specialist levels, between biology, biochemistry, and physics, in the multidisciplinary area of fluorescence. It is aimed at a postgraduate level, suitable also for those from outside of these fields of research. The book may be particularly useful to young researchers in need of texts introducing them to their new field of study.

We anticipate that it will also be of significant interest to a large number of academics, research staff, and professionals, especially those within life sciences and interested in embracing new fields of research. This is feasible and can be truly enriching; after all the disciplines of the natural sciences share the same empirical framework and rational approach, and it is only from this viewpoint that we can best appreciate the wholeness of the world.

The editor would like to express her gratitude to the individuals who made the book possible. Thanks are due to to all the above contributors: They have worked on this project with enthusiasm and efficiency, making the editorial effort truly enjoyable. We are all extremely sorry that Alan Hibbs was unable to see this project completed, he is sadly missed by our community. The editor would like to thank Anne Barnett, Ross Moore, and Hemant Bhatta, who were very kind to assist with book preparation; Anna Goldys, the author of the graphic concept and design for the book cover; and Mick Godlewski, who contributed the image used. The project would not be possible without the support of Thom Moore, Karen Chambers, and all staff from Wiley. We are sincerely grateful for their professionalism and encouragement.

EWA M. GOLDYS

ACKNOWLEDGMENTS

This volume has been compiled by the fluorescence community, mostly from Australia, brought together by the two leading funding agencies, Australian Research Council and National Health and Medical Research Council, which supported us in an effort to improve the linkages within the research community. It is a pleasure for us to acknowledge their support through grant RN460002.

E.M.G

ABOUT THE CONTRIBUTING AUTHORS

This book brought together key teams with world-class expertise in biological and biomedical sciences, chemistry, physics, and optoelectronics. Some authors concentrate on the development of novel fluorophores with optimized properties through chemical synthesis, bioprocesses, or identification of naturally occuring fluorescent compounds. Others specialize in the diagnostic use of fluorescence to elucidate molecular environments, especially in biological systems. Some groups utilize fluorophores in studies of molecular and cellular dynamics, biological/medical imaging, clinical applications, proteomics, genomics, and flow cytometry. The development of techniques (such as confocal FRET, FRAP, and time-resolved microscopy) for identification and localization of trace chemicals with high temporal and spatial resolution is also carried out within the present group of authors. Others focus on the development of industrially significant instrumentation for biotechnology as well as medical and bioengineering fields. This involves new applications in laser and microelectronics to produce instrumentation with lower cost, improved sensitivities, and new functionalities. Brief author biographies are included below.

Robert Learmonth is Associate Professor of Biochemistry in the Department of Biological and Physical Sciences at the University of Southern Queensland, Australia. His research in biotechnology has concentrated on the development and application of fluorescence techniques for analysis of the identity, vitality, and adaptability of microbial, plant, and animal cell systems, with major efforts in elucidating roles of cell membranes in environmental adaptation of yeasts. He currently focuses on fermentation processes in winemaking. His interests also include enhancement of biochemical and biophysical education.

Scott Kable is Professor of Chemistry at the University of Sydney, Australia. He specializes in fluorescence and phosphorescence spectroscopy with a particular focus on the structure and properties of free radicals. His interests also include photochemistry, astrophysics, and mass spectrometry.

Ken Ghiggino is Head of the School and Masson Professor of Chemistry at the University of Melbourne, Australia. His key field of expertise is ultrafast spectroscopy and photochemistry. With his group he investigates light-induced processes in a variety of molecular systems including synthetic polymers, biological macromolecules, and supramolecular assemblies.

Ian Harper is Director of Monash MicroImaging, a microscopy and imaging research facility for the life sciences at Monash University, Melbourne, Australia. He is also an Associate Professor and expert in optical microscopy and imaging, with special interests in quantitative imaging, fluorescence microscopy, live cell imaging, and various forms of three-dimensional microscopy.

Mark Prescott is Senior Lecturer in the Department of Biochemistry and Molecular Biology at Monash University, Melbourne, Australia. His interests include the structure, function, development, and application of novel genetically encoded fluorophores with a particular focus on the application of such probes to investigations into the role and mechanism of autophagy.

Anya Salih is Research Fellow and Manager of the Confocal Bio-Imaging Facility at the University of Western Sydney, Australia. She explores fluorescent proteins in corals and studies their properties and biological role.

Krystyna Tomsia is Senior Research Fellow in physics at Macquarie University, Sydney, Australia. She has been involved in semiconductor quantum dot research for electronic and biological applications over 10 years. She has expertise in materials synthesis, their optical and structural characterization, and imaging techniques, in both academia and industry.

Michal Godlewski is Assistant Professor in the Department of Physiological Sciences, Faculty of Veterinary Medicine, Warsaw University of Life Sciences in Poland, currently at Macquarie University, Sydney, Australia. In his work he focuses on scanning cytometry and a quantitative approach to confocal microscopy. He is involved in research projects on molecular mechanism of programmed cell death in cancer and tissue development, roadblocks in the secretory pathway of filamentous fungi, and processes involved in the remodeling of complex tissue of intestinal mucosa.

Pascal Vallotton leads the Biotech Imaging Group at the Mathematical and Information Sciences Division of CSIRO (Sydney), Australia's major government research organization. His interests include the extraction of quantitative information from digital images of biological origin and the development of new microscopy techniques.

Aloke Phatak is an applied statistician at CSIRO (Perth, Australia). He has a strong background in chemometrics and bioinformatics, and his current interests lie in several areas, including unmixing of hyperspectral images, analysis of microarray data, and biomarker discovery.

Mark Berman is Chief Research Scientist at CSIRO (Sydney, Australia). He has many years experience in developing and applying sophisticated unmixing algorithms for spectroscopic and hyperspectral data, initially for mineral exploration applications, but more recently in biological and pharmaceutical applications.

Marko Nykänen (Children's Hospital at Westmead, Sydney, Australia) develops advanced imaging technologies, especially for subcellular and molecular analyses. He has over 12 years hands-on experience in various light (LM) and electron (EM) microscopies. He has been involved with ultrastructural studies and biological imaging in both academia and industry.

Andrew Clayton is a NHMRC RD Wright Fellow and an Assistant Member at the Ludwig Institute for Cancer Research (LICR), Melbourne, Australia. He is Head of the Cell Biophysics Research Group at the LICR Melbourne Branch of Tumour Biology. His group concentrates on structure–function studies on the EGF/EGF receptor family and the development of fluorescence microscopy techniques.

Nectarios Klonis is Research Fellow and **Leann Tilley** is Professor of Biochemistry in the Department of Biochemistry at La Trobe University in Melbourne, Australia.

They are interested in various aspects of the cell biology of the malaria parasite during its intraerythrocytic life stage. They have utilized a variety of fluorescence-based live cell methods, including the photobleaching techniques to examine macromolecular dynamics and protein trafficking in these cells.

Trevor Smith is Associate Professor in the School of Chemistry, University of Melbourne, Australia. His research is concerned with chemical processes that occur on ultrafast (femtosecond, picosecond, and nanosecond) timescales. He develops ultrafast laser spectroscopic techniques that are applied to the study of photophysical processes occurring in macro- and supramolecular systems and adapted to microspectroscopic studies.

Craig Lincoln is Research Associate in the School of Chemistry, University of Melbourne, Australia. His research is concerned with developing new microscopy techniques for high-resolution imaging of biological samples. He is also involved in femtosecond spectroscopy experiments investigating the photophysics and photochemistry of many novel materials and biological samples.

Damian Bird is Research Fellow in the School of Chemistry, University of Melbourne, Australia. His research is directed at developing advanced optical imaging systems based on spectral and time-resolved techniques that are capable of extracting the most valuable diagnostic information possible from fluorescence signals. He applies these systems to studies of breast cancer and pharmaceutics with the ultimate aim of translating these devices into the clinical setting.

Jörg Enderlein is Professor of Biophysical/Complex Systems at the Institute of Physics at Georg August University, Göttingen, Germany. He has over 15 years experience in developing and applying advanced techniques of single-molecule fluorescence spectroscopy and imaging. In particular, his group has developed high-precision double focus fluorescence correlation spectroscopy, fluorescence lifetime correlation spectroscopy, and defocused image analysis of molecular orientation.

Russell Connally is Research Fellow at Macquarie University, Sydney, Australia. He is an acknowledged expert in the field of time-gated luminescence detection and its application in microscopy and flow cytometry. He holds key patents in flow cytometry, fluorophore chemistry, and biological instrumentation. A key aim of Connally's research is the development of ultrasensitive luminescence-based techniques for pathogen detection.

Graham Vesey is the founder and chief scientific officer at BTF, a Sydney-based biotechnology company specializing with precision solutions for microbiology testing. Flow cytometry is the underpinning technology for making most of the BTF products and Dr. Vesey with his team has considerable pushed its boundaries.

Charlotte Morgan is Senior Scientist at BTF. BTF provides the world's most precise reference standards for microbiological testing.

Morry Silberstein is Associate Professor in the Department of Medical Imaging and Radiation Sciences at Monash University, Melbourne, Australia. His research interests relate to the investigation of the pathophysiology of central nervous system cell injury, the use of MR spectroscopy in the investigation of the biochemistry of disease, and the development of outcome measures for the use of cross-sectional imaging.

Wouter Kalle is Lecturer in Molecular Biology in the School of Biomedical Sciences, Faculty of Health Studies at Charles Sturt University, Wagga-Wagga, Australia. His research interests are in detection and diagnosis of cancer on a molecular level with a strong focus on microscopy.

Phillip Taderera Bwititi is Lecturer in Biochemistry and Clinical Biochemistry in the School of Biomedical Sciences, Faculty of Health Studies at Charles Sturt University, Wagga-Wagga, Australia. His interest is in analytical biochemistry and endocrinology.

Todd Walker is a consultant cytologist and Associate Professor of Biomedical Science at the University of Ballarat (Australia), where he teaches and researches diagnostic cytopathology. He is a Fellow of the International Academy of Cytology and the Editor of the Journal of the Australian Society of Cytology. Dr Walker serves on the National Board of Education, Australian Society of Cytology and more recently was appointed to the Cancer Screening Advisory Committee, Cancer Institute of NSW.

Evgenia G. Matveeva is Research Assistant Professor at the Department of Molecular Biology and Immunology, Health Science Center, University of North Texas, Fort Worth, Texas. She has over 20 years experience in immunoassay development in academia and industry. Over the course of her career Matveeva has engaged in a number of cross-disciplinary projects. She has published widely in the areas of fluoroimmunoassays, metal enhanced fluorescence, and synthesis and characterization of small molecules conjugated to fluorescent labels.

Ignacy Gryczynski is Professor in the Department of Cell Biology and Genetics, Health Science Center at the University of North Texas, Fort Worth, Texas. He is renowned for his work in multiphoton spectroscopy and microscopy including the effect of metal nanoparticles. He has been involved with protein chemistry, protein-ligand interaction and protein thermodynamics, applications of advanced fluorescence spectroscopy to study molecular processes in biological systems.

Zygmunt Gryczynski is Professor at Department of Molecular Biology and Immunology, Health Science Center at the University of North Texas, Fort Worth, Texas. He pioneered the studies of fluorescence effects mediated by ultrathin metal films, fluorescence enhancement and the surface plasmon coupled emission (SPCE). These technologies create opportunities for designing fluorescence-based assays and detection systems with much higher sensitivity and minimal need for sample pre-purification. He holds several patents and has authored and co-authored in excess of a hundred publications in the area of advanced fluorescence technologies.

Katharina Gaus is a NHMRC RD Wright Fellow at the Centre for Vascular Research and Associate Professor at the University of New South Wales, Sydney, Australia. Her research focuses on unraveling the organization of the cell membrane and understanding the role of lipid raft domains in signal transduction processes. Her most important contribution to the field to date has been the establishment of fluorescent microscopy techniques to visualize and quantify lipid structure in cell membranes.

Ronald Clarke is Senior Lecturer at the School of Chemistry, University of Sydney, Australia, He specializes in biophysical chemistry. His research interests include biological membranes and membrane proteins, the regulation and mechanism of charge transport across biological membranes and voltage-sensitive fluorescent dyes.

The editor, Professor **Ewa M. Goldys** holds a Personal Chair in Physics at Macquarie University, Sydney, Australia. Her expertise spans the fields of biophotonics, optical characterisation, ultrasensitive detection of analytes, biosensing, bioimaging, materials synthesis and characterisation and cathodoluminescence. Her research lies at the interface of materials science, photonics and biotechnology drawing on her earlier achievements in materials science and ultrasensitive optical characterisation. Her past most significant body of work focused on the optical characterisation of trace impurities and defects in materials and the development and application of cathodoluminescence for quantitative analysis of a wide variety of materials. Current work focuses on ultrasensitive surface plasmon resonance sensing system for bioassays. She has published over 150 papers in refereed journals.

Ewa established and leads the ARC/NHMRC Research Network "Fluorescence Applications in Biotechnology and Life Sciences", to foster cooperation in biological and biomedical sciences, chemistry, physics and optoelectronics and to translate scientific advances into commercial technologies. The Network brings together over 500 academics and industry representatives. This book is the result of one of the Network teaching and training initiatives.

CHAPTER 1

Basics of Fluorescence

ROBERT P. LEARMONTH

Department of Biological and Physical Sciences and Centre for Systems Biology, University of Southern Queensland, Toowoomba, Queensland 4350, Australia

SCOTT H. KABLE

School of Chemistry, University of Sydney, Sydney, New South Wales 2006, Australia

KENNETH P. GHIGGINO

School of Chemistry, University of Melbourne, Melbourne, Victoria 3010, Australia

1.1 INTRODUCTION

The study of the way that matter interacts with light is called *spectroscopy*. The origins of spectroscopy as a practical scientific discipline can be traced back to Newton's famous experiments on the spectrum of sunlight using prisms in 1665. The inability of physicists in the nineteeth century to quantitatively explain and predict their spectroscopic observations led to the foundation of the theory of quantum mechanics. Quantum theory and spectroscopy have since envolve hand in hand and underpin the way we currently understand the structure of molecules. For example, electronic structure, as well as molecular size and shape, has been learned from quantum mechanical interpretation of experimental spectroscopy. Optical microscopy has likewise evolved over a period of many centuries, allowing us to elucidate physical structures down to the micrometer scale. More recently, advanced approaches have allowed resolution on the nanometer scale.

The fusion of the disciplines of microscopy and spectroscopy over the past three decades, spawning microscopy applications such as fluorescence lifetime imaging microscopy (FLIM), fluorescence resonance energy transfer (FRET), and fluorescence recovery after photobleaching (FRAP), has made both disciplines more powerful, more sensitive, and more selective, though more complicated. Researchers now must have a sound understanding of the physics of optics, spectroscopy, and nonlinear processes and the chemistry of dyes, antifade agents, and intermolecular interactions and yet somehow remain experts in their native discipline!

The objective of this chapter is to provide a simple understanding of molecular spectroscopy, with a focus on concepts and techniques relevant to microscopy. The

Fluorescence Applications in Biotechnology and Life Sciences, Edited by Ewa M. Goldys

inherently quantum mechanical concepts of phenomena, including *energy levels*, *radiative and nonradiative processes*, and *quantum yields*, will be developed from a nonmathematical framework that is often used by experts in spectroscopy when discussing general principles. This simplified framework is developed into a practical and useful understanding of optical spectroscopy aimed at nonspecialists. This groundwork supports the more detailed discussion of complex techniques in the following chapters.

To begin the chapter we will outline basic features and properties of light and energy states of molecules. We then connect the two by exploring the interaction of light with molecules, initially for an isolated molecule. We will consider the key properties of absorption and emission and also those properties that are the bane of microscopy—the so called nonradiative mechanisms. After considering the isolated molecule, we will discuss interactions of molecules with their environment, which develops the concepts underpinning photobleaching and quenching, and also the more recent techniques of FRET and FLIM. En route we will examine the excitation and emission spectra of typical dyes, which can be found in any dye catalogue (see also Jameson et al. [1] for further reading).

1.1.1 Properties of Light

Light as an Electromagnetic Wave Light is a form of electromagnetic (EM) radiation, consisting of an oscillating electric field with an oscillating magnetic field perpendicular to it (Figure 1.1). These oscillating fields behave like waves travelling in the direction of propagation at the speed of light (c), which in a vacuum is $c = 3.00 \times 10^8$ m/s. In optical spectroscopy and microscopy, the wavelength of the light (λ), measured typically in nanometers ($1\,\text{nm} = 10^{-9}$ m), is its most commonly used characteristic. Light can be distinguished by many other characteristics, including the frequency (ν), which is defined as the number of wavefronts passing a fixed point every second (Figure 1.1). The frequency is therefore inversely proportional to the wavelength; at a fixed speed, more wavefronts of shorter wavelengths will pass a fixed point in a given time than will wavefronts of longer wavelengths.

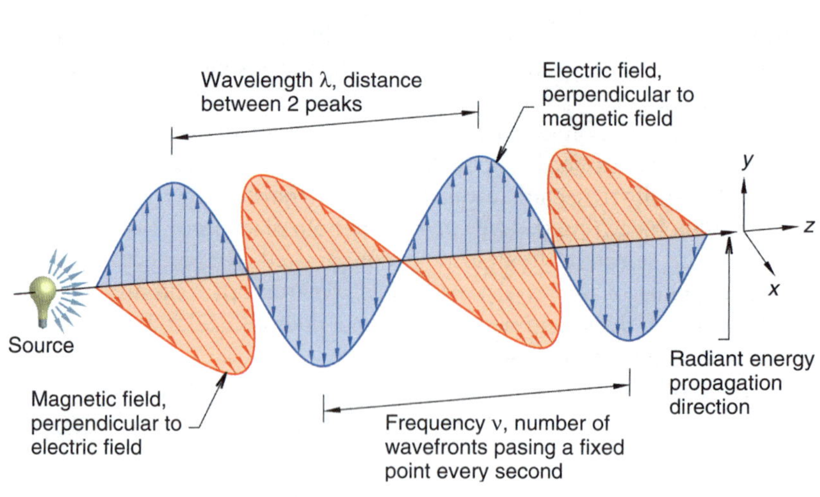

Figure 1.1 Electromagnetic ray showing wavelength and frequency.

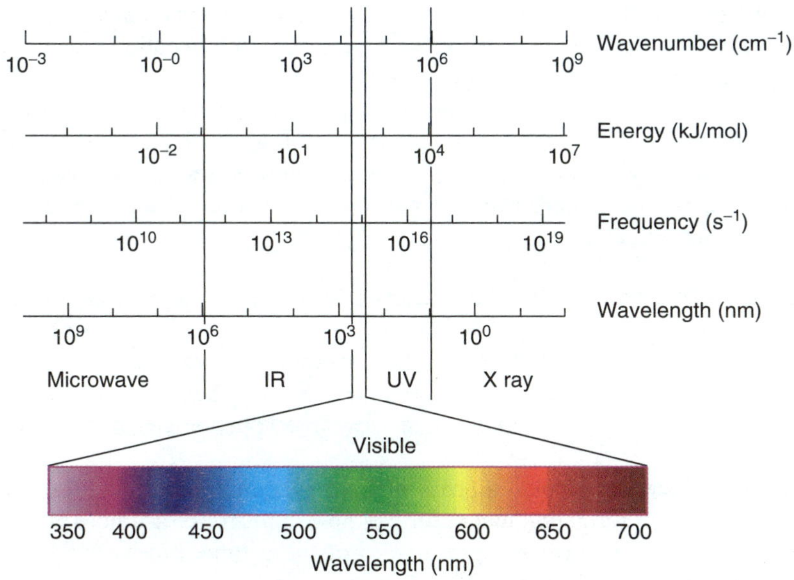

Figure 1.2 Different regions of the electromagnetic spectrum.

The mathematical relationship that defines these three properties is

$$\nu = \frac{c}{\lambda} \tag{1.1}$$

The wavelength of light can vary over many orders of magnitude, without limit, as illustrated in part in Figure 1.2. The optical, or visible, wavelengths form a narrow range, extending from approximately 400 to 750 nm. The wavelength range immediately following the longer wavelengths is called infrared (IR) while the adjacent region with shorter wavelengths is the ultraviolet (UV). Historically, although UV illumination has been used to excite fluorescence emission in the visible region, optical microscopy has dealt exclusively with the visible wavelength region because our eyes were the detectors. This was supplemented with emulsion film photography; furthermore, more recently, with the development of IR- and UV-sensitive detectors and the advent of nonlinear optical techniques, these neighboring wavelength regions have also become important.

Dual Nature of Light About one hundred years ago, Planck postulated that the *energy* of an EM wave could not have any value but was quantized. This smallest unit of energy is proportional to its frequency ν and has a magnitude

$$E = h\nu \tag{1.2}$$

where h is now called the *Planck constant*. This smallest amount, or quantum, of energy is associated with one *photon* of light. It is important to note that molecules usually absorb or emit one photon at a time. The exception to this rule is under conditions of very intense radiation, where two or more photons can be absorbed simultaneously, leading to multiphoton absorption (see Section 1.2.3).

The dichotomy of the two descriptions of light (the *wave* and *particle* descriptions) was the source of enormous debate for the first part of the twentieth century and was eventually united in quantum mechanics. Both definitions are helpful in different situations. For example, reflection, refraction, diffraction, and polarization are best described using wave properties. Absorption and emission of light by molecules are more intuitively described using the particle (photon) description. In the discussion and chapters that follow, we will use the wave and particle description of light interchangeably, depending on the process.

Reflection, Refraction, Diffraction, and Polarization Reflection, refraction, and diffraction of light are of obvious importance, especially when the instrumentation is considered. Although seemingly simple, these phenomena are actually quite complex, both in the intellectual sense and the mathematical sense of being described by complex numbers. Here, we will define and describe these three phenomena only in the simplest terms.

All of these processes involve a beam of light encountering a (nonabsorptive) substance with a different refractive index, for example, a mirror or a simple piece of glass. *Reflection* of light is the most straightforward of these three processes. As illustrated in Figure 1.3*a*, a beam of light striking a surface such as glass or water will reflect from that surface at the same angle as it is incident on the surface. Clearly, this is the process that underpins the behavior of all mirrors.

A spoon in a glass of water that is apparently bent is a good example of the second process, *refraction*. When light passes from one medium to another of a different refractive index, its speed changes. This causes it to bend if it enters the second medium at an angle, as shown in Figure 1.3*b*. The light always bends toward the medium of higher refractive index.

When light passes through a small opening, it diffracts from the edges of the hole, as shown in Figure 1.3*c*. When the hole approaches the same size as the wavelength of light, the *diffraction* becomes significant. This is the main phenomenon limiting the resolving power of a conventional light microscope. A conventional light or fluorescence microscope can only resolve features as small as the wavelength of light used to view the object. This is called the *diffraction limit*.

One of the complicating but powerful features of reflection, refraction, and diffraction is that the phenomena depend on many other factors, including the wavelength of light, the polarization of the light (see below), the refractive index of the materials, and the angles involved. These features are all used to advantage in the construction of a fluorescence microscope but are otherwise beyond the scope of this introductory chapter. The reader is referred to [2] for further information on these areas.

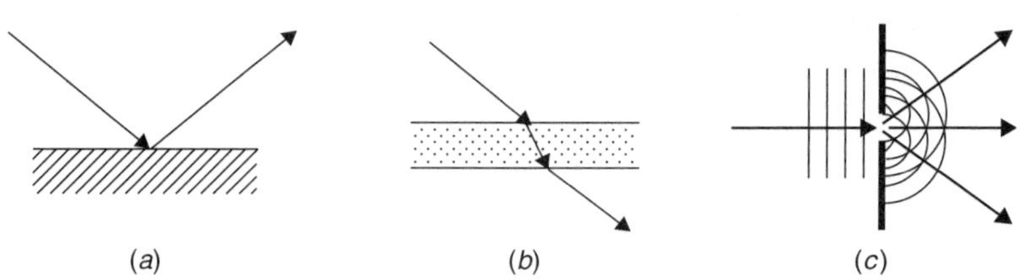

Figure 1.3 Simple depictions of (*a*) reflection of a beam of light from a surface; (*b*) refraction of light through a medium of higher refractive index; and (*c*) diffraction of light through a small hole.

The polarization of light also has important implications for some types of fluorescence spectroscopy and microscopy, for example, the determination of rotational mobility of components in biological systems, which is commonly assessed by measurement of fluorescence emission polarization. Briefly, polarization of light refers to the following characteristics. As noted above, EM radiation consists of oscillating electric and magnetic fields, each perpendicular to the other and also perpendicular to the direction of propagation (Figure 1.1). If we consider the electric field only (for simplicity), the electric field vector can assume any direction of oscillation perpendicular or normal to the light propagation direction. If one was to view the light "end on" (i.e., along the axis of propagation), then the electric vector could be found at any angle within 360° (as shown for the light at the left side of Figure 1.4). If all such angles are equally likely, then this is *unpolarized light*.

It is possible to use polarizing optics, including filters or prisms, to only pass light of one polarization (i.e., electric vector oscillating in only one plane), as shown in Figure 1.4. The light that passes through such a polarizing filter is now *linearly polarized*. Polarized sunglasses work in the same way and utilize the fact that unscattered light from the sun is randomly polarized. Reflections of a horizontal smooth surface such as water or the road are highly polarized, mostly horizontally (parallel to the reflective surface). The polarized sunglasses block this horizontally polarized light while passing vertically polarized light and therefore preferentially block the light scattered from horizontal surfaces. It is also possible, by turning the head on the side, to observe the reverse—we will then preferentially see the scattered light.

1.1.2 States of Molecules

When a molecule is placed in an electric field, any charged part of the molecule will experience a force. If the field is oscillating, as it is in light, then parts of the molecule will be pushed and pulled at that frequency. Just as in musical instruments, molecules

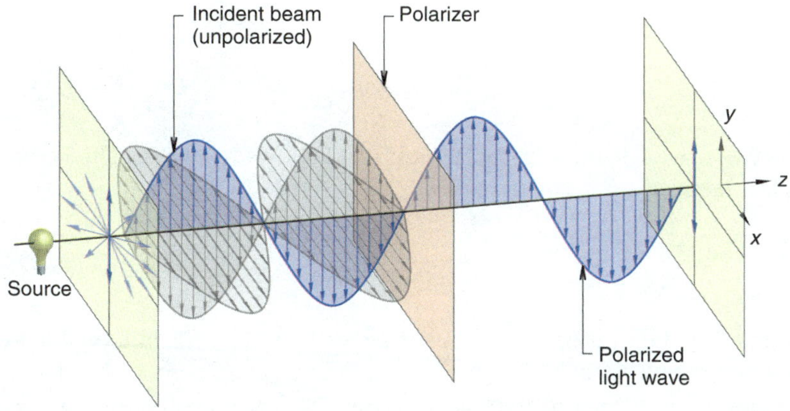

Figure 1.4 Representation of unpolarized and polarized light. In natural light, shown by a light bulb on the left, the electric field oscillation as seen along the direction of propagation can be aligned in any direction, as represented by the arrows on the plane next to the bulb. Using a polarizing device, light can be selected with electric field oscillation in a single plane, as shown propagating to the right of the polarizer and represented on the plane at the far right.

also have specific resonant frequencies at which they like to oscillate. Each of the resonant frequencies ν (or energies, as $E = h\nu$) is related to *states* of the molecule, each with an associated *energy level*. For example, *vibrational states* correspond to particular resonant frequencies of the atoms in a molecule vibrating together. Electrons in a molecule oscillating with a resonant frequency do so by making periodic transitions back and forth between two *electronic states* and the resonant frequency is given by the energy separation between these states. Because there are multiple atoms in a molecule, most with multiple electrons, there are a large number of energy levels; in fact, the number of each electronic and vibrational energy level is infinite. Fortunately, only a few are practically important.

There are many other states in molecules that give rise to different forms of spectroscopy, including nuclear spin [nuclear magnetic resonance (NMR) spectroscopy], rotation (microwave spectroscopy), and electron spin [ESR or electron paramagnetic (EPR) spectroscopy]. However, it is the interaction of light with the electrons and nuclei that is important in optical spectroscopy and microscopy, so we shall restrict our discussion to these interactions.

Vibrational States If a group of molecules is cooled to near absolute zero, then they will all have the minimum energy possible; that is, they will all be in their *ground state*. The concept of the ground state comes from the idea that an elevator at the ground level is at the lowest possible level. As the temperature is raised, some molecules will start to vibrate after collisions with the walls or each other or by absorbing background thermal radiation. Vibration of the atoms in a molecule is one means by which a molecule can store energy.

In a simple but accurate picture, the vibrating atoms in a molecule can be treated as balls joined by springs (the bonds). To take the simplest such example, consider two balls joined by one spring to represent a diatomic molecule. These two balls can vibrate with a characteristic frequency that depends on the mass of the balls and the "tightness" of the spring holding them together. Mathematically, the equation that describes the characteristic oscillation frequency ν and how it depends on mass μ and spring (or force) constant k is given by

$$\nu = \frac{1}{2\pi}\sqrt{\frac{k}{\mu}} \tag{1.3}$$

Note here that μ is called the "reduced mass" and allows for the balls to be of different masses. The reduced mass is defined as

$$\frac{1}{\mu} = \frac{1}{m_1} + \frac{1}{m_2} \tag{1.4}$$

According to Eq. 1.3, stiffer springs (or stronger bonds) result in a higher frequency. Heavier atoms result in a lower frequency. This is consistent with what we know about vibrations of strings in musical instruments: For example, the heavy E string on a guitar is a much lower note (82.4 Hz) than the lighter E string, which is four times higher in frequency (329.6 Hz), while tightening a string increases the pitch (frequency).

This simple system of either two balls and a spring or two atoms and a bond has a single characteristic frequency. The balls, or atoms, can only vibrate with this characteristic frequency or an integer multiple of this frequency. These integer-multiple frequencies are called *overtones*, both in music and spectroscopy.

A more complex molecule can still be modeled quite accurately as balls of different masses joined by springs of different tensions (representing different atoms with different bonds). Although it might not be as intuitively obvious, there are still a limited number of characteristic frequencies for a polyatomic molecule. For example, benzene has 30 characteristic vibrations, while MitoTracker red, a common fluorescent dye, has 243 (the number of characteristic frequencies is given by $3N - 6$, where N is the number of atoms in the molecule). While the number of characteristic vibrations increases only slowly with the size of the molecule, the number of overtones rises more rapidly. Additionally, now that there are different types of vibrations, these vibrations may occur together, giving rise to combination vibrations. The number of these combinations now increases almost exponentially with increasing energy. The result is that for spectroscopically "large" molecules, including all microscopy dyes, the number of vibrational states is too high to count or even to portray accurately in a diagram. This can be a significant complication for a spectroscopist, but for the purposes of this introductory chapter, we do not have to be concerned with the specifics of vibrational states and only need to recognize that there are an incredibly large number of vibrational states and that these states are a temporary store of energy in a molecule (see below).

Electronic States Electrons, being over 1000 times lighter than nuclei, oscillate at much higher frequencies. Oscillations of the valence electrons (those involved with chemical bonding) correspond to transitions between electronic states induced by EM waves with wavelengths in the ultraviolet and visible (UV/Vis) region of the spectrum. Oscillations (transitions) of the core electrons, which are bound very tightly to the nucleus, occur at a much higher frequency, corresponding to the X-ray region of the spectrum (remember a tight spring vibrates with a higher frequency than a loose spring). Optical spectroscopy and microscopy, involving radiation in the UV/Vis region of the spectrum, therefore involve the excitation of valence electrons in a molecule.

A property of electrons called *spin* is also associated with specific energetic states (spin represents a form of energy inherent in the spinning of a particle about an axis within itself, also called its *intrinsic angular momentum*). Most stable molecules have an even number of electrons. Because each electronic energy level (i.e., orbital) can only have two electrons with opposite spin (the *Pauli principle*), the lowest (ground) electronic state of most molecules has a zero total electron spin, as shown schematically in Figure 1.5. When an electron is excited to a higher electronic state, its spin is usually

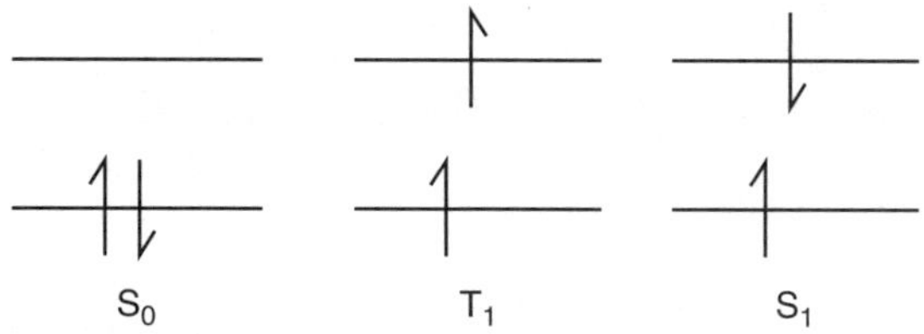

Figure 1.5 Electron spin for ground state, first singlet state, and first triplet states of the hydrogen molecule as a simple example.

unaffected. Therefore, although two of the electrons are now unpaired (the one excited to a higher orbital and the one left behind), the total electron spin on the molecule is still zero. All states with zero total electron spin are called singlet states and are given the label S. The labels are appended with a numerical subscript that simply counts from the ground state, S_0, through the first excited singlet state, S_1, and so on for higher states.

If the electron spin is flipped after being excited to a higher state, then the total electron spin on the molecule will be 1. In the same way that an orbital angular momentum of $l = 1$ gives rise to the three p orbitals, $S = 1$ in a molecule gives rise to three close-lying electronic states. This collection of states is called a *triplet* state and is given the label T. If more than one electron is excited, then more "unpairings" can occur, giving rise to quintet states, and so on. A molecule with an odd number of electrons will have a half integral total spin, which gives rise to doublet and quartet states, and so on. However, for most molecules used in practical UV/Vis spectroscopy and microscopy, only singlet and triplet states are important.

Depicting States and Transitions (Perrin–Jablonski Diagrams) When a molecule absorbs a photon of light, it gets excited to a higher energy state. Unless the absolute energies of the molecular states are particularly important, then the energy levels of a molecule are depicted in a diagrammatic way, often called a *Jablonski diagram* but more correctly termed a *Perrin–Jablonski diagram* in recognition that Perrin was the first to formalize this diagrammatic analysis [1], a simple example of which is shown in Figure 1.6. Energy in this diagram is increasing along the vertical axis. This axis is usually not depicted because the energies are not drawn to scale. The horizontal axis in this diagram is meaningless and never drawn. Electronic states are represented by thick lines. In Figure 1.6, only three such states are drawn: the ground state S_0 and two excited electronic states labeled S_1 and T_1. As discussed above, these latter two states are the lowest excited singlet and triplet states. Notice that T_1 is of lower energy than S_1. This is always the case and crucial to the fluorescence characteristics of various dyes (see below).

The vibrational states in a Perrin–Jablonski diagram are represented by lightweight lines. Although there are a multitude of vibrational states, the vibrational energy-level structure is only drawn in a cartoon fashion. Often this is just a set of equally spaced lines, or sometimes a set of lines that get closer together in spacing to represent that the density of vibrational states is increasing with energy.

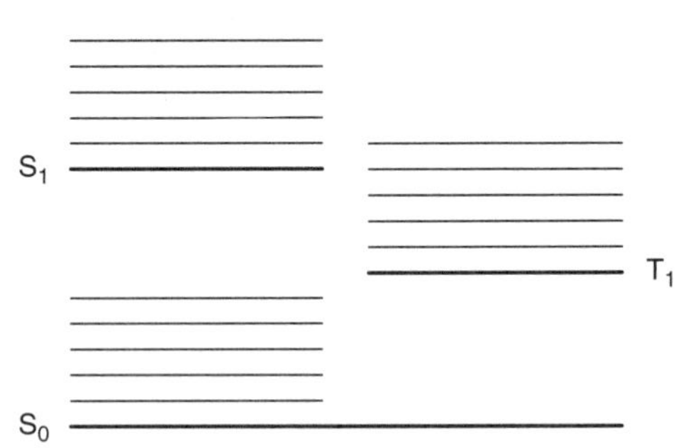

Figure 1.6 Simple Perrin–Jablonski diagram showing three electronic states (thick lines) and several vibrational states (thin lines).

One of the key aspects of a Perrin–Jablonski diagram is that it is only drawn as complicated as it needs to be to get across the concept under discussion. For example, if triplet states were unimportant to a topic, then they would be omitted.

1.2 ABSORPTION AND EMISSION OF LIGHT

1.2.1 Interaction of Light with a Molecule

When a molecule is placed in an oscillating EM field (i.e., light is shone on the molecule), the oscillating fields can push and pull the molecule around. In particular, charged parts of the molecule are affected by the oscillating *electric* field of light; the effect of the oscillating *magnetic* field is much weaker. If the charges on the molecule can oscillate in synchrony with the oscillating field (this is called *resonance*), then the molecule can absorb energy from the field. As a physical analogy, we can consider a child on a swing. If the child is randomly pushed, then the swing never really gets going. But if it is pushed *in resonance* with the oscillation of the swing, then the swing can absorb a lot of energy.

This concept of resonance is frequently encountered in our daily life, from musical instruments to radio reception. One thing we should notice is that there is often one specific resonant frequency for simple systems. We can only push the child on the swing at one frequency. If we play middle C on a piano, then the piano string vibrates 262 times per second. Molecules likewise have specific resonant frequencies. A typical C–H bond in a molecule vibrates about 10^{14} times per second (10^{14} Hz), while a C–C bond vibrates at about 3×10^{13} Hz. Although this is incredibly fast compared to middle C above, Eq. 1.3 provides the reason: H and C atoms are around 10^{24} times lighter than the piano string. This mass difference on its own causes a $\sqrt{10^{24}} = 10^{12}$ difference in vibrational frequency. An oscillating EM field at 10^{14} Hz corresponds to light in the mid-IR region of the spectrum (see Figure 1.2). The corresponding range of wavelengths is about to 3–30 μm (see Eq. 1.1). A molecule exposed to mid-IR radiation of the right frequency can therefore absorb one photon from the field to become vibrationally excited.

Electrons are over 1000 times lighter than nuclei and oscillate at even higher frequencies. Again, simple application of Eq. 1.3 suggests that this frequency is a factor of about 30 times higher. Indeed, a typical frequency of light absorbed by valence electrons is 10^{15} Hz, which is 30 times faster than the C–C bond vibration. Light with this frequency corresponds to the near-UV region of the spectrum. More generally, the range of wavelengths absorbed by valence electrons varies from about 1000 nm (near IR) through the visible and UV down to about 100 nm (far UV).

Absorption of EM radiation and excitation of electrons take place more or less instantaneously ($\sim 10^{-18}$ s) relative to nuclear motion ($\sim 10^{-15}$ s), according to the *Franck–Condon principle*. Despite this difference in time scales, excitation of electrons in a molecule can also cause a change in molecular structure. The absorbed energy leads to a redistribution of the electron cloud of the molecule, resulting in altered vibrational levels, an altered dipole moment, and a change in the shape of the molecule. Quite simply, the bonds are not the same after an electron has been removed and put into a different orbital. A consequence of this is that electronic absorption is often accompanied by vibrational motion as the atoms move to their new positions.

Excited states of molecules are unstable. They relax (lose their energy) by a number of mechanisms, including collisions with other molecules, for example, the solvent, or reaction with other species, for example, dissolved oxygen. The excited molecule may also relax by emitting a photon of light to return to a lower state, though not always the same lower state from which it came. The emitted photon will have an energy corresponding to the difference in energy between the initial and final states of the molecule. This emission of a photon is known as *fluorescence* or in some cases *phosphorescence*, as we shall see below.

1.2.2 Absorption and Emission of Light Depicted on a Perrin–Jablonski Diagram

An enduring picture that should be remembered for absorption and emission of radiation is that they occur in coincidence with a molecule undergoing a transition between two specific energy levels. On a Perrin–Jablonski diagram, these transitions are represented by arrows, as shown in Figure 1.7. At room temperature, molecules are almost always in their ground electronic state, S_0. Even for vibrational states, the ground state is still the most likely state of a molecule, although low-frequency vibrations may have significant population. Therefore, on the Perrin–Jablonski diagram, the absorption transition is shown as starting in the ground state. There is no such restriction on the excited state; therefore absorption may occur to a variety of vibrational states in the excited electronic states. The typical amount of vibrational excitation, as discussed above, depends on the change in geometry of the molecule between the two different electronic states. Small changes in geometry are accompanied by small vibrational excitation (arrow 1) whereas large changes in geometry are accompanied by large vibrational excitation (arrow 2). Essentially, to be absorbed, the energy of the incident radiation must exactly match one of the available energy-level transitions. Given the many possible combinations of electronic and vibrational energy levels for a polyatomic molecule, a range of light energies may be absorbed. As noted above (Eq. 1.2), the energy of the light is proportional to its frequency (thus inversely related to its wavelength), so a given molecule will absorb a specific set of wavelengths of light, giving rise to its absorption spectrum.

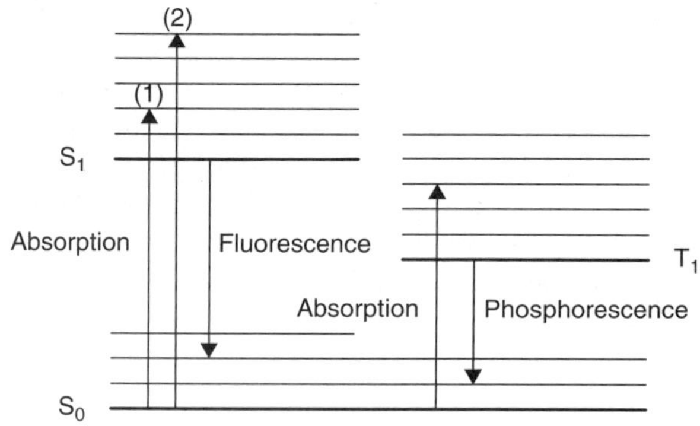

Figure 1.7 Simple Perrin–Jablonski diagram showing three electronic states, several vibrational states, absorption of EM radiation, and emission of fluorescence or phosphorescence.

The Perrin–Jablonski diagram in Figure 1.7 shows absorption to both S_1 and T_1. In reality, the transition from S_0 to T_1 is many orders of magnitude weaker than from S_0 to S_1. Absorption into triplets states, as shown in the figure, is therefore practically unimportant in most cases and is only observed in specialized situations in spectroscopy. However, this is not to say the population of triplet states is unimportant: quite the contrary. Population of triplet states is one of the main mechanisms for photobleaching, which will be discussed later. It is simply, and fortuitously, that triplets are not populated to any great extent by absorption of light by molecules commonly used in fluorescence spectroscopy and microscopy.

Emission of light is shown on a Perrin–Jablonski diagram as an arrow from the excited state back to the ground state. Emission that does not change electron spin, just like absorption, is much preferred over emission in which the electron spin is flipped. This spin-conserving emission is called *fluorescence*. Because the process is favorable, it happens readily and quickly with the result that excited electronic states survive for only a very short period of time, typically a few nanoseconds, before emitting. Emission between triplet and singlet states is called *phosphorescence*. Because this is a weak and therefore slow process, the molecule can remain excited much longer, typically milliseconds to seconds. Although this might seem still like a very rapid process, it is slow compared to molecular events and can give rise to unusual chemistry in the excited state leading to reduction in fluorescence efficiency, photobleaching, and other processes (see later).

1.2.3 Multiphoton Excitation

The discussion above on absorption of light and excitation of fluorescence could be termed "one-photon" excitation; that is, one photon is absorbed, leading to one photon being emitted. The reader may already have heard about laser-scanning microscopic techniques designated as "two photon" or more generally as "multiphoton." Such technology has several advantages and is becoming increasingly common. Multiphoton laser-scanning microscopy involves using pulsed (femtosecond, 1 fs $= 10^{-15}$ s) laser beams and optics to focus an intense incident beam of coherent photons to a precise spot. Using such intense radiation allows the possibility of more than one photon to (essentially) simultaneously excite a fluorophore.

A simple understanding of two-photon (or multiphoton) excitation can be achieved using either the particle or wave description of light. Consider first a photon (particle) with exactly half the energy required for a specific electronic transition. This photon, at the speed of light, will impinge upon the fluorophore, for approximately 10^{-18} s. If a second photon impinges on the molecule within this interaction time, then the molecule can absorb both photons together to impart twice the amount of energy into the molecule, as would be expected. The likelihood of two photons impinging on the molecule at the same time is proportional to the number of photons squared (akin to second-order kinetics for those familiar with kinetic theory). Therefore, the (very low) number of two-photon absorption events scales with the square of the laser power. Hence, two-photon microscopy is only possible with very intense lasers.

Above, we described the conventional absorption of light as arising from the interaction of the oscillating electric field of a wave of light with charged regions of the molecule. If the electric field becomes very intense, then the molecule will experience overtones of the field. To use a music analogy again, if you blow a recorder modestly, you should blow a fairly pure note. If you blow too hard, then you will also generate the next octave higher, which is exactly one overtone (twice the frequency). This is a convenient analogy for what a molecule experiences in a very intense laser field; it also experiences the overtone at twice the frequency of the field, which can then be absorbed. Again, it can be shown that the amount of overtone scales as the intensity squared, so the probability of two-photon absorption also scales as the laser intensity squared using the wave description of the process.

No matter which picture of two-photon absorption we are more comfortable with, the total energy of the two (or more) photons must still correspond to a difference of real energy levels of the molecule, as shown in the Perrin–Jablonski diagram in Figure 1.8. This diagram also shows that the resultant fluorescence emission, following two-photon absorption, is still the conventional one-photon emission. Two-photon spontaneous fluorescence has never been observed because the intensity of the fluorescence is much too weak.

The generalized term "multiphoton" refers to the fact that excitation can be effected by absorption of two or more photons; two-photon systems are now becoming common, and commercial three-photon systems are under development. Multiphoton excitation provides some interesting and useful variations from the one-photon case. If we consider as an example two-photon excitation, coincident absorption of two photons, each with half the energy required for single-photon excitation, results in the excited state. This produces the same fluorescence output, but at approximately double the wavelength of the incident light. Consider Eqs. 1.1 and 1.2; combining them gives

$$E = \frac{hc}{\lambda} \quad \text{or} \quad \lambda = \frac{hc}{E} \tag{1.5}$$

A practical consequence of this doubling of the wavelength of the incident light is that the energy of the illumination is reduced from the high-energy UV region to the lower energy red to near-IR region of the EM spectrum (700–1050 nm). This provides a number of advantages over conventional one-photon fluorescence excitation. Photobleaching is dramatically reduced by the use of lower energy red to near-IR

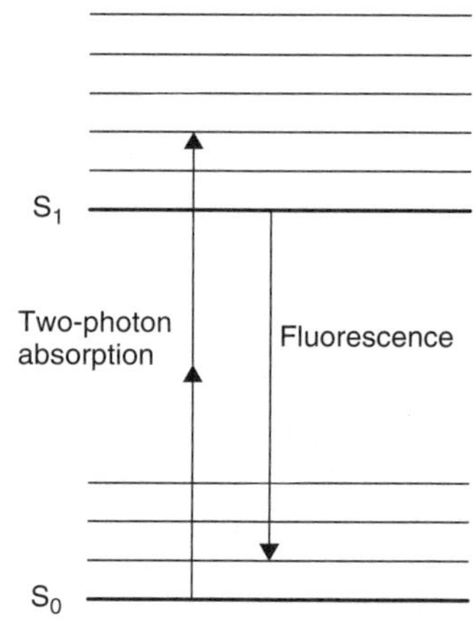

Figure 1.8 Perrin–Jablonski diagram showing two-photon absorption followed by conventional fluorescence.

irradiation, as excitation occurs only at the focal point of illumination of the specimen (only here is the laser intensity high enough for two-photon absorption). This also enables studies of UV-excitable dyes with red laser systems without the additional expense and maintenance of UV laser systems. In addition, due to reduced susceptibility to scatter, the penetration of longer wavelength radiation into turbid media such as biofilms of microorganisms and animal or plant tissues is much greater, allowing analysis of events at much greater depth.

1.3 NONRADIATIVE DECAY MECHANISMS

Excited molecules are inherently unstable. As noted above, fluorescence and phosphorescence are two *radiative* mechanisms for returning the molecule to a stable state. There are also a variety of *nonradiative* processes that can deactivate a molecule. As the name suggests, these processes do not result in the emission of light and therefore are not useful for fluorescence spectroscopy and microscopy. However, an understanding of them is essential to explain characteristics of fluorophores, including their optical properties, fluorescence efficiency, and bleaching.

1.3.1 Vibrational Relaxation

Molecules are continuously interacting with their surroundings by virtue of their translational, vibrational, and rotational motions. As the atoms collide with their neighbors, they can transfer vibrational energy to and from the vibrations of the surrounding molecules. This is an important process which leads to excitation of cold molecules until they react or deexcitation of hot molecules until they reach thermal equilibrium. The vibrational energy transfer process from hot molecules into their surroundings, called *vibrational relaxation (VR)* or *thermalization*, is very efficient and takes place on a picosecond (10^{-12} s) timescale.

Vibrational relaxation occurs in both the ground and excited electronic states. Recall that fluorescence occurs on a nanosecond scale and phosphorescence on an even longer scale, and thus VR will deexcite any excess vibrational energy caused by the absorption

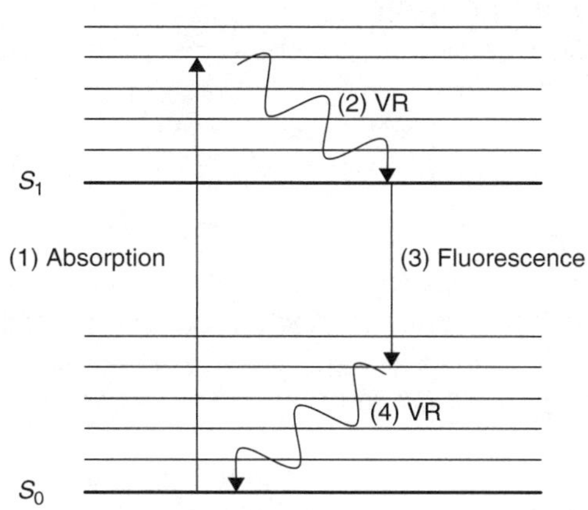

Figure 1.9 Perrin–Jablonski diagram showing four steps in absorption/reemission of light.

of light before the molecule has a chance to reemit as fluorescence or phosphorescence. Figure 1.9 shows this process in a Perrin–Jablonski diagram. Four processes are shown:

1. Absorption of light from S_0 to a high vibrational level in S_1.
2. Thermodynamics dictates that energy will flow from the vibrationally hotter molecule to the cooler surroundings. Therefore VR removes the excess vibrational energy, leaving the molecule in the lowest vibrational level of the S_1 state.
3. Fluorescence emission, decreasing the electron's energy to a high vibrational level in S_0. This is not a random choice of vibrational state; if a large change in geometry between S_0 and S_1 causes significant vibrational excitation upon absorption, then the reverse geometry change will occur upon emission, again causing significant vibrational excitation.
4. VR removes this excess energy, leaving the molecule back where it started.

1.3.2 Internal Conversion

An interesting question concerns why the electronic energy is not also removed by the solvent in the same way that vibrational energy is. In fact it is! The difference is that the relaxation of an excited electronic state requires a much larger energy exchange with the surroundings. It is well known in the energy transfer literature that larger energy exchanges between molecules are much more difficult than small exchanges of energy. A small exchange of energy can occur between an excited fluorophore and the solvent if the fluorophore swaps its electronic energy for the same amount of vibrational energy. This process is shown schematically in the left panel of Figure 1.10, where an excited molecule has undergone several VR steps until it is left in the lowest vibrational state of S_1—the same as Figure 1.9. Now, however, the excited state is converted to a high vibrational state of S_0—a state of similar total energy. This is indicated on the Perrin–Jablonski diagram by a horizontal (meaning energy is constant), wavy arrow. This process is called *internal conversion (IC)*. Although Figure 1.10 shows IC between S_1 and S_0, the process can occur between any states of the same multiplicity, that is, between singlet states or between triplet states. In fact, IC between higher states is even more likely and often occurs with a much faster rate than IC between S_1 and S_0. This is because higher electronic states lie closer in energy to each other than do the S_1 and S_0 state; the gap between S_0 and S_1 is usually the largest gap between any two electronic states. As a result, the energy exchange between fluorophore and solvent is less and the IC process is more efficient between higher states. The right-hand side of Figure 1.10 shows this other common fluorescence cycle: absorption to a higher electronic state, S_2, followed by IC to S_1, then fluorescence. This illustrates a process known variously as *Vavilov's law* or *Kasha's law*, which states that fluorescence only occurs from the lowest excited electronic state, irrespective of which state is initially excited. A consequence of this law combined with VR is that a fluorophore usually fluoresces at exactly the same wavelength, no matter which electronic or vibrational state is excited. This is shown in Figures 1.9 and 1.10. In both cases the fluorescence is exactly the same, even though S_1 is excited in one case and S_2 in the other. Specific examples of Vavilov's or Kasha's law are shown for fluorophores later in this chapter.

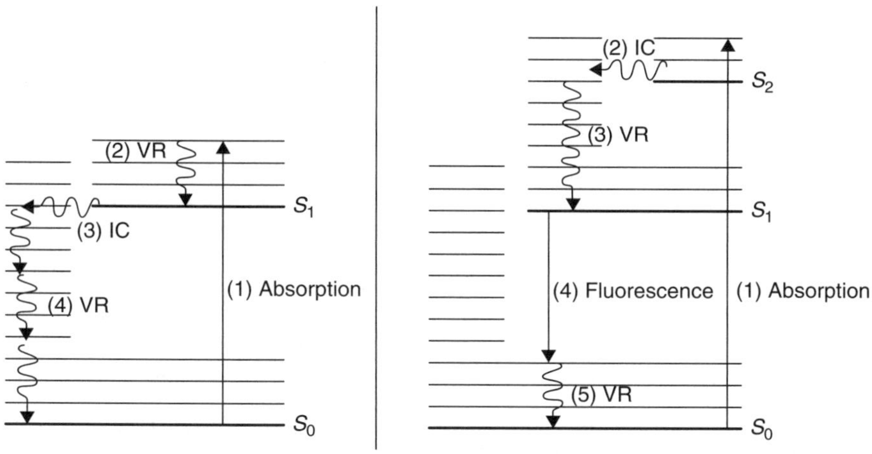

Figure 1.10 Perrin–Jablonski diagrams showing nonradiative loss of absorption energy (left) and excitation to higher electronic state but emission from lowest exited state (right).

1.3.3 Intersystem Crossing

We have already seen that singlet and triplet manifolds do not interconvert readily by absorption or emission of light. Collisions with surrounding molecules seem to be more efficient at flipping a molecule from singlet to triplet states (and vice versa). The nonradiative transfer between singlet and triplet states is called *intersystem crossing (ISC)*. Figure 1.11 shows how to represent ISC in a Perrin–Jablonski diagram. Once in the triplet manifold, all the normal processes occur with similar efficiency, including VR and IC. After the initial ISC event the molecule will usually relax downward in energy until it reaches the lowest vibration level of the lowest triplet state. This state is *metastable*, which means that there is no efficient process to remove energy, even though the molecule is still in an excited state. This is a dangerous place for a molecule to be! The lowest triplet state, remember, has two unpaired electrons, which makes for a very reactive molecule. One of the main decomposition (or photobleaching) mechanisms for fluorophores is to react from a triplet state.

1.4 PROPERTIES OF EXCITED MOLECULES

1.4.1 Quantum Yield

With so many processes that can occur after the absorption of one photon, it becomes crucial to know which are the most important. One measure of the importance of each process is the *quantum yield*. Mathematically, the quantum yield ϕ_i for a process i is

$$\phi_i = \frac{k_i}{\sum k} \tag{1.6}$$

where k_i is the rate of process i divided by the sum of all rates. Conceptually, the quantum yield is simply the fraction of times that a molecule undergoes a particular process. For example, a quantum yield for fluorescence, $\phi_f = 0.90$, means that after

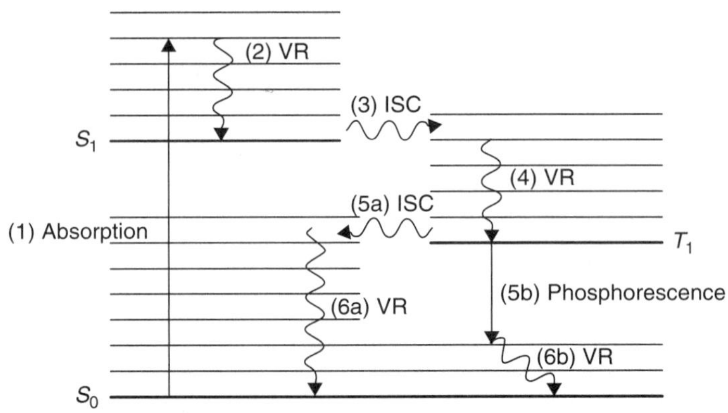

Figure 1.11 Perrin–Jablonski diagram showing production and relaxation from triplet states. The state at the end of process 4 is metastable and can undergo a variety of fates, two of which are shown here (chemical reaction is another possibility).

absorption of a photon, 90% of the molecules will reemit the energy as fluorescence. Clearly, the higher the quantum yield for fluorescence, the brighter a fluorophore will appear (more photons out for the same photons in). In terms of degradation of the fluorophore, the quantum yield for intersystem crossing, ϕ_{ISC}, is the important value, and clearly this should be as small as possible.

1.4.2 Excited-State Lifetime

The lifetime of fluorescence or phosphorescence is the time of persistence of electronic state excitation. The lifetime, denoted by the Greek letter tau (τ), is a practically important parameter that may be affected by changes in the environment of a fluorophore, thereby affecting other measured parameters such as polarization. The lifetime is specifically defined as the inverse of the sum of the rate constants that deplete the excited state, and thus for the singlet state the relative contributions of internal conversion, intersystem crossing, and the radiative process will determine the lifetime value. The magnitude of the rate constants that deplete S_1 is typically around 10^8 s^{-1}, indicating a fluorescence lifetime on the order of 10 ns (10×10^{-9} s), although known fluorophores have lifetimes varying from picoseconds to hundreds of nanoseconds. In the case of phosphorescence emission, the rate processes depleting the triplet state are generally slower (between 10^3 and 1 s^{-1}), leading to lifetimes around milliseconds to seconds.

1.5 SPECTROSCOPY AND FLUOROPHORES

1.5.1 Absorption, Excitation, and Emission Spectra

In this section we bring together all the earlier concepts into a concrete discussion of the spectra of dyes. Three different kinds of spectra are often reported, and the ability to interpret these spectra is crucial to the correct selection of instrumental parameters for fluorescence spectroscopy and microscopy and/or of an appropriate dye for the application at hand. These three spectra are the *absorption, emission*, and *excitation* spectra and we will deal with them separately.

1. *Absorption Spectra* The *absorption spectrum* of a dye is the most fundamental of the three spectra to the extent that all molecules will have an absorption spectrum, though they might not fluoresce. The innate strength with which a molecule absorbs light is characterized by the *absorption coefficient (or extinction coefficient*, ε). The amount of light absorbed (*absorbance* A) is described by the *Beer–Lambert law*, which relates this absorbance to the concentration of the compound (c) and the length of the path through which the light travels (l):

$$\text{Absorbance} = \log_{10}\frac{I_0}{I} = \varepsilon c l \tag{1.7}$$

As Eq. 1.7 shows, the absorbance is defined in terms of the intensity of incident light, I_0, and the intensity of transmitted light, I. The unit of the pathlength is usually the centimeter (indeed, the standard absorption cell is 1 cm in length). If the units of c are moles per liter or grams per liter, then ε has units of liters per mole per centimeter or liters per gram per centimeter. Figure 1.12 shows the absorption spectrum, in black, of the fluorophore pyrenesulfonic acid (PSA). The spectrum at first may appear complicated but can readily be understood using the discussion in the previous sections. The main peaks, labeled S_1, S_2, and S_3, are the transitions corresponding to the lowest three excited singlet states of PSA. A subsidiary peak, displaced about 20 nm to the shorter wavelength of each labeled peak (blue-shifted), is absorption to a specific vibrational level within each electronic state. In this case the assignment is quite straightforward based largely on the *emission spectrum*.

2. *Emission Spectra* The emission spectrum of PSA, excited by 347-nm light (i.e., the peak of the S_1 transition), is shown in blue in Figure 1.12. We should notice that the emission spectrum is shifted to a longer wavelength than the absorption spectrum. This is always true and Figure 1.9 shows why. Vibrational relaxation always removes some of the energy of the photon into the environment as heat. The energy of the emitting photon is therefore always lower than the photon that was absorbed (or at best the same energy). Lower energy corresponds to longer wavelength (Eq. 1.4). This difference between the absorption peak and the fluorescence peak is known as the *Stokes shift* (named after Sir George Stokes, who in 1852 described this phenomenon and also coined the term *fluorescence*). Different dyes have a different Stokes shift; this is related simply to the change in molecule geometry upon electronic excitation. As described above, a large change in geometry leads to a large vibrational excitation, which in turn leads to a large amount of VR both in S_1 and S_0 and ultimately to a large Stokes shift. Large Stokes shifts are very useful in microscopy and spectroscopy because it is easy to filter out the exciting light in favor of the fluorescence. However, large Stokes shifts are also associated with more energy dissipated as heat and therefore heating of the sample and faster degradation of the fluorophore.

The second thing to notice is that the emission spectrum has some structure to it. This structure must be a vibrational structure as there are no electronic states between S_1 and S_0, by definition (excluding triplet states, which, as discussed above, are very weak absorbers and emitters of light). In Figure 1.9, these fluorescence transitions would be indicated by arrows terminating in different vibrational states.

Finally, one should notice that the emission spectrum looks like a mirror image of the absorption spectrum, at least the part of the spectrum attributed to S_1. Again, Figure 1.9 shows the cause of this. The lowest energy (longest wavelength) transition would excite the $v = 0$ (lowest) level of the S_1 state. As the sample is scanned at increasing energies (shorter wavelength), the light becomes resonant with higher and higher lying vibrational states in S_1. The states that show up most clearly are those associated with any change in geometry of the molecule after electronic excitation. Vibrational relaxation quickly removes this excess vibrational energy. In emission, the highest energy transition is now the transition back down to the $v = 0$ level in S_0. Emission to higher and higher vibrational states now corresponds to lower energy photons or longer wavelengths. Therefore the absorption spectrum marches out to the blue with increasing vibrational energy, while the emission spectrum marches out to the red for the same reason.

3. *Excitation Spectra* The *excitation spectrum* is notionally much the same as the absorption spectrum. While the absorption spectrum measures the amount of light absorbed, the excitation spectrum measures the amount of fluorescence generated following absorption. The excitation spectrum is therefore an indirect measurement of the absorption process. The red-colored excitation spectrum of PSA in Figure 1.12 matches the absorption spectrum from 375 nm down to about 250 nm. Below 250 nm the two spectra deviate. The molecule is clearly absorbing strongly, but this is not showing up in the excitation spectrum. The reason is simple—at high energy (short wavelength) the molecule is not fluorescing any more. We can speculate about the reason; perhaps the molecule is undergoing a photochemical reaction at these energies and the photon is breaking a chemical bond rather than releasing the energy as fluorescence. In technical terms, the absorption and excitation spectra are identical as long as the fluorescence quantum yield remains the same (see Eq. 1.5). If the quantum yield drops off, so does the excitation spectrum compared to the absorption spectrum.

Figure 1.13 shows the absorption and three emission spectra of another fluorescent dye. Again, three different electronic states are evident. The three fluorescence spectra, which are color coded, were generated following excitation of the dye at the three color-coded wavelengths indicated by arrows, that is, excitation into the S_1, S_2, and

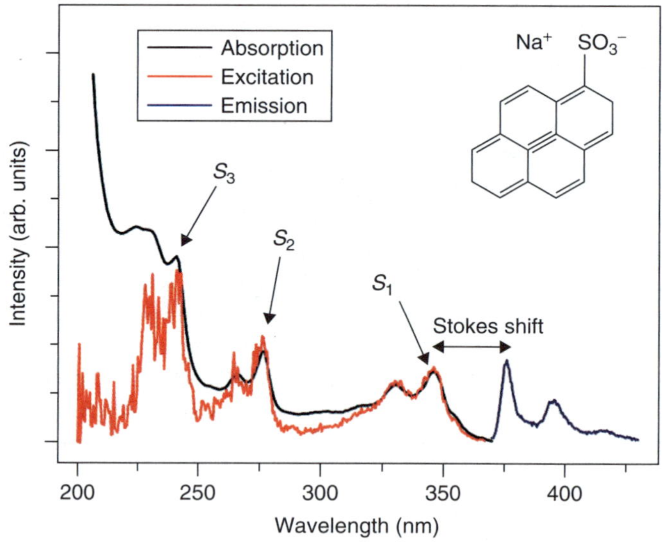

Figure 1.12 Absorption, excitation, and emission spectra for pyrenesulfonic acid (structure shown as inset).

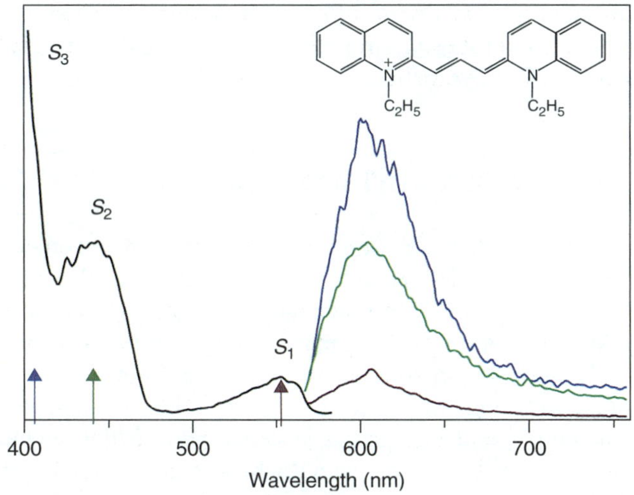

Figure 1.13 Absorption and fluorescence spectra of 1,1′-diethyl-2,2′-carbocyanine ion (structure shown as inset). Each colored fluorescence spectrum was generated following excitation at the three positions marked by arrow of the same color.

S_3 states. It is very clear that the emission spectrum is essentially the same in each case, with only the intensity changing. The difference in intensity is simply related to the difference in absorption coefficient at each wavelength. At first thought, it might seem strange that the emission spectrum does not depend on the excitation wavelength. On second thought, Figure 1.10 provides the explanation. Vavilov's law or Kasha's law says that whatever excited energy level is reached through absorption of light, energy loss via VR and IC means that the fluorescence emission always occurs from the lowest vibrational level of the first excited state (S_1). Remember here that VR and IC occur on a timescale of 10^{-12} s, at least three orders of magnitude faster than the fluorescence emission which typically occurs on a timescale of 10^{-9} s.

1.5.2 Basic Properties of Fluorophores

Fluorescence emission generally occurs from organic molecules with conjugated double-bond systems, such as aromatic molecules, which are called *fluorochromes* or *fluorophores*. The fluorophores in Figures 1.12 and 1.13 are good examples of this. In the study of biological systems, fluorophores may be naturally occurring molecules such as the amino acid tryptophan (and to a lesser extent tyrosine and phenylalanine), porphyrins, quinine, adenosine triphosphate (ATP), nicotinamide adenine dinucleotide (NADH), and other cofactors. In addition, a host of synthetic chemical fluorophores are available for specific labeling of biological systems (e.g., fluorescein, rhodamine, ethidium bromide) as well as fluorescent proteins which can be "genetically" attached to proteins of interest. Such fluorophores will be discussed in later chapters of this book, so only brief mention is made in this introductory chapter. Important considerations in selection of a fluorophore include its absorption coefficient and quantum yield (typically both as high as possible), Stokes shift (typically as large as possible), emission spectrum (and its differentiation from background autofluorescence), solubility, reactivity, and method of labeling. The basis of a commercial catalogue, *Molecular Probes Handbook of Fluorescent Probes and Research Products* (http://probes.invitrogen.com/), provides a very useful guide to the types and characteristics of synthetic fluorophores.

1.6 ENVIRONMENTAL SENSITIVITY OF FLUOROPHORES

It has long been known that the excitation or emission spectra and other parameters such as the lifetime of some fluorophores are sensitive to their local environment. Factors such as polarity and interaction with other molecules may affect the spectra. Various fluorophores are known to have such dramatic changes in fluorescence quantum yield that they effectively fluoresce in some environments but not in others. This has been utilized to advantage in a range of practical techniques. For example, ethidium bromide has a very low quantum yield in aqueous systems, with a high quantum yield when intercalated between the nucleotide bases in double-stranded nucleic acids. Thus, when incorporating ethidium bromide into agarose gels used for electrophoretic separation of DNA, upon illumination with UV light bands of DNA can be identified by their bright fluorescence against a low-fluorescence background. This classical approach in molecular biology is still in use, although newer fluorochromes with less toxicity are becoming more routinely employed. A second example is 1-anilinonaphthalene-8-sulfonic acid (1,8-ANS), which when dissolved in water emits only a very weak, yellow fluorescence with a quantum yield of 0.004. However, upon addition of a solution of protein, an immediate, dramatic increase in fluorescence is noted (with quantum yield of 0.75) as well as a "blue shift" in emission maximum (color change from yellow to blue-green). In similarity to ethidium bromide, the increase of emission reflects movement of ANS from water to a hydrophobic environment provided by the protein. In this case water molecules effectively lower the energy of the ANS excited state (hence the lower energy, yellow emission) and also quench the fluorescence. These features have been applied in numerous studies of protein-folding mechanisms. A further example of useful changes in fluorescence emission is provided by hydrophobic fluorophores that preferentially partition into membranes, for example, 1,6-diphenylhexatriene (DPH) and 6-dodecanoyl-2-dimethylamino naphthalene (laurdan). Since these probes effectively fluoresce in membranes but not in aqueous systems, membranes of whole cells can be analyzed by spectroscopy or microscopy without the complication of background probe fluorescence from aqueous compartments.

In addition to dramatic changes in emission quantum yield, more subtle effects of the environment on fluorophores may be utilized in experimental systems. For example, considering the amino acid tryptophan, upon excitation at an optimal wavelength of around 280 nm, while generally considered to emit at around 340 nm, tryptophan emission is sensitive to the polarity of its environment. This has been used to explore the microenvironment of tryptophan residues in proteins, thereby giving information on protein-folding states and interactions; for example, when buried in the hydrophobic core of a protein, tryptophan emits with maximum around 335 nm, but when the protein is unfolded, the emission "red shifts" to around 365 nm.

In addition to naturally occurring compounds, fluorophores have been produced to have large dipole moments and high sensitivity to their environment. A prime example is the membrane probe laurdan, which was designed and synthesized by Gregorio Weber in the 1970s. The large dipole moment leads to a large Stokes shift as well as high sensitivity to polarity. In membranes, laurdan shows a 50-nm red shift in emission spectrum over the gel to liquid crystalline phase transition. The spectroscopic property generalized polarization (GP), derived from fluorescence intensities at the red and blue edges of the laurdan emission spectrum, which represent gel (440 nm) and liquid crystalline (490 nm) phases, can be used as a membrane fluidity index. The GP is calculated in an analogous way to the polarization parameter (see Section 1.8) using the intensity at the critical wavelengths instead of polarization orientation. Further examples of environmentally sensitive probes which are analyzed by ratiometric techniques include probes to detect specific ions or indicate pH.

1.6.1 Quenching of Fluorescence

In addition to emission of light and nonradiative processes described above, interaction with a *quencher* is a further way in which a molecule can lose its excited-state energy. A quencher is a molecule which can deactivate the excited state either through a collisional process or by formation of a nonfluorescent complex. Quenchers that form complexes generally have very specific interactions with particular types of fluorophores. Many fluorophores are based on aromatic ring structures which potentially interact with other aromatic nonfluorescent molecules via weak van der Waals forces, forming nonfluorescent complexes. Quenching of ethidium bromide by caffeine is an example of this type of complexing interaction. Collisional quenchers, on the other hand, tend to be small molecules or ions. Common examples include oxygen (O_2), iodide (I^-), and heavy metals such as mercury (Hg^{2+}). Collisional quenching interactions can be described using the *Stern–Volmer equation*

$$\frac{F_0}{F} = 1 + k_+^*[Q]\tau_0 \tag{1.8}$$

where F_0 is the initial fluorescence intensity before addition of quencher, F is the fluorescence in the presence of quencher, k_+^* is the "bimolecular quenching rate constant," Q is the quencher concentration, and τ_0 is the fluorescence lifetime in the absence of quencher. The plus sign in the bimolecular quenching constant indicates that the process is an interaction between two molecules. Quenching studies can provide direct information on the diffusion of small molecules in solution and in cellular compartments, providing insights into solvent accessibilities and viscosities. However, in some practical situations quenching can be a problem, whereby the intensity of measured fluorescence is reduced by an undesirable component (such as heavy metal contamination) in the system being analyzed. For example, it is not feasible to measure *phosphorescence* emission in the presence of oxygen, as the latter effectively quenches the emission to a high degree. Therefore, when investigating phosphorescence emission in solutions, it is common practice to deoxygenate the solutions, for example, by utilizing the glucose oxidase reaction.

1.6.2 Photobleaching

As noted above, excited electronic states may have increased chemical reactivity, particularly if triplet states are formed. In their excited state, molecules may react with other molecules such as oxygen or heavy metals, leading to formation of transient or stable complexes that further lead to irreversible deactivation of the excited state without the emission of light. Note that, as outlined above, a consequence of loss of excited-state energy by VR leads to heating, which further increases the rate of potentially damaging photochemical reactions. Apart from the specialized case of some green fluorescent proteins, photobleaching is an irreversible process, leading to lowered fluorescence emission intensity as a function of time of illumination of the fluorophore. Practical solutions to this problem have included the use of antifade reagents (containing antioxidants and commonly used for fixed-specimen fluorescence microscopy but incompatible with live cell investigations), development of fluorophores less susceptible to photobleaching, and minimization of illumination intensity or duration. The latter has been achieved in spectroscopy by limiting the illumination wavelength bandwidth and intensity and minimizing the period that illumination shutters are open as well as stirring samples to prevent fluorophores from remaining in the illumination beam for long periods. Approaches in microscopy have included development of confocal laser-scanning microscopy systems which limit the illumination to a cone that is scanned across the specimen (as opposed to whole-specimen illumination by transmission or epifluorescence microscopy) as well as attenuation of the intensity of the illuminating beam. The situation may be improved further by multiphoton laser-scanning microscopy (see Section 1.2.3), which further limits photobleaching by minimizing the focal volume of excitation to a precise point as well as illuminating with wavelengths of half the incident energy.

In some cases, photobleaching has been used to advantage in experimental investigations and in fact is used in the FRAP or *fluorescence photobleaching recovery (FPR)* technique, as will be described in a later chapter. Laser-based microscopy systems allow high-intensity pulses of illumination to be focused on specific areas of a specimen, causing localized photobleaching. Subsequent observation of the bleached regions over time can elucidate whether fluorescently labeled molecules are able to move into the bleached area, the magnitude of this movement, and the diffusion coefficients of the labeled molecules.

1.6.3 Fluorescence Resonance Energy Transfer

Another process which can lead to nonradiative dissipation of the excited-state energy is transfer of this energy to another "acceptor" molecule in a process known as fluorescence (or *Förster*) resonance energy transfer. In some cases the acceptor molecule further dissipates this energy by VR mechanisms, although in most cases the transferred energy becomes the excitation of the acceptor molecule which subsequently emits fluorescence. Note this emission would necessarily be of lower energy, that is, of longer wavelength, than would be the emission of the initially excited molecule. The processes and application of FRET will be discussed further in a later chapter.

1.6.4 Solvent Relaxation

As discussed in Section 1.3.1, after excitation, a certain amount of the energy is lost by VR. In some cases, additional energy is lost during the excited-state lifetime by a process known as *solvent relaxation*, whereby solvent dipoles reorientate around the excited-state dipole. This reorientation favors new dipole–dipole interactions which lower the overall energy of the system. As the resultant "stabilized" S_1 level is of

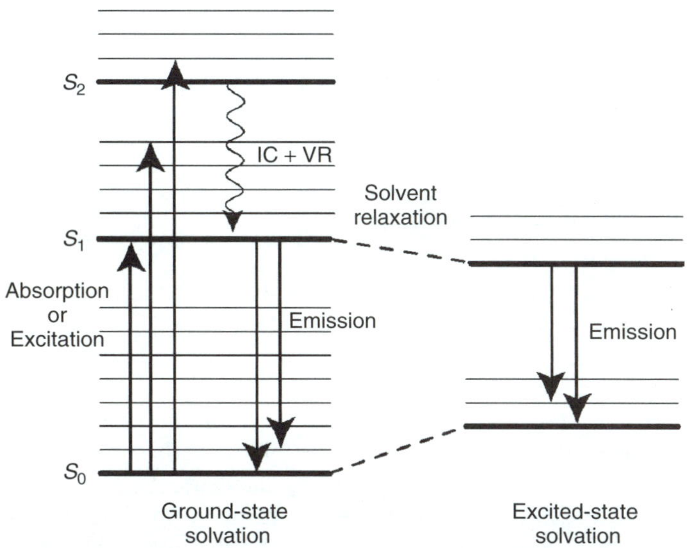

Figure 1.14 Perrin–Jablonski diagram representing absorption and emission of EM radiation and effect of solvent relaxation.

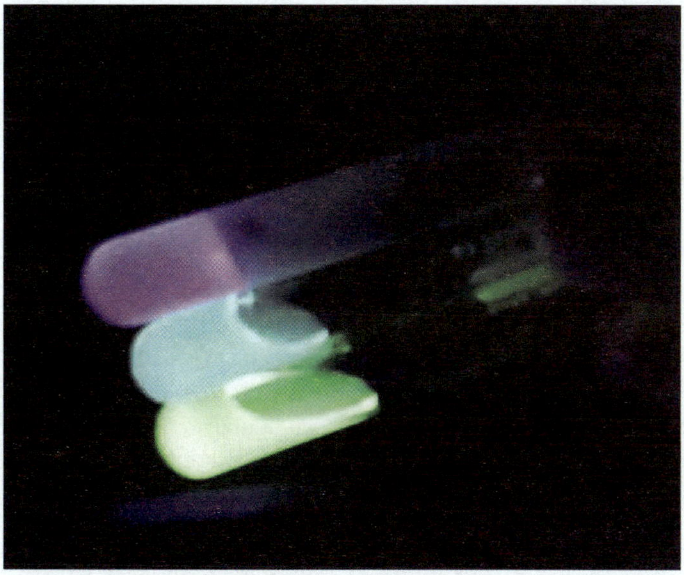

Figure 1.15 Test tubes containing laurdan in glycerol cooled to −70°C with dry ice/propanol (top) at room temperature (25°C) and heated to 80°C with hot water (bottom) under excitation at 366 nm by UV hand lamp.

lower energy, the emitted fluorescence will also be of lower energy, that is, longer wavelength. This phenomenon is represented in terms of a Perrin–Jablonski diagram in Figure 1.14.

Figure 1.15 shows a striking visual demonstration of the solvent relaxation phenomenon. Fluorescence emission of the fluorophore laurdan dissolved in glycerol is seen to red shift as solvent relaxation increases. The tubes are inclined to show the viscosity and flow properties of glycerol solutions at -70°C (solid, bluish fluorescence), 25°C (high viscosity, greenish fluorescence), and 80°C (low viscosity, high solvent relaxation, yellowish-green fluorescence).

1.7 POLARIZATION OF FLUORESCENCE

As noted above, rotational mobility in biological systems is commonly assessed by measurement of fluorescence emission polarization using instrumentation equipped with linearly polarizing filters or prisms. In this section we will briefly describe concepts underpinning the measurement of fluorescence polarization.

Put in the most simplistic terms, if a molecule is illuminated with polarized light and is able to rotate during the excited-state lifetime, then the fluorescence emission will become depolarized in relation to the incident illumination. The degree of depolarization will relate to the mobility of the emitting species; in other words, fluorescence polarization decreases as rotational mobility increases (in relation to the excited-state lifetime). Thus, the measured polarization of a molecule increases with increasing molecular size, increasing viscosity of the medium, and decreasing temperature, reflecting decreased rotational mobility. To this simplistic picture we need to add that there will be some depolarization of emission due to differences in angle between excitation and emission dipoles, and this can be accounted for in determining theoretical maximum polarization values.

As noted above, for unpolarized light the electric vector could be found at any angle but could be considered as a wave which has an average of half its vibrations in a horizontal plane and half of its vibrations in a vertical plane. This helps provide a rationale for simple measurement of the degree of polarization. Rather than sample all possible angles of polarization, a suitable estimate could be taken by considering the intensity of emission at two orientations perpendicular to each other, commonly denoted as vertical (or 0°) and horizontal (or 90°).

The calculated parameters denoted as *polarization* (P) and *anisotropy* (r) are given by the equations below, where I_{VV} is the fluorescence emission intensity measured in the plane parallel to the plane of vertically polarized excitation and I_{VH} is fluorescence emission intensity measured in the plane perpendicular to the plane of vertically polarized excitation (the first subscript refers to the orientation of the excitation polarizer while the second subscript refers to the emission polarizer orientation):

$$P = \frac{I_{VV} - I_{VH}}{I_{VV} + I_{VH}} \quad \text{(polarization)} \tag{1.9}$$

$$r = \frac{I_{VV} - I_{VH}}{I_{VV} + 2I_{VH}} \quad \text{(anisotropy)} \tag{1.10}$$

It should be noted that these equations need to be corrected by an instrument grating correction factor to account for differences in the efficiency of monochromators and detectors for the different polarization orientations. This is achieved by multiplying the I_{VH} values by the grating correction factor G, which is calculated from measurements taken with the excitation polarizer in the horizontal position (as opposed to the vertical orientation for the polarization measurements):

$$G = \frac{I_{HV}}{I_{HH}} \tag{1.11}$$

Anisotropy and polarization are both expressions of the same phenomenon and can be easily interconverted as follows:

$$r = \frac{2P}{3 - P} \tag{1.12}$$

However, the anisotropy expression is generally preferred as anisotropies of individual components are directly additive, making mathematical analyses of multicomponent systems much more straightforward. The anisotropy can be related to the rotational mobility of the fluorophore by the *Perrin equation*:

$$\frac{r_0}{r} = 1 + \frac{RT\tau}{\eta V} \tag{1.13}$$

where r_0 is the limiting anisotropy (in the absence of any fluorophore rotation), r is the measured anisotropy, η is the viscosity of the environment, V is the volume of the rotating molecule, R is the universal gas constant, T is the temperature (in degrees Kelvin), and τ is the excited-state lifetime. The Perrin equation is often simplified to express the time-dependent decay of anisotropy in terms of the rotational correlation time (θ, often denoted τ_c) of a fluorophore (assuming a spherical molecule rotating isotropically):

$$\frac{r_0}{r} = 1 + \frac{\tau}{\theta} \tag{1.14}$$

where $\theta = (\eta V)/(RT)$. If the rotational correlation time θ is much longer than the lifetime τ, then the measured anisotropy will approximate r_0, whereas if θ is much shorter than the lifetime τ, the measured anisotropy will approximate zero. The use of rotational correlation time might be confused with considerations from nuclear magnetic resonance, so an earlier term, the *Debye rotational relaxation time* ($\phi = 3\theta$), may be a more suitable term in these expressions.

Another way of expressing the anisotropy–mobility relationship is as follows:

$$\frac{r_0}{r} = 1 + 6D\tau \tag{1.15}$$

where D is the rotational diffusion coefficient. However, although rotational relaxation times or microviscosities can be calculated, in many studies it is considered that comparison of anisotropy data would be sufficient to estimate and compare relative mobility. It should be noted here that these analyses are simplified, and a full description will take into account the photoselection of fluorophores by polarized illumination, angles between absorption and emission dipoles, and further refinement of calculations to estimate rotational parameters of biological molecules which are nonspherical. An extension of the technique is to incorporate pulsed or modulated excitation sources in the experimental arrangement to determine the temporal decay of the fluorescence anisotropy.

1.8 CONCLUSION

This chapter has provided a basic introduction to fluorescence and has raised in a simplistic manner various issues that will be expanded in the following chapters. More detailed discussion of these issues may be found in the References.

REFERENCES

1. D. M. Jameson, J. C. Croney, and P. D. J. Moens, "Fluorescence: Basic concepts, practical aspects, and some anecdotes," *Methods Enzymol.* **360**, 1–43 (2003).
2. I. Parker, "Photonics for biologists," *Methods Enzymol.* **360**, 345–382 (2003).
3. J. C. Croney, D. M. Jameson, and R. P. Learmonth, "Fluorescence spectroscopy in biochemistry: Teaching basic principles with visual demonstrations," *Biochem. Mol. Biol. Ed.* **29**, 60–65 (2001).
4. R. P. Learmonth, "LASER-based fluorescence microscopy," *Microbiol. Austral.* **23**(1), 16–17 (2002).
5. J. R. Lakowicz (Ed.), *Principles of Fluorescence Spectroscopy*, 3rd ed., Springer, Singapore, 2006.
6. K. E. Van Holde, W. C. Johnson, and H. P. Shing, *Principles of Physical Biochemistry*, 2nd ed., Pearson Prentice-Hall, Upper Saddle River, NJ, 2006.
7. M. G. Gore (Ed.), *Spectrophotometry and Spectrofluorimetry: A Practical Approach*, Oxford University Press, Oxford, 2000.
8. D. E. Wolf, "Fundamentals of fluorescence and fluorescence microscopy," *Methods Cell Biol.* **72**, 157–184 (2003).
9. D. M. Jameson and S. E. Seifried, "Quantification of protein-protein interactions using fluorescence polarization," *Methods* **19**, 222–233 (1999).
10. W. H. Sawyer, "Fluorescence spectroscopy in the study of membrane fluidity: Model membrane systems," in *Advances in Membrane Fluidity*, R. C. Aloia, C. C. Curtain, and L. M. Gordon (Eds.), Alan R. Liss, New York, 1998, pp. 161–191.

CHAPTER 2

Labeling of Cells with Fluorescent Dyes

IAN S. HARPER

Monash Micro Imaging, School of Biomedical Sciences, Monash University, Clayton, Victoria 3800, Australia

2.1 INTRODUCTION

Fluorescence microscopy occupies a unique position in the life sciences as the specificity and sensitivity of fluorescence probes makes it possible to detect and analyze biochemical and biophysical properties as well as morphology of cells and tissues. The continuing and vigorous development of fluorescent probes (fluorophores) in conjunction with the analytical fluorescence-based imaging modalities such as confocal, deconvolution, multiphoton, 4Pi, stimulation-emission depletion fluorescence microscopy (STED), total internal reflection fluorescence microscopy (TIRF), and single plane illumination microscopy (SPIM), and spectral and structured light microscopy, among others, has been a major contributor to our understanding of dynamic processes and subcellular architecture of cells and tissue. A detailed discussion of all currently available fluorophores and their characteristics is not within the scope of this chapter, and for this the reader is referred to reviews [38, 73] and the very comprehensive handbook of fluorescent probes [33]. Additional help with selection of specific probes is available via applets that show spectra of filter sets and dye combinations available on some manufacturers' websites: for example, Invitrogen (Molecular Probes, http://probes.invitrogen.com/resources/spectraviewer/), BD (http://www.bdbiosciences.com/spectra/), Chroma (https://www.omegafilters.com/curvo2/index.php), Zeiss, Leica, Nikon, and Olympus. Fluorescent probes and reagents are available from Amersham Pharmacia Biotech, Calbiochem, Fluka, Jackson ImmunoResearch Laboratories, Invitrogen, Atto-Tec, Polysciences, Serotec, Sigma-Aldrich, and others. Fluorescent proteins and their vectors are available from Clontech Laboratories, Quantum Biotechnologies, Life Technologies, and others.

This chapter will therefore emphasize the general principles of fluorophore selection and loading for investigation of various biological signals. Furthermore, understanding that the list of fluorescence probes (and applications) grows on a daily basis, it is therefore not possible to provide an exhaustive and up-to-date list of fluorophores; however, tables are provided to illustrate some of the most commonly used probes with their spectral characteristics to assist choosing dyes for multiple-label experiments

Fluorescence Applications in Biotechnology and Life Sciences, Edited by Ewa M. Goldys

TABLE 2.1 Fluorescent Probes for Conjugation to Antibodies or Other Reagents

Emission Range	Fluorophore	Ex	Em
Blue	AMCA (aminomethylcourmarin)	350	450
	Cascade blue	400	420
	Alexa Fluor 350	346	442
Green	Alexa Fluor 488	491	515
	Atto 488	501	523
	Cy2 (cyanine)	489	505
	FITC	494	520
	FluoroGreen	490	520
	BODIPY FL	505	513
	Oregon green 488	496	524
	Oregon green 514	511	530
Yellow	Eosin	524	544
	Alexa Fluor 532	531	554
Orange	BODIPY TMR	543	569
	Alexa Fluor 546	553	569
	TRITC	554	576
	TMR (tetramethylrhodamine)	555	580
Orange–red	Cy3 (indocarbocyanine)	552	568
	R-phycoerythrin	565	578
	Atto 656	563	592
	Lissamine rhodamine	570	590
	Alexa Fluor 568	573	596
	Cy3.5	578	593
	Alexa 594	585	610
	BODIPY TR	592	618
	Texas red	595	615
Red–far red	Allophycocyanin	650	671
	Cy5 (indodicarbocyanine)	650	670
	Alexa Fluor 647	650	668
	Atto 655	663	684
	Cy5.5	678	698
	Alexa Fluor 700	702	723
	Cy7	747	768

Note: Fluorophores presented in Tables 2.1–2.4 should be considered as a guide only and are not comprehensive. For example Alexa and Atto dyes are available across the range of 350–700-nm emission. Peak excitation (Ex) and emission (Em) wavelengths may vary slightly since the data are derived from multiple sources and vary according to different procedures and apparatus.

(Tables 2.1–2.4). A listing of fluorescent labels currently available for protein and antibody conjugation is also included (see Table 2.1) for completeness and since it is common for investigators to chemically fix and stain tissue at the end of experiments for subsequent immunofluorescence.

A frequently exploited feature of fluorescence imaging is the ability to monitor a number of specific probes simultaneously, thus allowing colocalization or multiparameter imaging of structures within cells or tissues. Naturally, for general wide-field

TABLE 2.2 Fluorophores Used for Microscopy of Live Cells/Tissue: Permeant Probes for Specific Organelles

Parameter	Fluorophore	Ex	Em
Nucleus	DAPI	358	461
	Hoechst 33258	350	461
	Acridine orange	500	526
	Hexidium iodide	518	600
	Syto dyes	Various	
	7-Aminoactinomycin D	546	647
	DRAQ5™	647	670
Nuclear envelope	FM4-64	600–620	700
Mitochondrial localization	MitoFluor green	489	517
	MitoTracker green FM	490	516
	MitoTracker orange CMTMRos	551	576
	MitoTracker red CMXRos	578	599
	MitoTracker red CM-H_2XRos	578	599
	Rhodamine 123	507	529
	Rhodamine 6G	528	551
	$DiOC_6(3)$	484	519
	Rhodamine B hexyl ester	556	578
Mitochondrial membrane potential	TMRE	549	574
	TMRM	548	573
	JC-1	510	527/590
Golgi	NBD C6-ceramide	466	536
	BODIPY FL C5-ceramide	505	512
	BODIPY FL sphingomyelin	505	511
	BODIPY FL brefeldin A	505	511
	BODIPY FL cerebroside	505	511
Endoplasmic reticulum (ER)	ER Tracker blue-white DPX	374	575
	$DiOC_6(3)$	484	519
	Rhodamine B hexyl ester	556	578
Lysosomes	Fluorescent dextrans	Various	
	LysoTracker green	504	511
	LysoTracker yellow	534	551
	LysoTracker red	577	590
	LysoSensor dyes	Various	
Vacuoles	FM1-43	510	626
	MDY-64 (yeast)	456	505
	Carboxy DCFDA	490	520
Plasma (and other[a] membranes)	FM1-43	510	626
	FM4-64	515	640-700
	RH414	532	716
	Laurdan	364–390	440/500

Note: Fluorophores with two wavelengths for excitation (Ex) or emission (Em) are dual excitation or dual emission ratiometric indicators, and wavelengths cited are approximate, since different manufactures and authors provide different data.

[a]Plasma membrane specificity depends on labeling and incubation conditions.

TABLE 2.3 Fluorophores Used for Microscopy of Live Cells/Tissue: Cellular Activities

Parameter	Fluorophore	Ex	Em
Cell morphology: shape/volume	Calcein AM	495	520
	$DiOC_6(3)$	484	501
Cell viability			
Live	Most AM forms		
	FDA, CFDA, DCFDA	490	520
	Calcein AM	495	520
Dead (nuclear)	Sytox green	504	523
	TO-PRO-1, TOTO-1	513	530
	Ethidium homodimer-1	528	617
	Propidium iodide	530	615
	TO-PRO-3	631	661
Ion physiology			
Ca^{2+}	Indo-1	350	405/485
	Fura-2	335/362	505
	Fluo-3	506	526
	Fluo-4	494	516
	Fura red	458, 488	597
	Calcium green	506	526
	Calcium orange	550	580
	Calcium crimson	590	620
	Oregon green 488 BAPTA	488	520
	Rhod-2	553	576
	X-Rhod-1	580	602
pH	BCECF	439, 490	530
	Carboxy SNARF-1	488-568	580/640
	Carboxy SNAFL-2	514	546/630
Na^+	SBFI	340	410/590
	Sodium green	488	535
K^+	PBFI	340/380	505
Cl^-	SPQ	343	443
	Bis-DMXPQ	365	450/565
Mg^{2+}	Mag-Indo-1	343	405/485
cAMP	Cyclic AMP Fluorosensor®	488	520/580
Reactive oxygen species (probes nonfluorescent until oxidized)	Dihydrorhodamine 123	507	529
	Dihydrorhodamine 6G	528	551
	Dihydroethidium (oxidized probe binds to DNA)	488	610
	Tetramethylrosamine	578	599
	H_2DCFDA or DCFH (2′7′-dichlorofluorescin)	488	530
	Reduced MitoTracker probes	(see Table 2.2)	

Note: Fluorophores with two wavelengths for excitation (Ex) or emission (Em) are dual excitation or dual emission ratiometric indicators, and wavelengths cited are approximate, since different manufactures and authors provide different data.

TABLE 2.4 Fluorophores Used for Tracking Live Cells or Cellular Processes

Parameter	Fluorophore	Ex	Em
Tracking cells	CellTracker blue (CMHC)	372	470
	Lucifer yellow (and derivatives)	428	533
	CellTracker green (CMFDA)	492	516
	CFDA succinimidyl-ester (CFSE)	494	525
	CellTracker yellow-green (CMEDA)	524	544
	CellTracker orange (CMTMR)	541	565
	CellTracker CM-DiI	553	570
	MitoTracker probes		
	LavaCell™ (epicocconone)[a]	405, 488-520	610
Lipophilic tracers	CellTracker CM-DiI	553	570
	DiI[b]	549	565
	DiO [b]	484	501
	DiD [b]	644	655
	PKH26	551	567
	PKH2	490	504
Endocytosis	Fluorescent bacteria, spores, dextrans, or beads		
	FM1-43	510	626
	FM4-64	515	640
	PKH26	551	567
	PKH2	490	504
Receptor and peptide distribution and trafficking	Labelled Fluo-peptides™		
	BODIPY 576/589 neurotensin	576	589
	Fluo-NPY, -GHRH, -glucagon, etc.	494	520
Fluorescent proteins[c]	T-sapphire	399	511
	Cerulean	433	475
	eGFP	488	507
	Emerald	487	509
	EYFP	514	527
	mCitrine	516	529
	YPet	517	530
	mOrange	548	562
	mCherry	587	610
	mRFP1	584	607
	DsRed	556	586
	mPlum	590	649

[a]LavaCell shows two excitation peaks.

[b]New Vybrant™ formulations of these dyes (filtered solutions) have dramatically improved consistency, and efficiency of staining.

[c]This is a brief list of the more favored proteins.

fluorescence this requires that the probes are able to be distinctly resolved based on excitation and emission spectra. While the more modern spectral imaging confocal microscopes are able to unmix or deconvolve overlapping spectra, this is still a developing field and may be a hazardous choice for live imaging approaches where the spectra of some fluorophores may change in response to their environment or photoinduced changes due to laser/lamp excitation. On the other hand, spectral imaging is becoming increasingly important to investigate such changes (see later for membrane probes such laurdan, which undergo spectral shifts due to changes in phospholipid packing). Moreover, the ability to introduce multiple probes into live specimens presents an opportunity to investigate biological function and activity in a unique and dynamic way. The fluorophores and methods described in this chapter are relevant to both conventional (wide-field) fluorescence microscopy and confocal fluorescence microscopy, and much of this information (with the exception of the actual fluorophore excitation spectra) is also applicable to multiphoton microscopy.

2.2 FLUOROPHORE SELECTION

As there is now a vast array of fluorescence probes for most imaging applications, attested to by the very weighty handbook of fluorescence probes [33], the problem is often not so much about actually locating a probe as determining which is the most appropriate probe to use and how to optimize it for a given application. Choice of the probe may be determined in many cases both by the available instrumentation (i.e., the excitation source and detection filters available) and by the specific application. For example, while it is possible to analyze cell shape and volume using the probe calcein (which generally "fills the cell"), lipid-soluble dyes such as $DiOC_6$ which label cell membranes would also work given the appropriate labeling conditions and subsequent imaging. However, if one wished to measure shape/volume changes over time in living cells, this may not be a good choice, due to dye diffusion and phototoxicity. Hence, overall, the basic requirements of the ideal probe are that it should (a) specifically associate with the target molecule, structure, or cell; (b) be nontoxic; (c) be very bright (i.e., have a high quantum efficiency); (d) not photobleach, and (e) not dissociate or leach out of the cell. Cost of the fluorophore may also be a consideration, particularly when used in large amounts as for bulk samples or when a long workup is required to optimize a method.

Possibly the most important parameter for selection of label after target specificity is that of compatibility with the excitation source and emission filters available on the microscope. Mercury lamps have peak emissions at 366, 405, 436, 546, and 578 nm and a strong background continuum, whereas xenon lamps have a strong flat spectrum from about 350 to 700 nm with several more intense peaks in the 700–1000-nm range. In contrast, lasers emit monochromatic light of very high intensity, and various lasers are chosen for their specific emission characteristics. The most common lasers for confocal microscopy are generally Ar ion (457, 488, and 514 nm), green HeNe (543 nm), yellow HeNe (594 nm), and red HeNe (633 nm). Mixed-gas ArKr lasers (457, 488, 568, 647 nm) are becoming far less common now as diode and solid-state lasers improve and become more common. These compact lasers provide excitation lines at 405, 408, 440, 473, 488, 532, 561, and 635 nm and combinations of these lasers are now starting to replace other combinations such as Ar ion (488 nm) plus green and red HeNe lasers that have until now been the most common sources in confocal microscopes.

It is important to choose fluorophores that will be maximally excited by the lamp or laser line, thereby requiring less detector gain to achieve a reasonable image and hence less background noise. New hard-coated (ion-beam-sputtered) filters from companies such as Semrock and Chroma are displacing the previous generation of (soft-coated) narrowband interference filters and have significantly improved transmission or reflection because of very steep edges that define their spectral characteristics. This improved transmission results in more efficient excitation and detection and hence also less bleedthrough between channels in multiplexed experiments. Although it is possible to reassign or unmix bleedthrough and spectrally overlapping fluorophores, this is not advocated for those who are unaware of the potential pitfalls of such an approach. It is generally far more sensible to select fluorophores and systems for optimal excitation, sensitivity, and spectral separation. The past few years have seen the introduction of fluorophores aimed specifically at the laser-based flow cytometry and confocal microscopy markets where multiple labeling of specimens is common. Triple fluorophore labeling with excitation in the blue, green/yellow, and red regions can be accomplished with little overlap between regions. For example, probes such as Oregon green 488, Alexa 568, and Cy5 (Table 2.1) can now be employed with good spectral separation and should be used in preference, particularly when multiple labels over the visible light spectrum are required. Figure 2.1 illustrates osteosarcoma cells imaged with 405-, 488-, and 543-nm lasers after labeling the cytoskeleton (Alexa Fluor 488—phalloidin), Golgi (Alexa Fluor 568—secondary antibody against a golgi protein), and nuclei (DAPI). The fluorescence emission spectra are clearly separated, which can be checked by single-line excitation. Most of the automated multiuser confocal systems now also provide sequential scanning routines that will scan specific channels individually and then rapidly merge resultant images to provide a double- or triple-channel image.

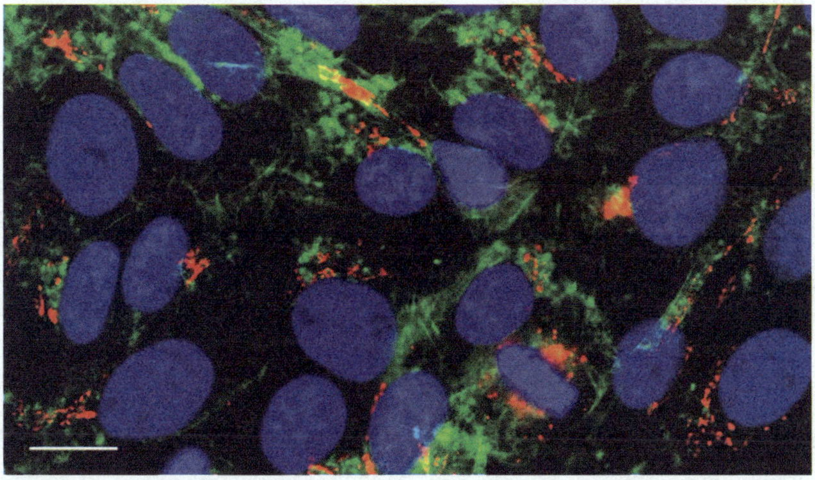

Figure 2.1 Multiple labeling of cultured osteosarcoma cells to illustrate optimal dye selection imaged on FV1000 confocal microscope. Nuclei are labeled with DAPI (blue) and excited by a 405 laser, actin (green) is directly labeled with Alexa Fluor 488–conjugated phalloidin (488 nm excitation), and Golgi (red) is labeled with Alexa Fluor 568–conjugated secondary antibody directed against anti-Golgin97 (543 nm excitation). Scale bar = 10 μm.

While many probes are not entirely selective for a specific organelle, for example, $DiOC_6(3)$ for ER [70] or calcein for mitochondria [45], careful selection and testing of probe concentrations and loading conditions and strategies such as selective quenching after loading can be effectively used to locate the fluorescence to the area of interest. This is discussed briefly in the following section.

Finally, selection of a probe should also take into account the possible need for localization, possibly even by electron microscopy, following chemical fixation. Many probes are now available in a modified form that can be crosslinked by formaldehyde or glutaraldehyde, commonly used in histology and electron microscopy. Modifications include the addition of amino groups (particularly lysine) to dextran, and thiol-reactive chloromethyl groups to a range of probes that are known as Tracker probes (e.g., MitoTracker®, CellTracker™). Probes such as propidium iodide and acridine orange that intercalate with DNA may also be retained after fixation, and some probes may also be retained during freeze substitution [36] so that there are increasingly more approaches for the cell biologist to track structure from live cell imaging through to high-resolution electron microscopy. Apart from direct observation of postfixation fluorescence, fluorescence can be tracked after fixation by photoconversion to a diaminobenzidine (DAB) product that is observable with light microscopy and, after further processing, with electron microscopy [58]. Fluorophores that have been shown to precipitate DAB when irradiated with light at their absorption peak include acridine orange, DAPI, DiI, DiO, and $DiOC_{18}(3)$ and their derivatives, eosin, ethidium bromide, fluorescein isothiocyanate (FITC), lucifer yellow, propidium iodide, and TRITC. Fluorescent proteins such as green and cyan fluorescent protein (GFP, CFP) have also been shown capable of photooxidation [28], and together with the approach of fluorescent protein immunocytochemistry, this gives a variety of tools for correlative microscopy discussed in more detail further in this volume.

2.3 LOADING AND LABELING LIVE CELLS

Methods for loading living cells with fluorophores differ depending on the number of parameters, some of which can be modified and manipulated to enhance the amount and specificity of loading, or to reduce possible toxicity or photoinjury. The exact loading conditions depend on the probe being used and the cellular or molecular target. A recent review [17] discusses probe selection and handling, so the following discussion is restricted to labeling procedures to target specific organelles, cells, or pathways.

In general, lipid-soluble dyes such as the carbocyanines (DiI, DiD, DiO) will associate with cell membranes. They may diffuse through the plasma membrane and stain all interior membranes or they may remain predominantly in the plasma membrane itself. New formulations of these dyes in the so-called Vybrant™ cell-labeling solution provide improved staining based on better dispersion of the dye in a specially filtered dye solution. On the other hand, nonlipophilic and free acid forms of fluorophores like Fura-2, Fluo-3, and BCECF will require special loading procedures such as eletroporation, scrape loading, microinjection, hypotonic shock, or osmotic lysis following pinocytotic loading [33]. One of the most common methods of introducing fluorophores into the cell is through incubation with the acetoxymethyl ester (AM) form of the probe. While this is one of the more variable procedures, it does provide potentially exploitable options for improving selectivity of fluorophore loading.

The main factors that affect fluorophore loading are fluorophore concentration, incubation time, temperature, and agitation. However, when larger amounts of tissue are being labeled, the surface area and mass of material should also be taken into consideration since effective dye concentration will become reduced as dye diffuses into the tissue. Labeling individual cells (either in suspension or attached to a coverslip) probably represents the most favorable situation for AM ester loading, as most of the parameters can be controlled with relative ease and loading strategies systematically tested. As tissue samples increase in size, a more complex situation arises, since both dye loading and microscopic resolution may attenuate with increasing distance from the periphery of the tissue. In this case, if possible, dye loading through perfusion should be attempted, as is done in whole organs such as the heart [19] or liver.

2.3.1 Loading AM Forms

This method is comparatively very simple, relying on the fact that the AM derivatives of fluorophores have ester moieties that mask the carboxy groups of the probes, making the compound permeant. Once inside the cell, endogenous esterases remove the ester groups, thus converting the probe to a nonpermeant salt or acid form that remains trapped within the cytosol. An additional advantage for some probes (such as calcein) is that they are not fluorescent in their AM form and hence do not contribute to an extracellular fluorescent signal. Successful loading of the cell with fluorophore depends on a combination of factors that influence the final destination of the probe. Generally, mammalian cells and tissues can be loaded with solutions of about 1–10 μM for 10–30 mins at temperatures ranging from ambient to 37°C. Under these conditions, it is estimated that intracellular concentrations of hydrolyzed probe may reach 30–50 μM. Changing these parameters tends to influence the final pattern of fluorophore distribution, and successful results depend very much on careful evaluation of the contribution of these parameters for each tissue or cell type.

For fluorophores used to report ion fluxes in the cytosol, it is usual to load for shorter times (i.e., 10–15 mins) at 37°C in order to ensure that most of the probe is hydrolyzed in the cytosol. Longer periods and/or lower temperatures tend to increase the organelle loading. Even under conditions favoring cytosolic loading, a significant proportion of the fluorophore might gain entry to other organelles [7, 47] and be a source of significant error [60], so careful evaluation of fluorophore distribution is required. Several possibilities exist for evaluating the contribution of fluorescence from noncytosolic compartments, including preferential quenching of cytosolic fluorescence using Mn^{2+} or Co^{2+} [29, 45] or differential permeabilization [39]. Microinjection of non-AM forms of the dyes can also be used to compare the effects with AM-loaded cells, or if only a few cells need to be analyzed, this can be the dominant approach to introduce the dye into the cell. Alternatively, in some cases when a dye is used to report on a specific compartment and does not load specifically into that compartment, it may be possible to extract nonspecific fluorescence based on the distribution of a second specific probe. For example, Fluo-3 loaded intracellularly in a nonspecific fashion can still be used to detect calcium fluxes in mitochondrial and cytosolic compartments based on the distribution of TMRM-loaded mitochondria [10, 52].

2.3.2 Leakage and Hydrolysis of AM Esters

Leakage of hydrolyzed AM derivatives is an acknowledged problem, but generally usually encountered only after extended periods (several hours) and is more prevalent in some tissues than in others. Several remedies are used to combat this. First, some probes have been modified by the addition of chloromethyl moieties that covalently bind to intracellular thiols and help retain the probes within the cells. These compounds, known as CellTracker probes, are able to persist for hours and even days within labeled cells. A second possibility to enhance probe retention in cells is to use, in millimolar amounts, an inhibitor of organic anion transport, such as probenicid or sulphinpyrazone [8, 29]. These inhibitors all attenuate rather than completely prevent dye leakage and in our laboratories have also been effectively used to reduce loading variation in chinese hamster ovary (CHO) cells. Anion transport inhibitors are also effective in reducing probe sequestration in cells [22], which may be a major cause of reduced and punctate loading in some cells.

On the other hand, probe leakage from the cytosol may be exploited to advantage. It is possible to utilize a regime of cold loading for Rhod-2 (4°C for 1 h) followed by an extended warm incubation period (several hours at 37°C) during which time the cytoplasmic concentration of the probe decreased substantially, leaving a predominantly mitochondrial distribution. This facilitated analysis of mitochondrial calcium in a probe which is not completely selective for mitochondria. While most probes that are loaded in the form of an AM ester are also available as carboxylic (free) acids, it is also possible to chemically hydrolyze AM esters in the laboratory using KOH. This is useful for checking hydrolysis rates and to produce free acids in small amounts as needed. To do this, a small amount of the ester is dissolved in dimethyl sulfoxide (DMSO) to make a 1 mM stock diluted to 0.5 mM with methanol and then hydrolyzed for several hours (preferably overnight) by addition of a drop of 2 M KOH (for a precise method see http://www.probes.com/media/pis/g002.pdf).

2.4 FLUOROPHORES FOR LIVE CELL IMAGING

2.4.1 Cell Viability

Cell viability might be monitored in several ways, but the most common procedure is to monitor probes that cross the cell membrane in injured, permeabilized, or ruptured cells. Probes such as propidium iodide, ethidium homodimer 1, and Sytox green will only enter the cell after significant membrane damage, at which time they then bind to nucleic acid, labeling the nuclei intensely (Table 2.3). These probes may be added in micromolar amounts to experimental media and buffers to allow continuous monitoring of viability. While leakage of a cytosolic located dye would occur during or after cell death, leakage may also occur in viable cells. It is thus common to determine the relative incidence of cell death using a combination of (live/dead) cell stains, such as calcein and ethidium homodimer 1, or other combinations [18].

2.4.2 General Morphology

Most of the probes used to stain specific organelles can be coloaded with a general cytoplasmic or membrane probe, such as calcein or $DiOC_6(3)$, which then acts as a more general stain for the whole cell body. These probes can also be used with optical sectioning techniques to reconstruct the entire cell and provide shape and volume information over time; see Table 2.2 for details.

2.4.3 Specific Organelles

Nucleus There are a number of fluorescent dyes that are membrane permeant and that will localize in the nucleus of living cells. These include DAPI and Hoechst 33258, which are excitable by UV and hence not always convenient, and hexidium iodide. Used at low concentrations, these dyes are nontoxic and can be used to study chromatin dynamics. The Syto dyes (eg., Syto 11 to 16) stain nucleic acids in general, and while they will thus differentiate nuclei, there is also a variable (sometimes high) amount of cytoplasmic staining. Other nuclear probes such as 7-aminoactinomycin D (7AAD), acridine orange, and DRAQ5 may also give variable results, but it is usually worth the effort to optimize staining conditions. While acridine orange binds to both DNA and RNA, it is possible to differentiate between these as the emission of the DNA-bound form is predominantly green and there is a significant red shift to 650 nm when it associates with RNA [38]. When staining the nuclear envelope, FM4-64 exhibits a strong red shift in its absorption peak from 520 nm (for all other membranes) to 600 nm [72] probably reflecting the different molecular composition and order of this membrane.

Injection of fluorescent-labeled DNA precursors such as Cy5-dUTP has been effectively used to image dynamics of chromosome assembly and movement [42]. Another widely used approach is to target nuclear structures such as histones or centromeres using GFP–fusion protein constructs [64].

Mitochondria and Mitochondrial Membrane Potential A fairly wide range of probes is available for localization of mitochondria (2.2), including the short-chained carbocyanine dyes, like $DiOC_6(3)$, DASPMI, Rhodamine 6G, Rhodamine 123, and the newer generation MitoTracker, and MitoFluor probes. The cationic probes, Rhodamine 123 and tetramethylrhodamine methyl and ethyl (TMRM and TMRE) esters, and MitoFluor all show intense select staining for mitochondria but are not retained after cell death or fixation. In contrast, the thiol-reactive chloromethyl moieties of the Tracker probes aid their retention in the organelle, even after aldehyde fixation. MitoTracker green will accumulate in mitochondria regardless of mitochondrial membrane potential and is hence considered to be a good general stain for mitochondria. In contrast, $DiOC_6(3)$ and the other lipophilic carbocyanine dyes stain most intracellular compartments, but selective mitochondrial staining can be achieved at low concentrations in several cell types [69].

MitoTracker orange and red are tetramethylrosamine dyes that redistribute across the mitochondrial membrane based on membrane potential [44] and are hence used as potentiometric indicators. However, there is some indication that retention of the Tracker probes occurs largely due to binding of the chloromethyl moieties to SH groups, and hence results should be carefully assessed [63]. Another useful potentiometric probe is JC-1, a green fluorescent cyanine dye which remains in the monomeric form in low concentrations or at low membrane potential and becomes aggregated in aqueous concentrations higher than 0.1 μM or at higher potentials. The so-called J-aggregate form is red shifted, and hence ratiometric measurement with 490 nm excitation and

530/590 nm emission has been found to be a sensitive indicator of mitochondrial membrane potential [21, 57]. The TMRM and TMRE esters are rapidly taken up by living cells in a manner dependent on membrane potential [24, 25] and can be calibrated to show membrane potential in live cells [11]. The latter dyes are cationic redistribution dyes with a nernstian accumulation in organelles, and hence the ratio of fluorescence intensities measured in two compartments separated by a membrane can be used to monitor mitochondrial membrane potential quantitatively. We have carried out tetramethylrhodamine loading by incubating cells briefly (10–30 min) in about 500 nM TMRM, with 50–150 nM added to all subsequent buffers during subsequent imaging and measurement [32, 39, 52]. Higher concentrations of TMRM and TMRE are reported to inhibit respiration, and some groups therefore use concentrations as low as 25–30 nM [23, 50]. For a detailed review of functional imaging of mitochondria, see Duchen et al. [23].

Several reduced forms of mitochondrial probes which require oxidation before becoming fluorescent are available for probing mitochondrial oxidation status and the presence of reactive oxygen species (ROS). These include dihydrorhodamine 123, dihydrorhodamine 6G, dihydrotetramethylrosamine, MitoTracker red CM-H2Xros, MitoTracker orange CM-H2TMRos [55].

Endoplasmic Reticulum (ER) and Golgi Most probes suitable for staining of the ER and Golgi are either lipids or chemical inhibitors of protein movement, such as Brefeldin A. Fluorescent ceramide or sphingolipid analogues are most commonly used for live cell imaging [3, 54], whereas the fluorescent-conjugated lectins concanavalin A (Con A) and wheat germ agglutinin (WGA), which bind to the ER and Golgi apparatus, respectively, have been more useful for localization after aldehyde fixation. ER-Tracker blue-white DPX is a highly selective and photostable stain for the ER in live cells. Unlike the conventional ER stain $DiOC_6(3)$, ER-Tracker blue-white DPX does not stain mitochondria, and staining at low concentrations does not appear to be toxic to cells. Fluorescent Brefeldin A (either as the green-fluorescent BODIPY FL or the red-orange-fluorescent BODIPY 558/568) has also been used to selectively localize ER and Golgi apparatus in several different cell lines [20]. The probes do not generally give an identical staining pattern, as there is some distortion of intracellular trafficking of protein through the ER and Golgi [15]. Brefeldin A also alters the morphology of endosomes and lysosomes so these probes should be used with appropriate controls.

2.4.4 Ionic Environment

The importance of measurement of intracellular ions is reflected in the number of fluorescent probes that are available for the principal ions, Ca^{2+}, Na^+, and H^+ (Table 2.3). Choice of indicators is dependent on whether intensometric or ratiometric analysis is required, fluorescence characteristics, binding affinity, or sensitivity range. Intensometric probes such as Fluo-3, Oregon green BAPTA-1, calcium green, and sodium green are single excitation/emission wavelength dyes which provide valuable data of relative intensities and which can also be calibrated [48, 66]. In contrast, ratiometric indicators may be dual emission (e.g., Indo-1 for calcium, SNARF-1 for pH) or dual excitation (e.g., Fura-2 for calcium, BCECF for pH). Tbese provide the ability to calibrate and exclude artefacts of loading, leaching, photobleaching, and movement. Fluorescent spectra are published for most indicators and are important data to have available as the excitation wavelength significantly affects the photochemistry and emission spectra for probes. For example, carboxy SNARF can be excited by 488-, 514-, 530-, or 568-nm light, yielding substantially different spectra [7, 11, 33].

While not widely used, it is also possible to use combinations of two dyes to effect a ratiometric dual-emission approach, for example, Fura red and Fluo-3 [40, 62]. In this instance great care must be taken to ensure that there is a similar loading and intracellular distribution of the dye. This can be overcome by use of dextrans double conjugated with calcium green 1 and a calcium-insensitive probe such as Texas red, providing that the cells/tissues are able to be loaded by microinjection, endocytosis or scrape loading, and so on. It is also possible to carry out simultaneous imaging of Ca^{2+} and pH by coloading with two indicators and measuring at multiple wavelengths [43, 53, 75] facilitating correction of pH-sensitive calcium indicators under conditions where changes in both pH and calcium occur.

On the other hand, dextrans conjugated to pH indicators like BCECF, SNARF, and SNAFL (pK_a 7.0–7.8 range) can be used to follow uptake into acidic organelles as their fluorescence is either quenched or significantly shifted under pH 5.5. Accurate measurement of pH in the region of 2–3 should be done with dextrans conjugated to probes such as Oregon green, Rhodol green, DM-NERF, or Cl-NERF, which have pK_a of 3.8–5.6.

The literature provides further details of methods and protocols available for imaging of Ca^{2+} [34, 61, 67], pH [14, 35, 53, 75], and Na^+ [30, 37, 59]. The reactive oxygen species (ROS) (including singlet oxygen, superoxides, and hydroxy radicals) can be detected using a number of probes (Tables 2.2 and 2.3) that react with ROS in the process being converted by oxidation from a nonfluorescent form (e.g., dichlorofluorescein, DCFH) to a fluorescent form (dichlorofluorescein, DCF). Recently DCFH has been used as a marker for oxidative stress in cardiac muscle [68]. Reduced forms of mitochondrial probes such as dihydrorhodamine 123 and MitoTracker red CM-H2XROS are also available for ROS detection.

2.4.5 Tracers for Membranes and Cells

A number of lipophilic fluorophores are available to facilitate probing membrane and lipid dynamics, endocytosis, and intracellular lipid trafficking and cell fusions. These fluorophores can also be used to examine neuronal development and morphology, and to track cells, see Table 2.4.

Fluorescently conjugated particles, bacteria (live or dead), latex spheres, and dextrans have all been used to study endocytotic uptake and intracellular movement. FM1-43 and similar styryl dyes are proven useful probes for membrane trafficking because they reversibly stain membranes, are impermeable to membranes, and are more fluorescent when bound to membranes than when in solution. FM1-43 has been used to study endocytosis, trafficking, and recycling in synaptic nerve terminals [16, 16], and selective quenching of background (nonendocytosed) membrane signals can be achieved by bathing in another fluorophore, sulf-rhodamine [56]. Similarly, trypan blue can be used to quench extracellular fluorescence after internalization of FITC-dextran. Ligands can also be labeled and then used to study receptor location, density, internalization, and trafficking. This has been effectively done using fluoresceinylated or BOPIDY-labeled neurotensin, somatostatin, and mu- and delta-selective opioid peptides in live cells and tissue slices [4].

Pagano and co-workers have pioneered the use of lipid analogues to study membrane dynamics and trafficking in living cells [54]. NBD and BODIPY-conjugated lipids and lipid analogues not only are effective in tracking intracellular distribution and movement of lipids, but also, since emission characteristics change with fluorophore-lipid packing, may be used to indicate selective internalization and possibly lipid sorting [12]. The membrane dye laurdan reports on phospholipid packing also as it undergoes a shift in its peak emission from 500 nm in fluid membranes to 400 nm in ordered membranes [2] and is well suited to multiphoton imaging where it has been used to detect local concentration of lipids in T-lymphocyte signaling [27].

Probes for tracking cells may be cell impermeant and bind irreversibly to the membrane (PKH2, PH26, CM-DiI), cell impermeant and require loading by physical means such as microinjection (fluorescent-labeled dextrans, lucifer yellow), or membrane permeant (chloromethyl CellTracker probes). Recently, a natural compound (epicocconone) isolated from the fungus *Epicoccum nigram* has been found to be a very useful and nontoxic label for cells which readily absorb the compound: Epicocconone is weakly fluorescent in the green (520) but on binding to protein (inside the cell) fluoresces bright orange and is further enhanced in lipophilic environments [13]. It is therefore a convenient fluorophore to facilitate tracking specific cell populations or as a general cellular stain. Lucifer yellow has long been a favorite probe for studying neuronal morphology and pathways [6] because it contains a carbohydrazide group that is linked to intracellular molecules during aldehyde fixation. The long-chain carbocyanines such as DiI, DiO, and DiD, although not cell impermeant, have similarly been used to trace cells, cell contacts, and membrane cell continuity. These dyes diffuse readily through the cell membrane but are hydrophobic [74]. CM-DiI has been used as a marker in lymphocyte migration and can be recovered after 40 h [1]. It is better retained than DiI after fixation, and because the probe has increased solubility in aqueous solutions, it is an attractive choice for labeling cells in solution. CellTracker green (CMFDA), on the other hand, labels the cytosol and has been used to label mast cells and then track them from the blood circulation to the brain [65]. We have used CMFDA to label rat platelets which are then reintroduced to the circulation of an animal with carotid artery injury. Fixation and dissection of the vessel allow subsequent analysis of morphology and size of thrombus formation (shown in [31]) which, because of retention of the fluorophore in the fixed tissue, can be carried out after a few days in storage. PKH2 and PKH26, which bind irreversibly to the membrane, have been used extensively for tracking cells over the long term (up to 60 days) with subsequent analysis by flow cytometry [5] and histology [26]. However, it is important to distinguish between fluorophores that are used to track cells by recovering labeled cells at an end point and those that allow repeated or continual imaging in live cells. Thus, while PKH2 and PKH26 are suitable for recovering cells after several days, repetitive imaging over 5 min is sufficient to cause phototoxicity [51]. It is thus advisable to include appropriate controls and probes to monitor cell viability when dynamic imaging is required.

2.4.6 Fluorescent Proteins

Genetically encoded fluorescent proteins (FPs) will be covered in greater detail in Chapter 3, but for completeness and cross referencing of spectral peaks, they are briefly included in Table 2.4. While CFP, GFP, yellow FP (YFP), and DsRed have been commonly used over approximately the past decade, there is now a considerable choice for probes with the best characteristics of brightness, photostability, resistance to oligomerization, and reduced sensitivity to environmental conditions (unless specifically programmed to report that environment, as with the chameleons and pH-sensitive forms of GFP [46, 49]. As many of these forms are now encoded into living organisms (especially mice) to establish models of disease or development, there is a significant effort to develop even more red-shifted probes (e.g., mCherry, mPlum) responding to the need for deep-tissue imaging (less scatter and enhanced penetration) and discrimination of signal over autofluorescence. Finally, although not specifically related to fluorescent proteins, HaloTag™ (Promega) technology should also be mentioned. HaloTag is a nonfluorescent genetic construct that can be introduced into cells by standard transfection techniques. A HaloTag ligand is then applied in an incubating solution and it readily diffuses across the cell membrane to covalently bind with HaloTag, rendering it fluorescent. Cells or tissues expressing this tag can be imaged live over long periods of time with little background. Applications include protein translocation, cell tracking, and cell cycle analysis, with fusion proteins able to be retrieved for protein analysis via conventional techniques.

REFERENCES

1. W. Andrade, T. J. Seabrook, M. G. Johnston, and J. B. Hay, "The use of the lipophilic fluorochrome CM-DiI for tracking the migration of lymphocytes," *J. Immunol. Methods* **194**, 181–189 (1996).
2. L. A. Bagatolli, S. A. Sanchez, T. Hazlett, and E. Gratton, "Giant vesicles, laurdan, and two-photon fluorescence microscopy: Evidence of lipid lateral separation in bilayers," *Methods Enzymol.* **360**, 481–500 (2003).
3. J. Bai and R. E. Pagano, "Measurement of spontaneous transfer and transbilayer movement of BODIPY-labeled lipids in lipid vesicles," *Biochemistry* **36**, 8840–8848 (1997).
4. A. Beaudet, D. Nouel, T. Stroh, F. Vandenbulcke, C. Dal-Farra, and J. P. Vincent, "Fluorescent ligands for studying neuropeptide receptors by confocal microscopy," *Braz. J. Med. Biol. Res.* **31**, 1479–1489 (1998).
5. A. J. Beavis and K. J. Pennline, "Tracking of murine spleen cells in vivo—Detection of PKH26-labeled cells in the pancreas of non-obese diabetic (NOD) mice," *J. Immunol. Meth.* **170**, 57–65 (1994).
6. P. V. Belichenko and A. Dahlstrom, "Confocal laser scanning microscopy and 3-D reconstructions of neuronal structures in human brain cortex," *Neuroimage* **2**, 201–207 (1995).
7. P. S. Blank, H. S. Silverman, O. Y. Chung, B. A. Hogue, M. D. Stern, R. G. Hansford, E. G. Lakatta, and M. C. Capogrossi, "Cytosolic pH measurements in single cardiac myocytes using carboxy-seminaphthorhodafluor-1," *Am. J. Physiol.* **263**, H276–H284 (1992).
8. M. D. Bootman, K. W. Young, J. M. Young, R. B. Moreton, and M. J. Berridge, "Extracellular calcium concentration controls the frequency of intracellular calcium spiking independently of inositol 1,4,5-triphosphate production in HeLa cells," *Biochem. J.* **314**, 347–354 (1996).
9. J. L. V. Broers, B. M. Machiels, G. J. J. M. van Eys, H. J. H. Kuijpers, E. M. M. Manders, R. van Driel, and F. C. S. Ramaekers, "Dynamics of the nuclear lamina as monitored by GFP-tagged A-type lamins," *J. Cell Sci.* **112**, 3463–3475 (1999).

10. E. Chacon, H. Ohata, I. S. Harper, D. R. Trollinger, B. Herman, and J. J. Lemasters, "Mitochondrial free calcium transients during excitation-contraction coupling in rabbit cardiac myocytes," *FEBS Lett.* **382**, 31–36 (1996).

11. E. Chacon, J. M. Reece, A.-L. Nieminen, G. Zabhrebelski, B. Herman, and J. J. Lemasters, "Distribution of electrical potential, pH, free Ca^{2+} and volume inside cultured adult rabbit myocytes during chemical hypoxia: A multiparameter digitized confocal microscopic study," *Biophys. J.* **66**, 942–952 (1994).

12. C. S. Chen, O. C. Martin, and R. E. Pagano, "Changes in the spectral properties of a plasma membrane analoque during the first seconds of endocytosis in living cells," *Biophys. J.* **72**, 37–50 (1997).

13. H.-Y. Choi, D. A. Veal, and P. Karuso, "Epicocconone, a new cell-permeable long Stokes' shift fluorescent stain for live cell imaging and multiplexing," *J. Fluoresc.* **16**, 475–482 (2005).

14. S. H. Cody, P. N. Dubbin, A. D. Beischer, N. D. Duncan, J. S. Hill, A. H. Kaye, and D. A. Williams, "Intracellular pH mapping with SNARF-1 and confocal microscopy. 1. A quantitative technique for living tissues and isolated cells," *Micron* **24**, 573–580 (1993).

15. L. Cole, D. Davies, G. J. Hyde, and A. E. Ashford, "ER-Tracker dye and BODIPY-brefeldin A differentiate the endoplasmic reticulum and golgi bodies from the tubular-vacuole system in living hyphae of *Pisolithus tinctorius*," *J. Microsc.* **197**, 239–249 (2000).

16. M. A. Cousin and P. J. Robinson, "Mechanisms of synaptic vesicle recycling illuminated by fluorescent dyes," *J. Neurochem.* **73**, 2227–2239 (1999).

17. C. Cullander, "Fluorescent probes for confocal microscopy," in *Methods in Molecular Biology* S. W. Paddock (Ed.), Humana Press, Totowa NJ, 1999, pp. 59–73.

18. P. Decherchi, P. Cochard, and P. Gauthier, "Dual staining assessment of Schwann cell viability within whole peripheral nerves using calcein-AM and ethidium homodimer," *J. Neurosci. Meth.* **71**, 205–213 (1997).

19. P. J. Delnido, P. Glynn, P. Buenaventura, G. Salama, and A. P. Koretsky, "Fluorescence measurement of calcium transients in perfused rabbit heart using Rhod-2," *Am. J. Physiol.* **43**, H728–H741 (1998).

20. Y. P. Deng, J. R. Bennink, H. C. Kang, R. P. Haugland, and J. W. Yewdell, "Fluorescent conjugates of brefeldin A selectively stain the endoplasmic reticulum and golgi complex of living cells," *J. Histochem. Cytochem.* **43**, 907–915 (1995).

21. F. Di Lisa, P. S. Blank, R. Colonna, G. Gambassi, H. S. Silverman, M. D. Stern, and R. G. Hansford, "Mitochondrial membrane potential in single living adult rat cardiac myocytes exposed to anoxia or metabolic inhibition," *J. Physiol. Lond.* **486**, 1–13 (1995).

22. F. Di Virgilio, T. H. Steinberg, and S. C. Silverstein, "Inhibition of Fura-2 sequestration and secretion with organic anion transport blockers," *Cell Calcium* **11**, 57–62 (1990).

23. M. R. Duchen, J. Jacobson, J. Keelan, M. H. Mojet, and O. Vergun, "Functional imaging of mitochondria within cells," in *Methods in Cellular Imaging*, A. Periasamy (Ed.), Oxford University Press, New York, 2001, pp. 88–111.

24. B. Ehrenberg, V. Montana, M. D. Wei, J. P. Wuskell, and L. M. Loew, "Membrane potential can be determined in individual cells from the nernstian distribution of cationic dyes," *Biophys. J.* **53**, 785–794 (1988).

25. D. L. Farkas, M. Wei, P. Febbroriello, J. H. Carson, and L. M. Loew, "Simultaneous imaging of cell and mitochondrial membrane potential," *Biophys. J.* **56**, 1053–1069 (1989).

26. J. W. Ford, T. H. Welling, J. C. Stanley, and L. M. Messina, "PKH26 and I-125-PKH95—Characterization and efficacy as labels for in vitro and in vivo endothelial cell localization and tracking," *J. Surg. Res.* **62**, 23–28 (1996).

27. K. Gaus, E. Chklovskaia, B. F. de St. Groth, W. Jessup, and T. Harder, "Condensation of the plasma membrane at the site of T lymphocyte activation," *J. Cell Biol.* **171**, 121–131 (2005).

28. M. Grabenbauer, W. J. C. Geerts, J. Fernadez-Rodriguez, A. Hoenger, A. J. Koster, and T. Nilsson, "Correlative microscopy and electron tomography of GFP through photooxidation," *Nat. Methods* **2**, 857–862 (2005).

29. E. J. Griffiths, M. D. Stern, and H. S. Silverman, "Measurement of mitochondrial calcium in single living cardiomyocytes by selective removal of cytosolic Indo 1," *Am. J. Physiol.* **273**, C37–C44 (1997).

30. A. T. Harootunian, J. P. Y. Kao, B. K. Eckert, and R. Y. Tsien, "Fluorescence ratio imaging of cytosolic free Na in individual fibroblasts and lymphocytes," *J. Biol. Chem.* **264**, 19458–19467 (1989).

31. I. S. Harper, "Fluorophores and their labeling procedures for monitoring various biological signals," in *Methods in Cellular Imaging*, A. Periasamy (Ed.), Oxford University Press, New York, 2001, pp. 20–39.

32. I. S. Harper, J. M. Bond, E. Chacon, J. M. Reece, B. Herman, and J. J. Lemasters, "Inhibition of Na^+/H^+ exchange preserves viability, restores mechanical function, and prevents the pH paradox in reperfusion injury to rat neonatal myocytes," *Basic Res. Cardiol.* **88**, 430–442 (1993).

33. R. P. Haugland, *The Handbook. A Guide to Fluorescence Probes and Labeling Technologies*, 10th ed., Molecular Probes, Eugene, OR, 2005.

34. A. Hayes, S. H. Cody, and D. A. Williams, "Measuring cytosolic Ca^{2+} in cells with fluorescent probes: An aid to understanding cell pathophysiology," *Int. Rev. Exp. Pathol.* **36**, 197–212 (1996).

35. C. R. House, "Confocal ratio-imaging of intracellular pH in unfertilised mouse oocytes," *Zygote* **2**, 37–45 (1994).

36. G. J. Hyde, D. S. Davies, L. Cole, and A. E. Ashford, "Retention of fluorescent probes during aldehyde-free anhydrous freeze-substitution," *J. Microsc.* **210**, 125–130 (2003).

37. D. W. Jung, L. M. Apel, and G. P. Brierley, "Transmembrane gradients of free Na^+ in isolated heart mitochondria estimated using a fluorescent probe," *Am. J. Physiol.* **262**, C1047–C1055 (1992).

38. F. H. Kasten, "Introduction to fluorescent probes: Properties, history and applications," in *Fluorescent and Luminscent Probes for Biological Activity: A Practical Guide to Technology for Quantitative Real-Time Analysis*, W. T. Mason (Ed.), Academic, Cambridge, 1999, pp. 17–39.

39. J. J. Lemasters, A. L. Nieminen, E. Chacon, J. M. Bond, I. Harper, J. M. Reece, and B. Herman, "Single cell microscopic techniques for studying toxic injury," *Meth. Toxicol.* **1**(B.1), 438–455 (1994).

40. P. Lipp and E. Niggli, "Ratiometric confocal Ca^{2+}-measurements with visible wavelength indicators in isolated cardiac myocytes," *Cell Calcium* **14**, 359–372 (1993).

41. K. Lubyphelps, S. Mujumdar, R. B. Mujumdar, L. A. Ernst, W. Galbraith, and A. S. Waggoner, "A novel fluorescence ratiometric method confirms the low solvent viscosity of the cytoplasm," *Biophys. J.* **65**, 236–242 (1993).

42. E. M. M. Manders, H. Kimura, and P. R. Cook, "Direct imaging of DNA in living cells reveals the dynamics of chromosome formation," *J. Cell Biol.* **144**, 813–821 (1999).

43. R. Martinezzaguilan, M. W. Gurule, and R. M. Lynch, "Simultaneous measurement of intracellular pH and Ca^{2+} in insulin-secreting cells by spectral imaging microscopy," *Am. J. Physiol.* **39**, C1438–C1446 (1996).

44. A. Mathur, Y. Hong, B. K. Kemp, A. A. Barrientos, and J. D. Erusalimsky, "Evaluation of fluorescent dyes for the detection of mitochondrial membrane potential changes in cultured cardiomyocytes," *Cardiovasc. Res.* **46**, 126–138 (2000).
45. T. Minamikawa, A. Sriratana, D. A. Williams, D. N. Bowser, J. S. Hill, and P. Nagley, "Chloromethyl-X-rosamine (MitoTracker Red) photosensitizes mitochondria and induces apoptosis in intact human cells," *J. Cell Sci.* **112**, 2419–2430 (1999).
46. A. Miyawaki, O. Griesbeck, R. Heim, and R. Y. Tsien, "Dynamic and quantitative Ca^{2+} measurements using improved cameleons," *Proc. Natl. Acad. Sci.* **96**, 2135–2140 (1999).
47. E. D. W. Moore, P. L. Becker, K. E. Fogarty, D. A. Williams, and F. S. Fay, "Ca^{2+} imaging in single living cells: Theoretical and practical issues," *Cell Calcium* **11**, 157–179 (1990).
48. A. J. Morgan and A. P. Thomas, "Single cell and subcellular measurement of intracellular Ca^{2+} concentration ($[Ca^{2+}_{(i)}]$) calcium," *Signal. Protocol* **114**, 93–123 (1999).
49. Y. Nagai, M. Miyazaki, R. Aoki, T. Zama, S. Inouye, K. Hirose, M. Iino, and M. Hagiwara, "A fluorescent indicator for visualizing cAMP-induced phosphorylation in vivo," *Nature Biotechnol.* **18**, 313–316 (2000).
50. E. M. O'Reilly, K. E. Fogarty, R. M. Drummond, R. A. Tuft, and J. V. Walsh, "Quantitative analysis of spontaneous mitochondrial depolarizations," *Biophys. J.* **85**, 3350–3357 (2003).
51. D. J. Oh, G. M. Lee, K. Francis, and B. O. Palsson, "Phototoxicity of the fluorescent membrane dyes PKH2 and PKH26 on the human hematopoietic KG1a progenitor cell line," *Cytometry* **36**, 312–318 (1999).
52. H. Ohata, E. Chacon, S. A. Tesfai, I. S. Harper, B. Herman, and J. J. Lemasters, "Mitochondrial Ca^{2+} transients in cardiac myocytes during the excitation-contraction cycle: Effects of pacing and hormonal stimulation," *J. Bioenerg. Biomembr.* **30**, 207–222 (1998).
53. M. Opas, "Measurement of intracellular pH and pCa with a confocal microscope," *Trends Cell Biol.* **7**, 75–80 (1997).
54. R. E. Pagano and C. S. Chen, "Use of BODIPY-labeled sphingolipids to study membrane traffic along the endocytic pathway," *Ann. N. Y. Acad. Sci.* **845**, 152–160 (1998).
55. M. Poot, Y. Z. Zhang, J. A. Kramer, K. S. Wells, L. Jones, D. K. Hanzel, A. G. Lugade, V. L. Singer, and R. P. Haughland, "Analysis of mitochondrial morphology and function with novel fixable fluorescent stains," *J. Histochem. Cytochem.* **44**, 1363–1372 (1996).
56. J. L. Pyle, E. T. Kavalali, S. Choi, and R. W. Tsien, "Visualization of synaptic activity in hippocampal slices with FM1-43 enabled by fluorescence quenching," *Neuron* **24**, 803–808 (1999).
57. M. Reers, S. T. Smiley, C. Mottolahartshorn, A. Chen, M. Lin, and L. B. Chen, "Mitochondrial membrane potential monitored by JC-1 dye," *Methods Enzymol.* **260**, 406–417 (1995).
58. J. H. Sandell and R. H. Masland, "Photoconversion of some fluorescent markers to a diaminobenzidine product," *J. Histochem. Cytochem.* **36**, 555–559 (1988).
59. H. Satoh, H. Hayashi, N. Noda, H. Terada, A. Kobayashi, Y. Yamashita, T. Kawai, M. Hirano, and N. Yamazaki, "Quantification of intracellular free sodium ions by using a new fluorescent indicator, sodium-binding benzofuran isophthalate in guinea pig myocytes," *Biochem. Biophys. Res. Commun.* **175**, 611–616 (1991).
60. M. Scanlon, D. A. Williams, and F. S. Fay, "A Ca^{2+}-insensitive form of fura-2 associated with polymorphonuclear leukocytes. Assessment and accurate Ca^{2+} measurement," *J. Biol. Chem.* **262**, 6308–6312 (1987).
61. D. Schild, "Laser scanning microscopy and calcium imaging," *Cell Calcium* **19**, 281–296 (1996).
62. D. Schild, A. Jung, and H. A. Schultens, "Localization of calcium entry through calcium channels in olfactory receptor neurones using a laser scanning microscope and the calcium indicator dyes Fluo-3 and Fura- Red," *Cell Calcium* **15**, 341–348 (1994).

63. L. Scorrano, V. Petronilli, R. Colonna, F. Di Lisa, and P. Bernardi, "Chloromethyltetramethylrosamine (Mitotracker Orange) induces the mitochondrial permeability transition and inhibits respiratory complex I. Implications for the mechanism of cytochrome c release," *J. Biol. Chem.* **274**, 24657–24663 (1999).

64. R. D. Shelby, K. M. Hahn, and K. F. Sullivan, "Dynamic elastic behavior of alpha-satellite DNA domains visualized in situ in living human cells," *J. Cell Biol.* **135**, 545–557 (1996).

65. A. J. Silverman, A. K. Sutherland, M. Wilhelm, and R. Silver, "Mast cells migrate from blood to brain," *J. Neurosci.* **20**, 401–408 (2000).

66. A. W. M. Simpson, "Fluorescent measurement of $[Ca^{2+}]_{(c)}$—Basic practical considerations," *Calcium Signal. Protocol* **114**, 3–30 (1999).

67. S. A. Stricker and M. Whitaker, "Confocal laser scanning microscopy of calcium dynamics in living cells," *Microsc. Res. Tech.* **46**, 356–369 (1999).

68. L. M. Swift and N. Sarvazyan, "Localization of dichlorofluorescin in cardiac myocytes: Implications for assessment of oxidative stress," *Am. J. Physiol.* **278**, H982–H990 (2000).

69. M. Terasaki and M. E. Dailey, "Confocal microscopy of living cells," in *Handbook of Biological Confocal Microscopy*, 2nd ed., J. B. Pawley (Ed.), Plenum, New York, 1995, pp. 327–346.

70. M. Terasaki and T. S. Reese, "Characterization of endoplasmic reticulum by co-localization of BiP and dicarbocyanine dyes," *J. Cell Sci.* **101**, 315–322 (1992).

71. L. Tiano, P. Ballarini, G. Santoni, M. Wozniak, and G. Falcioni, "Morphological and functional changes of mitochondria from density separated trout erythrocytes," *Biochim. Biophys. Acta* **1457**, 118–128 (2000).

72. T. Zal, M. A. Zal, C. Lotz, C. J. Goergen, and N. R. J. Gascoignel, "Spectral shift of fluorescent dye FM4-64 reveals distinct microenvironment of nuclear envelope," *Traffic* **7**, 1607–1613 (2006).

73. R. Y. Tsien and A. Waggoner, "Fluorophores for confocal microscopy: Photophysics and photochemistry," in *Handbook of Biological Confocal Microscopy*, 2nd ed., J. B. Pawley (Ed.), Plenum Press, New York, 1995, pp. 267–279.

74. A. Vercelli, M. Repici, D. Garbossa, and A. Grimaldi, "Recent techniques for tracing pathways in the central nervous system of developing and adult mammals," *Brain Res. Bull.* **51**, 11–28 (2000).

75. M. Weinlich, U. Heydasch, M. Starlinger, and R. K. Kinne, "Intracellular pH-measurements in rat duodenal mucosa in vitro using confocal laserscan microscopy," *Z. Gastroenterol.* **35**, 263–270 (1993).

76. T. B. Wiegmann, L. W. Welling, D. M. Beatty, D. E. Howard, S. Vamos, and S. J. Morris, "Simultaneous imaging of intracellular $[Ca^{2+}]$ and pH in single MDCK and glomerular epithelial cells—Special communication," *Am. J. Physiol.* **265**, C1184–C1190 (1993).

CHAPTER 3

Genetically Encoded Fluorescent Probes: Some Properties and Applications in Life Sciences

MARK PRESCOTT

Department of Biochemistry and Molecular Biology, School of Biomedical Sciences, Monash University, Clayton, Victoria 3800, Australia

ANYA SALIH

Confocal Bio-imaging Facility, School of Natural Sciences, University of Western Sydney, Sydney, New South Wales 1797, Australia

3.1 INTRODUCTION

The green fluorescent protein (GFP) was first isolated from the bell margin tissue of the bioluminescent jellyfish, *Aequorea victoria* [1, 2], where it is found in close proximity to the chemoluminescent protein aequorin. The gene encoding this protein known as *av*GFP was subsequently cloned [3] and now represents the founding member of an enormously powerful technology that has revolutionized the way in which the life scientist carries out research on living cells [4]. Often referred to as the "paint-in-a-can" or the "genetic code for fluorescence," the outstanding feature of this family of proteins is their remarkable ability to form an optically active chromophore in the absence of any cofactors, requiring only the presence of oxygen. Some key advantages for using fluorescent protein (FP) technology are highlighted in Table 3.1.

Tissues of many of nonbioluminescent marine organisms—reef corals, sea anemones, and zoanthids—are often brightly pigmented with purple-blue or intensely fluorescent homologues of *av*GFP, with fluorescence emissions in cyan (470–499 nm), green (500–520 nm), yellow, and red (<520 nm) wavelengths (Figure 3.1). Intensely colored but weakly fluorescent homologs are often referred to as chromoproteins (CP). These FP and CP pigments are particularly abundant in reef corals [5, 6] and constitute a large proportion of total tissue protein [7]. Accordingly, a spectacular variety of fluorescent and colored proteins have been cloned from various marine organisms such as cnidarians and even several marine copepods (e.g., see [8]). Many novel proteins have spectral, molecular, and chemical properties distinct from *av*GFP and provide cell biologists, medical researchers, and biotechnologists with a diverse choice of multicolored fluorescent labels for imaging or screening.

Fluorescence Applications in Biotechnology and Life Sciences, Edited by Ewa M. Goldys

TABLE 3.1 Advantages and Features of FPs

Genetically encoded
Optical properties can be readily tuned and optimized using molecular biological techniques
Readily fused to individual proteins
Accessible N- and C-termini for expression fused to target proteins
Can be readily targeted to different locations and compartments of cell
Other than molecular oxygen, no cofactors for chromophore formation required
Noninvasive
Fluorescence emissions covering visible spectrum (450–650 nm)
Variety of different photoswitchable variants available
Instrumentation suitable for fluorescence detection commonly available in molecular cell biology laboratories
Can be configured to sense a wide range of cellular parameters

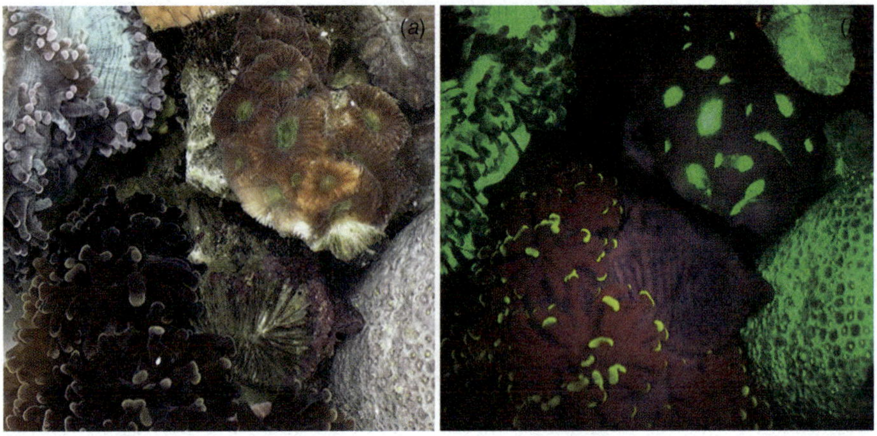

Figure 3.1 Colors due to GFP-like proteins in tissues of different species of reef corals: (*a*) corals viewed in daylight; (*b*) same corals imaged in the dark using blue excitation light.

Significant effort has been expended to develop particular proteins into sophisticated and invaluable tools. However, the biological function of these proteins in marine organisms remains unclear, although many suggestions have been made. For example, *av*GFP is thought to act as a secondary light emitter to transduce the calcium-dependent blue emissions of aequorin into green fluorescence [9] which may have a role in predator–prey behavior. GFP-like proteins in *Anthozoa* are thought to help modulate the cellular light environment and to optimize it for the photosynthesis carried out by symbiotic microalgae (zooxanthellae) that reside in cells of these marine animals as well as to protect the animal host [6]. By screening the symbionts and coral tissues from solar radiation, GFPs reduce coral mortality following bleaching events that are now known to be linked to global warming.

Other suggested functions of GFP-type proteins include photosensing of the light environment by the coral host (Salih, A., unpublished data); regulating the relationships between the coral host and its symbiont microalgae via GFP photosensors analogous to phytochromes and cryptochromes of higher plants [10]; providing secondary antioxidant cellular protection [10]; and even portable cellular proton pumps [11]. It is perhaps worth noting that the G2F domain of human nidogen, a nonpigmented extracellular matrix protein, bears a striking three-dimensional (3D) structural similarity to the GFP β-can [12]. Clearly, the biological functions of GFP-like proteins are both important and diverse, even if only some of the hypothesized functions will be eventually validated in future studies. As our understanding of the diversity and the biology of GFP-like proteins in various organism increases, our ability to develop novel applications of these unique proteins will also be enhanced.

FP technology is some 13 years old but continues to evolve through both engineering of existing proteins and the discovery of new members of the family. In this chapter we highlight some of their key properties and the conceptual approaches and their application. Of course, FP technology is not without its limitations and we also bring into focus some of the problems associated with the technology. Given the broad scope of this book, we hope it will be informative for those with limited awareness of research in the life sciences.

3.2 CHROMOPHORE AND ITS FORMATION

Many hundred complementary DNAs (cDNAs) encoding GFP-like proteins have been isolated, and we now have a reasonably good picture of the GFP protein family and the underpinning genes. A search of the Protein Database (www.rssb.org) indicates that GFP-like proteins form a diverse range but each have the same basic structure—an 11-stranded β-barrel with a threaded α-helix from which, in a solvent-protected environment, the chromophore is suspended (Figures 3.2*a*,*b*). A typical member of this family, such as *av*GFP, contains 238 amino acids. The N- and C-termini are freely accessible for fusion to other proteins. With the exception of several amino acids at the N- and C-termini which can be deleted, further truncations are not tolerated. Nevertheless, the protein will accept the insertion of domains into the β-barrel or relocation of its N- and C-termini to form useful biosensors. Three consecutive amino acids (XXG) in the primary sequence give rise, through a series of posttranslational modifications (see below), to an optically active chromophore in a process termed maturation. Most proteins, due to the presence of tryptophan residues, show an intrinsic fluorescence in the ultraviolet. The chromophore extends the emission into the visible spectrum and into the far red. Fluorescent proteins with fluorescence emissions throughout the visible range of wavelengths (450–650 nm) have been found and many are commercially available (Table 3.2).

The posttranslational steps leading to the formation of an FP chromophore are outlined in Figure 3.3. In *av*GFP the chromophore amino acids are serine 65, tyrosine 66, and glycine 67. The first step in the maturation process is believed to be a series of rearrangements that allow nucleophilic attack of the carboxyl carbon of the serine residue (Ser65) on the amide nitrogen of glycine 67. This is followed by a dehydration step and the formation of an imidazolin-5-one heterocyclic ring system. Oxidation of the tyrosyl-α,β carbon by molecular oxygen extends the imdidazolinone conjugation system to include the phenyl ring to form the chromophore characteristic of GFP.

The identities of the amino acids that contribute to the chromophore largely determine the optical properties of an FP. For example, the chromophore peptide XYG *av*GFP gives rise to green emission, while GFP variants containing XWG or XHG give rise to chromophores with cyan or blue emissions, respectively (Figure 3.4). Interestingly, although XXG motifs can form functional chromophores, only XYG motifs

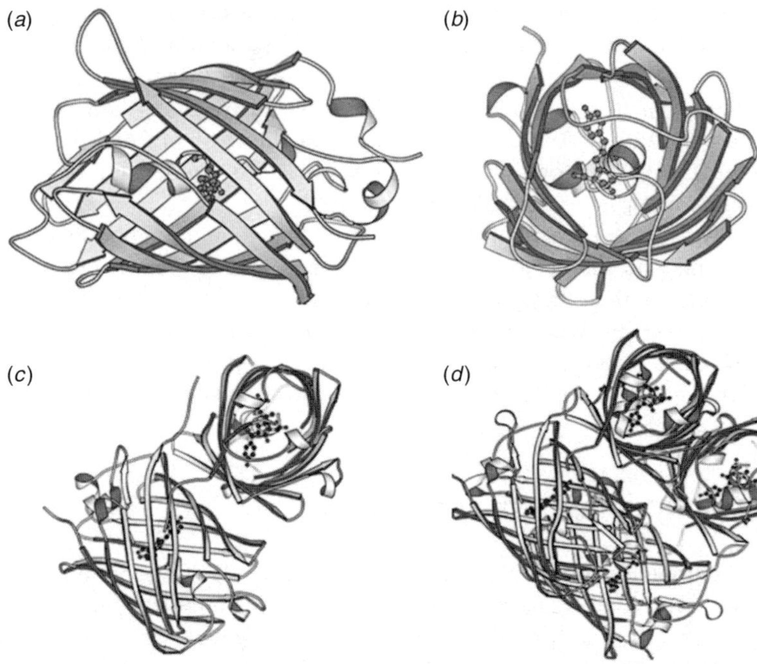

Figure 3.2 Secondary, tertiary, and quartenary structure of GFP-like proteins. The primary amino acid structure of FPs and CPs are organized into 11 β-strands (ribbons) with interconnecting loops to form highly stable β-barrel structure (*a*,*b*). The chromophore (shown in ball-and-stick form), derived from three consecutive amino acids in the primary sequence, can be seen suspended from an α-helix threaded through the center of the β-barrel where it is well protected from the external environment. The positions of the N- and C-termini to which proteins can be fused are shown. Many proteins have been engineered to behave as monomers as indicated for the individual protomers shown in (*a*) and (*b*). Naturally occurring proteins through a defined interface can form weak dimers (e.g., avGFP) or obligate dimers (eg., HcRed or Renilla GFP) (*c*) or obligate tetramers (*d*) (e.g., DsRed). Oligomerization of FPs can adversely affect function of proteins to which they are fused.

are encountered in nature. Amino acids absent in nature or other substitutions in the chromophore motif corresponding to position 66 can lead to proteins with novel properties, one example being GdFP, in which the chromophore tryptophan is substituted by (4-amino)tryptophan [13] (Figure 3.4).

Some of the different chromophore structures identified in GFP-like proteins are illustrated in Figure 3.4. Members of the protein family with significantly red-shifted optical properties, such as DsRed and EqFP611 (Table 3.2), undergo additional posttranslational steps that extend the conjugation system of the chromophore [14] (Figure 3.3). In DsRed, the peptide bond immediately preceding the first amino acid of the chromophore sequence is oxidized to an acylimine. It is has been proposed for particular proteins that the acylimine represents a "cross-road" in the formation of other chromophore structures. Thus, the formation of the triple-ring chromophore of the yellow fluorescent zFP538 and orange fluorescent mOrange (Figure 3.3) proceeds through an acylimine intermediate. Furthermore, cleavage during maturation at the position of the acylimine is also believed to lead to the formation of the chromophore

TABLE 3.2 Selected Properties of Useful GFP-Like Proteins

Protein	λ_{max}^{ex} (nm)	λ_{max}^{em} (nm)	EC (M^{-1} cm^{-1})	QY	pK_a	State	References	Relative Brightness
Blue fluorescent proteins								
EBFP	377	446	30,000	0.31	6.3	M	83	0.28
SBFP2	380	446	34,000	0.47	5.5	M	84	0.48
Azurite	384	450	22,000	0.59	5	M	36	0.39
mKalama1	385	456	36,000	0.45	5.5	M	35	0.48
mBlueberry2	402	467	51,000	0.48	<2.5	M	35	0.73
Cyan fluorescent proteins								
mTFP1	462	492	64,000	0.85	4.3	M	85	1.62
CyPet	435	477	35,000	0.51	5	M	29	0.53
ECFP	439	476	32,500	0.4	4.7	M	83	0.39
Cerulean	433	475	43,000	0.62	4.7	M	86	0.79
mCFP	433	475	32,500	0.4	4.7	M	87	0.39
SCFPA	433	474	30,000	0.51	4.7	M	88	0.46
Green fluorescent proteins								
Sapphire	399	511	25,000	0.64	4.9	M	89	0.47
T-sapphire	399	511	44,000	0.6	4.9	M	89	0.79
EGFP	484	507	56,000	0.6	6.2	M	90	1
Yellow fluorescent proteins								
Topaz	514	527	94,500	0.6	ND	M	91	1.7
Venus	515	528	92,200	0.57	6	M	92	1.56
mCitrine	516	529	77,000	0.76	5.7	M	93	1.74
YPet	517	530	104,000	0.77	5.6	M	29	2.38
TagYFP	508	524	64,000	0.62	5.5	M	Evrogen	1.18
mBanana	540	553	6,000	0.7	6.7	M	26	0.13
mHoneydew	487/ 504	537/ 562	17,000	0.12	<4	M	26	0.06
SYFP2	515	527	101,000	0.68	6	M	88	2.04
Orange fluorescent proteins								
Kubisara-Orange (mKO)	548	559	51,600	0.6	5	M	94	0.92
mOrange	548	562	71,000	0.69	6.5	M	26	1.45
Red fluorescent proteins								
DsRed	558	583	75,000	0.79	4.7	T	8,30	1.76
DsRed2	561	587	43,800	0.55	ND	T	95	0.72
DsRed dimer2	552	579	60,000	0.69	4.9	pM	30,96	1.23
DsRed T3	560	587	49,500	0.59	ND	T	96	0.87
DsRed T4	555	586	30,300	0.44	ND	T	96	0.4
DsRed tdimer2	552	579	120,000	0.36	4.9	pM	30	1.28
EqFP611	559	611	78,000	0.45	ND	D	97	1.04
EqFP611 dimerV124T	559	611	74,000	0.42	ND	D	98	0.93
mKeima	440	620	14,400	0.21	6.5	m	99	0.09
HcRed	598	645	125,000	0.05	ND	D	21	0.19
HcRed dimer	590	637	160,000	0.04	ND	pM	100	0.19
mRFP1	584	607	50,000	0.25	4.5	M	30	0.37
Tomato	554	581	69,000	0.69	4.7	D	26	1.41
tdTomato	554	581	138,000	0.69	4.7	pM	26	2.83

Note: This table presents a wide variety of available proteins but is in no means an exhaustive list. Some of those indicated are available commercially but most are available for the laboratories in which they were developed. Brightness is defined as the product of the quantum yield (QY) and the extinction coefficient (EC). The brightness of EGFP is defined as M, monomer; T, tetramer; D, dimer; pM, pseudomonomer (expressed as tandem dimer).

λ_{max}^{ex}, wavelength at which excitation is at maximum.

λ_{max}^{em}, wavelength at which emission is at maximum.

in asCP595 and the commercially available kindling fluorescent protein KFP1 [15]. Conversion of the green-emitting Kaede protein to the red-emitting form is believed to involve reactions involving the acylimine (Figure 3.3).

The optical properties of FPs are the result of a complex interplay between the amino acid side chains that contribute to the chromophore environment (protein matrix) and the chromophore itself. Alterations in this protein matrix can have a profound influence upon the optical properties of FPs and CPs. For example, introducing the substitution T203Y into GFP results in a yellow FP having significantly red-shifted optical properties while introduction of the additional substitution, Y145W, essentially eliminates fluorescence emission without compromising light absorption properties [16, 17].

Naturally occurring chromoproteins have been an important source of raw material for the engineering far-red fluorescent proteins such as HcRed [21] or the photoactivatable KFP [15]. The chromophores in highly fluorescent proteins are generally coplanar.

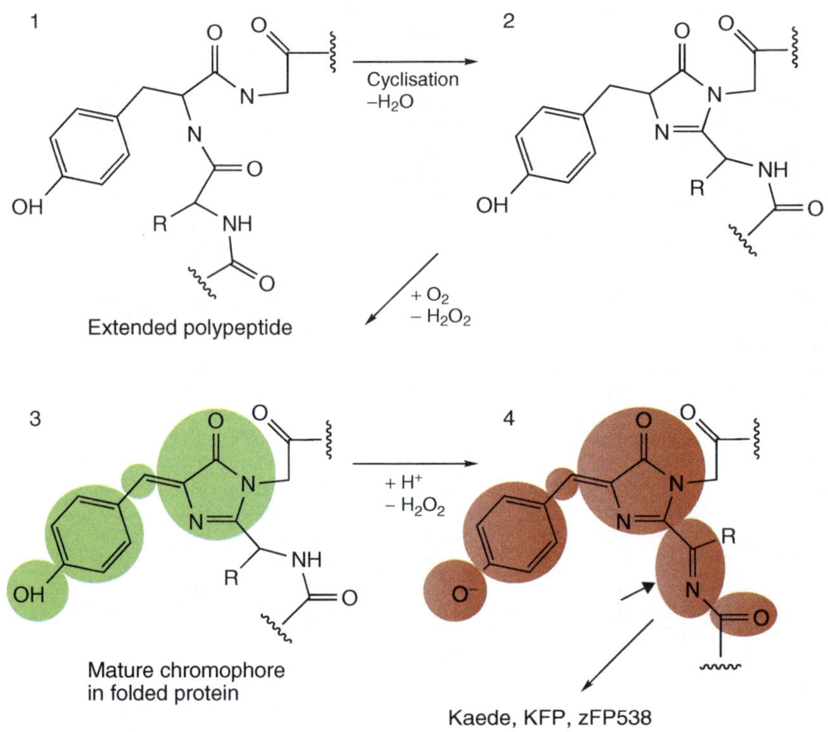

Figure 3.3 Chromophore maturation. Shown are steps leading to formation GFP-like chromophore (3). Subsequent steps involving the addition of an acylimine bond (open arrow) result in formation of a DsRed-like chromophore (4). The extent of the conjugation is shown in green or red shading. The acylimine can be considered the crossroads in the formation of other novel chromophore structures with significantly different optical properties. Correct folding of the polypeptide is essential to provide the necessary 3D arrangement of amino acid side chains catalyzing the chromophore chemistry. Glycine in the chromophore peptide (XYG) is an absolute requirement for chromophore formation. Although XXG can lead to functional a chromophore, only XYG motifs are found in nature.

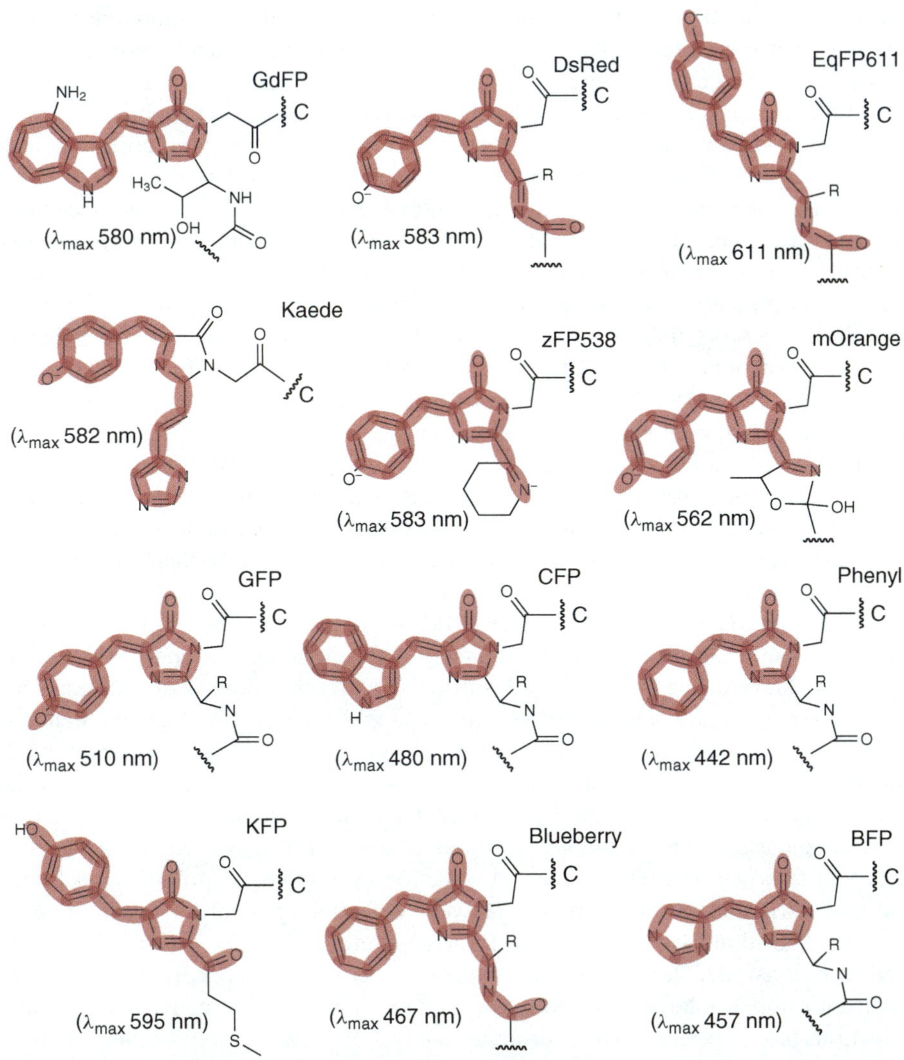

Figure 3.4 Selection of chromophore structures encountered in GFP-like proteins. The chromophore of DsRed and EqFP611 are extended by an acylimine bond and are distinguished by their respective cis and trans conformations with respect to the imidazole ring. Kaede requires UV illumination to generate the red-emitting chromophore by cleavage of the polypeptide backbone. zFP538 and mOrange undergo backbone cleavage during maturation without illumination to generate a second heterocyclic. The chromophore of KFP shown in trans configuration and noncoplanar (not illustrated) isomerizes to a fluorescent cis coplanar configuration upon illumination with intense light. The chromophore structure of some GFP variants is shown in which the tripeptide tyrosine in GFP is substituted by a tryptophan (CFP), histidine (BFP), or phenylalanine (here denoted phenyl). Although a blue fluorescent, the chromophore of Blueberry is extended by an acylimine. GdFP contains the nonnatural amino acid 4-amino tryptophan. The trans noncoplanar tyrosyl ring is responsible for the nonfluorescent properties of KFP and other related chromoproteins. The extent of conjugation in each chromophore is highlighted by shading. The fluorescence emission maximum shown in parentheses for each chromophore type can vary depending on the protein variant. The polypeptide continuing toward the C-terminus (C) is shown. Amino acid side chains are shown (R).

It turns out that fluorescence emission from CPs in which the chromophore is held by the protein matrix in a noncoplanar trans configuration is dramatically reduced [18–20] (Figure 3.3). The biotechnological value of such nonfluorescent proteins or CPs may not be immediately obvious, but such CPs can also be useful. Their high absorbance (large extinction coefficients) enables them to serve as excellent nonfluorescent acceptors for a range of fluorescent acceptors in Förster resonance energy transfer (FRET) applications. For example, Ultramarine, a monomeric CP, can act as an acceptor for donor FP variants emitting in the spectral region from cyan into the orange (Prescott, M., 2008, unpublished data). A nonfluorescent, genetically encoded "dark acceptor," REACh, has recently been developed from yellow fluorescent protein (YFP) [16]. These dark acceptors help to overcome problems of spectral bleed-through between the emission of donor and acceptor FPs and also make available additional spectral bandwidth for monitoring the emissions of other probes that would otherwise have been occupied by the emission of the acceptor.

There is an enormous range of FPs available and space constraints prevent us from covering the various properties of these proteins or their suitability for particular applications. The reader is referred to a number of excellent recent reviews on this subject [22–24]. However, we show a selection of the proteins and their properties in Tables 3.2 and 3.3. The availability of this rainbow of complimentary FPs, with different emission and excitation spectra, allows great flexibility in their application. In suitable combinations they can be used to simultaneously follow multiple events in populations of cells by fluorescence activated cell sorting (FACS) analysis or in individual cells through imaging approaches. Protocols are available for the simultaneous analysis of ternary and quaternary combinations of ECFP/EGFP/EYFP/DsRed by means of flow cytometry [25]. A combination of EGFP, citrine, mBanana, mOrange, mStrawberry, and mCherry were analyzed by flow cytometry using a single excitation at 514 nm and detection using three suitable emission channels [26]. The emission spectra of FPs are quite broad and require careful selection of excitation and emission filters to avoid unwanted spectral bleed-though between detection channels. The use of spectral unmixing algorithms have been useful for separating strongly overlapping fluorescence emissions [27, 28]. These approaches are covered elsewhere in this volume. Significant effort has been invested in optimising FPs for fluorescence energy transfer applications (e.g., see [29]). These proteins can be introduced into live cells, where they allow monitoring of protein interactions, and an increasing range of cellular events and metabolites, through clever design and implementation of biosensors. Some of these biosensors are considered in more detail in a later section (see below).

3.3 "LIFE AND DEATH" OF FLUORESCENT PROTEIN

The literature contains numerous examples describing the successful application of FP technology. Such outcomes are founded upon the considerable effort expended by a number of research groups to overcome inherent problems and generally improve our understanding of their properties. It is important to recognize that, although many of the issues arising from the application of FP technology have been satisfactorily resolved (e.g., oligomerization or slow maturation), commercially available products for one reason or another do not always incorporate the latest advances. Alternately, it is possible that the user may wish to apply some of the latest FPs described in the

TABLE 3.3 Selected Photoactivatable GFP-like Proteins Isolated from Marine Organisms

PAFP Name	Structure	Activation/ Quenching	λ_{max}^{abs} or $\lambda_{max}^{ex}/\lambda_{max}^{em}$ (nm) Before PA	After PA	Fluorescence Change	Fluorescence Contrast	QY Before PA	QY After PA	Source Organism	Supplier
PA-GFP	Monomeric	UV-violet	400/515	504 /517	Increase in green	100	0.13	0.79	*Aequorea victoria* (jellyfish)	
PAmRFP1-1	Tetrameric	UV-violet	578/605	Increase in both	Increase in red	>400	0.2	0.23	*Discosoma* sp. (zoanthid)	Evrogen
PS-CFP	Monomeric	UV-violet	402/468	490/511	Cyan to green	300	0.16	0.23	*Aequorea coerulescens* (jellyfish)	Evrogen
Kaede	Tetrameric	UV-violet	508/518	572/580	Green to red	800	0.88	0.62	*Trachyphyllia geoffroyi* (coral)	MBL Int.
EosFP	Tetrameric	UV-violet	506/516	571/581	Green to red	2000	0.7	0.55	*Lobophyllia hemprichii* (coral)	University of Ulm
mEosFP	Monomeric	UV-violet	505/516	569 /581	Green to red	—	0.64	0.62	*L.* hemprichii (coral)	University of Ulm
lhemOFP	Tetrameric	UV-violet	507/517	542/572	Green to red	—	0.58	0.65	*L.* hemprichii (coral)	University of Ulm
KikGR	Tetrameric	UV-violet	507/517	583/593	Green to red	>2,000	0.7	0.65	*Favia favus* (coral)	MBL Int.
mcavRFP	Tetrameric	UV-violet	504/517	571/582	Green to red	—	0.6	0.6	*Montastrea cavernosa* (coral)	
Dendra2	Monomeric	UV-violet	486/507	553/573	Green to red	350	0.5	0.55	*Dendronephthya* sp. (soft coral)	Evrogen
KFP1	Tetrameric	Green/Blue	Increase at 590	Increase at 600	Kindling	70	<0.001	0.07	*Anemonia sulcata* (jellyfish)	Evrogen
Dronpa	Monomeric	UV-violet/blue	503/518	On/off 503/517	Photoswitching	N/A	N/A	0.85	*Pectinia* sp. (coral)	MBL Int.
mTFP0.7	Monomeric	UV-violet/458	453/488	On/off 453/488	Photoswitching	N/A	N/A	0.5	*Clavularia* sp. (soft coral)	

Note: PA, photoactivation.
λ_{max}^{abs}, wavelength at which absorbance is at maximum.

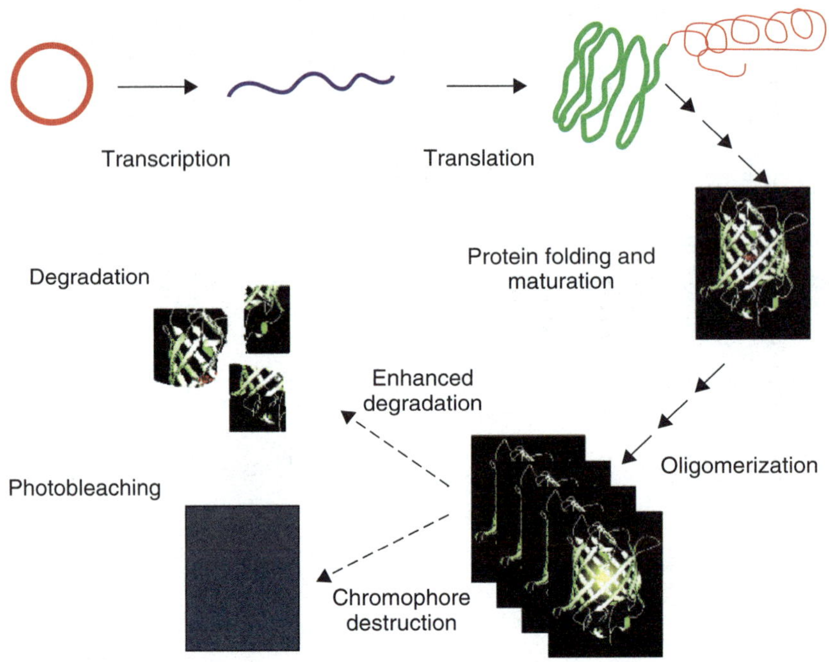

Figure 3.5 Life and death FP. Problems with the application of FPs can arise at each stage in the life and death of a GFP-like protein. Cryptic nuclease recognition sites in the transcribed message can lead to unwanted cleavage loss of mRNA in plants (blue). The use of codons inappropriate for the organism in which it is expressed can result in poor protein expression levels (green). Protein folding can be inefficient at elevated temperatures. Fusion to another protein (red) may also influence the efficiency of folding and maturation. Oligomerization can severely affect the function of fusion proteins. Photobleaching due to excessive illumination can result in destruction of the chromophore. The addition of degradation signals may be required in particular applications to accelerate degradation rates within the cell.

literature whose unique and useful properties have yet to be refined. Therefore, as with any technology, it is useful to have some understanding of the complicating issues.

There are a number of steps leading to the formation of a functional chromophore that must take place in an ordered, efficient, and correct manner. Some of these steps relate to those that are common to all proteins within a cell, while others are unique to GFP-like proteins (e.g., chromophore maturation). Problems can arise at each of the many different steps involved, some of which are summarized in Figure 3.5.

In contrast to the synthetic fluorescent probes which are used after they have been completely synthesized and do not undergo further changes, the GFP-like proteins used as probes undergo an evolution and it makes sense to talk about their "life." The FP molecules must first be synthesized within the cell. Thus, the life of an FP starts with the transcription of a DNA expression cassette encoding the protein to produce a messenger RNA (mRNA). Early investigations identified inappropriate splicing of the FP mRNA in certain organisms, such as plants, and this can prevent proper translation of the message. Fortunately, this is generally no longer a problem. In relation to expression level, it is desirable that the expression of an FP is controlled and driven in an appropriate manner. If possible, the promoter belonging to the gene product to which it is fused should be used to drive expression of the gene cassette. This helps avoid artefacts in localization and function of fusion proteins due to their overexpression.

Translation of the mRNA encoding an FP can, in cells, be inefficient, leading to a dim fluorescence signal. However, this can often be improved by ensuring correct codon use for the organism in which the protein is to be expressed (e.g., yeast or human). Most commercially available expression cassettes are supplied in a "humanized" format, and it is now feasible to have expression cassettes optimally synthesized for a selected expression system. Following translation of the mRNA to form a nascent polypeptide, it must then traffic to the desired subcellular location (e.g., mitochondrion) and assume the β-barrel fold providing the optimal environment for the chemical transformations which occur later. These transformations characterize the process of maturation which encompasses the numerous steps that result in the formation of a functional chromophore.

Researchers hope for the brightest fluorescence signal when labeling their biological samples. Brightness can be considered an operational parameter that is dependent on a number of factors that include the rate of chromophore maturation, the level of protein expression and QY, and molar extinction relevant to fluorescence emission. The detection regime also strongly influences the apparent brightness of the sample. The "true" brightness of an FP (measured in units of millimolars per centimeter) is the product of the EC and the QY. The relative brightness of some FPs is shown in Table 3.2. Brightness can be affected if the protein does not fold correctly or the chromophore maturation is incomplete. Those proteins which are able to absorb photons efficiently and have high fluorescence efficiency will appear the brightest. A high QY is not necessarily sufficient if the EC is low compared to proteins with high QY and high EC.

For quantitative experiments it is vital that a functional chromophore is generated within a timescale consistent with the process being monitored. Some of the early developed FPs, such as DsRed, took many hours or even days for maturation to reach an endpoint as a result of improper or poor folding rates at 37°C [8]. Variants are now available that mature with an average time $t_{1/2}$ for maturation of less than 30 min [22]. Nevertheless, the protein environment remains an important consideration as FPs have been reported to mature at different rates depending on the type of cell in which they are being expressed. Issues of poor or no maturation of the chromophore often arise if attempting to engineer FPs for particular attributes; for example, due to this problem, a significant effort was required to properly engineer mRFP, a fluorescent monomeric variant of DsRed [30].

3.3.1 Oligomerization

Many FPs and CPs are isolated as obligate oligomers and, in addition, can form aggregates (Figure 3.2, Tables 3.2 and 3.3). These properties can result in unwanted oligomerization of the protein to which it is fused, often disrupting its distribution and function and critically affecting the biological phenomenon under investigation (see, e.g., [31]). It is important, where possible, to use FPs that do not oligomerize. Strategies have been developed for generating fluorescent monomers of many such proteins and, in most emission and functional classes, FPs are now available as monomers (Table 3.2). The *av*GFP and many of its variants are often assumed to be monomers but do in fact form weak dimers. From this point of view mCFP and mCitrine represent better choices. Tandem dimers of some dimeric FPs such as HcRed [32] or

Tomato [26] have also been successful in overcoming the problem of oligomerization [33].

3.3.2 Fusion Proteins

In order to facilitate targeting of an FP to a particular cellular location or compartment (e.g., the mitochondrion), the FP is often expressed fused to a relatively short polypeptide of several amino acids. However, many applications require the FP to be expressed fused to a full-length functional protein. While it would appear the majority of proteins can be successfully expressed fused to a particular FP, one must be aware that fusion proteins that fail to express correctly are rarely highlighted in the literature. Failure might be manifested as aggregation in the cell, lack of fluorescence, or an altered biological function. Indeed, FPs have been used as a folding reporter to follow and optimize folding of the protein to which it is fused [34]. In the absence of any prior knowledge about your protein of interest, a useful strategy to consider is expression of alternative constructs in which the FP is fused to either the N- or C-terminus of the protein. The polypeptide linking the two proteins should also be given some consideration. A long linker might help promote folding of the FP and protein to which it is fused and perhaps facilitate interactions with yet other proteins important for its subsequent function once folded. Linker design can be critical for FRET applications. One should be careful to use linkers that do not have protease recognition sites. Finally, although FPs are particularly stable once correctly folded, particular variants sometimes better tolerate fusions to one of its termini [26].

3.3.3 Photobleaching

Not all the light absorbed by a fluorophore is emitted as useful fluorescence. A proportion of the excitation energy may lead to the generation of heat, which in extreme cases can produce significant localized heating of the sample. For live biological specimens this may alter the biology being visualised or, worse, lead to cell death. Alternatively, the excited electron associated with the chromophore may not return to the ground state and its excess energy instead can be channelled into chemical reactions that can lead to the irreversible destruction of the chromophore in a process referred to as photobleaching. This process in FPs is often complex, showing multicomponent decay rates, and its chemistry and precise mechanism remain poorly understood. Photobleaching is also intensity dependent and appears to vary with the type of illumination, such as its wavelength range.

Although the bleaching rate can be much lower than in other commonly used fluorescent labeling reagents, FPs undergo photobleaching in a similar manner, and the selection and the use of FPs need to be carefully considered. For example, some of the early versions of the blue fluorescent proteins (BFPs), such as EBFP (Table 3.2), were notorious for their high photobleaching rates and soon fell out of use to be replaced by the more stable alternative colors such as the significantly more photostable cyan fluorescent protein (CFP) and YFP. This problem now appears to have been overcome with the recent development of new photostable and brighter FPs such as Azurite and Blueberry [35, 36]. It should be noted, however, that the wavelengths of light in the UV used to excite these FPs can be toxic to live cells if exposure is not limited.

There is considerable variation in photostability covering an order of magnitude. A number of commonly available proteins have been compared and a recent review should be consulted for further information [22]. Photobleaching can be a particular problem when the level of fluorescence emission is low and long-term observations of the same subject lasting hours or days are required. The bleaching rate can vary depending upon the type of illumination (arc lamp versus laser) and the efficiency of the detection system. Pulsed illumination featuring temporal pulse separation $>1\mu s$ has been reported to reduce photobleaching to a significant extent through the process of dark-state relaxation [37]. Promising results have also been reported using an approach called controlled light exposure microscopy [38]. Careful attention to the selection of correct and efficient light filters is important in addition to limiting excitation light. Nevertheless, photobleaching is often not under the control of the experimenter but is dictated by the expression level of the FP in the cell. Photoxicity due to the generation of reactive oxygen species (ROS) by the excitation of FPs is also an important consideration in live cell experiments. On the other hand, if carefully controlled, as in the process of chromophore-assisted light inactivation (CALI), ROS production can be a very useful tool [39, 40] (see Section 3.4).

Moreover, it has been demonstrated recently that the experimental settings commonly used during routine imaging experiments may induce a phenomenon of reversible photobleaching of a number of GFP-like proteins, including such commonly used FPs as eCFP or eYFP [41]. The resulting steady-state fluorescence reflects a variable equilibrium between reversible photobleaching, spontaneous recovery, and light-induced recovery. The mechanism of the reversible photobleaching is linked to avGFP's complex photochromic behavior and can cause significant artifacts in commonly applied imaging techniques that utilize photobleach-based FRET determinations and FRAP assays.

3.3.4 Destabilization

The fluorescence emission of GFP-like proteins once they are correctly folded and fully matured has been shown to be remarkably stable when exposed to a number of different harsh treatments, including denaturants, temperature, and proteases [42]. Their optical properties are often maintained despite months or even years of storage on the laboratory bench, even in the presence of bacterial contamination. Their robust nature in part explains their remarkable general applicability. However, this increased stability has proven to be a problem in certain applications. For example, if attempting to follow the dynamics of promoter activity, the persistence of the fluorescence signal can mask subsequent reductions in expression. Destabilized forms of GFP have been generated through the addition of appropriate degradation signals that deliver the protein to the proteasome for degradation [43, 44]. The half-life in vivo could be reduced from 26 h to between 2 and 10 h depending on the application. This generally applicable strategy for reducing stability has been applied to a number of proteins such DsRed and HcRed to reportedly yield proteins with reduced half-lives [45].

The structural stability of FPs and CPs can be a distinct advantage when monitoring the events in organelles such as mammalian lysosome or vacuole of yeast. Proteins in these organelles are exposed to low pH ($\sim$5.0) and a cocktail of hydrolases. FPs have been particularly important for elucidating the mechanism of autophagy, an evolutionarily conserved process that delivers cellular constituents to these organelles for recycling [46]. Remarkably, FP emission is readily observed in these organelles when these proteins are targeted to the organelle for degradation.

3.4 APPLICATIONS

GFP-like proteins can be considered as tools that are passive, active, or interactive (Figure 3.6). The majority of applications fall into the passive group, examples of which are protein trafficking studies, monitoring promoter activity, and labeling of organelles. Also included in this category are applications of photactivatable proteins. The active category is a rapidly expanding group of applications that encompasses FPs that have been configured as biosensors to report on some aspect of their environment. Finally, the interactive group is a relatively new and exciting group of applications that allows for the manipulation of events in the cell by using light. For many applications unwanted fluctuations in the fluorescence emission of an FP, say due to pH variations, might be considered by some to be a nuisance. However, sensitizing FPs to particular aspects of their environment is the key to developing an ever-increasing range of useful and remarkable biosensors. Several approaches have been adopted for developing such tools, and some of these are summarized schematically in Figure 3.7. FP biosensors can be based on a single β-barrel or a combination of suitable FPs that are linked by some functional groups. Examples of the former are sensors for pH and redox equilibrium (Figure 3.7, 1–2). In each case the binding of ligands to these biosensors alters fluorescence emission in a predictable manner. The insertion into key regions of the β-barrel of specific effector domains borrowed from other proteins (Figure 3.7, 1–2) extends greatly the possibilities. HyPer, a reporter for hydrogen peroxide, is a recent example of this class of biosensor [47]. Biosensors containing more than one FP usually rely on the phenomenon of FRET. In general, the distance between the donor and acceptor FPs is controlled by a functional group (Figure 3.7, 4–7). Some examples of biosensors and their applications are shown in Table 3.4.

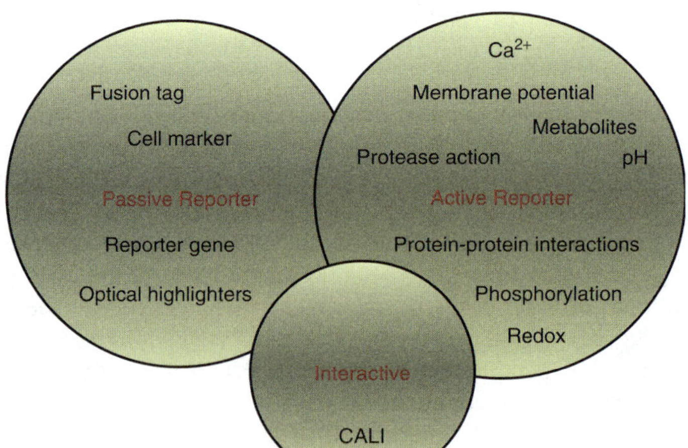

Figure 3.6 Applications of GFP-like proteins may be divided into three categorises. Active reporters alter their optical properties in response to a cellular parameter such as pH or metabolite. The optical properties of passive reporters are expected to be stable, but in the case of optical highlighters they can be altered by illumination with light of specific wavelengths. Particular GFP-like proteins when strongly illuminated can interact with and usefully perturb their cellular environment in a CALI process.

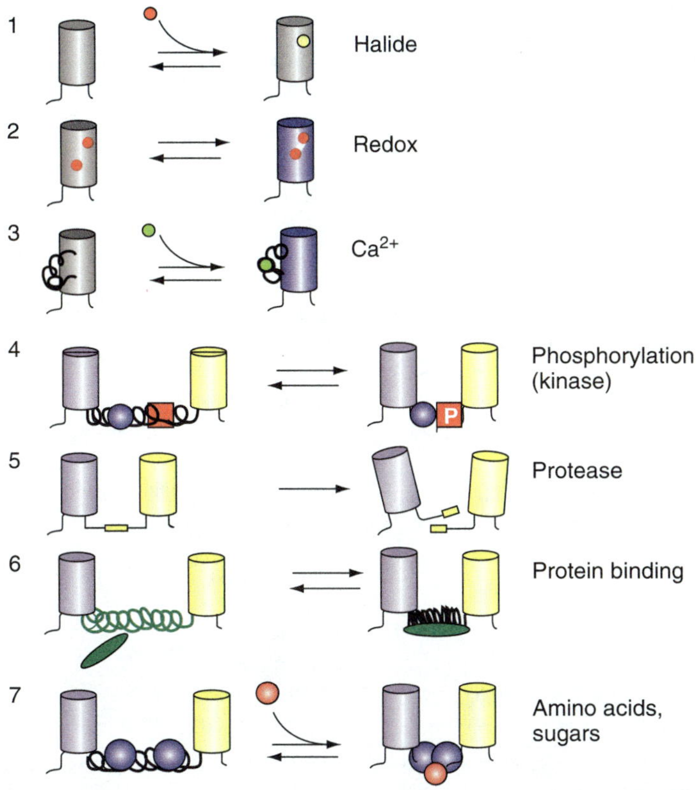

Figure 3.7 Example biosensors based on single or two linked FPs. The N- and C-termini are shown extending from the β-can of each FP. Chromophore ionization and fluorescence emission of particular FPs can be sensitive to pH or the binding of halides (yellow circle) (1). The strategic introduction of a pair of redox-active cysteines (red circles) (2) or Ca^{2+} binding motifs (black loop) (3) can, upon reduction or binding of Ca^{2+} (green circles), respectively, lead to measurable changes in fluorescence emission (shown as the grey-to-blue color change). Linking two FPs (cyan and yellow) suitable for fluorescence energy transfer expands the range of cellular processes that can be monitored. The distance between FPs and FRET efficiency can be modulated by including functional protein domains in the polypeptide linker (black spiral). Example are biosensors for (4) phosphorylation (kinase activity) which contain protein domains (blue circle and red square) in the linker that interact when phosphorylated (P); (5) protease activity in which the linker contains a protease recognition site (yellow oblong); (6) protein–protein interactions where a domain in the linker interacts with other proteins (green elipse); or (7) metabolites such as sugars and amino acids (red polygon) that interact allosterically with the linker containing their cognate binding proteins (blue circles).

3.5 PASSIVE APPLICATIONS

Photoactivatable fluorescent proteins (PAFPs) either alter their fluorescence intensity without extensive photodestruction or switch from one color to another. They have been variably referred to as photoactivatable, photoswitchable, or photoconvertible proteins [48–50]. The development of the use of PAFPs in optical marking technology for differentially highlighting and tracking cells, organelles, and fusion proteins represents

TABLE 3.4 Selected FP Configurations and Applications

Biosensor or Configuration	Substrate/Phenomenon	References
Monomolecular sensors		
rxYFP149/202	Redox (nonratiometric)	79
roGFP	Redox (ratiometric)	103
Hyper	Hydrogen peroxide	47
YFP^{H148Q}	Chloride	77
FlaSH	Voltage	104
Camgaroo	Calcium	70
Pericam	Calcium	71
Phluorins (ratiometric and ecliptic, superecliptic) and other GFP variants	pH	75,105
Timer	Temporal events	61
Biomolecular sensors		
Cameleon	Calcium	106
CyPet-Ypet	Caspase 3 (protease activity)	29
GFP-DsRed.T3 fusion	Autophagy (pH)	107
Rango	RanGTP	108
AKAR	cAMP kinase activity (PKA)	109,110
Cygnet	cGMP	111
FLIPglu	Glucose	72
FLIIPE	Glutamate	72
FLIPmal	Maltose	72
FLIPPi	Phosphate	74

Note: Examples are included to the range of events that may be monitored. The list is not intended to be comprehensive and there are many other examples in the literature.

the "second generation" of GFP-based tools [48] as they enable direct photolabeling. They are now replacing the more traditional technology of indirect analysis of fluorescence kinetics in or out of a photobleached region, as in the technique of fluorescence recovery after photobleaching (FRAP) discussed elsewhere in this book. The advantage of photoactivation is that it requires less energy than bleaching. In FRAP, subpopulations of molecules, proteins, or organelles that move rapidly and have a short residence time are bleached and therefore often undetectable, whereas by using PAFPs these can be monitored. PAFPs allow the spatial detection of the successive translocations of proteins in a cell and therefore provide a visual, pulse-chase, real-time view of protein dynamics. There are several types of PAFPs grouped on the basis of their behavior in response to light of specific wavelengths (Figure 3.8, Table 3.3).

3.5.1 Photoamplifying PAFPs

These variants increase their fluorescence intensity following photoactivation by light and include PA-GFP, an optimized variant of *av*GFP [51]. Irradiation with UV (400-nm) light results in stabilization of the bright-emitting anionic (λ_{max}^{ex} 504 nm, λ_{max}^{em} 517 nm) chromophore state through irreversible decarboxylation of an amino acid side chain contacting the very dim neutral chromophore (λ_{max}^{ex} 400 nm). Fluorescence emission at 517 nm is consequently increased ~100-fold.

(a)
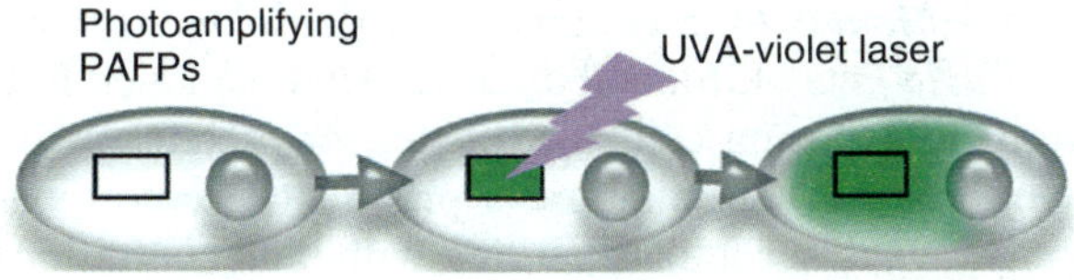

(b)
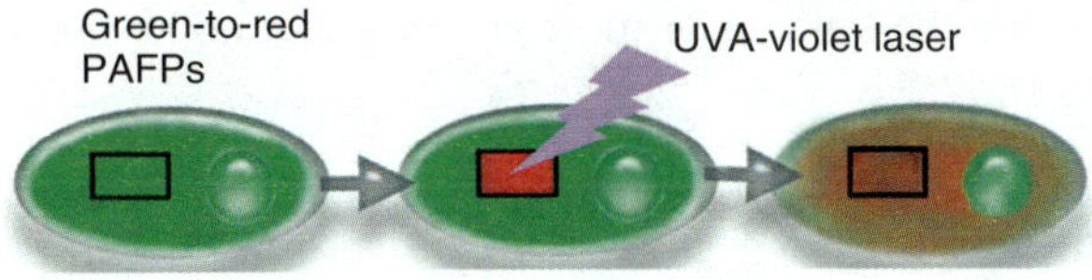

(c)
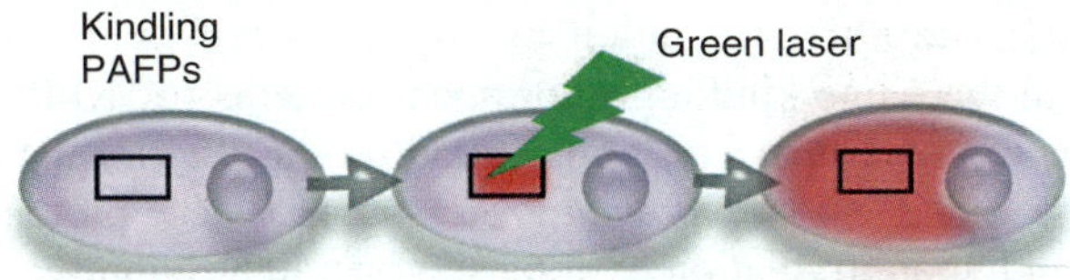

(d)
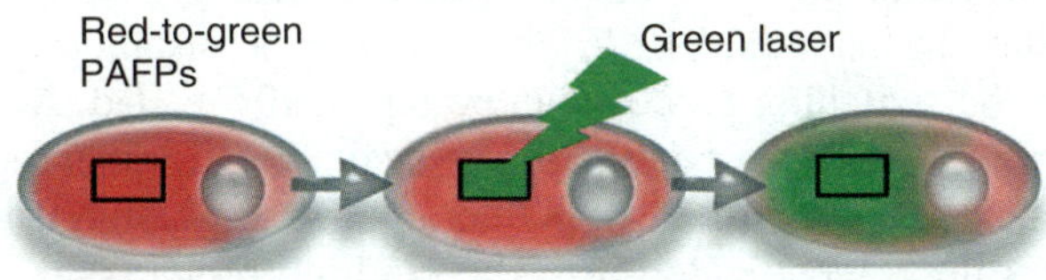

Figure 3.8 Applications of different types of photactivatable FPs. The square in a cell, which is shown with a circular nucleus, represents an area of interest (AOI) irradiated (arrow) by a selected laser line and causing irradiated molecules to become fluorescent or to change color. (*a*) PAFPs, such as PA-GFP, change from a dim (504-nm) to a bright (517-nm) form upon irradiation by 405-nm laser, showing that movement of fluorescently labeled molecules is restricted by the nuclear membrane. (*b*) Green-to-red PAFPs convert to a red form by UV-violet light irradiation, converting to a red form. (*c*) Kindling PAFPs convert from a purple-blue nonfluorescent form to a bright red fluorescent form at green light irradiation. (d) Red-to-green PAFPs convert to a bright and stable green form after irradiation by certain wavelengths, in this case by green light.

3.5.2 Photoconverting PAFPs

In these variants, irradiation by light of specific wavelength, most commonly by near UV, causes a change of color. The *cyan-to-green*-converting PS-CFP was developed from the jellyfish *Aequorea coerulescens* and is believed to have a similar mechanism of photoactivation to PA-GFP [52]. Photoconversion is irreversible and causes an ~300-fold increase in green and a corresponding 5-fold decrease in cyan fluorescence (resulting in green-to-cyan fluorescence ratio of 1500-fold).

The *green-to-red* PAFPs are an even more exciting type of photoconverters, at first accidentally discovered by the Japanese researchers when a GFP cloned from the coral *Trachyphylia geoffroyi* was accidentally exposed to sunlight and turned red after exposure to UV. They called the protein Kaede after maple leaves [53]. This group includes the green-to-red converters, such as tetrameric EosFP, and the monomeric mEosFP, from *Lobophyllia hemprichii*, named after the Greek goddess of dawn [54];

mcavRFP from coral *Montastraea cavernosa* [55]; *Ricordea florida* (rfloRFP) [55]; KikGR from coral *Favia favus* [56]; and dimeric Dendra, cloned from *Dendronephthya* sp. [57]. By selectively exposing cells, organelles, or proteins of interest labeled with green-to-red converters to UV irradiation, a pronounced color change from green to red occurs, enabling advanced cellular marking with high contrast. These proteins were shown to be good trackers of cellular dynamics where a small cell area is color changed by UV irradiation and the kinetics of molecule or protein diffusion can thus be studied (Figure 3.8).

3.5.3 Kindling PAFPs

These proteins are homologous to GFP, but surprisingly they were found to acquire bright red fluorescence after irradiation by intense green light, which is referred to as kindling, hence the name kindling fluorescent proteins (or KFPs). Kindling optical behavior was first discovered in a protein asFP595 (or asulCP), isolated from the purple tentacle tips of the sea anemone, *Anemonia sulcata* [15]. The protein asFP595 absorbs light at 568 nm and upon irradiation by intense green light fluoresces at $\lambda_{em} = 595$ nm. Kindling is a reversible process—the fluorescent state gradually relaxes back to a nonfluorescent state in the dark. The bright form can be instantly quenched by a flash of blue light and the switching process can be repeatedly cycled. An enhanced form of asulFP595, known as KFP1, is commercially available (from Evrogen). A model for kindling mechanism proposed that it was due to cis–trans isomerization of the excited chromophore to a fluorescent state [58]. The kindling proteins are nonfluorescent but strongly light absorbing and, consequently, are brightly colored.

Red-to-green photoconverters convert from a red to a green form following irradiation at a specific wavelength. The best known example is DsRed, which requires femtosecond irradiation ($\lambda < 760$ nm) that bleaches the red species of the tetramer and causes the fluorescence of the green species, which is normally quenched by FRET, to be enhanced (Figure 3.8*d*). Other GFP-type proteins may require different wavelengths of single- and multiphoton excitation to achieve conversion and may use different mechanisms of returning to green, referred to as greening. This greening property is used as a powerful technique for selective optical marking of specific regions of cells and protein layers. The greening method can be used to label entire cells expressing DsRed protein as well as optical labeling of defined subcellular regions and fusion proteins restricted within discrete organelles [59]. Another type of reversibly photoswitching PAFP, such as Dronpa, convert from a bright fluorescent green to a very low fluorescent form after irradiation by blue light that quenches fluorescence, while irradiation by UV (~400 nm) reswitched fluorescence [60]. The on–off switching process can be repeated many times in a single cell thanks to a molecular mechanism similar to kindling. Although the above methods of optically marking cells are very useful, many have drawbacks, including dimness, photoconversion instability, and oligomerization. Consequently, the search for GFP-like proteins with novel and optimized photoproperties is currently of great scientific interest.

3.5.4 Fluorescent Timers

The passage of time is fundamental to all biological systems fluorescent timers. A group of recently found GFP-like proteins that change color from green to red during maturation or green to yellow (due to a mix of green and red forms), such as DsRed (drFP583), zoan2RFP, mcavRFP, and rfloRFP, are known as fluorescent timers [55]. The fluorescence emission of E5, a mutant of the red fluorescent protein drFP583, was found to change from green to red with a rate that was independent of protein concentration [61]. It can be used to monitor both activation and down regulation of target promoters on the whole-organism scale. The ratio of green to red emission has been used to track expression from the heat-shock-dependent promoter in *Caenorhabditis elegans* and from the *Otx*-2 promoter in developing *Xenopus* embryos.

3.6 ACTIVE APPLICATIONS

3.6.1 Protein–Protein Interactions

Protein–protein interactions underpin the architecture, structure, and activity of the cell, and understanding the temporal and spatial distribution of such interactions in living cells is the key to understanding cellular function. Fluorescent proteins, including the photoactive FPs, can be used in one of two techniques to report on protein–protein interactions: fragment complementation and FRET-based applications.

Fragment Complementation FPs derived from *A. victoria* can be expressed individually as two defined fragments neither of which possess a functional chromophore [62, 63]. If association of these fragments is promoted through their expression fused to interacting proteins, a functional chromophore will be formed which is optically active (Figure 3.9). Combinations of fragments from different FP variants can recombine to produce different colors. This approach can be multiplexed so that one can optically differentiate between different reaction outcomes. This method has very high signal-to-noise ratio but is not suited for monitoring reversible reactions.

FRET When two fluorophores or, in this case FPs, are brought into close proximity, nonradiative energy transfer (FRET) can take place between the donor and acceptor fluorophore molecules. This process has been described elsewhere in this volume (Chapter 8). The efficiency of FRET is dependent on a number of parameters including spectral overlap, relative dipole orientation, and molecular distance. There are a number of different donor/acceptor pairs suitable for FRET, and they continue to be developed and optimized. Most recently a coevolution strategy has led to the development of an optimized cyan–yellow combination, Cy-Pet and Y-Pet, with very high FRET efficiency [29]. It is likely the newly available BFPs such as Azurite and Blueberry 2 will be useful for FRET applications when partnered with suitable FP acceptors.

The photophysical consequences of FRET allow the phenomenon to be monitored in a number of different ways discussed in a separate chapter concerned with FRET. For example, monitoring the fluorescence lifetime (FLIM) of donor emission alone eliminates the problem of donor/acceptor crosstalk. In this case the acceptor need not be fluorescent; an example here is a genetically encoded nonfluorescent acceptor such as REACh [16].

Monitoring FRET between an FP and another organic dye can be useful for monitoring interaction between proteins and other molecules. For example, the interaction of DNA-binding proteins with nuclear DNA labeled with the Sytox dyes is readily followed [64].

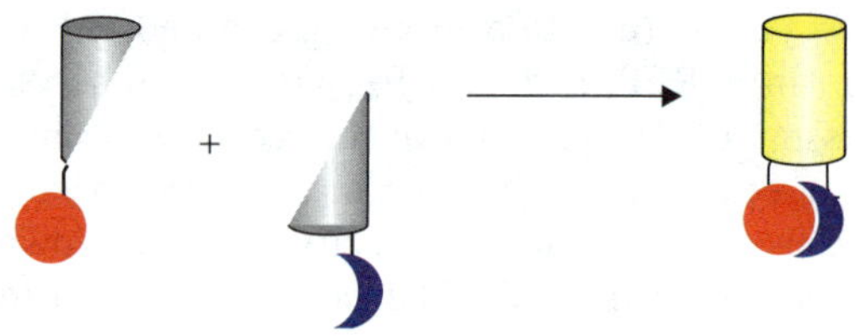

Figure 3.9 Bimolecular fluorescence complementation. Variants of GFP can be separately expressed as two nonfluorescent but complementary fragments (grey sectors) that when combined will produce a functional chromophore. Expressing each complementary fragment fused to one of a pair of interacting proteins (red circle or blue crescent) can promote the correct assembly of the fluorescent protein barrel (yellow barrel) to form a functional chromophore.

3.6.2 Monitoring Enzyme Activity

Translocation The fusion of FPs to domains that upon modification undergo translocation to different regions of the cell has been used with great success for following enzyme activities. Autophagy is a process that involves the sequestration of cellular components in a specialized vesicle or autophagosome for delivery to the lysosome for degradation. LC-3, a marker for the autophagosome, is recruited to the developing autophagosome from the cytosol after proteolytic processing and lipidation. This translocation event is readily observed in cells expressing GFP-LC3 [65]. There are many other examples of this strategy, particularly in studies of cellular signalling. Examples include translocation sensors for Rho small guanosine triphosphatases (GTPases) and G-protein activation [66] or translocation of pleckstrin homology domains to the plasma membrane as sensors of phospholipase activity [67].

FRET Biosensors The inclusion between FPs suitable for FRET of domains that when modified alter the efficiency of FRET between the donor and the acceptor extends the number of different activities that can be monitored. The inclusion of a Caspase 3 protease recognition site (DEVD) in the linking polypeptide allows enzyme activation to be monitored during apoptosis or cell death due to cleavage of the linker, separation of the donor and acceptor, and loss of FRET [29]. Since proteolysis is irreversible, the signal from these biosensors once activated cannot be readily turned off. Other FRET sensors are fully reversible. The inclusion of a polypeptide domain(s) that when phosphorylated undergo conformational rearrangements allows a range of different phosphorylation events or protein kinase activity to be monitored via alterations in FRET [68].

3.6.3 Monitoring Small Molecules and Metabolites

Many biosensors for following intracellular levels of key metabolites rely on allosteric binding of molecules to effector domains. Conformational alterations in calmodulin upon binding calcium have been used to alter the FRET between suitable pairs of FPs. This has been achieved by using conformational changes in calmodulin to alter the distance between FRET pairs [69] (Figure 3.7). Alternatively, single-FP biosensors have been developed where the binding domain is inserted at key positions in the β-barrel of the FP [70, 71].

Bacteria periplasmic binding proteins (bPBPs) represent a diverse superfamily whose members undergo significant conformational change when binding their cognate ligand. Such ligands include amino acids, sugars, and ions. A range of FRET-metabolite sensors have been developed using bPBPs as their binding domain. These include sensors for glucose, sucrose, maltose, glutamate, and most recently phosphate [72–74] (Figure 3.7).

3.6.4 Monitoring pH and Other Small Molecules

The pH and its variations over physiological values can affect the emission of FPs if the pK_a governing ionization of the chromophore falls within a suitable range. Such proteins include the commonly used EGFP and YFP (Table 3.2). One can avoid these effects by using FPs with fluorescence emission which is relatively insensitive to pH, such as DsRed, with stable emission over the pH range between 4 and 11. The use of these proteins is desirable if one wishes to monitor acidic compartments of cells such as the lysosome (pH $\sim$ 5.0). On the other hand, these apparent disadvantages of pH sensitivity can be usefully employed to follow alterations in pH in different compartments of live cells by selecting an FP with a suitable pK_a (Table 3.2). A number of FP variants are available that have been optimized for monitoring pH [75, 76].

It is useful to note that halides are able to gain access to the chromophore of particular FPs and alter their optical properties. A variant YFP has been successfully employed to monitor halide concentrations in cells [77]. Halides can also alter the optical properties of chromoproteins such as Rtms5 but have yet to be developed into useful probes [78].

3.6.5 Monitoring Redox

Redox equilibrium is a key cellular parameter. Changes in redox state of the cell are implicated in many key cellular processes, including growth, stress response, and gene transcription. The introduction of pairs of redox-active cysteines into the structure of the β-barrel makes fluorescence emission sensitive to the redox activity (Figure 3.7). The formation of a disulfide bond results in a localized distortion of the β-barrel and useful alterations in fluorescence emission due to changes in the chromophore environment [79]. Improved sensors, roGFPs, based on GFP, have been developed that have ratiometric dual-excitation/single-emission output overcoming the artefacts associated with probes having nonratiometric outputs (Table 3.4) [80].

3.7 INTERACTIVE APPLICATIONS

One of the key advantages of FP technology (Table 3.1) is the ability to monitor in a noninvasive manner specific events in living cells. Cells contain many endogenous chromophores (e.g., nucleotides and aromatic amino acids) that can interact with light, particularly in the UV, and lead to unwanted photochemistry and cellular damage due to the production of ROS, which are highly reactive, have very short half-lives, and travel only short distances in cells. The illumination of exogenous fluorescent probes such as FPs may also have undesirable phototoxic effects. Well-designed live cell experiments limit the exposure of cells to the intense excitation light. However, if the light source is sufficiently intense and focused ($\sim 10^6$ greater than used in conventional confocal imaging applications), significant quantities of ROS may be produced whose level is dependent on the concentration of the fluorophore, illumination intensity, and efficiency of ROS production by that fluorophore. The highly reactive nature of the ROS can be usefully employed to inactivate targets within their sphere of influence in the CALI process, one of the few viable methods capable of modulating target protein function in a spatial and temporal manner in the cell. Organic dyes, such as malachite green, are particularly efficient at ROS production. The expression of EGFP fused with proteins of interest allows ROS production to be temporally and spatially localized to specific biological processes in living cells [39]. The efficiency of ROS by particular FPs upon illumination is determined by the chromophore environment in a way which has yet to be systematically investigated. For example, "Killer Red" (KR), a red fluorescent protein developed from a chromoprotein, yields in excess of 100-fold greater quantities of ROS compared to other commonly available FPs such as DsRed [40]. The biological activity of proteins expressed fused to KR can be readily inactivated in living cells on illumination with light of an appropriate wavelength (Figure 3.10). KR is an example of a new class of tool: genetically encoded photosensitizers that will be extremely important for investigation of molecular networks. Variants that are monomeric with alternative excitation wavelengths and yet more efficient ROS producers are eagerly awaited by the research community.

3.8 CONCLUSIONS

Although most researchers will, to some extent, be familiar with GFP technology, it is likely many will not be aware of how extensive are its capabilities. In this brief overview we have attempted to demonstrate the enormous range of GFP-like proteins that are now available and some different ways in which they are being applied. We have also attempted to provide some idea of the complexity underlying their structure and some issues relating to their applications.

The technology continues to evolve and would appear that applications are limited only by the imagination and, of course, hard work and persistence of the researcher.

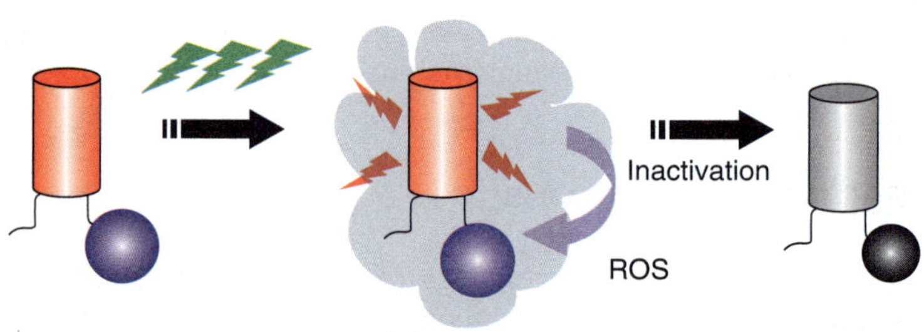

Figure 3.10 Chromophore-assisted light inactivation using FP. The red FP, KillerRed (KR; red barrel) yields significantly more ROS than other commonly used FPs. The "cloud" of ROS (blue shading) produced upon illumination of KR chromophore with intense light (green lightning bolts) can inactivate (blue arrow) the biological activity of a target protein (blue sphere) to which KR is fused or otherwise in close proximity. The process results in destruction of the KR chromophore (grey shading).

We are set to witness, in the coming years, the application of optimized versions of these proteins for imaging events in cells at superresolution, as was foreshadowed in recent publications [81, 82].

REFERENCES

1. F. H. Johnson, O. Shimomura, Y. Saiga, G. Gershman, G. T. Reynolds, and J. R. Waters, *J. Cell. Comp. Physiol.* **60**, 85–103 (1962).
2. O. Shimomura, F. H. Johnson, and Y. Saiga, *J. Cell. Comp Physiol.* **59**, 223–240 (1962).
3. D. C. Prasher, V. K. Eckenrode, V. W. Ward, F. G. Prendergast, and M. J. Cormier, *Gene* **111**(2), 229–233 (1992).
4. M. Chalfie, Y. Tu, G. Euskirchen, W. W. Ward, and D. C. Prasher, *Science* **263**(5148), 802–805 (1994).
5. S. G. Dove, O. Hoegh-Guldberg, and S. Ranganathan, *Coral Reefs* **19**, 197–204 (2001).
6. A. Salih, A. Larkum, G. Cox, M. Kuhl, and O. Hoegh-Guldberg, *Nature* **408**(6814), 850–853 (2000).
7. F. Oswald, F. Schmitt, A. Leutenegger, S. Ivanchenko, C. D'Angelo, A. Salih, S. Maslakova, M. Bulina, R. Schirmbeck, G. U. Nienhaus, M. V. Matz, and J. Wiedenmann, *FEBS J.* **274**(4), 1102–1109 (2007).
8. M. V. Matz, A. F. Fradkov, Y. A. Labas, A. P. Savitsky, A. G. Zaraisky, M. L. Markelov, and S. A. Lukyanov, *Nat. Biotechnol.* **17**(10), 969–973 (1999).
9. J. G. Morin and J. W. Hastings, *J. Cell Physiol.* **77**(3), 313–318 (1971).
10. S. F. Field, M. Y. Bulina, I. V. Kelmanson, J. P. Bielawski, and M. V. Matz, *J. Mol. Evol.* **62**(3), 332–339 (2006).
11. N. Agmon, *Biophys. J.* **88**(4), 2452–2461 (2005).
12. M. Hopf, W. Gohring, A. Ries, R. Timpl, and E. Hohenester, *Nat. Struct. Biol.* **8**(7), 634–640 (2001).
13. H. J. Bae, M. Rubini, G. Jung, G. Wiegand, M. H. Seifert, M. K. Azim, J. S. Kim, A. Zumbusch, T. A. Holak, L. Moroder, R. Huber, and N. Budisa, *J. Mol. Biol.* **328**(5), 1071–1081 (2003).
14. L. A. Gross, G. S. Baird, R. C. Hoffman, K. K. Baldridge, and R. Y. Tsien, *Proc. Natl. Acad. Sci. USA* **97**(22), 11990–11995 (2000).
15. D. M. Chudakov, V. V. Belousov, A. G. Zaraisky, V. V. Novoselov, D. B. Staroverov, D. B. Zorov, S. Lukyanov, and K. A. Lukyanov, *Nat. Biotechnol.* **21**(2), 191–194 (2003).
16. S. Ganesan, S. M. Ameer-Beg, T. T. Ng, B. Vojnovic, and F. S. Wouters, *Proc. Natl. Acad. Sci. USA* **103**(11), 4089–4094 (2006).
17. M. Ormo, A. B. Cubitt, K. Kallio, L. A. Gross, R. Y. Tsien, and S. J. Remington, *Science* **273**(5280), 1392–1395 (1996).
18. M. Prescott, M. Ling, T. Beddoe, A. J. Oakley, S. Dove, O. Hoegh-Guldberg, R. J. Devenish, and J. Rossjohn, *Structure* **11**(3), 275–284 (2003).
19. P. G. Wilmann, J. Petersen, R. J. Devenish, M. Prescott, and J. Rossjohn, *J. Biol. Chem.* **280**(4), 2401–2404 (2005).
20. P. G. Wilmann, J. Petersen, A. Pettikiriarachchi, A. M. Buckle, S. C. Smith, S. Olsen, M. A. Perugini, R. J. Devenish, M. Prescott, and J. Rossjohn, *J. Mol. Biol.* **349**(1), 223–237 (2005).
21. N. G. Gurskaya, A. F. Fradkov, A. Terskikh, M. V. Matz, Y. A. Labas, V. I. Martynov, Y. G. Yanushevich, K. A. Lukyanov, and S. A. Lukyanov, *FEBS Lett.* **507**(1), 16–20 (2001).

22. N. C. Shaner, P. A. Steinbach, and R. Y. Tsien. *Nat. Methods* **2**(12), 905–909 (2005).
23. B. N. Giepmans, S. R. Adams, M. H. Ellisman, and R. Y. Tsien, *Science* **312**(5771), 217–224 (2006).
24. S. G. Olenych, G. K. Claxton, G. K. Ottenberg, and M. W. Davidson, *Curr. Protocols Cell Biol.* **21.5**(33), 1–33 (2006).
25. T. S. Hawley, D. J. Herbert, S. S. Eaker, and R. G. Hawley, *Methods Mol. Biol.* **263**, 219–238 (2004).
26. N. C. Shaner, R. E. Campbell, P. A. Steinbach, B. N. Giepmans, A. E. Palmer, and R. Y. Tsien, *Nat. Biotechnol.* **22**(12), 1567–1572 (2004).
27. T. Zimmermann, J. Rietdorf, and R. Pepperkok, *FEBS Lett.* **546**(1), 87–92 (2003).
28. T. Zimmermann, J. Rietdorf, A. Girod, V. Georget, and R. Pepperkok, *FEBS Lett.* **531**(2), 245–249 (2002).
29. A. W. Nguyen and P. S. Daugherty, *Nat. Biotechnol.* **23**(3), 355–360 (2005).
30. R. E. Campbell, O. Tour, A. E. Palmer, P. A. Steinbach, G. S. Baird, D. A. Zacharias, and R. Y. Tsien, *Proc. Natl. Acad. Sci. USA* **99**(12), 7877–7882 (2002).
31. P. D. Gavin, M. Prescott, S. E. Luff, and R. J. Devenish, *J. Cell Sci.* **117**(Pt. 11), 2333–2343 (2004).
32. M. E. Bulina, V. V. Verkhusha, D. B. Staroverov, D. M. Chudakov, and K. A. Lukyanov, *Biochem. J.* **371**(Pt. 1), 109–114 (2003).
33. J. Zhang, R. E. Campbell, A. Y. Ting, and R. Y. Tsien, *Nat. Rev. Mol. Cell Biol.* **3**(12), 906–918 (2002).
34. G. S. Waldo, B. M. Standish, J. Berendzen, and T. C. Terwilliger, *Nat. Biotechnol.* **17**(7), 691–695 (1999).
35. H. W. Ai, N. C. Shaner, Z. Cheng, R. Y. Tsien, and R. E. Campbell, *Biochemistry* **46**(20), 5904–5910 (2007).
36. M. A. Mena, T. P. Treynor, S. L. Mayo, and P. S. Daugherty, *Nat. Biotechnol.* **24**(12), 1569–1571 (2006).
37. G. Donnert, C. Eggeling, and S. W. Hell, *Nat. Methods* **4**(1), 81–86 (2007).
38. R. A. Hoebe, C. H. Van Oven, T. W. Gadella, Jr., P. B. Dhonukshe, C. J. Van Noorden, and E. M. Manders, *Nat. Biotechnol.* **25**(2), 249–253 (2007).
39. T. Surrey, M. B. Elowitz, P. E. Wolf, F. Yang, F. Nedelec, K. Shokat, and S. Leibler, *Proc. Natl. Acad. Sci. USA* **95**(8), 4293–4298 (1998).
40. M. E. Bulina, D. M. Chudakov, O. V. Britanova, Y. G. Yanushevich, D. B. Staroverov, T. V. Chepurnykh, E. M. Merzlyak, M. A. Shkrob, S. Lukyanov, and K. A. Lukyanov, *Nat. Biotechnol.* **24**(1), 95–99 (2006).
41. D. Sinnecker, P. Voigt, N. Hellwig, and M. Schaefer, *Biochemistry* **44**(18), 7085–7094 (2005).
42. W. W. Ward and S. H. Bokman, *Biochemistry* **21**(19), 4535–4540 (1982).
43. X. Li, X. Zhao, Y. Fang, X. Jiang, T. Duong, C. Fan, C. C. Huang, and S. R. Kain, *J. Biol. Chem.* **273**(52), 34970–34975 (1998).
44. X. Zhao, T. Duong, C. C. Huang, S. R. Kain, and X. Li *Methods Enzymol.* **302**, 32–38 (1999).
45. *Clontechniques*, BO Biosciences **17**(4) (2002).
46. D. J. Klionsky, A. M. Cuervo, and P. O. Seglen, *Autophagy* **3**(3), 181–206 (2007).
47. V. V. Belousov, A. F. Fradkov, K. A. Lukyanov, D. B. Staroverov, K. S. Shakhbazov, A. V. Terskikh, and S. Lukyanov, *Nat. Methods* **3**(4), 281–286 (2006).
48. G. H. Patterson and J. Lippincott-Schwartz, *Methods* **32**(4), 445–450 (2004).

49. K. A. Lukyanov, D. M. Chudakov, S. Lukyanov, and V. V. Verkhusha, *Nat. Rev. Mol. Cell Biol.* **6**(11), 885–891 (2005).

50. J. N. Henderson and S. J. Remington, *Physiol. (Bethesda)* **1**, 162–170 (2006).

51. G. H. Patterson and J. Lippincott-Schwartz, *Science* **297**(5588), 1873–1877 (2002).

52. D. M. Chudakov, V. V. Verkhusha, D. B. Staroverov, E. A. Souslova, S. Lukyanov, and K. A. Lukyanov, *Nat. Biotechnol.* **22**(11), 1435–1439 (2004).

53. R. Ando, H. Hama, M. Yamamoto-Hino, H. Mizuno, and A. Miyawaki, *Proc. Natl. Acad. Sci. USA* **99**(20), 12651–12656 (2002).

54. J. Wiedenmann, S. Ivanchenko, F. Oswald, F. Schmitt, C. Rocker, A. Salih, K. D. Spindler, and G. U. Nienhaus, *Proc. Natl. Acad. Sci. USA* **101**(45), 15905–15910 (2004).

55. Y. A. Labas, N. G. Gurskaya, Y. G. Yanushevich, A. F. Fradkov, K. A. Lukyanov, S. A. Lukyanov, and M. V. Matz, *Proc. Natl. Acad. Sci. USA* **99**(7), 4256–4261 (2002).

56. H. Tsutsui, S. Karasawa, H. Shimizu, N. Nukina, and A. Miyawaki, *EMBO Rep.* **6**(3), 233–238 (2005).

57. N. G. Gurskaya, V. V. Verkhusha, A. S. Shcheglov, D. B. Staroverov, T. V. Chepurnykh, A. F. Fradkov, S. Lukyanov, and K. A. Lukyanov, *Nat. Biotechnol.* **24**(4), 461–465 (2006).

58. D. M. Chudakov, A. V. Feofanov, N. N. Mudrik, S. Lukyanov, and K. A. Lukyanov, *J. Biol. Chem.* **278**(9), 7215–7219 (2003).

59. J. S. Marchant, G. E. Stutzmann, M. A. Leissring, F. M. LaFerla, and I. Parker, *Nat. Biotechnol.* **19**(7), 645–649 (2001).

60. S. Habuchi, R. Ando, P. Dedecker, W. Verheijen, H. Mizuno, A. Miyawaki, and J. Hofkens, *Proc. Natl. Acad. Sci. USA* **102**(27), 9511–9516 (2005).

61. A. Terskikh, A. Fradkov, G. Ermakova, A. Zaraisky, P. Tan, A. V. Kajava, X. Zhao, S. Lukyanov, M. Matz, S. Kim, I. Weissman, and P. Siebert, *Science* **290**(5496), 1585–1588 (2000).

62. S. Cabantous, J. D. Pedelacq, B. L. Mark, C. Naranjo, T. C. Terwilliger, and G. S. Waldo, *J. Struct. Funct. Genomics* **6**(2/3), 113–119 (2005).

63. T. K. Kerppola, *Nat. Protocals* **1**(3), 1278–1286 (2006).

64. F. G. Cremazy, E. M. Manders, P. I. Bastiaens, G. Kramer, G. L. Hager, E. B. van Munster, P. J. Verschure, T. J. Gadella, Jr., and R. van Driel, *Exp. Cell Res.* **309**(2), 390–396 (2005).

65. N. Mizushima, A. Yamamoto, M. Matsui, T. Yoshimori, and Y. Ohsumi, *Mol. Biol. Cell* **15**(3), 1101–1111 (2004).

66. O. Pertz and K. M. Hahn, *J. Cell Sci.* **117**(Pt. 8), 1313–1318 (2004).

67. S. R. Nahorski, K. W. Young, R. A. John Challiss, and M. S. Nash, *Trends Neurosci.* **26**(8), 444–452 (2003).

68. M. T. Kunkel, Q. Ni, R. Y. Tsien, J. Zhang, and A. C. Newton, *J. Biol. Chem.* **280**(7), 5581–5587 (2005).

69. T. Nagai, S. Yamada, T. Tominaga, M. Ichikawa, and A. Miyawaki, *Proc. Natl. Acad. Sci. USA* **101**(29), 10554–10559 (2004).

70. D. Yu, G. S. Baird, R. Y. Tsien, and R. L. Davis, *J. Neurosci.* **23**(1), 64–72 (2003).

71. T. Nagai, A. Sawano, E. S. Park, and A. Miyawaki, *Proc. Natl. Acad. Sci. USA* **98**(6), 3197–3202 (2001).

72. K. Deuschle, S. Okumoto, M. Fehr, L. L. Looger, L. Kozhukh, and W. B. Frommer, *Protein Sci.* **14**(9), 2304–2314 (2005).

73. S. Okumoto, L. L. Looger, K. D. Micheva, R. J. Reimer, S. J. Smith, and W. B. Frommer, *Proc. Natl. Acad. Sci. USA* **102**(24), 8740–8745 (2005).

74. H. Gu, S. Lalonde, S. Okumoto, L. L. Looger, A. M. Scharff-Poulsen, A. R. Grossman, J. Kossmann, I. Jakobsen, and W. B. Frommer, *FEBS Lett.* **580**(25), 5885–5893 (2006).

75. G. Miesenbock, D. A. De Angelis, and J. E. Rothman, *Nature* **394**(6689), 192–195 (1998).
76. G. T. Hanson, T. B. McAnaney, E. S. Park, M. E. Rendell, D. K. Yarbrough, S. Chu, L. Xi, S. G. Boxer, M. H. Montrose, and S. J. Remington, *Biochemistry* **41**(52), 15477–15488 (2002).
77. R. M. Wachter, D. Yarbrough, K. Kallio, and S. J. Remington, *J. Mol. Biol.* **301**(1), 157–171 (2000).
78. P. G. Wilmann, J. Battad, T. Beddoe, S. Olsen, S. C. Smith, S. Dove, R. J. Devenish, J. Rossjohn, and M. Prescott, *Photochem. Photobiol.* **82**(2), 359–366 (2006).
79. H. Ostergaard, A. Henriksen, F. G. Hansen, and J. R. Winther, *EMBO J.* **20**(21), 5853–5862 (2001).
80. C. T. Dooley, T. M. Dore, G. T. Hanson, W. C. Jackson, S. J. Remington, and R. Y. Tsien, *J. Biol. Chem.* **279**(21), 22284–22293 (2004).
81. M. Hofmann, C. Eggeling, S. Jakobs, and S. W. Hell, *Proc. Natl. Acad. Sci. USA* **102**(49), 17565–17569 (2005).
82. E. Betzig, G. H. Patterson, R. Sougrat, O. W. Lindwasser, S. Olenych, J. S. Bonifacino, M. W. Davidson, J. Lippincott-Schwartz, and H. F. Hess, *Science* **313**(5793), 1642–1645 (2006).
83. G. H. Patterson, S. M. Knobel, W. D. Sharif, S. R. Kain, and D. W. Piston, *Biophys. J.* **73**(5), 2782–2790 (1997).
84. G. J. Kremers, J. Goedhart, D. J. van den Heuvel, H. C. Gerritsen, and T. W. Gadella, Jr., *Biochemistry* **46**(12), 3775–3783 (2007).
85. H. W. Ai, J. N. Henderson, S. J. Remington, and R. E. Campbell, *Biochem. J.* **400**, 531–540 (2006).
86. M. A. Rizzo, G. H. Springer, B. Granada, and D. W. Piston, *Nat. Biotechnol.* **22**(4), 445–449 (2004).
87. D. A. Zacharias, J. D. Violin, A. C. Newton, and R. Y. Tsien, *Science* **296**(5569), 913–916 (2002).
88. G. J. Kremers, J. Goedhart, E. B. van Munster, and T. W. Gadella, Jr., *Biochemistry* **45**(21), 6570–6580 (2006).
89. O. Zapata-Hommer and O. Griesbeck, *BMC Biotechnol.* **3**, 5 (2003).
90. R. Heim, A. B. Cubitt, and R. Y. Tsien, *Nature* **373**(6516), 663–664 (1995).
91. A. B. Cubitt, L. A. Woollenweber, and R. Heim, *Methods Cell. Biol.* **58**, 19–30 (1999).
92. T. Nagai, K. Ibata, E. S. Park, M. Kubota, K. Mikoshiba, and A. Miyawaki, *Nat. Biotechnol.* **20**(1), 87–90 (2002).
93. O. Griesbeck, G. S. Baird, R. E. Campbell, D. A. Zacharias, and R. Y. Tsien, *J. Biol. Chem.* **276**(31), 29188–29194 (2001).
94. S. Karasawa, T. Araki, T. Nagai, H. Mizuno, and A. Miyawaki, *Biochem. J.* **381**(Pt. 1), 307–312 (2004).
95. Y. G. Yanushevich, D. B. Staroverov, A. P. Savitsky, A. F. Fradkov, N. G. Gurskaya, M. E. Bulina, K. A. Lukyanov, and S. A. Lukyanov, *FEBS Lett.* **511**(1–3), 11–14 (2002).
96. B. J. Bevis and B. S. Glick, *Nat. Biotechnol.* **20**(1), 83–87 (2002).
97. J. Wiedenmann, A. Schenk, C. Rocker, A. Girod, K. D. Spindler, and G. U. Nienhaus, *Proc. Natl. Acad. Sci. USA* **99**(18), 11646–11651 (2002).
98. J. Wiedenmann, B. Vallone, F. Renzi, K. Nienhaus, S. Ivanchenko, C. Rocker, and G. U. Nienhaus, *J. Biomed. Opt.* **10**(1), 14003 (2005).
99. T. Kogure, S. Karasawa, T. Araki, K. Saito, M. Kinjo, and A. Miyawaki, *Nat. Biotechnol.* **24**(5), 577–581 (2006).
100. A. F. Fradkov, V. V. Verkhusha, D. B. Staroverov, M. E. Bulina, Y. G. Yanushevich, V. I. Martynov, S. Lukyanov, and K. A. Lukyanov, *Biochem. J.* **368**(Pt. 1), 17–21 (2002).

101. L. Wang, W. C. Jackson, P. A. Steinbach, and R. Y. Tsien, *Proc. Natl. Acad. Sci. USA* **101**(48), 16745–16749 (2004).

102. M. A. Shkrob, Y. G. Yanushevich, D. M. Chudakov, N. G. Gurskaya, Y. A. Labas, S. Y. Poponov, N. N. Mudrik, S. Lukyanov, and K. A. Lukyanov, *Biochem. J.* **392**(Pt. 3), 649–654 (2005).

103. G. T. Hanson, R. Aggeler, D. Oglesbee, M. Cannon, R. A. Capaldi, R. Y. Tsien, and S. J. Remington, *J. Biol. Chem.* **279**(13), 13044–13053 (2004).

104. G. Guerrero, M. S. Siegel, B. Roska, E. Loots, and E. Y. Isacoff, *Biophys. J.* **83**(6), 3607–3618 (2002).

105. M. Kneen, J. Farinas, Y. Li, and A. S. Verkman, *Biophys. J.* **74**(3), 1591–1599 (1998).

106. O. Griesbeck, *Curr. Opin. Neurobiol.* **14**(5), 636–641 (2004).

107. K. Nowikovsky, S. Reipert, R. J. Devenish, and R. J. Schweyen, *Cell Death Differ*. **14**(9), 1647–1656 (2007).

108. P. Kalab, A. Pralle, E. Y. Isacoff, R. Heald, and K. Weis, *Nature* **440**(7084), 697–701 (2006).

109. M. D. Allen and J. Zhang, *Biochem. Biophys. Res. Commun.* **348**(2), 716–721 (2006).

110. Q. Ni, D. V. Titov, and J. Zhang, *Methods* **40**(3), 279–286 (2006).

111. A. Honda, S. R. Adams, C. L. Sawyer, V. Lev-Ram, R. Y. Tsien, and W. R. Dostmann *Proc. Natl. Acad. Sci. USA* **98**(5), 2437–2442 (2001).

CHAPTER 4

Nanoparticle Fluorescence Probes

KRYSTYNA DROZDOWICZ-TOMSIA and EWA M. GOLDYS

Division of Information and Communication Sciences, Macquarie University, Sydney, New South Wales 2109, Australia

4.1 INTRODUCTION

This chapter is concerned with nanoparticle fluorescent probes, which are based on semiconductor quantum dots (QDs). Other types such as magnetic nanoparticles or colloidal metals, mainly gold and silver, some of which have been recently investigated for surface-enhanced Raman spectroscopy (SERS) and fluorescence enhancement, will not be discussed. These are mostly used in other applications, such as scanning electron microscopy (SEM) imaging, or their commercial availability may be limited. This chapter aims to provide an understanding of the basic physics of QDs, their synthesis and optical characterization, and their biofunctionalization and use for biological and biomedical applications. We will also discuss selected examples, where due to their unique spectral and structural properties the QDs have advantages over other fluorescent probes. It should be noted that QDs have other important applications in the areas of optoelectronics, telecommunication, and X-ray imaging which are beyond the scope of this book.

4.2 NANOMATERIALS FOR BIOLOGICAL APPLICATIONS

The last two decades witnessed the rapid development of new nanoscale technologies (nano $= 10^{-9}$ m). With recent advances in nanobiotechnology and nanoengineering it has become possible to create artificial inorganic nanocrystals (NCs) made of inorganic semiconductor materials called quantum dots. These can be integrated with biomolecules for specific tasks such as drug delivery and act as robust contrast agents, fluorescence probes, and sensing enhancers. From a structural point of view, the NCs most frequently used in biological applications have the dimensions of 2–10 nm; such NCs comprise 200–10,000 atoms. In order to make them highly luminescent and biocompatible, additional layers such as an inorganic confinement shell, polymer coating, and biofunctional groups are added to produce structures with a final diameter of 15–20 nm. This size (Figure 4.1) is comparable with biological molecules such as

Fluorescence Applications in Biotechnology and Life Sciences, Edited by Ewa M. Goldys

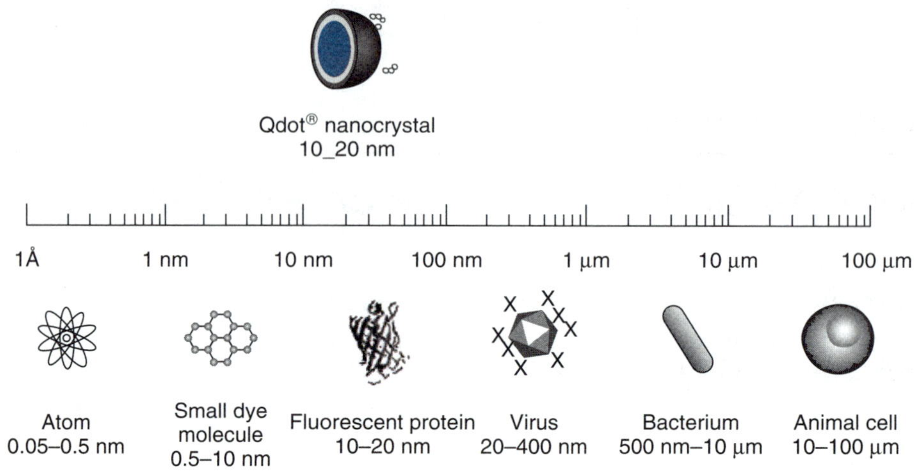

Figure 4.1 Relative size of quantum dot nanocrystals. (Reproduced with permission from Invitrogen).

proteins and DNA. With proper NC surface bioengineering, they can be attached to the surface or incorporated into cells and tissues. QD bioconjugates, that is, materials comprising luminescent colloidal QDs conjugated with biomolecules, can be used in applications such as molecular detection, bioimaging, and future diagnostics applications.

Biological tagging with fluorophores is used in many areas, including immunoassays, microarray-based gene analysis in genomics, flow cytometry, disease diagnostics, drug development, and cell and tissue imaging in both simple and multiplex approaches. Such multiplex detection relies on using a single-wavelength excitation to detect various molecular components labeled with different, spectrally distinguishable tags. Fluorescence microscopy imaging has become one of the most useful techniques to assess the activity of individual cells and at a subcellular level. This requires robust, stable, and bright fluorescent probes. Organic fluorophores, the most commonly used probes may have limitations such as narrow excitation bands and broad emission spectra with a red tail, small Stokes shift, low resistance to photobleaching, self-quenching at high concentrations, and pH dependence of the optical properties. These affect their performance in imaging over extended periods of time and multicolor detection. The interest in inorganic QDs has been stimulated by their optical properties, which are very different from conventional fluorophore molecules. The wavelengths of light emitted by the QDs strongly depend on the material used as well as the NC size due to quantum confinement of the charge carriers on a nanometer scale. It is also attractive that QDs can be excited with a much broader range of wavelengths than conventional fluorophores. Owing to the tunability of emission by QD size, QDs are well suited to be used as highly multiplexed labels, where for example different parts of cells are tagged with QDs emitting at different colors. It is important to note that, by using a few different semiconductor materials and a range of different sizes, it is possible to create QDs with colors which span the entire visible spectrum from ultraviolet to infrared. It was demonstrated that QD emission wavelength can be continuously tuned from 400 to 2000 nm by changing both nanocrystal size and their composition [2–7, 13].

Notably, QDs can be engineered with the excitation and emission band maxima in the near-infrared (NIR) range (650–900 nm); such fluorophores have significant advantages for deep-tissue imaging. This is because the NIR light is capable of penetrating much deeper (up to several centimeters) into the soft tissues and bones [1] due to the low absorption of the tissue components (water and hemoglobin) in the NIR range.

Advances in synthesis and biofunctionalization of colloidal semiconductor NCs during the past two decades have led to a development of commercially available fluorescent probes based on these materials. They are now offered, for example, by Evident Technologies (www.evidenttech.com) and Invitrogen Corporation (www.invitrogen.com). These new probes have generated a widespread interest among investigators as they offer an advanced alternative in certain bioanalytical and imaging applications [8, 9]. We now give a brief description of photophysical properties of the semiconductor QDs and a wide range of synthesis approaches suitable for core and core/shell nanocrystals. We also discuss the surface modification of the nanocrystals and their application for in vitro and in vivo detection in biological cells.

4.3 INORGANIC QUANTUM DOTS: PHYSICS AND OPTICAL PROPERTIES

QDs are inorganic semiconductor nanocrystals which exhibit quantum confinement effects once their dimensions become smaller than a characteristic nanoscale length, called the *Bohr's radius*. The emission properties of semiconductors in bulk form are defined by their bandgap, which is the energy-level separation between the group of very close energy levels occupied by electrons only in part, called the conduction band, and another group of very close levels occupied by electrons and located just below the conduction band called the valence band. The absorption of light transfers electrons from the valence band to the conduction band leaving behind holes in the valence band. Their recombination with excited electrons leads to the emission of light at characteristic wavelengths corresponding to the energy gap. The optical properties of semiconductor NCs retain some characteristics of the constituent bulk materials but are dominated by new effects referred to as the quantum confinement. These effects originate from the tight, nanoscale spatial localization of electrons and holes within the QD. The localization shifts the electronic energy levels so that the apparent semiconductor bandgap energy increases with decreasing NC size. This manifests itself as a size-dependent blue shift of the spectral features in absorption and fluorescence emission with decreasing NC size. The size-dependent relationship can be explained by using a simple mathematical model of the particle-in-a-box. This elementary approximate model predicts, in agreement with experimental observations, that the emitted light by the quantum dots can be continuously tunable by varying nanoparticle size [8, 10].

A wide spectral emission range from ultraviolet to NIR can be obtained by appropriate selection of the materials with different bandgaps and varying the size of the nanocrystals. The QD materials may belong to groups II–VI, such as ZnSe, CdS, CdSe, CdTe, and CdHgTe, but also to groups III–V, such as GaAs, InAs, InP, GaP, or IV-VIs (PbS, PbSe, PbTe) (Figures 4.2*a*,*b*). Fluorescence of semiconductor QDs is characterized by a a narrow and symmetric spectral emission band with typically 25–35 nm full width at half maximum (FWHM) and a comparatively long lifetime ($>$10 ns) [11]. The emission band may exhibit a significant blue shift with respect to

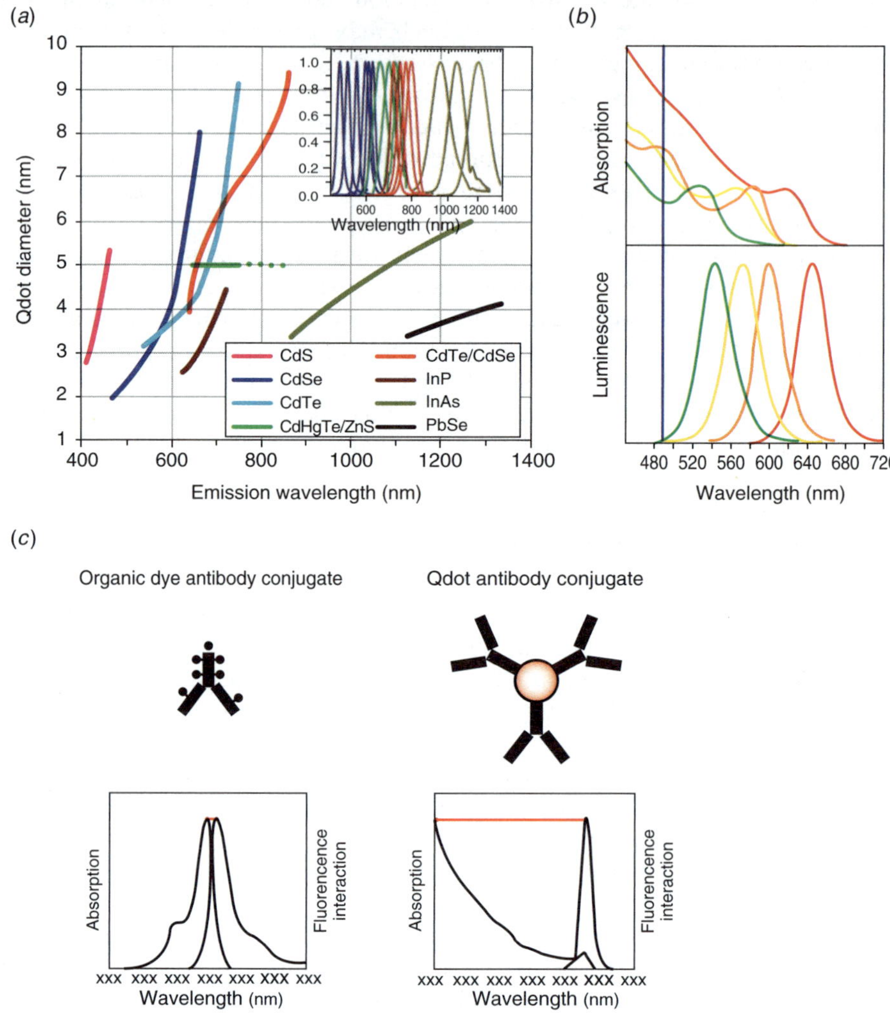

Figure 4.2 (*a*) Emission maxima and sizes of QDs with different compositions. The curves represent experimental data from the literature relating the peak emission wavelength to QD diameter. The range of emission wavelengths is from 400 to 1350 nm for sizes varying from 2 to 9.5 nm. (*b*) Absorption (upper curves) and emission (lower curves) spectra of four CdSe/ZnS QD samples. The blue vertical line indicates the 488-nm wavelength of an argon–ion laser, which can be used to efficiently excite all four types of QDs simultaneously. (*a*, *b*: Reprinted with permission from [14].) (*c*) Comparison of absorption and emission spectra of QDs and common fluorescent dyes. Left: The fluorescence spectrum of a typical organic fluorophore (Texas Red® dye) is shown below a schematic of an organic fluorophore-labeled IgG antibody with a typical number of dye molecules per a single IgG molecule. Right: The fluorescence spectra of the Qdot® 605 nanocrystal are shown below a schematic of a Qdot nanocrystal–labeled IgG antibody with a typical number of antibody molecules per nanocrystal. Both antibody conjugates are drawn roughly to scale. (Reprinted with permission from Invitrogen).

the band edge of the corresponding bulk material (Figure 4.2*b*). For example, in the case of CdSe, which has a bandgap of 1.7 eV (corresponding to 730 nm), the emission peak can be centered anywhere within the visible range between 460 to 650 nm by simply changing the nanocrystal diameter from 2 to 8 nm. In addition to their desirable emission properties, QDs have advantageous absorption properties. Unlike organic dyes, which show large absorption cross section only across a narrow spectral band, the QDs have broad absorption spectra, with an onset near the high-energy edge of the QD emission which increases steadily toward the ultraviolet (UV). Quantum dots show high molar absorptivities and their molar extinction coefficients are 10–100 $\times$ larger than those of conventional dyes. Large effective Stokes shifts make it possible to efficiently excite a mixed population of QDs at a single wavelength far away ($\sim$100 nm) from their cumulative emissions (Figure 4.2*b*). This indicates that QDs are well suited for multiplexing or simultaneous detection of multiple fluorescent signals. It should be noted that the efficiency of excitation increases strongly toward shorter excitation wavelengths. Thus much shorter wavelengths than those used for organic fluorophores may be preferred for excitation; such wavelengths may not always be available with older instrumentation.

QDs are also very stable light emitters owing to their inorganic composition and crystalline character, making them much less susceptible to photobleaching and chemical degradation than organic dyes [8, 14]. This was shown in a number of biological experiments, one of them illustrated in Figure 4.3, where the photostability of samples labeled with QDs was compared with common fluorophores such as Alexa-Fluor [35]. As a result QDs remain a very attractive alternative for real-time monitoring of biological processes or multiple sectioning in confocal microscopy imaging of thick specimens over long periods of time with minimal specimen damage. As the QDs have much longer lifetimes than native biological fluorescent components and one order of magnitude longer than the fluorescence dyes, they are also very well suited for time-correlated lifetime imaging spectroscopy. This allows the improved and effective separation of QD fluorescence from the background fluorescence, resulting in better image contrast by reducing the signal-to-noise ratio [15] in the time-delayed data acquisition mode.

Despite many advantages, QDs possess some photophysical properties that can in some cases limit their applicability. One of these is the property called "blinking," that is, random alternation between an emitting and nonemitting state, observed for single QDs irrespective of their size and composition [16, 17]. This intermittence in emission of QDs is often attributed to the presence of nonradiative recombination, especially at the surface, which is strong in most types of QDs. Not only blinking but also emission quantum yield (QY) (which is the ratio of the amount of light emitted from a sample to the amount of light absorbed) depends critically on the conditions on the QD surface, such as the degree of passivation of unsaturated bonds. This passivation can be significantly improved by using appropriate organic ligands or by the controlled growth of a crystalline shell of a wider bandgap semiconductor material [18, 19]. It was also reported that the fluorescence intensity of QDs may increase upon excitation, a phenomenon referred to as photobrightening [9, 20]. Although this property can be advantageous, it presents problems in quantitative studies. Both blinking and photobrightening are linked with mobile charges on the surfaces of QDs. The properties of QDs and their comparison with fluorescent dyes are summarized in Table 4.1 [21].

TABLE 4.1 Comparison of Properties of QDs and Organic/Protein Fluorophores

Property	Fluorophores (Dyes)	Quantum Dots
Photophysical		
Absorption spectra	Variable/narrow, generally a mirror image of emission spectra	Broad spectra, steadily increase toward UV from first absorption band edge
Molar extinction coefficients	Variable, generally $<200{,}000\ M^{-1}\ cm^{-1}$	High, 10–100 × that of fluorophores
Emission spectra	Broad, asymmetric red-tailed emission	Narrow–full width at half maximum, 25–40 nm for CdSe core materials
Maturation time	Needed for fluorescent proteins	NA
Effective Stokes shift	Generally <100 nm	>200 nm possible
Tunable emission	NA	Unique to QDs, can be size tuned from UV to IR
Quantum yield	Variable, low to high	Generally high, 0.2–0.7 in buffer depending on surface coating
Fluorescence lifetime	Short, <5 ns	Long, 10–20 ns or greater
Spectral range	Necessitates different dye every 40–60 nm	UV–IR depending upon binary/ternary material Vis—CdSe
Photostability	Variable to poor	Excellent, strong resistance to photobleaching several orders of magnitude that of dyes
Multiphoton cross section	Variable to poor	Excellent, >2–3 orders of magnitude that of dyes
Single-molecule capabilities	Variable	Excellent
Fluorescence resonance energy transfer capabilities	Variable, mostly single donor–single acceptor configuration	Excellent donors, size-tuned emission to improve overlap with acceptor dye, single donor–multiple acceptor configurations possible
Multiplexing capabilities	Rare	Excellent, largely unexplored
Intermittency (blinking)	Negligible	May be problematic in isolated circumstances (single-molecule tracking)
Chemical		
Chemical resistance	Variable	Excellent
Reactivity	Multiple reactivities commercially available	Limited conjugations chemistries available
Monovalent attachment	Easy	Difficult
Multivalent attachment	Rare, mostly bis-functional	Good possibilities, can attach several molecules to QDs depending upon size
Other		
Physical size	<0.5 nm	4–7 nm for CdSe core material
Electrochromicity	Rare	Largely untapped
Cost effectiveness	Very good/multiple suppliers	Poor, two commercial suppliers

Source: Sapsfold et al. [22].

(*a*)

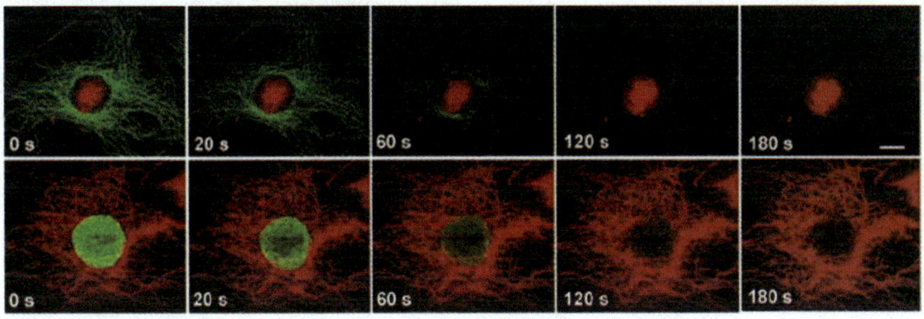

(*b*)

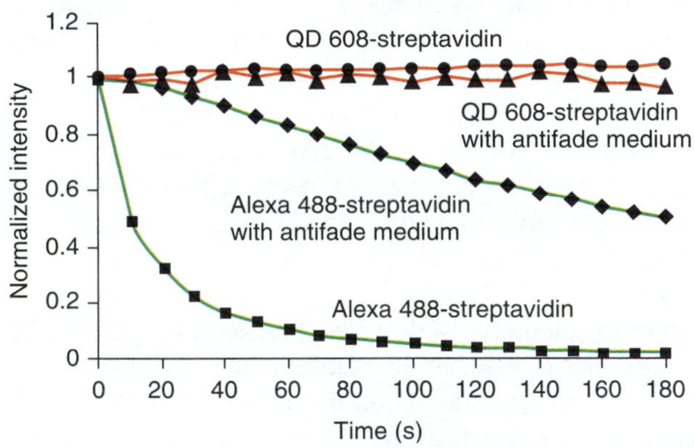

Figure 4.3 Comparison of photostablility between QDs and Alexa 488. (*a*) Top row: A QD labeled cell. The nucleus is labeled with QD 630–streptavidin (red) and microtubules are labeled with Alexa 488 conjugated to antimouse IgG (green). Bottom row: Microtubules were labeled with QD 630–streptavidin (red) and the nucleus was stained green with Alexa 488 conjugated to antihuman IgG. The specimens were continuously illuminated for up to 3 min. (*b*) Quantitative analysis of intensity changes of QD 608–streptavidin (stained microtubules) and Alexa 488-streptavidin (stained nucleus). (Reprinted with permission from [36].)

4.4 SYNTHESIS OF MONODISPERSE COLLOIDAL QUANTUM DOTS FOR BIOLABELING APPLICATIONS

Several methods of preparation have been developed for highly fluorescent QDs. They can be broadly classified into methods which produce powders or agglomerated NCs and those resulting in colloidal NCs. Only methods producing colloidal, well-dispersed QDs are useful for biological applications. These methods include high-temperature synthesis in high-boiling-point, nonpolar solvents/ligands and growth at low temperatures within inverse micelles (also called a water-in-oil microemulsion system). Generally, syntheses at higher temperatures offer the advantage of improved nanocrystal quality with lower defect density as the defects formed during crystal growth can be easily annealed. In addition, at higher temperatures both the nucleation and growth stages can be controlled and tuned more easily. The nanocrystals grown in such conditions require postsynthesis treatments to make them water soluble and biocompatible. The synthesis can proceed either by dispersion (continuous division) or by reduction (controlled growth of the constituents starting from atoms). High-temperature synthesis methods in the high-boiling-point, nonpolar solvent/ligand belong to the class of reduction methods.

In the following section we will describe the synthesis and postprocessing with emphasis on nanocrystals of group II–VI compounds. Similar general concepts are also applicable to group III–V nanocrystals. We will also discuss the modification of the NC surface to enable the attachment of biological molecules.

4.4.1 Quantum Dot Synthesis

A large number of different synthesis methods for QDs of groups II–VI have been described in the literature. They can be easily formed as free particles in solutions following simple chemical exchange reactions at room temperature. The reactants may include soluble salts of metal (M) from group II and compounds containing chalcogenide (E) from group VI (M = Zn, Cd, Hg) and chalcogenides (E = S, Se, Te), but such synthesis leads to production of poorly fluorescent powders or nanoparticle agglomerates. They typically have broad spectral features and inadequate structural quality even with the addition of colloidal stabilizers. Consequently the commercially available QDs currently used for biological applications are exclusively produced by high-temperature methods.

High-temperature synthesis methods in selected high-boiling-point, nonpolar solvents/ligands can produce monodisperse, highly luminescent and stable colloidal NCs. In addition, the nucleation and growth stages can be controlled and tuned more easily. Classic studies by La Mer and Dinegar [23] and Murray et al. [24] show that production of monodisperse colloids requires an instantaneous nucleation event followed by slower controlled growth on the existing nuclei. By rapid addition of reagents to the reaction vessel, it is possible to raise the concentration of reaction precursors above the nucleation threshold. A short nucleation burst which follows relieves the supersaturation and, as long as the consumption of reagents by the growing colloidal NCs is not exceeded by the delivery rate of the precursors to the solution, no new nuclei are formed. The initial size and size distribution of the NCs are then largely determined by the temperature and the formation and growth time of the nuclei. A general overview of synthesis techniques is given in the literature [25, 29].

For growth of group II–VI NCs the preferred method is based on an airless pyrolysis technique of organometallic compounds (dimethylcadmium, diethylzinc, dibenzylmercury) as a source of group II metal and organophosphine (TOP: tri-*n*-octyl phosphine), chalcogenides (e.g., TOPSe, TOPTe), or bis-trimethylsilylchalcogenides TMS_2E (TMS, trimethylsilyl, E = S, Se, Te) [23] as a source of group VI atoms. The synthesis is carried out in high-boiling-point, nonpolar organic solvent/ligand at high temperatures in the range 250–350°C (see Figure 4.4). In the case of Cd atoms it is now possible, following the recent advances in CdSe synthesis, to replace organometallic Cd compounds with less hazardous precursors such as CdO or Cd^{2+} complexes with alkyl-phosphonic or carboxylic acids [25].

The nonpolar organic solvent/surfactant molecules most frequently used for growth of group II–VI NCs include phosphines and phosphine oxides: TOP and tri-*n*-octylphosphine oxide (TOPO) [23, 26]. The reaction mixture can also be more complex and include alkyl amines (e.g., hexadecylamine) and phosphonic and carboxylic acids. The group III–V NCs have also been grown using a similar

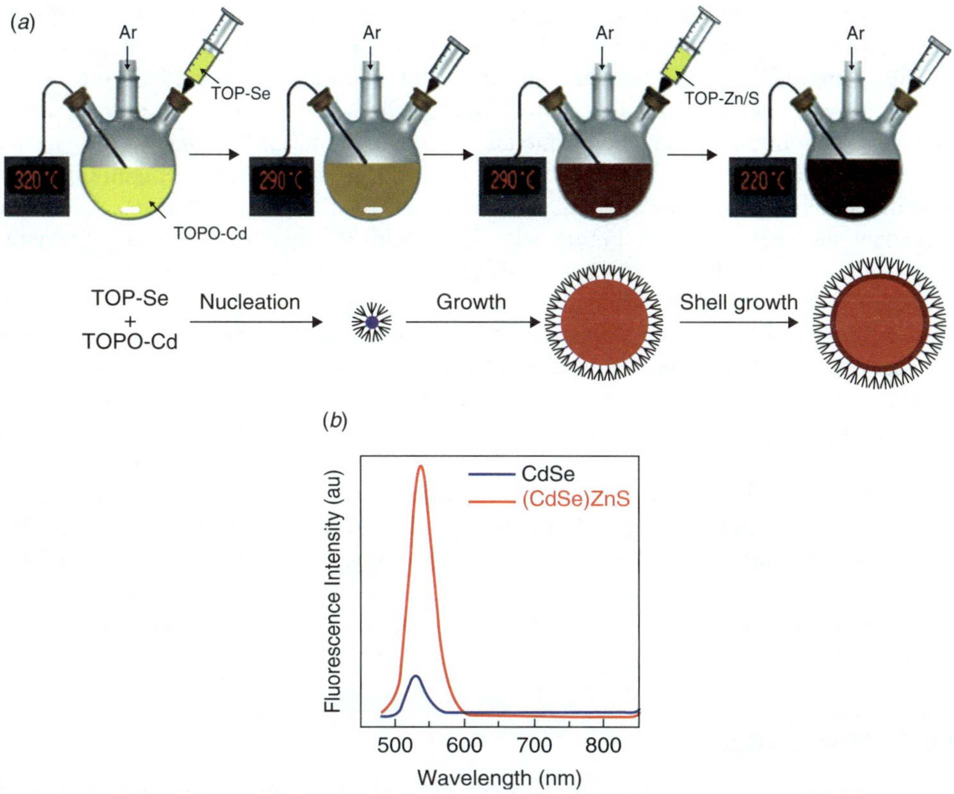

Figure 4.4 High-temperature synthesis of colloidal CdSe/ZnS quantum dots in coordinating solvent. (*a*) Synthesis of core-shell QDs. In a typical reaction, a three-necked flask is placed in a heating mantle equipped with a thermocouple and temperature controller. A cadmium precursor (e.g., cadmium oxide or cadmium acetate) is dissolved in the TOPO coordinating solvent in an inert atmosphere (argon or nitrogen flow). Under continuous stirring at high temperature (320°C) a selenium precursor dissolved in TOP (TOP–Se) is quickly injected into the flask, initiating rapid nucleation of CdSe nanoparticles. Nucleation ceases quickly, partially due to the rapid decrease in temperature (to 290°C) caused by the injection of the room temperature solution, and particle growth commences. When the desired size has been obtained, the solution may be cooled (220°C) to prevent further particle growth. A passivating layer of ZnS may then be grown epitaxially by injection of zinc and sulfur precursors dissolved in TOP. Upon cooling to room temperature, these core-shell QDs may be isolated via precipitation. (Reprinted with permission from [30].) (*b*) Introduction of ZnS shell around CdSe significantly increases NC fluorescence emission and only marginally red shifts emission wavelength.

approach. In this case, a metal precursor such as $InCl_3$ is complexed to either TOPO or TOP producing a poorly defined precursor, which is reacted with a silylated pnictide, typically $E(SiMe_3)_3$ (E = As, P) at temperatures of up to 265°C to form InP or InAs NCs dispersed in TOPO [28]. The organic molecules play a key role in controlling this synthesis. First, they serve as a solvent for growing NCs; second they act as the surfactants and third as capping agents, passivating surface defects. At high growth temperature they bind dynamically to the surface of the NCs. Additionally, they form complexes with the atomic species in solution, thus controlling the reactivity and the diffusion rates of the elemental species to the surface of the growing NCs. As such they control the growth kinetics. When the synthesis is interrupted by lowering the reaction temperature, such molecules form a stable monolayer around NCs preventing further growth and stabilize their monodisperse character (minimize size variations). In a very simplified model, the surfactant molecules bind and unbind to the surface of the NCs, and the rates of these two processes are controlled by temperature. The growth of the crystals can only take place at the available surface sites, where the surfactant molecules are competing with ions/atoms of precursors coming from the bulk of the solution. In order to have sufficient control over the growth dynamics, the surfactant with optimum binding properties for the growth of particular NCs system must be found. For other systems the reaction temperatures and the optimal choice of reagents and surfactants are usually different, but general principles of nucleation, growth, and stabilization are still the same. The reaction is interrupted before the "Oswald ripening" stage by rapid lowering of temperature. Oswald ripening is a process in which smaller nanocrystals which are less thermodynamically stable start to dissolve and release free atomic species into solution, thus allowing acceleration in the growth of larger, more stable nanocrystals. If not prevented, Oswald ripening leads to an overall broadening of NC size distribution. By removing aliquots from the reaction vessel at various time intervals after the initial injection of precursors, fractions of different size NCs emitting at different colors can be extracted for further modifications.

4.4.2 Shell Synthesis

The quantum yield responsible for fluorescence brightness of "core" QDs (made up of a single inorganic compound) is typically of the order of up to a few percent only. Such poor quantum yield is related to the presence of surface defects, most notably dangling bonds. These may be passivated by the application of various procedures aimed at creating a coating over the nanocrystals. The most common organic capping molecules such as TOPO (and TOPSe in CdSe synthesis) can only passivate one type of dangling bonds which originate from cadmium by forming TOP–O–Cd or TOP–Se–Cd bonds but not those related to the other type of dangling bonds (e.g., from Se). Fortunately, there is a method able to passivate both types of dangling bonds in NCs at the same time. Such passivation of surface defects is achieved by growing a lattice-matched, higher bandgap material over the nanocrystal cores. This is done by high-temperature pyrolysis in a similar process as discussed previously (Figure 4.4). This "shell" layer serves two purposes: It eliminates core surface traps and confines the excitation into the NC core [14]. For example, the shells made from CdS ($E_g =$ 2.49 eV) and ZnS ($E_g = 3.8$ eV) are used for CdSe ($E_g = 1.75$ eV) cores. CdS is better lattice matched to CdSe, but ZnS, with its higher bandgap, gives better confinement. Growing a thin, few-monolayer shell surrounding the CdSe core dramatically increases quantum yield, up to the value of about 85%. The core/shell arrangement also increases photochemical stability, so the photobleaching is reduced. The addition of shell to the core/shell NCs slightly shifts the absorption edge and emission peak toward red as compared with core-only structures (shown in Figure 4.4*b*). So far a wide range of core/shell NCs, such as CdSe/ZnS, CdSe/CdS, and CdTe/CdSe but also InAs/GaAs and InP/GaP, have been synthesized and all have improved stability and fluorescence quantum yield.

4.4.3 Water Solubilization and Functionalization

High-quality core, core/shell, or more recently developed alloyed QDs are typically synthesized at elevated temperatures in organic solvents, such as TOPO and hexadecylamine (HDA). This automatically leads to NC capping with a monolayer of hydrophobic organic molecules, which prevents them from aggregation. In order to make the NCs water soluble, the amphiphilic molecules (molecules having both hydrophilic and hydrophobic properties) must be introduced, and NC agglomeration in the new medium needs to be prevented. In general, there are two strategies to stabilize nanoparticles in an aqueous solution. The first is based on the introduction of charge. Nanoparticles of similar charge repel each other, which prevents aggregation. However, in electrolytic solutions charges are screened by ions of opposite charge and electrostatic repulsion is weakened, which, at high NC concentrations, can lead to their agglomeration. Additionally, the charge of stabilizing molecules usually very strongly depends on the pH value of the solution. An alternative method of stabilization is through steric repulsion. The introduction of ligand molecules, which form hydrophilic "brushes" around the nanoparticle surface, prevent contact between inorganic NCs [31]. Typical molecules used for this purpose are polyethylene glycol (PEG) and dextran. The next challenge is coating these initially hydrophobic nanoparticles with a hydrophilic ("water-liking") shell to make them water soluble. This quality is essential for biological labeling, and different strategies to produce such QDs have been described in the literature, as recently summarized by Michalet et al. [32] (see Figure 4.5).

The TOPO-passivated CdSe/ZnS QDs can be solubilized in aqueous buffers by the addition of a layer of amphiphilic molecules containing hydrophilic and hydrophobic moieties. An alternative approach is by exchange of TOPO with molecules with a Zn-coordinating end [such as, e.g., a thiol group (–SH) and a hydrophilic end group (–COOH)]. The MAAs are possible exchange ligands which meet these criteria. Nanocrystals can be dispersed in water after deprotonation of the carboxylic acid group by increasing the pH. The disadvantages of this procedure are the pH sensitivity of the colloidal dispersion and high tendency for nonspecific interactions of the (charged) carboxylate groups with biomolecules such as proteins or DNA. Also, since binding affinity of thiols to ZnS surface is only moderate, these nanoparticles are not stable in aqueous solutions for long periods. Such an exchange method was also demonstrated using DTT, DHLA, oligomeric phosphines, crosslinked dendrons, and peptides. More elaborate protocols are based on ligand exchange of the stabilizing molecules but with the possibility of crosslinking of these molecules. Growth of an additional silica shell (surface silanization) over the inorganic semiconductor shell can also be regarded as a method based on exchange of the TOPO cap [9]. The first step of this process involves exchanging the surface ligand with thiol-derived silane such as mercaptotrimethoxysilane (MPS). The trimethoxylane groups can be crosslinked by the formation of siloxane bonds. During further silica shell growth, other types of silanes can be added to confer charge and provide different functional groups on the surface. This method, though leading to very high stability of nanocrystals, requires a rather complicated series of synthesis and purification steps. Its major drawback is difficult control of the resulting surface chemistry. On the other hand, various functional groups such as thiol –SH, amino $-NH_2$, or methyl-phosphate $-PO-(O^-)CH_3$ can be incorporated into the shell during this step, which may help tailor the nanocrystal functionality. The most successful "addition" method is based on encapsulating the nanocrystals with a crosslinked polymer such as PEG-derivatized phospholipids.

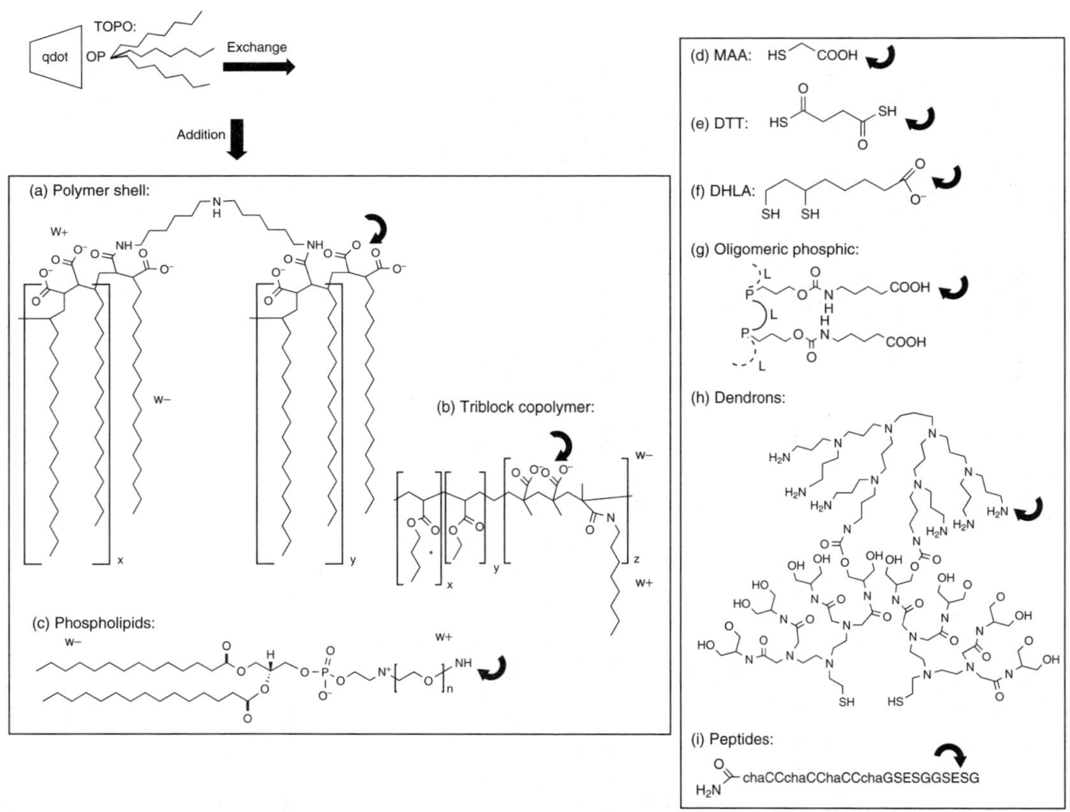

Figure 4.5 QD solubilization and functionalization. (*a*) Surface chemistries. TOPO-passivated QDs can be solubilized in aqueous buffer by addition of a layer of amphiphilic molecules containing hydrophilic (w^+) and hydrophobic (w^-) moieties or by exchange of TOPO with molecules that have a Zn-coordinating end (usually a thiol group, SH) and a hydrophilic end. Examples of addition include (*a*) formation of a crosslinked polymer shell, (*b*) coating with a layer of amphiphilic triblock copolymer, and (*c*) encapsulation in phospholipid micelles. Examples of exchange include (*d*) mercaptoacetic acid (MAA), (*e*) dithiothreitol (DTT), (*f*) dihydrolipoic acid (DHLA), (*g*) oligomeric phosphines, (*h*) crosslinked dendrons, and (*i*) peptides. The curved arrow indicates sites available for further functionalization. (Reprinted with permission from [32].)

It leads to the coating of the nanocrystals with a layer of amphiphilic triblock copolymer or charged proteins. This procedure does not replace ligands but adds another layer on top of the original surface ligands such as TOPO. All molecules used here contain both a hydrophobic segment or a side chain (mostly hydrocarbons) and a hydrophilic segment or group (such as PEG or multiple carboxylate groups). As illustrated in Figure 4.6, the hydrophobic domains strongly interact with TOPO on the QDs' surface, whereas the hydrophilic groups face outward and make the QDs water soluble. Therefore, the same procedure can be applied to almost any TOPO-capped particle, regardless of the material of inorganic core. This provides additional benefits such as essentially preserving the initial fluorescence quantum yield, shielding the core from the outside environment, and preventing QD agglomeration. It also allows incorporation of different functionalities directly into the surrounding shell. On the other hand, following this procedure the diameter of the QDs increases significantly, typically within the range of 15–25 nm. This can be disadvantageous for certain applications due to the reduced ability of the QDs to access some intracellular targets. To achieve binding specificity or targeting abilities, such polymer-coated QDs are linked to affinity ligands such as peptides, oligonucleotides, DNA, monoclonal antibodies, or small-molecule inhibitors. This process is called functionalization of QDs. Linking to polyethylene glycol or similar ligands can also lead to improved biocompatibility and reduced nonspecific binding [33].

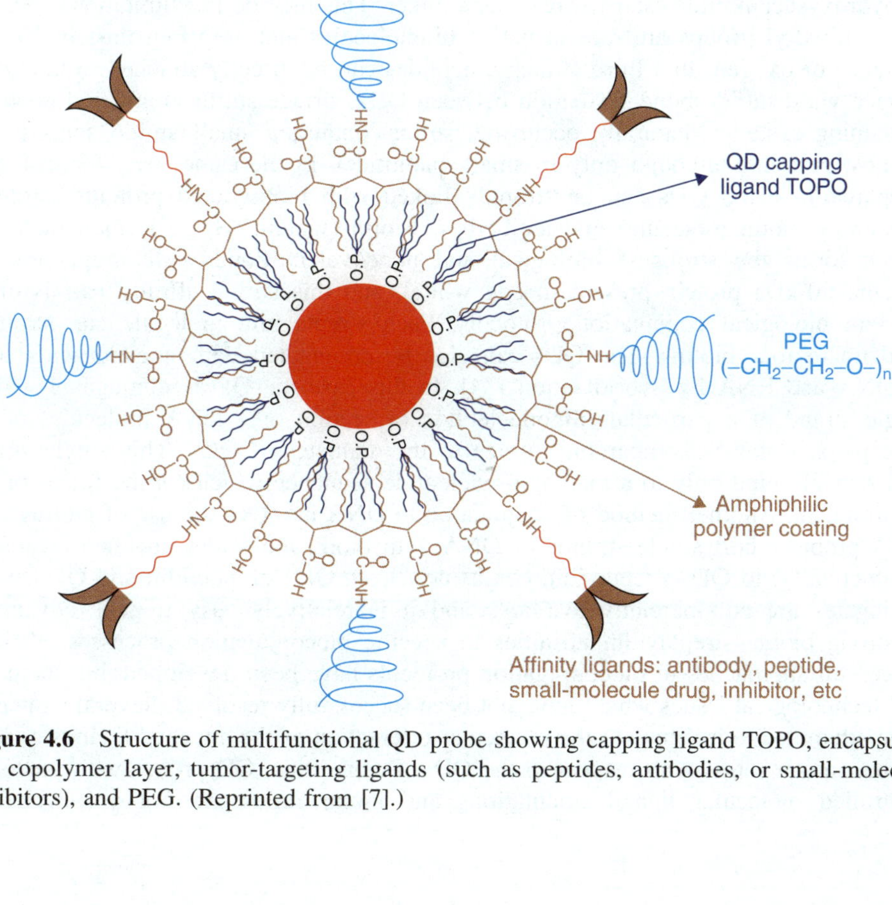

Figure 4.6 Structure of multifunctional QD probe showing capping ligand TOPO, encapsulating copolymer layer, tumor-targeting ligands (such as peptides, antibodies, or small-molecule inhibitors), and PEG. (Reprinted from [7].)

4.4.4 Quantum Dot Bioconjugation

The purpose of water solubilization and functionalization of the QDs is to enable QD binding to specific molecules or cells in an environment abundant in water without disturbing the biological function of these molecules. This process is called bioconjugation. Such molecules can then be observed or detected by fluorescence emitted by attached QDs. Sometimes nonspecific binding only may be required. However, for most applications, such as in targeted fluorescence imaging or detection, specific linker molecules are needed. Such linker molecules can selectively interact with target molecules inside the cells in cell-imaging studies or bind to specific proteins, antibodies, peptides, or fragments of DNA in immunoassays or other studies.

The QD bioconjugation can be achieved by several methods, including passive adsorption, multivalent chelation, or covalent bond formation. Biomolecules can be bound covalently by employing crosslinkers, which crosslink the functional groups such as $-COOH$, $-NH_2$, or $-SH$ introduced in functionalization steps on the QDs' surface with the functional groups present in the biomolecules. There are several principal approaches to attach proteins to QDs surface. One strategy uses N-ethyl-N'-(3-diethylaminopropyl) carbodiimide (EDC) as a heterocrosslinker, which mediates stable amide formation by crosslinking the carboxylate group to the amine group. This method can be used to bind QDs to proteins without any further chemical modification as most of the proteins contain primary amines. Another strategy is based on the active ester maleimide–mediated reaction to crosslink amine $-NH_2$ and sulfhydryl group $-SH$ using 4-(N-maleimidomethyl)-cyclohexanecarboxylic acid N-hydroxysuccinimide ester (SMCC) as a linker. This method has limitations because free sulfhydryl groups are rare in native biomolecules and are often unstable in the presence of oxygen. In a third strategy, peptides can be directly attached to the QDs' surface via disulfide bond formation between QDs surface sulfur atoms and peptides containing cysteine (naturally occurring, sulfur-containing small amino acids found in most proteins, although only in small quantities). In the same way, for instance, streptavidin-coated QDs can be strongly linked with biotinylated proteins (proteins containing biotin molecule) and antibodies. Biotin (vitamin H) is a small molecule which forms the strongest biological and noncovalent bond with streptavidin (a specific 60-kDa protein present in egg white), and this strong affinity pair is often used in biological conjugation protocols. Each streptavidin molecule can strongly bind up to four biotins. The QDs can also be conjugated with nucleic acids such as DNA and RNA by hybridization [34]. In this case the QD is conjugated with a single strand of a particular oligonucleotide (a section of a DNA molecule) of 12 base pairs, which is comparable in size to the diameter of QDs. This single strand will strongly bind only to a matching nucleotide sequence which can be found in the environment. Another method of conjugation to DNA involves the use of biotinylated DNA probes (short single strands of DNA with biotin molecules attached, available commercially) to QD–streptavidin conjugates. Both QD–streptavidin and QD–biotin conjugates are commercially available and it is relatively easy to take advantage of strong biotin–streptavidin affinities in specific bioconjugation processes. Various successful approaches to bioconjugation protocols have been developed, but there are still technological issues which have not been successfully resolved. Several strategies were attempted to manipulate the molecular orientation of the attached ligands as well as their molar ratios with respect to the QDs. Despite this, QD probes with precisely controlled molecular ligand orientations and molar ratios are not yet available.

Another critical aspect of QD probes such as specificity (percentage of specifically bonded probes to total number of probes used), which is one of the most important criteria for assessing applicability of labeling probes, needs further improvement.

4.5 QUANTUM DOTS AS IN VITRO PROBES

Over the past few years, QDs have been tested in most biotechnological applications that use fluorescence, including DNA array technology, immunofluorescence assays, and studies of cell and animal biology. These are extensively discussed in the literature.

QDs can be used either as fluorescent probes or fluorescent labels (markers) in various cell and tissue examinations in fixed and living specimens. For example, they can be used to locate specific molecules, detect signaling pathways, establish cell lineage (cell lineage of an organism is the pattern of cell divisions during its development), and cell motility [35]. In all such studies, it has been proven that specifically functionalized QDs can target and label biological material within cells due to their bioconjugation abilities based on specific antibody-binding techniques. Subsequently they can be imaged or detected using their advantageous optical characteristics, especially high brightness, multiplexing, and single-molecule detection capabilities. Numerous cellular components and proteins have been labeled and visualized with functionalized QDs, such as nuclei, mitochondria, microtubules, actin filaments, cytokeratin, endocytic compartments, and numerous specific proteins. High resistance of QDs to photobleaching enables observation of cell changes over extended time periods, even weeks or months, which is not possible with conventional dyes.

The first milestone biological application of QDs as fluorescent markers was reported by Alivisatos' group [8], who demonstrated multicolour labeling of fixed mouse 3T3 fibroblasts (see Figure 4.7). In this process biotinylated QDs with red photoluminescence selectively stained cytoskeletal filaments modified with streptavidin and green-emitting QDs with trimethoxysilylpropyl urea and acetate groups showed high affinity to the nucleus. These authors presented, for the first

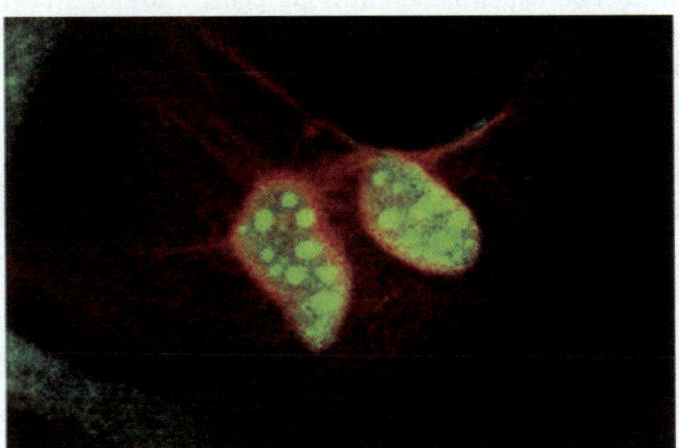

Figure 4.7 Mouse 3T3 fibroblasts labeled selectively with two color CdSe quantum dots. Red-emitting QDs stain cytoskeletal filaments and green-emitting QDs are located in nucleus. (Reprinted from [8].)

time, that with single excitation wavelength, multicolor and high-resolution imaging could be achieved using QDs emitting at two different wavelengths. Simultaneously, Chan and Nie [10] showed that QDs labeled with the protein transferrin underwent receptor-mediated endocytosis in cultured HeLa cells (stored and immortal cervical cancer cells from patient Henrietta Lacks now routinely used by biologists), and those QDs that were labeled with immunomolecules recognized specific antibodies and antigens allowing for their localization and imaging. These two papers reported in 1998 laid the foundation for the application of QDs as biolabels and, more generally, opened the field of biological application of QD nanoparticles. In the following years impressive progress has been achieved, especially in cancer imaging studies using QDs. In 2003, Wu and coworkers [36] developed reliable and highly specific QD probes to localize the breast cancer cell surface marker Her2, cytoskeleton fibers, and antigens in fixed cells, live cells, and tissue sections, with a substantial increase in brightness and photostability as compared to organic dyes. Different cell lines which were successfully studied using specifically targeted QD probes include human mammary epithelial tumor, different human breast cancers, human prostrate cancers, squamous carcinoma, human neuroblastoma, colon tumor, and lung tumor and bone tumor cells [37].

Research of signaling pathways between and within cells also relies heavily on bright and sensitive fluorophores. QDs have begun to play a major role in this field. Rosenthal et al. [38] reported using serotonin-linked QDs to target the neurotransmitter receptor on the cell surface. The QD conjugates not only recognized and labeled serotonin-specific neurotransmitters on cell membranes but also inhibited the serotonin transportation in a dose-dependent manner, similarly to that of free serotonin, making QDs a valuable probe for exploring the serotonin transport mechanism. Dahan and co-workers [39] similarly reported that glycine receptors on the membranes of living neurons could be stained with QDs coupled to an antibody fragment specific for the receptor. Single receptors were identified, and tracking of single QDs on the membranes allowed discovery of three different locations of glycine receptors and calculation of respective protein diffusion constants. Being more photostable than organic dyes and much smaller than fluorescent beads, QDs proved to be suitable probes for single-molecule detection experiments in living cells. Thus QDs have been shown to bridge the gap between labeling using large beads (typically 1 μm in diameter) and small organic fluorophores.

Other signaling pathways were also quantitatively characterized using QDs, providing essential background information for future use in receptor-targeted therapeutics and drug delivery. These included the study of epidermal growth factor (EGF)–conjugated QD probe behavior and receptor-mediated signal transduction as well as binding and internalization kinetics of this process in different cancer cell lines.

In another application the saccharide-coated QDs, forming spheres of different sizes, were used for cell endocytosis studies and provided very useful information for the design of artificial molecule delivery systems for gene and drug delivery. These studies suggested that endocytosis is highly size dependent and the optimum size for most efficient endocytosis is around 50 nm [40].

Another area of QD applications as cell markers is in long-term studies of cell–cell interactions, cell differentiation, and cell lineage tracking. It has been discovered that QDs can be internalized by cells, by either receptor-mediated or nonspecific endocytosis, and, in most experiments, do not interfere with normal cell physiology and differentiation [41]. Once QDs enter cells by nonspecific endocytosis, they accumulate in vesicles in the perinuclear region, in the endosomes and lysosomes, and divide with the daughter cells at cell divisions. Mattheakis and co-workers [42] using a peptide-mediated transportation method were able to incorporate different-colored QDs, targeting specifically a variety of live mammalian cells. They generated unique and easily spectrally resolvable barcodes for each cell types (up to 100), which was possible due to the multiplexing capabilities of QDs. Dubertret et al. [43] opened new research possibilities by tracking the embryogenesis of *Xenopus* (carnivorous frog native to Africa) using fluorescence imaging of early-stage embryos with microinjected phospholipid-coated QDs, tracking their development to the tadpole age. A recent study showed that the microinjection method overcomes earlier difficulties in intercellular delivery of QDs functionalized with appropriate peptide sequences targeted to cell organelles such as mitochondria and nucleus and allows us to optimize protocols leading to highly efficient delivery [44].

Alivisatos and his group proved that internalized QDs can be very effective in long-term studies of cell–cell interactions. Using QDs as cell-type identification markers they were able to examine in-time interaction between normal and cancerous cells and visualize and better understand how breast tumor cells undergo apoptosis [45].

Other characteristics important in cancer research include the motility and migration patterns of cancer cells as they are associated with metastases (spread of cancer) and the formation of secondary tumors. The movement of the individual cell on a cell culture substrate can be followed by using the so-called phagokinetic track method. Using the natural ability of cells to uptake the QDs by nonspecific endocytosis as they crawl over them, it is possible to observe by fluorescence the cell movement specific to a particular cell type. This is done by observing the QD free track on uniformly QD coated substrates. This process applied, for example, in cancer research not only provides insight into the invasive potential of different cancer cells but also, by adding to such prepared samples different potential cancer treatment drugs, makes it possible to measure the effect of chemotherapeutic agents on normal and cancerous cell motility. In comparison with other methods, which normally use fixed cells, QDs give more sensitive, reliable, and quantitative data with less sample preparation. The procedures using QDs can also be highly automated. Additionally, with fluorescence microscopy, the intensity levels characteristic to varying QD intake among different cancer cell types can be quantified, allowing for rapid identification of the type of cancers and assessment of their ratio to normal cells.

QDs as probes were also found to be more photostable, as such giving more flexibility with respect to analysis time and yielding higher signal-to-noise ratio than organic dyes in the procedure called fluorescent in situ hybridization (FISH). This method utilizes DNA or oligonucleotides conjugated to QDs for gene mapping and can be used, for example, for the identification of chromosomal abnormalities. Recently researchers from Quantum Dot Corporation [46] developed a new method using the Qbead™ system for high-throughput genotyping of single-nucleotide polymorphisms (SNPs). The Qbead system employs polystyrene microspheres containing three colors of fluorescent Qdots™ in controlled ratios. Each type of QD in the bead has 10 intensity levels, creating a quantum-dot-based nanobarcode with ~1000 combinational possibilities. Because of the unique spectral properties of QDs, this technology has tremendous multiplexing capability and may provide a powerful future tool for genomics and high-throughout screening. In the demonstration experiment, they applied the Qbead system to SNP genotyping by encoding microspheres conjugated to allele-specific oligonucleotides. After hybridization of oligonucleotides to amplicons (fragments of DNA produced in amplification techniques) produced by multiplexed PCR (polymerase chain reaction) of genomic DNA, individual microspheres were analyzed by flow cytometry and each SNP distinguished by its unique spectral barcode.

We described here only selected examples of the use of QDs in in vitro studies and the list of applications is continuously increasing with new discoveries as the technology improves. It seems that the ability to image single-cell migration and differentiation in real time over long periods possible with QDs is expected to play a very important role in several research areas, including embryogenesis, cancer metastasis, stem cells, and lymphocyte immunology.

4.6 QUANTUM DOTS AS IN VIVO PROBES

One of the greatest advantages of QDs for imaging in living tissue is that their emission wavelength can be tuned throughout the NIR spectrum by adjusting their composition and size. Fluorescence at such NIR wavelengths is less absorbed by tissues. They also produce intense two-photon fluorescence as their two-photon absorption cross sections are about two to three orders of magnitude larger (see Table 4.1) compared with organic dyes [47, 51]. QDs used in multiphoton microscopy enable the imaging of structures deep within biological specimens or living organisms with minimum photobleaching and photodamage.

Owing to these properties, the QD technology is intensely studied in the context of applications in cancer detection and for assisting treatment. In this context the research has shown that nanoparticles in the size range of 10–100 nm are accumulated preferentially at tumor sites through an effect called enhanced permeability and retention (EPR) [49–51]. This effect is believed to arise from two factors: Growing tumors produce vascular endothelial growth factor that promotes angiogenesis and many tumors lack an effective drainage system, which leads to subsequent nanoparticle accumulation. This causes tumor-associated neovasculature to be highly permeable, allowing leakage of circulating nanoparticles into the tumor tissue. These effects were observed, for example, by Gao and co-workers (2004) [33] when they used multifunctional QDs for simultaneous targeting and imaging of tumors in vivo in living animals. A highly stable QD conjugate was synthesized with functionalization layer consisting of amphiphilic triblock copolymer (for in vivo protection) and different targeting ligands (for specific tumor antigen recognition) and multiple PEG molecules (for improved biocompatibility and circulation). Their in vivo targeting studies of human prostrate cancer growing in nude mice indicated that the QD probes easily accumulate at tumors by both the passive targeting mechanism, due to enhanced permeability and retention of tumor sites, and the active targeting mechanism, due to antibody binding to target-specific cell surface biomarkers. Because their QD probes were emitting in the visible spectrum, a special spectral unmixing algorithm was used to separate autofluorescence from QD signals to give improved visualization of the tumor sites.

Gao et al. [33] and Kim and co-workers [51] demonstrated the use of the NIR-emitting QDs for sentinel lymph node (SLN) mapping, a procedure aimed at detecting the spread of cancer cells in the lymph node closest to the affected organ. The QDs injected intradermally into the animal (mouse and pig) (see Figure 4.8) were

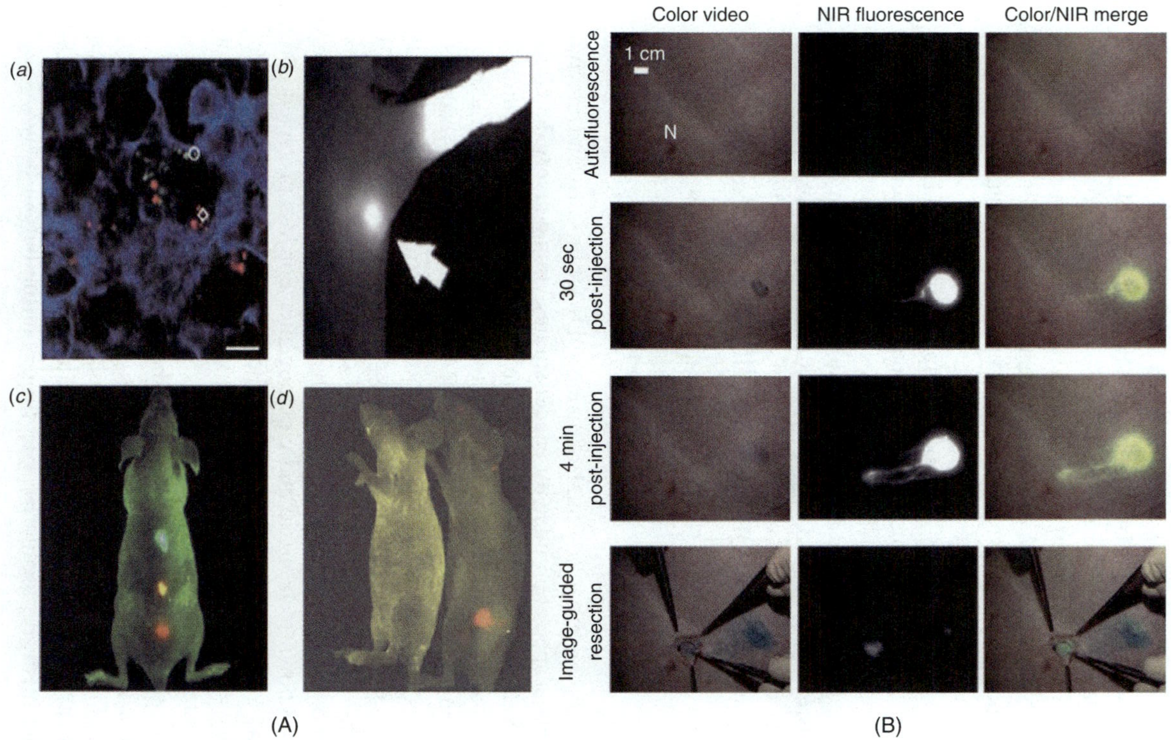

Figure 4.8 NIR QD sentinel lymph node mapping in mouse (A) and pig (B). A: (*a*) Ex vivo tissue examination of QD-labeled cancer cells trapped in a mouse lung. (*b*) Near-infrared fluorescence of water-soluble type II QDs taken up by sentinel lymph nodes. (*c*) In vivo simultaneous imaging of multicolor QD-encoded microbeads injected into a live mouse. (*d*) Molecular targeting and in vivo imaging of a prostate tumor in mouse using a QD–antibody conjugate (red). (Reprinted with permission from [33].) B: Images of the surgical field in a pig injected intradermally with 400 pmol of NIR QDs in the right groin. Four time points are shown from top to bottom: before injection (autofluorescence), 30 s after injection, 4 min after injection, and during image-guided resection. For each time point, color video (left), NIR fluorescence (middle), and color–NIR merge (right) images are shown. Fluorescence images have identical exposure times and normalization. To create the merged image, the NIR fluorescence image was pseudocolored lime green and superimposed on the color video image. The position of a nipple (N) is indicated. (Reprinted with permission from [51].)

followed by the surgeon using an intraoperative imaging system. The detection was possible in real time and at depths even up to 1 cm below the skin in the sentinel lymph node. This was a major breakthrough as, with the NIR QD guidance, rapid in situ visual identification of the position and size of affected SLN or even small lesions (e.g., metastatic tumors), which may be difficult or impossible to identify otherwise, was achieved, leading to more precise surgical procedures.

Most recently, So and co-workers from Stanford University proposed a very promising method for in vivo imaging by using self-illuminating QD probes based on bioluminescence resonance energy transfer (BRET) [52]. The group developed an eight-mutation variant of *Renilla reniformis luciferase* (Luc8) (protein present in marine organisms from the same group as jellyfish that catalyze a light-producing reaction), which has improved catalytic efficiency. The luciferase and antibodies against the cancer biomarkers to be detected were conjugated using an EDC linker (see Section 4.4.4) to QDs forming QD–Luc8–antibody complex probe. Such probes were intravenously injected into a cancerous mouse for the detection of cancer biomarkers. After the injection of coelenterazine, which is a substrate for Luc8 (initiator of bioemission), the emission from Luc8 and a strong emission from QDs in the NIR were observed as a result of BRET from Luc-8 to QDs. The tumor sites were imaged with greatly enhanced sensitivity and increased brightness (less background luminescence), as compared to targeting with standard QD protocols with external illumination.

4.7 CYTOTOXICITY

The above studies have shown great potential of using QDs as in vitro and in vivo probes for cell imaging and a special promise for cancer studies, drug delivery, and non-invasive body imaging. Still they require more extensive investigations to be routinely used. Cytotoxicity and potential interference of QD labeling with cellular processes are of primary concern in any live cell experiment. Most of the reports discussed above did not find adverse effects on cell viability, morphology, function, or development over the duration of the experiment at optimized concentrations of QDs. At higher concentrations, however, the effects on embryo development were noticeable. The most common QD composition, CdSe/ZnS, contains a core of cadmium and selenium, both of which are known to be toxic and carcinogenic. For less protected core or core/shell material and at larger QD concentrations more pronounced signs of interference with cell viability and function were observed [53]. The QDs therefore cannot be assumed to be completely innocuous, but it appears a relatively safe range exists, and with further technological improvements of core/shell protection, they are likely to find broader use. There are reports that injected QDs can accumulate in the kidney, liver, and spleen [33], and it is not known whether they can be ultimately fully cleared out. More investigation is required to understand degradation and metabolism of QDs before implementation in medical procedures or as probes in the human body.

4.8 FUTURE DIRECTIONS

Although the case for using QD-based fluorescent labels is compelling, it should be noted that QDs are not likely to replace organic dyes in all biological applications.

Some of the challenges that have still to be overcome include practical issues such as cost. QDs are much more expensive in comparison to organic dyes, and there is an initial investment required for researchers and instrument suppliers to produce systems optimized for use in labeling with QDs. Their detection specificity depends on the specific and nonspecific interactions of QD probes with target molecules and the surrounding environment. Specific biomolecular interactions are determined by conjugated ligands such as antibodies, peptides, nucleic acids, or small molecules. By maximizing biomolecular binding affinity and minimizing cross-reactivity, the QD probes can have highly specific interactions. However, because QDs are nanoparticle colloids, they have higher degree of nonspecific interactions also caused by steric hindrance than smaller molecules like fluorescence dyes. More improvement is still required to reduce the size of QD probes and their nonspecific binding.

Some promising applications of QDs have recently begun to emerge. They have recently been proposed as energy donors for photodynamic therapy, a process in which a photosensitizer within cells adsorbs light and transfers this absorbed energy to generate a reactive, cytotoxic oxygen species able to kill cancer cells [54]. This concept, combined with the potential innate cytotoxity of QDs, could result in dual-modality QD conjugates that are both targeted imaging contrast agents and therapeutic agents [54].

REFERENCES

1. C. Bremer, V. Ntziachristos, and R. Weissleder, "Optical-based optical imaging: Contrast agents and potential medical applications," *Eur. Radiol.* **13**, 231–243 (2003).
2. L. H. Qu and X. G. Peng, "Control of photoluminescence properties of CdSe nanocrystals in growth," *J. Am. Chem Soc.* **124**, 2049–2055 (2002).
3. X. H. Zhong, Y. Y. Feng, W. Knoll, and M. Y. Han, "Alloyed $Zn_xCd_{1-x}S$ nanocrystals with highly narrow luminescence spectral width," *J. Am. Chem. Soc* **125**, 13558–13563 (2003).
4. R. E. Bailey and S. Nie, "Alloyed semiconductor quantum dots: Tuning the optical properties without changing the particles," *J. Am. Chem. Soc.* **125**, 7100–7106 (2003).
5. R. E. Bailey, S. Kim, B. Fisher, H. J. Eisler, and M. Bawendi, "Type-II quantum dots: CdTe/CdSe(Core/Shell) and CdSe/ZnTe(Core/Shell) heterostructures," *J. Am. Chem. Soc.* **125**, 11466 (2003).
6. B. L. Wehrenberg, C. J. Wang, and P. Guyot-Sionnest, "Interband and intraband optical studies of PbSe colloidal quantum dots," *J. Phys. Chem. B* **106**, 10634–10640 (2003).
7. X. Gao, L. Yang, J. A. Petros, F. F. Marshall, J. W. Sinons, and S. Nie, "In vivo molecular and cellular imaging with quantum dots," *Curr. Opin. Biotechnol.* **16**, 63–72 (2005).
8. M. Bruchez, Jr., M. Moronne, P. Gin, S. Weiss, and A. P. Alivisatos, "Semiconductor nanocrystals as fluorescent biological labels," *Science* **281**, 2013–2015 (1998).
9. D. Gerion, F. Pinaud, S. C. Williams, W. J. Parak, D. Zanchet, S. Weiss, and A. P. Alivisatos, "Synthesis and properties of biocompatible water-soluble silica-coated CdSe/ZnS semiconductor quantum dots," *J. Phys. Chem. B* **105**, 8861–8871 (2001).
10. W. C. W. Chan and S. Nie, "Quantum dot bioconjugates for ultrasensitive nonisotopic detection," *Science* **281**, 2016–2018 (1998).
11. A. L. Efros and M. Rosen, "The electronic structure of semiconductor nanocrystals," *Annu. Rev. Mater. Sci.* **30**, 475–521 (2000).

12. C. A. Leartherdale, W. K. Woo, F. V. Mikulec, and M. G. Bawendi, "On the absorption cross section of CdSe nanocrystal quantum dots," *J. Phys. Chem. B* **106**, 7619–7622 (2002).
13. B. O. Dabbousi, J. Rodriguez-Viejo, F. V. Mikulec, J. R. Heine, H. Mattoussi, R. Ober, K. F. Jensen, and M. G. Bawendi, "(CdSe)ZnS core-shell quantum dots: Synthesis and characterization of a size series of highly luminescent nanocrystallites," *J. Phys. Chem. B* **101**, 9463–9475 (1997).
14. X. Michalet, F. F. Pinaud, L. A. Bentolila, J. M. Tsay, S. Doose, J. J. Li, G. Sundaresan, A. M. Wu, S. S. Gambhir, and S. Weiss, "Quantum dots for live cells in vivo imaging, and diagnostics," *Science* **307**, 538–544 (2005).
15. R. Peperkok, A. Squire, S. Geley, and P. I. H. Bastiaens, "Simultaneous detection of multiple green fluorescent proteins in live cells by fluorescence lifetime imaging spectroscopy," *Curr. Biol.* **CB 9**, 269–272 (1999).
16. M. Kuno, D. P. Fromm, H. F. Hamann, A. Gallagher, and D. J. Nesbitt, "Nonexponential 'blinking' kinetics of single CdSe quantum dots: A universal power law behavior," *J. Chem. Phys.* **112**, 3117–3120 (2000).
17. K. T. Shimizu, R. G. Neuhauser, C. A. Leatherdale, S. A. Empedocles, W. K. Woo, and M. G. Bawendi, "Blinking statistics in single semiconductor nanocrystal quantum dots," *Phys. Rev. B* **63**, 205316 (2001).
18. D. E. Gomez, J. van Embden, J. Jasieniak, T. A. Smith, and P. Mulvaney, "Blinking and surface chemistry of single CdSe nanocrystals," *Small* **2**, 204–208 (2006).
19. M. A. Hines and P. Guyot-Sionnest, "Synthesis and characterization of strongly luminescing ZnS-capped CdSe nanocrystals," *J. Phys. Chem.* **100**, 468–471 (1996).
20. D. V. Talapin, A. L. Rogach, A. Kornowski, M. Haase, and H. Weller, "Highly luminescent monodisperse CdSe and CdSe/ZnS nanocrystals synthesized in a hexadecylamine-trioctylphospine oxide-trioctylphospine mixture," *Nano Lett.* **1**, 207–211 (2001).
21. J. A. Kloepfer, R. E. Mielke, M. S. Wong, K. H. Nealson, G. Stucky, and J. L. Nadeau, "Quantum dots as strain- and metabolism specific microbiological labels," *Appl. Env. Microbiol.* **69**, 4205–4213 (2003).
22. K. E. Sapsford, T. Pons, I. L. Medintz, and H. Mattoussi, "Biosensing with luminescent semiconductor quantum dots," *Sensors* **6**, 925–953 (2006).
23. V. K. La Mer and R. H. Dinegar, *J. Am. Chem. Soc.* **72**, 4847–4854 (1950).
24. C. B. Murray, D. J. Norris, and M. G. Bawendi, "Synthesis and characterization of nearly monodisperse CdE (E = sulfur, selenium, tellurium) semiconductor nanocrystallites," *J. Am. Chem. Soc.* **115**, 8706–8715 (1993).
25. C. B. Murray, C. R. Kagan, and M. G. Bawendi, "Synthesis and characterization of monodisperse nanocrystals and close-packed nanocrystal assemblies," *Annu. Rev. Mater. Sci.* **30**, 545–610 (2000).
26. Z. A. Peng and X. Peng, "Formation of high-quality CdTe, CdSe, and CdS nanocrystals using CdO as precursor," *J. Am. Chem.* **100**, 468–471 (1996).
27. P. Reiss, J. Bleuse, and A. Pron, "Highly luminescent Cdse/Znse Core/Shell nanocrystals of low size dispersion," *Nano Lett.* **2**, 781–784 (2002).
28. A. A. Guzelian, J. E. B. Katari, A. V. Kadavanich, U. Banin, K. Hamad, E. Juban, A. P. Alivisatos, R. H. Wolters, C. C. Arnold, and J. R. Heath, "Synthesis of size-selected, surface passivated InP nanocrystals," *J. Phys. Chem.* **100**, 7212–7219 (1996).
29. O. Masala and R. Seshadri, "Synthesis routes for large volumes of nanoparticles," *Annu. Rev. Mater. Sci.* **30**, 41–81 (2004).
30. R. E. Bailey, A. M. Smith, and S. Nie, "Quantum dots in biology and medicine," *Phys. E* **25**, 1–12 (2004).

31. T. Pellegrino, S. Kudera, T. Liedl, A. Munoz Javier, L. Manna, and W. J. Parak, "On the development of colloidal nanoparticles towards multifunctional structures and their possible use for biological applications," *Small* **1**, 48–63 (2005).
32. X. Michelet, F. F. Pinaud, L. A. Bantolia, J. M. Tsay, S. Doose, J. J. Li, G. Sandaresan, A. M. Wu, S. S. Gambhir, and S. Weiss, "Quantum dots for live cells in vivo imaging, and diagnostics," *Science* **307**, 538–544 (2005).
33. X. Gao, X. Cui, R. M. Lavenson, L. W. K. Chung, and S. Nie, "In vivo cancer targeting and imaging with semiconductor quantum dots," *Nat. Biotechnol.* **22**, 969–976 (2004).
34. D. Gerion, W. J. Parak, S. C. Williams, D. Zanchet, C. M. Micheel, and A. P. Alivisatos, "Sorting fluorescent nanocrystals with DNA," *J. Am. Chem. Soc.* **124**, 7070–7074 (2002).
35. A. P. Alivisatos, W. Gu, and C. Larabell, "Quantum dots as cellular probes," *Annu. Rev. Biomed. Eng.* **7**, 55–76 (2005).
36. X. Wu, H. Liu, J. Liu, K. N. Haley, J. A. Treadway, J. P. Larson, N. Ge, F. Peale, and M. P. Bruchez, "Immunofluorescent labeling of cancer marker Her2 and other cellular target with semiconductor quantum dots," *Nature Biotechnol.* **21**, 41–46 (2003).
37. S. Sandra, D. Dutta, A. W. Glenn, and M. M. Brij, "Fluorescent nanoparticle probes for cancer imaging," *Techn. Cancer Res. Treat.* **4**, 593–602 (2005).
38. S. J. Rosenthal, A. Tomlinson, E. M. Adkins, S. Schroeter, S. Adams, et al., "Targeting cell surface receptors with ligand-conjugated nanocrystals," *J. Am. Chem. Soc.* **124**, 4586–4594 (2002).
39. M. Dahan, S. Levi, C. Luccardini, P. Rostaing, B. Riveau, and A. Triller, "Diffusion dynamics of glycine receptors revealed by single-quantum dot tracking," *Science* **302**, 442–445 (2003).
40. F. Osaki, T. Kanamori, S. Sando, T. Sera, and Y. Aoyagi, "A quantum dot conjugated sugar ball and its cellular uptake. On the side effects of endocytosis in the subviral region," *J. Am. Chem. Soc.* **126**, 6520–6521 (2004).
41. W. J. Parak, R. Boudreau, M. Le Gros, D. Gerion, D. Zanchet, et al., "Cell motility and metastatic potential studies based on quantum dot imaging of phagokinetic tracks," *Adv. Mater.* **14**, 882–885 (2002).
42. L. C. Mattheakis, J. M. Dias, Y. J. Choi, J. Gong, and M. P. Bruchez, "Optical coding of mammalian cells using semiconductor quantum dots," *Anal. Biochem.* **327**, 200–208 (2004).
43. B. Dubertret, P. Skourides, D. J. Norris, V. Noireaux, A. H. Brivanlou, and A. Libchaber, "In vivo imaging of quantum dots encapsulated in phospholipid miscelles," *Science* **298**, 1759–1762 (2002).
44. A. M. Derfus, W. C. W. Chan, and S. N. Bhatia, "Intercellular delivery of quantum dots for live cell labeling and organelle tracking," *Adv. Mater.* **16**, 961–966 (2004).
45. A. P. Alivisatos, W. Gu, and C. Larabell, "Quantum dots as cellular probes," *Annu. Rev. Biomed. Eng.* **7**, 55–76 (2005).
46. H. Xu, M. Y. Sha, A. Y. Wong, J. Uphoff, Y. Xu, et al., "Multiplexed SNP genotyping using the Qbead system: A quantum dot encoded microsphere-based assay," *Nucleic Acid Res.* **31**, e43 (2003).
47. D. R. Larson, W. R. Zipfel, R. M. Williams, S. W. Clark, M. P. Bruchez, F. W. Wise, and W.W. Webb, "Water-soluble quantum dots for multiphoton imaging In vivo," *Science* **300**, 1434–1436 (2003).
48. R. Duncan, "The dawning area of polymer therapeutics," *Nat. Rev. Drug Discov.* **2**, 195–208 (2003).
49. R. K. Jain, "Transport of molecules, particles, and cells in solid tumors," *Annu. Rev. Biomed. Eng.* **1**, 241–263 (1999).

50. R. K. Jain, "Delivery of molecular medicine to solid tumors: Lessons from in vivo imaging of gene expression and function," *J. Control. Relase* **74**, 7–25 (2001).

51. S. Kim, Y. T. Lim, E. G. Soltesz, A. M. De Grand, J. Lee, et al., "Near infrared fluorescent type II quantum dots for sentinel lymph node mapping," *Nat. Biotech.* **22**, 93–97 (2004).

52. M. K. So, C. Xu, A. M. Loening, S. V. Gambhir, and J. Rao, "Self-illuminating quantum dot conjugates for in vivo imaging," *Nat. Biotech.* **24**, 339–343 (2006).

53. A. M. Derfus, W. C. W. Chan, and N. Bhatia Sing, "Probing the cytotoxicity of semiconductor quantum dots," *Nano Lett.* **4**, 11–18 (2004).

54. R. Bakalova, H. Ohba, Z. Zhalev, M. Ishkawa, and Y. Baba, "Quantum dots as photosensitizers?" *Nat. Biotechnol.* **22**, 1360–1361 (2004).

55. A. M. Smith, G. Ruan, N. Rhyner, and S. Nie, "Engineering luminescent quantum dots for in vivo molecular and cellular imaging," *Ann. Biomed. Eng* **34**, 3–14 (2006).

CHAPTER 5

Quantitative Analysis of Fluorescent Image: From Descriptive to Computational Microscopy

MICHAL MAREK GODLEWSKI

Department of Chemistry and Biomolecular Sciences, Division of Environmental and Life Sciences, Macquarie University, Sydney 2109, Australia

Department of Physiological Sciences, Faculty of Veterinary Medicine, Warsaw University of Life Sciences – SGGW, Warsaw 02-786, Poland

AGNIESZKA TUROWSKA

Department of Preclinical Sciences, Faculty of Veterinary Medicine, Warsaw University of Life Sciences – SGGW, Warsaw 02-786, Poland

PAULINA JEDYNAK

Department of Physiological Sciences, Faculty of Veterinary Medicine, Warsaw University of Life Sciences – SGGW, Warsaw 02-786, Poland

DANIEL MARTINEZ PUIG

Bioiberica S.A., Pol. Ind. "Mas Puigvert" Ctra., Palafolls, Barcelona 80029, Spain

HELENA NEVALAINEN

Department of Chemistry and Biomolecular Sciences, Division of Environmental and Life Sciences, Macquarie University, Sydney 2109, Australia

5.1 INTRODUCTION

The application of fluorescence in microscopy has led to a considerable breakthrough in biochemical sciences by facilitating a new way of observing complex biological processes, structures, and interactions and locating them in particular parts of the cell. Today, fluorescent imaging is widely applied as a tool to confirm research hypotheses. However, very few publications provide supporting information for the observations based on fluorescence through computational analysis of the acquired images. Instead, single "best" images are selected which may not be representative and thus may not be able to provide reliable information. Given that cell populations are typically quite diverse, it is very likely that a selected cell ("the cell") will be found that confirms

Fluorescence Applications in Biotechnology and Life Sciences, Edited by Ewa M. Goldys

a particular theory, although many others are contradictory. While cellular analysis requires a great deal of caution, descriptive tissue analysis is even more subjective and interpretations are highly dependent on the personal experience of the observer. Baak [2] addressed difficulties in qualitative assessment of microscopic samples in pathology. The reliability was acceptable when a sample was assessed by at least three specialists, but consistency was low, especially in more complex analyses. Comparison of the data between different laboratories is also difficult considering the simplicity of observations made and the complexity of the pathological processes.

Modern imaging methods which use charged-coupled devices (CCDs) or photomultipliers (PMTs) provide the possibility to capture the visual observations in a numerical, digital form. In this format reliable quantitative data can be extracted which open new ways of understanding the examined cells and tissues and support the qualitative observation process. In physiological studies, the aim is to observe and relate a process/pattern representative of the whole population or compare acquired results with the population average established during different experiments. Automated quantitative analysis of the data allows rapid and precise assessment of the development process (understanding growth, differentiation, and maturation of complex tissues), also providing the possibility to easily compare data between experiments and laboratories. In this chapter, various methods of quantitative analysis applicable to studies of a single cell as well as whole populations and tissues will be presented and discussed.

5.2 ADVANTAGES OF QUANTITATIVE ANALYSIS

Descriptive microscopy is able to provide limited information only, for example, on the presence or absence and localization of a particular process or phenomenon. This relative quantification, often expressed as $-/+/++$ (as accepted in pathology), can be easily improved through quantitative analysis. The diagnostic possibilities that lie in the combination of descriptive and quantitative assessment of biological samples are best seen in cancer diagnostics. Identification of cancer is mostly carried out by the means of descriptive analysis; however, in the case of leukemia, scanning cytometry provide an alternative with its ability to rapidly differentiate the cancer type based on 16 tumor-specific antigens [3, 4]. The amount of biological material needed for quantitative assessment by this method is minimal when compared to other techniques, including flow cytometry, thus allowing the whole analysis to be carried out on a single thin-needle biopsy. Finally, as the sample is analyzed on a microscope slide, the same material can be later used for traditional staining procedures.

When carrying out tumor analysis, we must be aware that cancerogenesis is a very complicated process, where multiple mutations are generated in various cells. During growth and spread of the disease, the cells differentiate into a variety of phenotypes that form the tumor. These clones vary, often significantly with respect to the expression level of various proteins, and therefore their response to an antitumor agent may be different. To prevent the selection of the resistant and therefore more dangerous cancer cell clones in the course of therapy, simple detection of the presence of antigens is insufficient. As indicated by Preston [16], traditional approaches to quantify the level of protein expression, such as real-time polymerase chain reaction (PCR) or Western and Northern blotting, give only the average expression level for the whole sample. The variability in the phenotypes of cells forming the tumor may introduce a serious possibility of misinterpretation when using these methods. In the worst-case scenario the majority of cells with low or no expression decrease the overall average expression to an insignificant level, hiding the small, highly aggressive population of cancer cells. This is dangerous, especially in the course of assessment of cell susceptibility to therapeutic agents and monitoring during the course of therapy.

Quantitative analysis based on a selection of markers answers several fundamental questions such as the percentage of the tumor cells expressing these markers, the level of expression, and any association between the expression of different proteins in various cell phenotypes. Figure 5.1 shows examples of a quantitative approach to evaluation of a cell culture and in tissue analysis. Quantification based on parameters of a large number of individual cells (measured by scanning cytometry, discussed below) showed significant differences ($p < 0.01$) between proapoptotic protein (Bax) expression levels, indicating that there were two phenotypes present in COLO 205 cells (Figure 5.1*a*) of otherwise uniform appearance. On the other hand, there were no differences in Bax aggregation, the parameter describing protein oligomerization and aggregation on cell organelles. Further experiments with an anticancer agent showed that response of COLO 205 cells to proapoptotic treatment was bimodal, with more sensitive cells dying earlier. Similar results were obtained in cells within tissues. In our experiments the extent of the apoptotic process in the duodenum of healthy young wistar rats was analyzed (Figure 5.1*b*). It was found that variations between groups with high and low apoptosis were significant ($p < 0.05$, asterisks). These variations were related to changes in the digestive juice flow and acidity (pancreatic juice, bile and hydrochloric acid) as they disappeared further along the gut [11].

5.3 METHODS OF QUANTITATIVE ANALYSIS

Single-cell analysis usually carried out by confocal microscopy provides deep insights into various processes occurring in the cell. However, observations performed on a single object cannot be assumed to be representative for the whole population. Thus repetitive experiments are required when a number of (randomly selected) cells are observed and the data compared. Quantification of the data facilitates the comparison process, as sets of numerical data are easier to manipulate than a collection of images. Furthermore, statistical data can be easily acquired from such quantitative measurements.

Currently an increasing number of researchers create and validate methods for data processing to support their experiments. Our analysis of protein translocations within the cell on the basis of fluorescence integrated optical density provides a good example. The fluorescence integrated optical density (IOD) is a parameter describing average fluorescence intensity multiplied by fluorescence area or volume. Using IOD, we analyzed interactions of the proapoptotic protein (Bax and Smac/DIABLO) with mitochondria [7, 12] and their translocation between cytoplasmic and nuclear compartments of the living cell (Figure 5.2). By trying different approaches, we found that only the whole volume cell analysis [three dimensional (3D) in time] gives accurate description of the pattern of changes. The analysis of a single-cell cross section, although quick and relatively easy, was not very accurate, as the expression varied in different layers of the cell and living cells were never entirely stationary throughout the entire experiment. Quantification of the data by using IOD allowed us to compare the results between a large number of experiments and present them graphically [7]. By comparing the temporal evolution of changes, we postulated the coincidence between Bax translocation

(*a*)

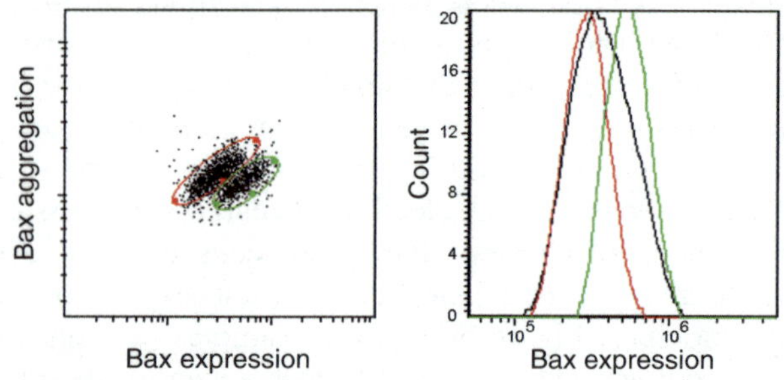

Bax expression

Rgn.#	Count	Pct.	Mean
1	1218	57.2%	0.34*
2	746	35.0%	0.63
Total	2129		0.45

Bax aggregation

Rgn.#	Count	Pct.	Mean
1	1218	57.2%	1384
2	746	35.0%	1224
Total	2129		1331

(*b*)

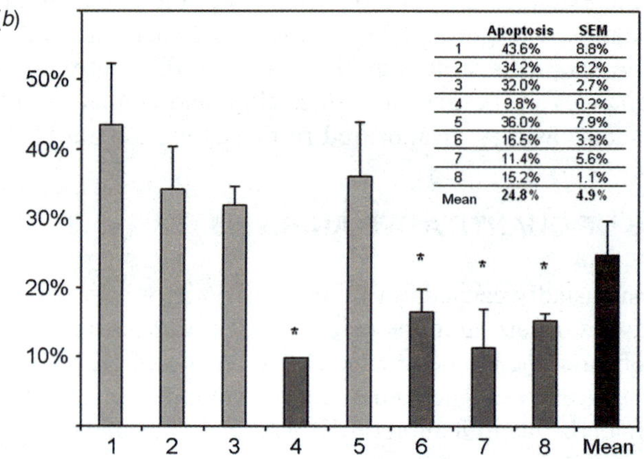

Figure 5.1 (*a*) Phenotype diversity in expression of proapoptotic protein Bax in genetically uniform human adenocarcinoma COLO 205 cell line measured by scanning cytometry. In the cytogram of Bax expression vs. aggregation (top left), the two subpopulations of cells were differentiated. The subpopulation with a higher average expression proved more susceptible to apoptosis induction (as confirmed by later experiments). Bax aggregation, a parameter describing protein oligomerization and translocation to cell organelles, however, remained similar. Bax expression histograms for the populations with higher (red) and lower (green) expression levels, respectively, were plotted against the population average (black line) (top right). The table shows numerical data from the analysis. The expression levels in single cells were statistically evaluated by a nonparametric Mann-Whitney test and a significant difference ($p < 0.01$) was found between low- and high-expression groups. (*b*) Differences in apoptosis index (percentage of apoptotic cells) evaluated by confocal-based image analysis of active caspase 3 expression in duodenum mucosa of healthy young (8-week-old) wistar rats. Caspase 3 is the major executor caspase in the late, irreversible phase of apoptosis. There were significant differences ($p < 0.05$ by nonparametric Mann-Whitney test) between groups with low (dark grey) and high (light grey bars) apoptotic index. The table (insert) shows the average results for different rats [± standard error of the mean (SEM)] and the black bar represents the average in the entire experiment.

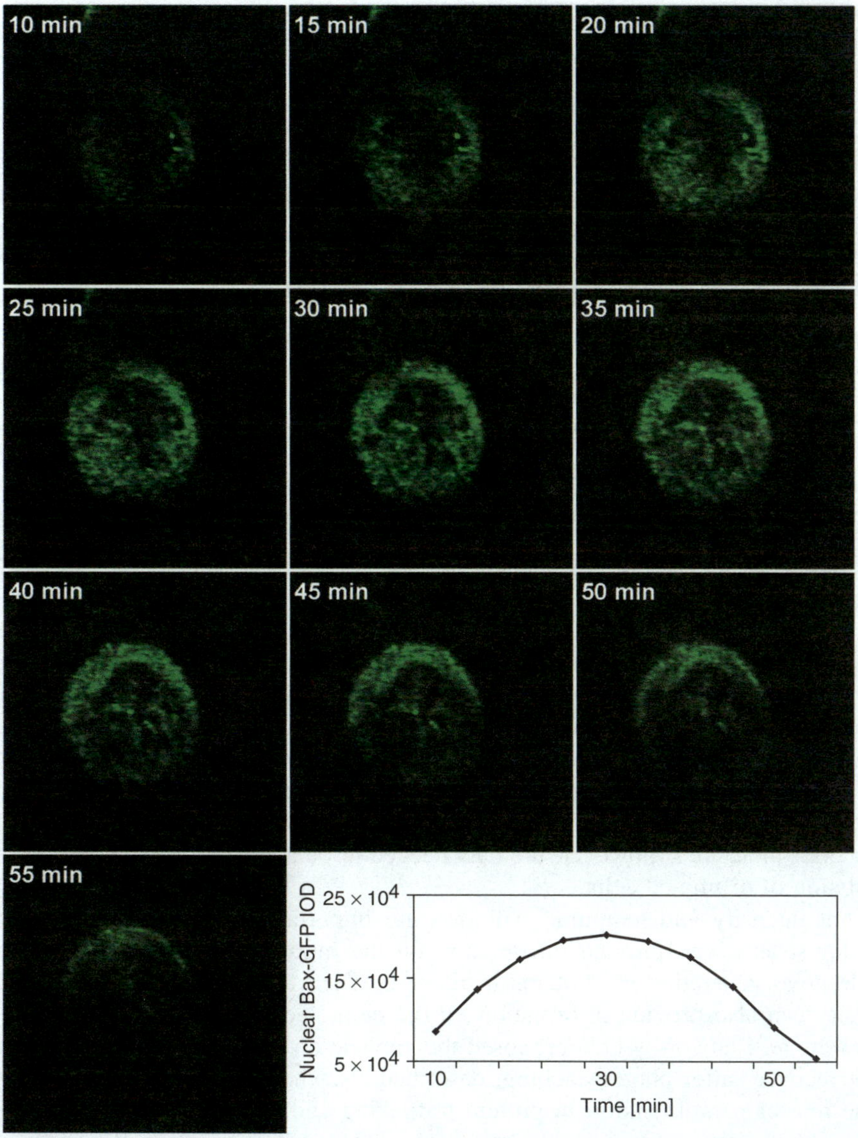

Figure 5.2 Four-dimensional (3D in time) analysis of Bax–green fluorescent protein (GFP) translocation to nucleus in living human adenocarcinoma COLO 205 cell. Subsequent images show the 3D reconstruction of a single COLO 205 cell incubated with the anticancer agent nimesulide (1 μm) at 5-min intervals. The graph shows the results of IOD volumetric analysis of Bax in the nuclear area, showing the peak of translocation 30 min after proapoptotic stimuli.

and Smac/DIABLO efflux to and from the mitochondria, which was later confirmed by immunogold electron microscopy. Digital analysis of the data also made it possible to compare experiments performed in living cells with those carried out on fixed cell populations, which can be seen by comparing Figures 5.2 and 5.3.

IOD is related to the total amount of protein in the observation volume, while fluorescence intensity is related to another parameter of interest, protein concentration.

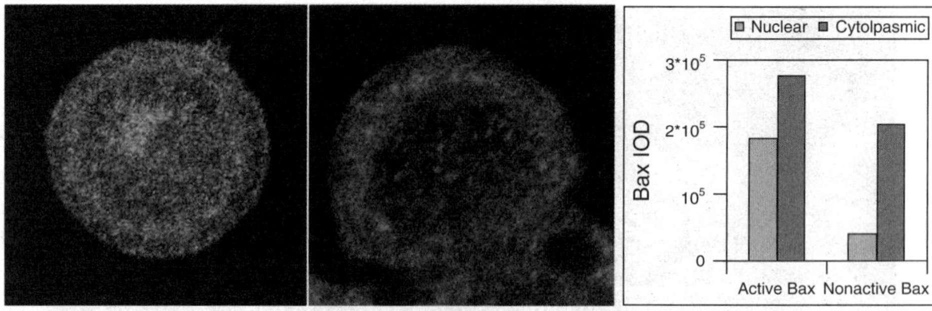

Figure 5.3 Differences in distribution of active (left) and inactive (middle) form of Bax within human adenocarcinoma COLO 205 (fixed) cells stimulated to apoptosis by 30-min incubation with anticancer agent camptothecin (0.15 μm) measured by confocal microscopy. The active form of Bax was labeled with antibodies recognizing the 44–63 amino acid (AA) sequence within the death domain responsible for protein oligomerization and activity. The inactive form of Bax was labeled by antibodies against the 11–30 AA sequence of the N-terminal part of the protein that is cleaved upon Bax activation. The graph (right) shows differences in the active and nonactive Bax-related IOD in the nuclear and cytoplasmic compartments of the cell, determined from the area where DNA-related fluorescence was observed (not shown).

A significant challenge in the quantitative analysis of fluorescent images is to relate the fluorescence intensity to protein concentrations in the cell. A recent technique proposed for data interpretation uses an external calibration and is based on the intensity curves for a series of dilutions of recombinant proteins, which is then compared to the fluorescence intensity observed in the cell [6, 18]. This approach has given satisfactory results in studies with yellow fluorescent protein (YFP)–tagged fusion proteins and transporter molecules; however, the data needed to be averaged over a relatively large population of examined cells.

Light intensity and temporal evolution are important quantitative parameters for a biologist as it can provide information on the intracellular transport patterns and the de novo generation of proteins in the cell. The varying patterns of fluorescence intensity can also provide information on the biomolecular processes within the cell. For example, Kenworthy [13] proposed the application of quantitative FRAP (fluorescence recovery after photobleaching, described elsewhere in this volume) for a study of the role of palmitoylation in protein trafficking and recycling within the cell. Her results showed that protein recirculation was a dynamic process, as it took less than a minute for a full recovery of the fluorescence in the photobleached area. Furthermore, experiments conducted with cycloheximide (a nonspecific inhibitor of protein synthesis) showed that proteins were recirculated to the Golgi complex from the cell membrane. A different approach to the quantification of protein dynamics was proposed for the study of association and disassembly of actin filaments within the cell. For this purpose, fluorescence speckle microscopy (FSM) was combined with mathematical computational models to recognize different patterns of fluorescence of the actin filaments which were later associated with biological activity [1, 5]. The movement of the molecules could also be analyzed by tracking the speckle flow through multiframe correlation [5].

Automated, fluorescence-based analysis of large populations of cells is the backbone of a computational approach in biology. The most popular approach in this field of research is flow cytometry. Its major limitation is that cells must be examined in suspension. It is a major disadvantage of the method, as the majority of cells grow attached to a surface and when removed tend to undergo considerable structural and/or biochemical changes; in some cases the detachment alone can trigger apoptosis. Tissue analysis is also very difficult as the tissue needs to be digested before experiments, leaving cells isolated but otherwise undamaged. Another problem is that cells in suspension (even dead, fixed ones) tend to aggregate, and this may produce misleading results. Finally, the cells after experiment cannot be retrieved, which removes the possibility for time evolution studies of the dynamic processes in the living cell population since single cells are identified separately. Two methods of analysis are able to overcome these problems, these are digital imaging using a confocal or fluorescence microscope and scanning cytometry. Both are used to analyze cells or tissue cross sections attached to the surface of a microscope slide or placed in a special chamber where live cell analysis can be performed. In scanning cytometry the slide is placed in a fluorescence microscope with a motorized stage which enables the entire slide to be scanned automatically with repeated focusing in each scanning step. The objects are identified based on either their higher than background fluorescence intensity or their edges. This produces a set of cellular images accompanied by cell coordinates and a number of quantitative parameters such as cell number and distribution combined with average, maximum, and minimum fluorescence intensities in designated observation areas. The fluorescence parameters may be measured separately over the nucleus and cytoplasmic area in each cell. Other analyses such as fluorescence in situ hybridization (FISH) are also possible as well as colony cell counts. The most popular form of studies by scanning cytometry performed on cell cultures is the cell cycle analysis. The cell position in the proliferation cycle can be established from the three measured parameters: the nucleus size, DNA-related fluorescence, and DNA aggregation pattern [8, 10, 14]. Another possibility is the observation of protein-related fluorescence. Compared to flow cytometry, scanning cytometry produces much more information concerning every single cell. Not only can the protein content and dispersion be measured but also we can also distinguish between subcellular compartments. The usual targets for analysis are the nuclear and cytoplasmic compartments of cells; however, organelles can also be differentiated from the rest of the cell by using specific organelle-targeting dyes (for details see [9]). On this basis, protein expression, localization, and translocation between different cellular compartments can be quantitatively analyzed in large-cell populations (Figures 5.4–5.6) [8, 10]. Based on the fluorescence intensity in single pixels and differences between neighboring pixels, the pattern and intensity of protein aggregation within the cell can also be studied [8, 10, 15]. Another unique feature of scanning cytometry is the ability to store X and Y coordinates of each cell along with the fluorescence-related data (Figure 5.5). This makes it possible to localize and identify them on a slide for further comparison between the biochemistry and morphological features of the cell (Figure 5.6).

In contrast to the "tidy" and "well-organized" cell cultures where all cells and nuclei are localized in the same plane, the analysis of tissues presents a major problem. Tissue architecture is much more complex and compact than that of individual cells. The nuclei are usually smaller and arranged randomly with respect to the dissection plane, and they often overlap. The tissues are also composed of a variety of cell types with different characteristics, and these assemblages can further be embedded in different types of extracellular matrices (Figure 5.7).

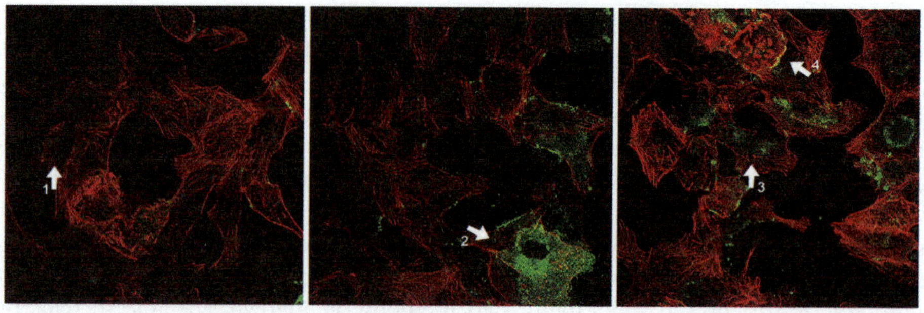

Figure 5.4 Equine herpesvirus (JanE EHV-1)–induced changes in actin cytoskeleton of horse epithelial ED cells visualized by confocal microscopy. F-actin was labeled with Alexa Fluor 633 (red fluorescence), virus antigen by fluoroscein isothiocyanate–conjugated gamakon. Confocal images present the pattern of F-actin organization in healthy cells where no virus antigenrelater fluorescence was observed (arrow 1) and in cells infected by the virus with low (arrow 2), normal (arrow 3), and increased (arrow 4) actin-related fluorescence intensity. Arrow numbers relate cells to quadrants presented on cytogram in Figure 5.6.

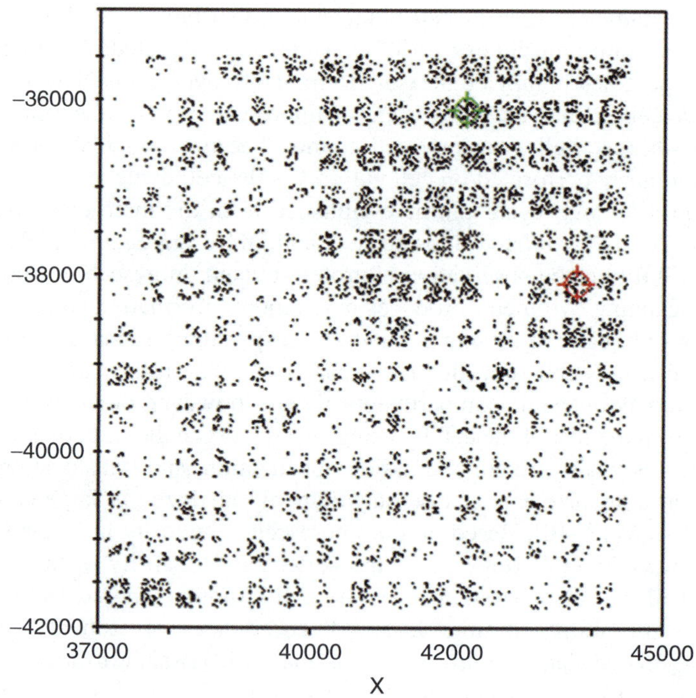

Figure 5.5 Map of cell distribution of horse epithelial ED cells generated by scanning cytometry from 195 randomly selected microscope fields of view. The 195 different fields of view are arranged in rows/columns and are variously filled with dots. Each dot represents cell nuclei recognized on the basis of nuclear-related HOECHST 33342 fluorescence intensity. Note the differences in cell density between the analyzed areas.

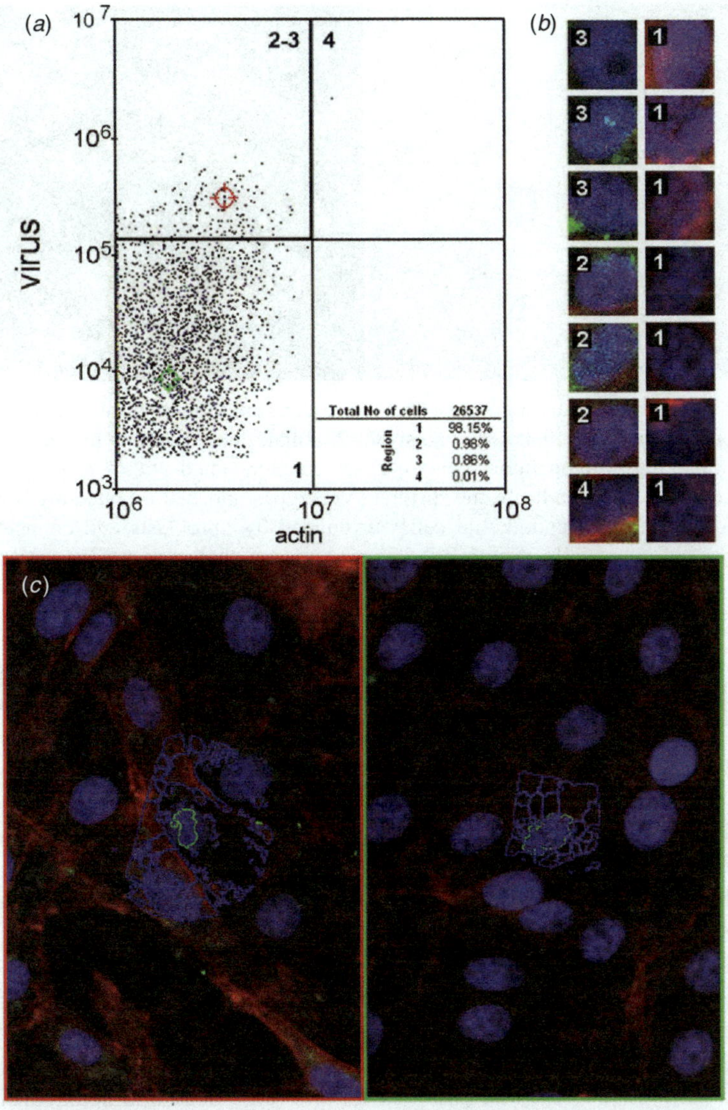

Figure 5.6 Equine herpesvirus (JanE EHV-1)–induced changes in actin cytoskeleton of horse epithelial ED cells quantitatively analyzed by scanning cytometry. F-actin was labeled with Alexa Fluor 633 (red fluorescence), virus antigen by FITC-conjugated gamakon, and cell nuclei were counterstained by HOECHST 33342. This analysis showed that the majority (over 98%) of the cells remained uninfected [(*a*) lower quadrant], and only around 2% of the infected cells remained attached to the slide (top quadrants). The cells with high gamakon and actin-related fluorescence have the lowest abundance (only 0.01%, top right quadrant). The gallery (*b*) shows randomly selected cells from the cytogram areas, labeled according to the region. Two cells from healthy (green crosshair on the quadrant cytogram) and virus-infected (red crosshair) cells were randomly selected and relocated (*c*) showing cell recognition (green outline) based on high intensity of DNA-related fluorescence with the related actin pattern (blue outline).

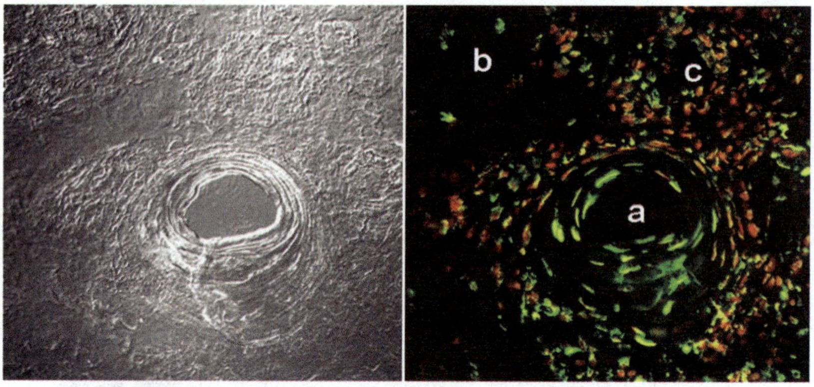

Figure 5.7 Confocal Nomarski contrast and fluorescent microphotographs of human head and neck carcinoma cross section labeled against Bcl-2, a major antiapoptotic protein overexpressed in a variety of tumors (green fluorescence); DNA counterstained with 7 aminoactinomycin-D (red fluorescence). Letters indicate the different cell types and cell architecture within the tissue: (*a*) blood vessel with endothelial cells surrounded by fibroblasts and connective tissue; (*b*) necrotic loci of a few cells of high Bcl-2 expression and characteristic distorted arrangement observed under Nomarski contrast; (*c*) solid tumor area with large number of compacted cells with variable Bcl-2 expression.

For the optimal observation conditions, a tissue sample should be cut in such a way as to consist only of a single layer of whole nuclei—a task which is near impossible. Therefore the common practice is to cut the slice as thin as possible (4–5 μm for paraffin-embedded and 10 μm for frozen tissues) to minimize the occurrence of overlapping nuclei (see Figures 5.8*a* and Figure 5.9). This is crucial for quantitative analysis, where nuclei-related fluorescence is the only method able to distinguish between cells. Unfortunately, thin slices only reduce the problem, but there are two ways in which it can be overcome. The first option is to increase the analyzed area and lens magnification so that a larger number of cells can be scanned with greater precision (Figure 5.10). The second option is to use a confocal aperture to dissect the tissue section into thinner slices (Figures 5.8*b* and 5.11*a*). Confocal imaging greatly increases the readout accuracy but at a cost of considerable increase of the analysis time. In our practice, we carry the analysis of complicated and variable tissues, such as gut cross sections [11, 19] and complex tumors (e.g., head and neck carcinomas) by confocal imaging, while uniform tissues (e.g., pancreas, solid tumors) can be analyzed with great accuracy by scanning cytometry.

Another source for serious problems in tissue analysis originates from the preparation and fixing method. Figure 5.12 shows three intestine cross sections labeled against MAP I LC3 (programmed cell death II marker) and DNA. In this image the staining and imaging procedures were the same; the only difference was the preparation technique. The high background-to-signal ratio observed in the case of Bouine solution fixing (Figure 5.12*b*) obscured the image, rendering automated analysis extremely difficult if not impossible. In contrast, a perfect background-to-signal ratio was obtained with the frozen tissues (Figure 5.12*c*). This kind of preparation requires confocal-based imaging as frozen specimens cannot be cut as thin as paraffin-embedded ones. For scanning cytometry and fluorescent microscopy, however, the best method seems to be *para*-formaldehyde fixing combined with paraffin embedding (Figure 5.12*a*). This

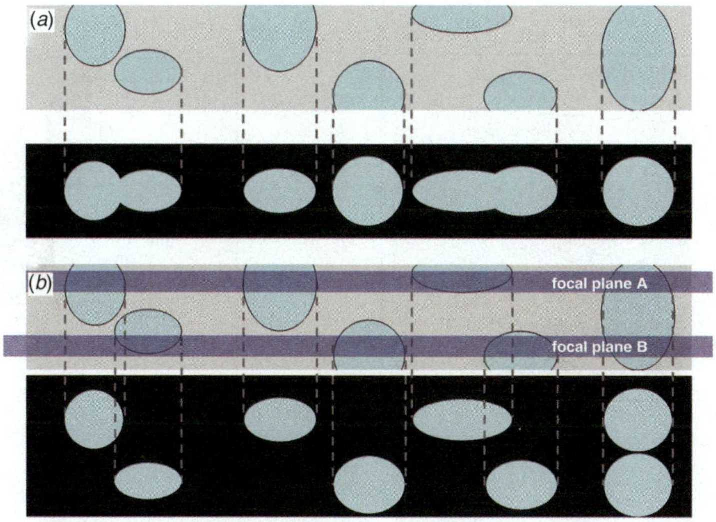

Figure 5.8 Schematic showing advantage of confocal imaging over fluorescence imaging in tissues. Cell nuclei are aligned in a relatively random pattern at different depths in the slice. When observed by fluorescent microscopy, they often overlap, providing misleading information about the DNA content and nucleus area (*a*). By "dissecting" the tissue into even thinner slices (focal planes) by using the confocal aperture, the architecture of the tissue can be resolved in much greater detail (b).

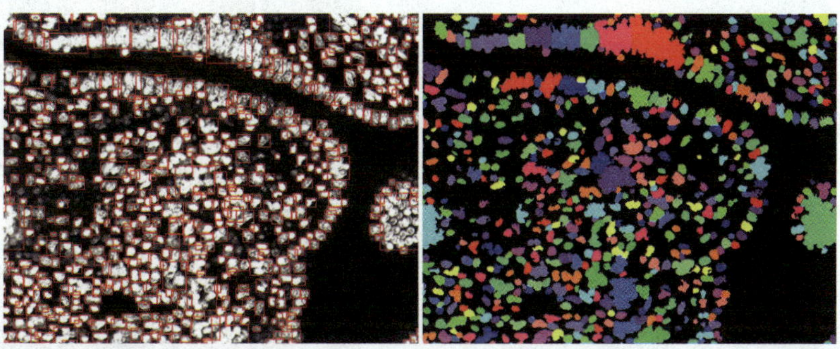

Figure 5.9 Scanning cytometry analysis of same cross sections of piglet midjejunum as presented in Figure 5.11. Fluorescent intensity–based automated nuclei recognition was done on the basis of DNA-related fluorescence of 7 aminoactinomycin-D. We draw attention to the large number of overlapping nuclei counted as a single object that had to be later removed by gating the DNA cytogram (see Figure 5.10).

method allows thin cross sections to be made from the fixed tissue (4–6 μm), minimizing the possibility of nuclei overlap, while the immunospecificity of the tissue is altered only slightly. We emphasize the need to acquire a large number of images in tissue analysis. In in-tissue cytometry (confocal-based image analysis) of protein expression indices (percentage of cells expressing the studied protein), at least 14 images were randomly acquired from the mucosa of every single intestine cross section and at least three cross sections per specimen were quantified. Random image selection of different

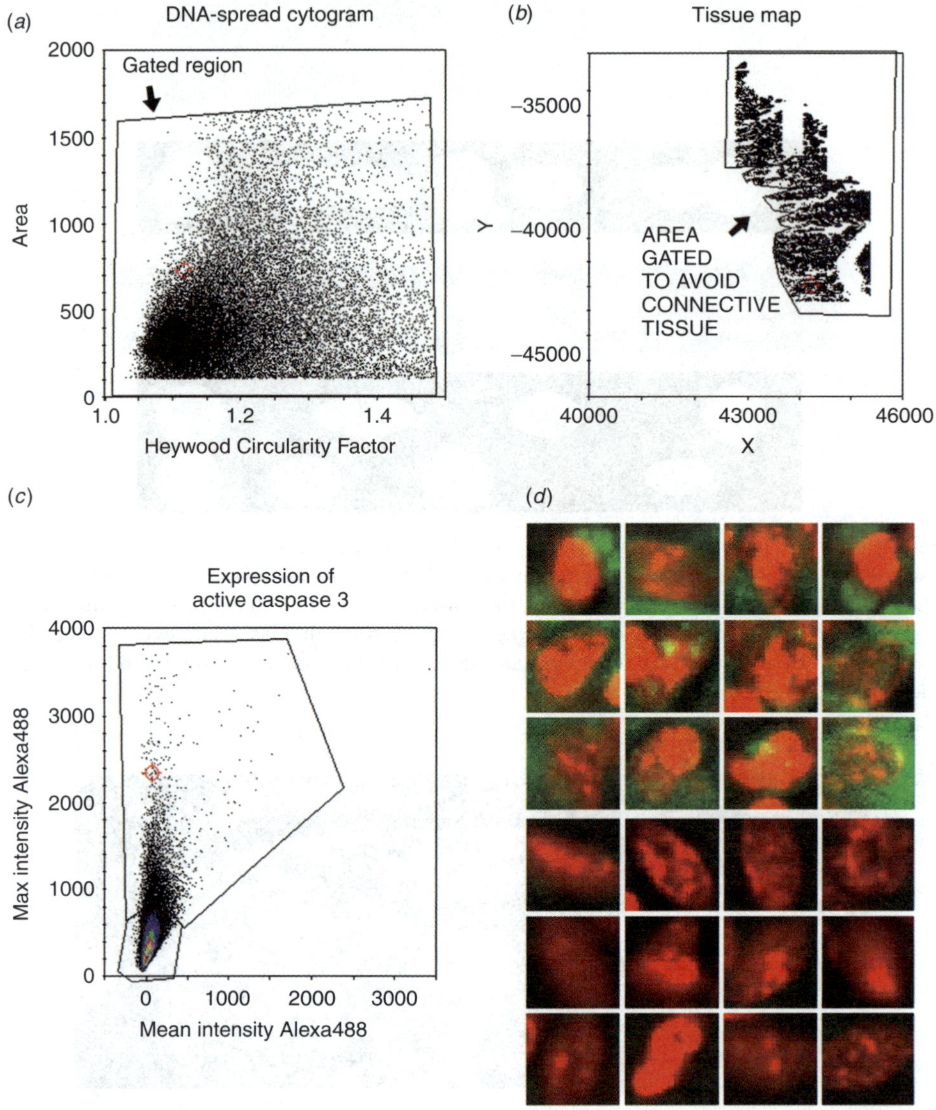

Figure 5.10 Scanning cytometry analysis of same cross sections of piglet midjejunum presented in Figure 5.11. Alexa Fluor 488 anti-active caspase 3 labeling (green fluorescence) combined with 7 aminoactinomycin-D DNA counterstaining (red fluorescence). The overlapping nuclei were eliminated from the DNA spread cytogram by initial gating based on the nucleus area and circularity factors (*a*). The tissue map of the whole scanned cross section was additionally gated to avoid connective tissue (*b*). Also shown is the active caspase 3 cytogram (*c*) gating cells with low (region in bottom right corner) and high caspase-related fluorescence. The red crosshair indicates localization of a single cell with high caspase 3 expression on the tissue map and within cytograms. Finally we show a gallery of randomly selected cells with high (upper) and low (lower) active caspase 3 expression (d).

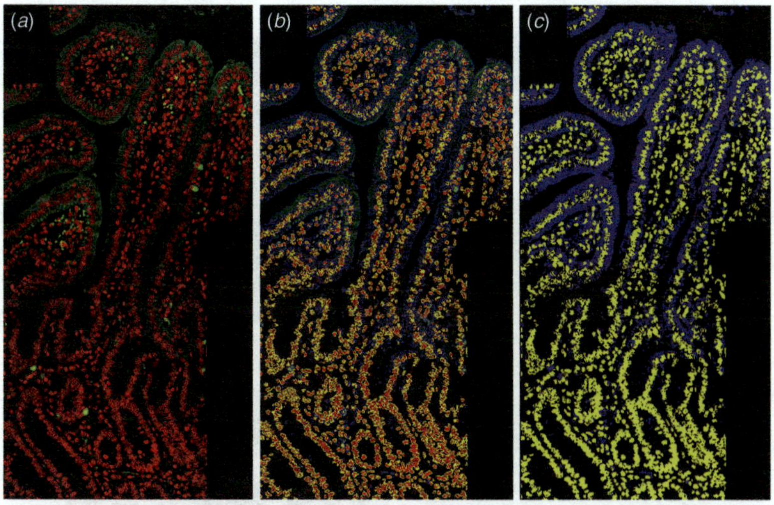

Figure 5.11 In-tissue cytometry analysis of apoptosis index in mucosa of piglet midjejunum labeled against active caspase 3 with Alexa Fluor 488 (green fluorescence); DNA counterstained with 7 aminoactinomycin-D. Multiple image reconstruction showing the whole depth of the mucosa layer from villi on the top to the crypt region at the bottom (*a*). Automated, fluorescence intensity–based recognition of cell nuclei (outlined in yellow) and active caspase 3–expressing cells (outlined in blue) carried out with image analysis system (*b*). Masking of cell nuclei (yellow) and caspase-positive cells (blue) as detected by the counting software (*c*).

areas in tissue analysis is also crucial since the areas may vary significantly in their protein expression level. This can be seen in Figure 5.11*a*, where we can compare active caspase 3 expression on the villi (top) and in the crypts (bottom). In this case, the object recognition was performed on the basis of fluorescent intensity; objects under 50 pixels in size were automatically eliminated and the remaining cells were counted (Figure 5.11). The number of objects, total fluorescence IOD, and fluorescent area were determined to provide the index, total protein expression level, and process intensity, respectively. The staining and image acquisition parameters were kept uniform in all experiments to achieve reproducibility between different specimens and experiments. The same intestine cross sections were also analyzed by scanning cytometry. At least three whole cross sections were analyzed per specimen with nuclei recognition based on the DNA-related fluorescence intensity. The system implemented the watershed method of mathematical separation which was carried out to separate the overlapping nuclei (Figure 5.9). All the remaining overlapping nuclear conglomerates were automatically eliminated from the readout by gating (see Figure 5.10*a*). From the tissue map reconstructed from the X and Y positions of the nuclei, all areas with connective tissue were manually gated out (see Figure 5.10*b*) and active caspase 3 expression was measured in the remaining cells (see Figure 5.10*c*). The picture gallery (Figure 5.10*d*) shows the cells from the regions of high and low caspase 3–related fluorescence relocated from the image of the slide on the basis of their stored $X–Y$ coordinates. The results obtained by the two methods discussed above were comparable, although the actual readout was higher in the case of scanning cytometry. Overall, no significant differences were found between the methods (Table 5.1).

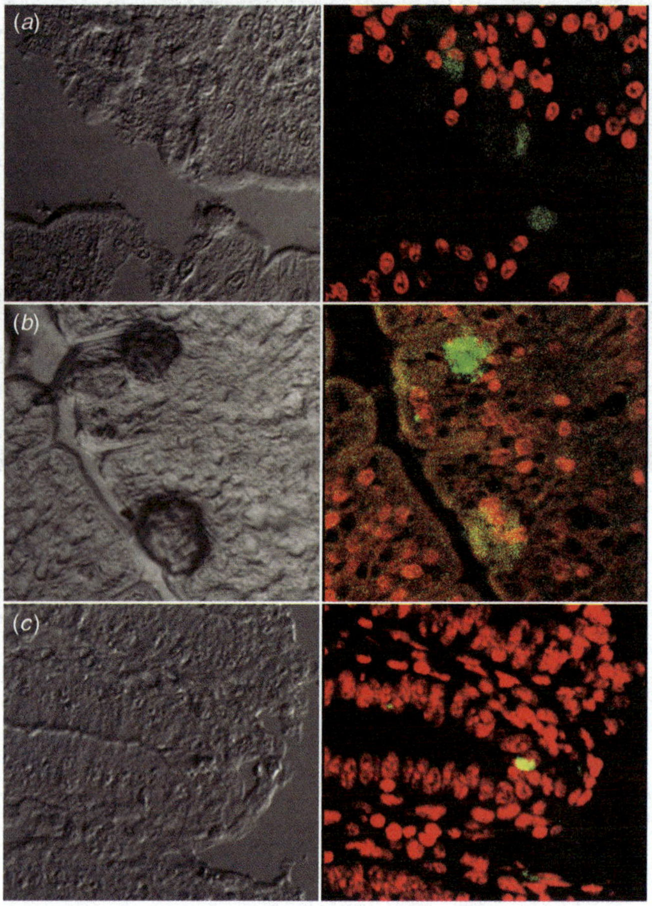

Figure 5.12 Cross-sections of piglet midjejunum labeled against MAP I LC-3 protein, marker of programmed cell death II (green fluorescence); nuclei were counterstained by 7 aminoactinomycin-D (red fluorescence). The tissues were prepared by three different techniques. (*a*) *para*-Formaldehyde-fixed, paraffin-embedded tissue shows good nuclei counterstaining, but the antibody-related labeling gives some background fluorescence. The advantage of the method is that samples can be cut into very thin (4–6-μm) slices, minimizing the risk of nuclei overlap in the acquired fluorescent image. This is our preferred method for scanning cytometry and fluorescence microscopy–based image analysis. (*b*) Bouine-fixed, paraffin-embedded tissue. The technique is widely used for morphometry studies and classical histochemical staining because it does not alter tissue dimensions. It gives strong background in both fluorescent channels, simultaneously significantly decreasing specific binding of both antibodies and DNA probes due to the presence of picric acid, making it unsuitable for image analysis. (*c*) Liquid nitrogen–frozen tissue gives the best background-to-signal ratio; however it requires confocal-based image acquisition because frozen samples cannot be cut as thinly as paraffin-embedded ones and the risk of nuclei overlap is increased.

TABLE 5.1 Comparison of Confocal-Based Image Analysis and Scanning Cytometry Performed on Cross Sections of Intestine.

	Percentage of Cells with High Expression of Active Caspase 3	
Specimen Number	Confocal-Based Image Analysis	Scanning Cytometry Analysis
1	22.48	25.17
2	19.03	20.02
3	7.7	15.3
4	20.83	36.3
5	15.09	15.04
6	23.96	30.47
Geomean	17.08	22.46
SEM	2.68	3.83
t student	0.111586444	

Note: Geomean, geometric mean; SEM, standard error of mean, *t*-student, results of t-student test.

5.4 IMAGE PROCESSING

Due to the digital form of the acquired image, one is tempted to try postcapture modification by various software packages. Most commonly, the authors tend to enhance the image contrast and correct the background-to-signal ratio to make sure that the presented data are clearly visible and optimized for the printing process. While in the case of descriptive microscopy this kind of image processing may be justifiable, there are some issues concerning analyses based on the processed image. The question one must ask is what kind of information is to be gathered and how does image processing affect interpretation of the data. Image processing greatly influences the brightness level of each pixel, thus altering fluorescent intensity readouts. Furthermore, the ability to vary the change between color ranges and tones to improve the image quality results in an even greater modification of the original data and significant loss of data fidelity. Thus the images processed in any manner cannot be used for expression-level analysis based on optical density (Figure 5.13). However, in the case of index analysis where simply the number of objects matters, image processing can be used to some extent to facilitate the recognition based on the difference between background and signal. Postcapture modification of the data in the case of index analysis offers significant advantages over precapture offsetting. Precapture offsetting removes all weak fluorescence from the image as a background regardless of its localization. Thus, a low-protein-expressing profile manifested by this weak, yet specific fluorescence may be irretrievably lost from the image. In the case of tissue analysis where uniformity in sample preparation as well as staining and scanning protocols are critically required to allow comparison between specimens, the differences in the expression level are often clearly visible (compare Figures 5.13*a* and 5.13*c*). Both background and intensity correction as presented in Figures 5.13*b* and 5.13*d* provide some advantages for the intensity histogram–based automated object recognition (Figure 5.13, white arrows). However, some artifacts are also generated (Figure 5.13, red arrows) and this fact needs to be strongly emphasized.

The volume analysis of the reconstructed confocal image presents different kinds of problems. Due to optical limitations, the acquired voxel (three-dimensional pixel) is different from its original form. An image is always distorted along the *Z* axis and the

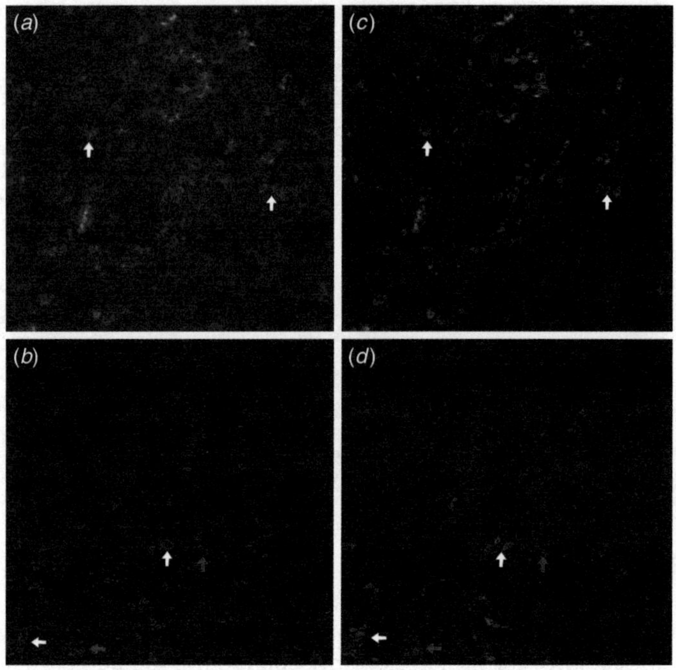

	Area	OD	IOD	Objects	Index
a	3455	3546.312	131276	96	41.38%
b	4416	2135.413	95801.34	106	45.69%
c	2320	443.1928	13111.33	79	25.40%
d	791	812.7293	20490.33	32	10.29%

Figure 5.13 Influence of postacquisition image processing on image analysis data. The background correction (*a*,*b*) increased the fluorescent intensity–based object recognition due to better resolved differences between objects (white arrows), but it also generated some artifacts (red arrows). The enhancement of very weak positive fluorescence (*c*,*d*) reduced the number of unspecific objects found and increased resolution between the cells (white arrows) at a cost of some positive objects (red arrows). Both methods significantly altered the integrated optical density of analyzed images, making it unsuitable for protein expression analysis (see the table).

fluorescence intensity is also slightly altered. Moreover, the smaller is the object being analyzed, the more it is distorted along all three axes (Figure 5.14) [9]. The interpretation of these images may be misleading, especially when the analysis is carried out on the basis of fluorescent spectra overlap during protein colocalization studies. The imperfections in fluorescent image can sometimes generate the overlap pattern that can be mistaken for the actual result. This is the reason why the colocalization experiments need to always be validated by other experimental techniques (fluorescence resonance energy transfer, coimmunoprecipitation, or immunogold electron microscopy). Some authors suggested using mathematical spatial deconvolution models to correct the problem [17]. Deconvolution is widely used to correct the image clarity, especially in 3D reconstructions. However, along with the increase of the number of deconvolutions, there is a danger of altering the image far beyond the original one and create artifacts. We therefore suggest restraint in any image correction before the analysis to minimize the risk of data misinterpretation.

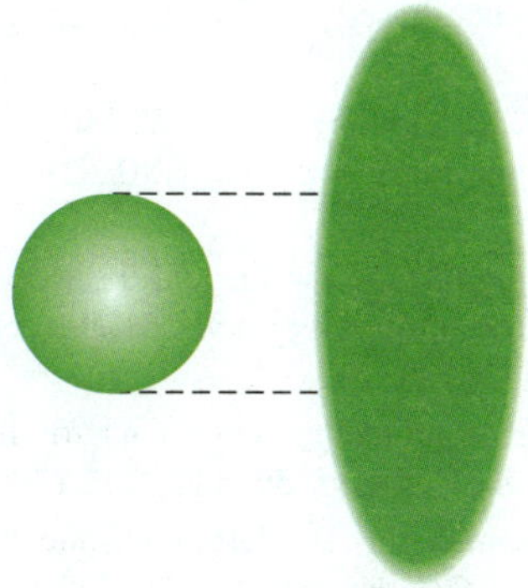

Figure 5.14 Differences between physical object dimensions (left) and its optical representation (right) when scanned along the $X-Z$ axes.

REFERENCES

1. M. C. Adams, W. C. Salmon, S. L. Gupton, C. S. Cohan, T. Wittmann, N. Prigozhina, and C. M. Waterman-Storer, "A high-speed multispectral spinning-disk confocal microscope system for fluorescent speckle microscopy of living cells," *Methods* **29**, 29–41 (2003).
2. J. P. A. Baak, "The framework of pathology: Good Laboratory Practice by quantitative and molecular methods," *J. Pathol.* **198**, 277–283 (2002).
3. R. J. Clatch, J. R. Foreman, and J. L. Walloch, "Simplified immunophenotypic analysis by laser scanning cytometry," *Cytometry* **34**, 3–16 (1998).
4. R. J. Clatch, J. L. Walloch, M. M. Zutter, and L. A. Kamentsky, "Immunophenotypic analysis of hematologic malignancy by laser scanning cytometry," *Am. J. Clin. Pathol.* **105**, 744–755 (1996).
5. G. Danuser and C. M. Waterman-Storer, "Quantitative fluorescent speckle microscopy of cytoskeleton dynamics," *Annu. Rev. Biophys. Biomol. Struct.* **35**, 361–387 (2006).
6. R. Fernández-González, A. Muñoz-Barrutia, M. H. Barcellos-Hoff, and C. Ortiz-de-Solorzano, "Quantitative in vivo microscopy: The return from the 'omics,' " *Curr. Opin. Biotechnol.* **17**, 501–510 (2006).
7. M. M. Godlewski and M. Gorka, "Quantitative analysis of fluorescent data from four-dimensional confocal studies," *Cell Proliferation* **39**, 341 (2006).
8. M. M. Godlewski, B. Gajkowska, M. Lamparska-Przybysz, and T. Motyl, "Colocalization of BAX with BID and VDAC-1 in nimesulide-induced apoptosis of human colon adenocarcinoma COLO 205 cells," *Anti-Cancer Drugs* **13**, 1017–1029 (2002).
9. M. M. Godlewski, M. Gorka, B. Gajkowska, and U. Wojewodzka, "Dissecting the pathways of doom—Application of spectroscopy in the study of cell death and survival," *Optica Applicata* **36**, 257–270 (2006).
10. M. M. Godlewski, M. A. Motyl, B. Gajkowska, P. Wareski, M. Koronkiewicz, and T. Motyl, "Subcellular redistribution of BAX during apoptosis induced by anticancer drugs," *Anti-Cancer Drugs* **12**, 607–617 (2001).
11. M. M. Godlewski, P. Slazak, R. Zabielski, A. Piastowska, and M. A. Gralak, "Quantitative study of soybean-induced changes in proliferation and programmed cell death in the intestinal mucosa of young rats," *J. Physiol. Pharmacol.* **57**, 125–133 (2006).
12. M. Gorka, M. M. Godlewski, B. Gajkowska, U. Wojewodzka, and T. Motyl, "Kinetics of Smac/DIABLO release from mitochondria during apoptosis of MCF-7 breast cancer cells," *Cell. Biol. Int.* **28**, 741–754 (2004).

13. A. K. Kenworthy, "Fluorescence-based methods to image palmitoylated proteins," *Methods* **40**, 198–205 (2006).
14. O. Kolek, B. Gajkowska, M. M. Godlewski, and T. Motyl, "Antiproliferative and apoptotic effect of TGF- 1 in bovine mammary epithelial BME UV1 cells," *Comp. Biochem. Physiol.* **134**, 417–430 (2003).
15. O. Kolek, B. Gajkowska, M. M. Godlewski, and T. Motyl, "Co-localization of apoptosis regulating proteins in mouse mammary epithelial HC11 cells exposed to TGF-β1," *Eur. J. Cell Biol.* **82**, 1–10 (2003).
16. R. J. Preston, "Quantitation of molecular endpoints for the dose-response component of cancer risk assessment," *Toxicol. Pathol.* **30**, 112–116 (2002).
17. P. Roux, S. Munter, F. Frischknecht, P. Herbomel, and S. L. Shorte, "Focusing light on infection in four dimensions," *Cell Microb.* **6**, 333–343 (2004).
18. J. W. Schwartz, D. Piston, and L. J. DeFelice, "Molecular microfluorometry: Converting arbitrary fluorescence units into absolute molecular concentrations to study binding kinetics and stoichiometry in transporters," *Handb. Exp. Pharmacol.* **175**, 23–57 (2006).
19. A. K. Strzalkowski, N. Hallay, M. M. Godlewski, G. Kulasek, Z. Gajewski, and R. Zabielski, "The effect of supplementing sow with bioactive substances on neonatal small intestinal epithelium," *J. Physiol. Pharmacol.* **58**, 115–122 (2007).

CHAPTER 6

Spectral Imaging and Unmixing

PASCAL VALLOTTON, ALOKE PHATAK, and MARK BERMAN

CSIRO, Mathematical and Information Sciences, North Ryde, New South Wales 1670, Australia

6.1 INTRODUCTION

Spectral imaging combines the advantages of both spectroscopy and imaging by acquiring spectral information at every pixel in an image. Given the orientation of this book, we will be mostly concerned with the situation where fluorescence emission spectra are recorded using a specialized fluorescence or laser scanning microscope. However, it is important to realize that the concepts and methods of spectral imaging are applicable to a great range of experimental techniques, from energy-dispersive X-ray spectroscopy (EDS), electron energy loss spectroscopy (EELS), and infrared (IR) spectroscopy to Raman spectroscopy, cathodoluminescence (CL) spectroscopy, scanning tunneling spectroscopy (STS), and mass spectrometry (MS). Spectral imaging is also referred to as hyperspectral imaging, imaging spectroscopy, or multipixel spectroscopy when the number of wavelengths at which the spectra are recorded is large. For a small number of wavelengths, the term *multispectral imaging* is also used.

The fluorescence spectra contain information about the chemistry of samples. Therefore, spectral imaging may give insights as to the chemical composition across the sample. Typically, the spectral signal measured at each pixel will result from contributions from multiple chemical species. Sometimes, this heterogeneity is due to the limited size of pixels, for example, when multiple regions such as small grains of different chemical nature are imaged into the same pixel. Sometimes, the species are mixed so thoroughly that even with very small pixels the heterogeneity would persist.

Central to spectral imaging is the ability to "unmix" the observed composite spectra of the sample in terms of the spectra of a finite set of pure species (so called end members) that is used to interpret the data. In the context of live cell imaging, these pure species could, for example, consist of several different variants of the green fluorescent protein (GFP), tagging several proteins of interest.

A set of data representing a spectral image can be regarded either as a collection of P rectangular images (often called bands or channels), measured at wavelengths λ_i, $i = 1, 2, \ldots, P$, or as a single image where a spectrum $I_j(\lambda_i)$ is measured at P wavelengths at each of $j = 1, 2, \ldots, N$ pixels. In principle, a standard RGB image

Fluorescence Applications in Biotechnology and Life Sciences, Edited by Ewa M. Goldys

can be thought of as an elementary spectral image, but in most modern applications, spectra are measured at tens, hundreds, and sometimes thousands of wavelengths.

When we refer to an entire spectrum, we will henceforth drop the subscript i and just write $I_j(\lambda)$, which is a vector of length P, the number of wavelengths in the image. For a modest size image of 512×512 pixels and the spectra measured at hundreds of wavelengths, very large sets of hundreds of megabytes of data need to be acquired, stored, and analyzed. This is a significant computing challenge that commercial microscope systems have become able to tackle only recently. This difficulty is compounded by the desire to observe live, dynamic samples in many applications, where numerous images must be taken. This introduces a need for trade-off between spatial, spectral, and temporal resolutions. Improving on current compromises is one of the main drivers of innovation for instrument manufacturers.

To better understand the need for spectral imaging, it is useful to consider the limitations of conventional fluorescence microscopy, where the choice of fluorescent probes and filter sets is critical for a successful experimental outcome. When taking a fluorescence microscope image, one needs to identify a fluorophore and a filter set such that only the emission of that fluorophore is measured in its associated channel (a channel refers to the signal measured by the instrument in a certain configuration of filters, laser lines, etc.). In the presence of several fluorescing species, this condition becomes very difficult to achieve due to spectral overlap. Usually, no more than four or five probes can be monitored in the same experiment without significant crosstalk between channels. The development of dyes such as quantum dots featuring very narrow emission spectra somewhat mitigates these limitations, but due to their toxicity and the difficulty of introducing them into live samples, their use is still limited (see Chapter 4 in this volume). Spectral imaging overcomes the limitations of conventional fluorescence microscopy, making possible the resolution of tens of probes in a single experiment. For example, Schrock et al. [1] were able to resolve 24 different probes in a karyotyping experiment, but even much greater levels of multiplexing are possible. In the pharmaceutical industry, where spectral imaging is increasingly used to inspect the homogeneity and composition of tablets, it is quite common to deal with hundreds of materials. Spectral imaging also extends considerably the precision and usefulness of fluorescence resonance energy transfer (FRET, see Chapter 8 in this volume) studies as well as other fluorescence techniques [2].

The development of fluorescent proteins and other tagging technologies made it possible to specifically label and monitor multiple proteins in their native cellular environments. Biologists wish to be able to dissect whole signaling pathways involving numerous different molecules with great spatial and temporal accuracy. Spectral imaging promises to translate this vision into reality, thus opening a window into highly multiplexed and dynamic cellular processes such as apoptosis, mitosis, or metastasis. This explains much of the excitement around the new instruments that have become available commercially.

This chapter is structured as follows. We start by describing possible configurations of hyperspectral microscopes. We then introduce the mathematics and practice of spectral unmixing, including both supervised/informed unmixing (where a library of the spectra of the pure materials present in the image—a spectral library—is available) and unsupervised/blind unmixing (where no a priori information on the fluorescent species is available). We give three examples of applications. The first concerns tablet inspection, the second features fluorescent microspheres, and in the third we present insights into molecular imaging of a mouse lung cancer. We conclude this chapter with some general remarks.

6.2 INSTRUMENTATION AND CONFIGURATIONS FOR HYPERSPECTRAL MICROSCOPES

Astronomical and airborne applications of spectral imaging have predated by many years the applications in the area of biological imaging [3]. While the design of spectral microscopes, particularly confocal microscopes, poses specific difficulties, these early technologies have inspired and are still inspiring instrument designers today.

One can distinguish three main types of configuration for spectral microscopes:

- *Category 1* Designed to acquire an entire image frame at a specified wavelength. The wavelength is scanned across the range of interest step by step (e.g., see Figure 6.1).
- *Category 2* Designed to acquire a full spectrum at each point or each line of a sample (e.g., confocal microscopes).
- *Category 3* Those that depend on a mathematical transformation to recover spectral information (e.g., Fourier transform interferometer microscopes).

The selection of an optimal instrument for a specific application is driven by photobleaching issues, by the required spectral and temporal resolution, and by cost considerations.

Figure 6.1 is a schematic of an instrument in the first category. In this simplest form, a spectral microscope is a standard wide-field epifluorescence microscope with

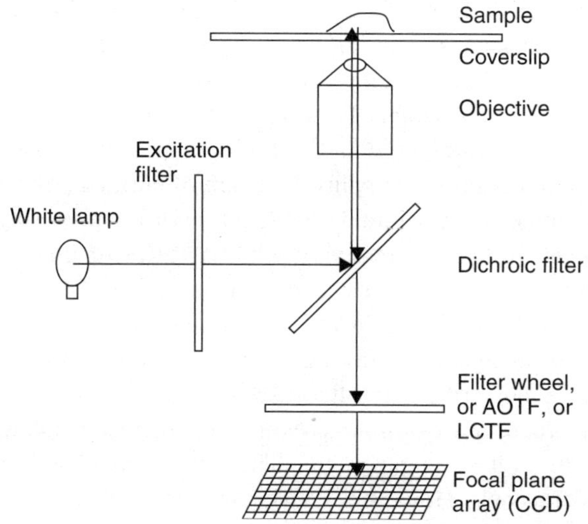

Figure 6.1 Elementary spectral microscope. Compared to a standard epifluorescence microscope, a dispersive element, such as a filter wheel, an acousto-optical tunable filter (AOTF), or a liquid crystal tunable filter (LCTF) allows selecting among a number of different emission wavelengths.

a rotating filter wheel which makes it possible to select various barrier filters. The barrier filter is located in front of the eyepiece or the camera. It takes as many as 20 filters to cover an emission spectrum extending over 200 nm if sampling is performed every 10 nm. It should be borne in mind that while the notation $I_j(\lambda_f)$ indicates that the signal is measured precisely at wavelength λ_f, in reality, $I_j(\lambda_f)$ is a convolution of the signal with the spectral profile of the filter. The width of the profile at half its maximum value is called the spectral resolution of the instrument (at the corresponding wavelength). Filter-based instrument configurations are almost never used in practice because of the high cost of interference filters and of further limitations, as discussed below.

An important limitation of such instruments is that switching between filters takes a few hundred milliseconds. If faster speeds are required, the filter wheel can be replaced by an AOTF or an LCTF. In an AOTF, a diffraction grating is created by a stationary sound wave in a crystal. The wave creates a periodic modulation of the refraction index. This diffracts the incident light, thereby allowing spatial selection of the wavelength of interest. The LCTF is a sandwich structure composed of polarizers, birefringent crystals, and a liquid crystal layer whose optical retardation is controlled electrically to select the transmitted wavelength. Both AOTFs and LCTFs offer much better spectral resolutions than filter-based instruments and provide precise and fast wavelength control [4].

A major shortcoming of instruments of the first category is photobleaching. Intense sample illumination is required because only a small fraction of the emitted fluorescence is collected. Assuming a spectral resolution of 10 nm for every filter, only about 5% of light (5% = 10 nm/200 nm) may be collected. Confocal microscopes, which belong to the second category of instruments, perform much better in this regard. Because each point (or line for certain instruments) in the sample is scanned successively, a prism or a grating can be placed just in front of the photomultiplier tube (PMT) detector to disperse the polychromatic fluorescence emission beam. By using a sensitive multichannel PMT consisting of an array of detectors, all emission wavelengths of interest can be acquired simultaneously, thereby considerably limiting photobleaching issues.

Among instruments in category 3 is the Fourier transform imaging interferometer [1]. In this design, an interferometer splits the beam of emitted polychromatic light into two arms and recombines them with a variable phase difference using a mobile mirror. The mobile mirror is shifted progressively while a series of images of the sample is recorded. These data can be transformed back to a series of monochromatic images using the Fourier transform. These instruments allow the acquisition of all emission wavelengths simultaneously while offering narrow spectral widths. In reality, excellent spectral resolution is not critical for fluorescence applications because fluorescence spectra tend to be broad and featureless. Moreover, precision interferometers for the visible range are difficult to manufacture. Thus, this design is not commonly used in fluorescence microscopy. However, Fourier transform instruments are widespread in infrared applications, where sharp spectral features carrying important information need to be resolved. These features (bands) are typically so narrow that they can be used independently of the rest of the signal to quantify the molecular species of which they are characteristic (spectral fingerprinting).

6.3 SUPERVISED AND UNSUPERVISED UNMIXING

Most published unmixing research can be found in either the remote-sensing or the chemometrics literature. An extensive review of unmixing methods in the remote-sensing literature is given by Keshava et al. [5], while a review of the chemometrics methods (where unmixing is often called multivariate curve resolution) is given by Jiang et al. [6].

The fundamental assumption in most unmixing procedures is that the observed spectrum $I_j(\lambda)$ at every pixel in an image is a linear combination of the spectra of the individual constituents in the image. This is a safe assumption in fluorescence applications. In other domains, such as remote sensing, the assumption does not always hold and appropriate care must be exercised. The use of nonlinear models taking into account the physics of light absorption is an active research field [7].

In the linear case, the *weights* c_{jk} are proportional to the concentrations of the individual species. Consider, for example, an idealized sample with $k = 1, 2, \ldots, D$ different species, each having a spectrum denoted by $E_k(\lambda)$. At each of the j pixels, the measured spectrum can be expressed as

$$I_j(\lambda) = \sum_{k=1}^{D} c_{jk} E_k(\lambda) \tag{6.1}$$

The objective of unmixing is to recover the weights c_{jk} of the individual constituents given only the measured signal $I_j(\lambda)$ at each pixel. The methods that are used can be divided into two broad groups—supervised/informed and unsupervised/blind unmixing—depending on whether the pure spectra $E_k(\lambda)$ are known or not.

6.4 SUPERVISED OR INFORMED UNMIXING

Supervised unmixing refers to the situation where a spectral library of pure constituents is available, of which all or only some are present in the image. Using matrix notation and including additive noise, we can write Eq. 6.1 above for the entire image as

$$\mathbf{I} = \mathbf{CE} + \mathbf{F} \tag{6.2}$$

where $\mathbf{I}$ is an $N \times P$ matrix containing, rowwise, the spectra at each of the N pixels in the image; $\mathbf{C}$ is an $N \times D$ matrix whose N rows contain the (unknown) concentrations of the D constituents in each of the N pixels; $\mathbf{E}$ is a $D \times P$ matrix whose rows are the pure spectra $E_k(\lambda)$ and $\mathbf{F}$ is an $N \times P$ matrix error term. It is common to minimize

$$(\mathbf{I} - \mathbf{CE})^{\mathrm{T}}(\mathbf{I} - \mathbf{CE}) \tag{6.3}$$

subject to the constraint that the c_{jk} are nonnegative. Minimization of a quadratic function subject to linear inequality constraints (e.g., nonnegativity) is performed using quadratic programming techniques [8].

Implicit in the minimization of Eq. 6.3 is the assumption that the covariance matrix of the noise is proportional to the "identity" matrix (i.e., the variance of the noise is the same in each band and it is uncorrelated between bands). However, because spectra are typically smooth curves, they are in fact highly correlated locally, so it is generally better to minimize

$$(\mathbf{I} - \mathbf{CE})\boldsymbol{\Sigma}^{-1}(\mathbf{I} - \mathbf{CE}) \tag{6.4}$$

where $\boldsymbol{\Sigma}$ is the covariance matrix of the errors. Minimization of Eq. 6.4 with the nonnegativity constraint on the c_{jk} can still be solved using quadratic programming techniques. When $\boldsymbol{\Sigma}$ is known or at least well estimated, minimization of Eq. 6.4 usually produces more accurate estimates of the c_{jk} than minimization of Eq. 6.3 does.

The situation where *all* the constituents in an image are known (and a spectral library of them is available) often occurs in manufacturing, where controlled quantities of different ingredients are mixed and then imaged. This is the case, for example, with pharmaceutical tablets (see application section). Alternatively, in biological applications, one typically uses a known set of fluorescent proteins to label different regions.

When there are many pure sample spectra of each constituent available and provided that the number of constituents, D, and the dimensionality of the data, P, are not too large, $\boldsymbol{\Sigma}$ can usually be well estimated using the average within-class covariance matrix of the pure samples [9]. However, when P is very large, this becomes problematic. One solution is to penalize the usual estimator of Σ toward one that is more suitable for smooth curves [10].

When the number of constituents, D, is large (often the case in pharmaceutical applications), a single pixel will usually contain only a small subset of them. Better estimates of the c_{jk} are usually obtained by variable-selection techniques. Efficient algorithms for obtaining these are available [11].

We have developed a package called The Spectral Assistant [12], which minimizes Eq. 6.4 subject to nonnegativity constraints on the c_{jk} and includes (i) penalized estimation of $\boldsymbol{\Sigma}$, (ii) fast subset selection, and (iii) simultaneous estimation of the background with the c_{jk}. The use of this package is illustrated in Section 6.7.1. A number of similar tools have been developed. In particular, most spectral microscope manufacturers, including Leica, Zeiss, and Olympus, provide unmixing capabilities within their own dedicated software that will satisfy the needs of most users. More specialized tools are also available, many of which are available as Matlab™ toolboxes. As a starting point we suggest exploring The Multivariate Image Analysis (MIA) toolbox (Eigenvector Research, http://software.eigenvector.com/); GUIPRO (Paul J. Gemperline, http://personal.ecu.edu/gemperlinep/Research/gemper_software.html); MCR-ALS (Tauler R., http://www.ub.es/gesq/mcr/mcr.htm); and the CenSSIS hyperspectral image analysis toolbox (http://www.censsis.neu.edu/software/hyperspectral/hyperspectral.html). These websites also contain a wealth of information on the topic of unmixing.

6.5 UNSUPERVISED OR BLIND UNMIXING

In unsupervised unmixing, neither the number nor the nature of the constituents in a spectral image is known a priori. Correspondingly, the algorithms are more complex than those used in supervised unmixing. Users need to be aware of indeterminacies that are inherent in all such unmixing methods. Algorithms for unmixing have been independently developed in many fields, including remote sensing [5] and chemometrics [6]. Different methodologies reflect differences in the nature of the images typical of the different application areas. Remotely sensed images tend to be very large, on the order of millions of pixels, and the spectra contain a modest number of bands, between 10 and 200. By contrast, the images obtained in chemical applications tend to be smaller, but the spectra may contain many hundreds of wavelengths.

Below, we outline a particularly robust method that we have developed for the unsupervised unmixing of hyperspectral data.

6.5.1 Iterated Constrained End-Members Algorithm

The iterated constrained end-Members (ICE) algorithm was originally developed for unmixing remotely sensed images [13], but it has also been successfully used to unmix a range of different types of images [14, 15]. As with most unmixing methods, the ICE algorithm assumes the linear mixture model of Eq. 6.1 or 6.2. There is a basic indeterminacy in the linear mixture model which stems from the fact that in Eq. 6.2, if $\hat{\mathbf{C}}$ and $\hat{\mathbf{E}}$ are solutions, then so too are $\hat{\mathbf{C}}\mathbf{Q}$ and $\mathbf{Q}^{-1}\hat{\mathbf{E}}$, where $\mathbf{Q}$ is any $D \times D$ invertible matrix. Hence, even when no noise is present, Eq. 6.2 does not have a unique solution. Indeterminacies of particular significance are *scale* (where $\mathbf{Q}$ is a diagonal matrix) and *rotation* (where $\mathbf{Q}^{T}\mathbf{Q} = \mathbf{I}_D$, the identity matrix).

Because of these indeterminacies, additional constraints are required to obtain a unique solution. In the ICE algorithm, the indeterminacy is resolved by imposing a convex geometry constraint, that is, we assume that, at each of the j pixels, the prefactors c_{jk} are *proportions*: Not only are they nonnegative but they sum to 1:

$$\sum_{k=1}^{D} c_{jk} = 1 \qquad c_{jk} \geq 0 \qquad k = 1, 2, \ldots D \tag{6.5}$$

When there is no error term in Eq. 6.2, the convex geometry constraint implies that the data lie inside a simplex generated by D vertices (the pure components, or "end members") within a subspace of dimensionality $D - 1$. For example, if there are only three pure materials in the image, the simplex is a triangle in a two-dimensional subspace; if $D = 4$, the simplex is a tetrahedron (pyramid) in a three-dimensional subspace. In any real example, however, the data will not be noise free. Additionally, some pure components may never appear in their pure form in the image. Thus, the true simplex must be inferred. Clearly, noise complicates the inference.

The steps in the ICE algorithm can be summarized as follows:

1. Preprocess the spectra to identify and remove noisy pixels, possibly normalize the data, determine the baseline, remove lighting gradients, and so on.
2. Reduce the dimensionality P of the problem by determining the dimension M of the subspace in which the simplex lies using the minimum-noise-fraction (MNF) transform [16].
3. Estimate the number of pure materials, D, in the image and then fit a simplex with D vertices in the M-dimensional subspace obtained in step 2 using a penalized alternating least-squares procedure. The simplex is penalized such that smaller simplexes are preferred to larger ones.
4. Once the algorithm has converged, the estimate of the pure materials will lie at the vertices of the fitted simplex, and the final step is to visualize the results by

calculating and displaying (a) the estimated spectra and (b) the proportion maps, which show the proportion of each of the D estimated end members at every pixel in the image.

It is worth emphasizing at this point the distinction between M, the dimensionality of the subspace in which we believe the simplex to lie (and which is obtained by carrying out the MNF transform in step 2), and D, the number of pure materials we believe to be present in the hyperspectral image. Note that M must be greater than or equal to $D - 1$ [e.g., a triangle ($D = 3$) only exists in a two- or higher dimensional space]. In practice, we use several diagnostic tools to help determine both M and D, as the examples below will demonstrate.

The MNF transform is a linear transformation similar to the well-known principal-component (PC) transform, and it includes the PC transform as a special case. Like the PC transform, the MNF transform is obtained from an eigenvector/eigenvalue decomposition, but it is of the more general form

$$\boldsymbol{S}_I \boldsymbol{a}_j = \mu_j \boldsymbol{S}_F \boldsymbol{a}_j \qquad \boldsymbol{a}_j^{\mathrm{T}} \boldsymbol{S}_I \boldsymbol{a}_j = 1 \qquad \boldsymbol{a}_j^{\mathrm{T}} \boldsymbol{S}_F \boldsymbol{a}_k = 0 \qquad k \neq j \tag{6.6}$$

where $\mathbf{S}_I$ is an estimate of the data covariance matrix, $\mathbf{S}_F$ is an estimate of the common noise covariance matrix of the errors $\mathbf{f}_j$, and $\mathbf{a}_j$ is the vector of weights used in the jth transformation. The eigenvalues μ_j can be interpreted as signal-to-noise ratios (SNRs). The number of eigenvalues significantly different from zero provides a rough indication of the value of M, the dimensionality of the subspace in which the simplex lies. Note that when $\mathbf{S}_F$ is a scalar multiple of the identity matrix, the MNF transform reduces to the PC transform. Methods for estimating $\mathbf{S}_I$ and $\mathbf{S}_F$ are outlined in Green et al. [16] and Nielsen [17]. The ICE algorithm is based on relatively advanced mathematics. However, as the examples below will demonstrate, it is not necessary to understand every technical detail in order to extract informative results from spectral data. Additionally, while the ICE algorithm is a particular embodiment of blind unmixing technology, it is representative of a number of alternative solutions that exploit similar methods and the same terminology. Again, most spectral microscope manufacturers offer blind unmixing capabilities within their dedicated software. A number of other organizations also offer blind unmixing software, including the Technical University of Delft (Hypertools, http://www-ict.et.tudelft.nl/ pavel/spectra/hypertools.html) and ITT (ENVI, http://www.ittvis.com/envi/index.asp).

6.6 SPECTRAL CLUSTERING

While the emphasis of this chapter is geared toward linear unmixing as a method of choice for quantitative analysis of spectral data, a number of alternative mathematical techniques are in use. In that respect, cluster analysis is especially interesting because it is not based on an explicit statistical model. Rather, spectral clustering identifies a set of pure species by grouping together pixels that exhibit similar spectral properties. As in linear unmixing, the number of species is not determined directly by the algorithm but rather inferred by the user based on domain knowledge. The development of an automated method for identifying the optimal species number is still an area of active research.

A number of clustering methodologies can be applied directly to spectral imaging. In the K-means (KM) algorithm of MacQueen [18], a set of K points is chosen randomly in P-dimensional space, where P is the number of wavelengths. The algorithm iteratively updates the position of these points until they represent the optimal centers of K clusters. At each loop of the algorithm, all image pixels are assigned to the nearest of the K points currently representing the set of pure species. The distance used in making this decision can be any of the Euclidean, city-block, or chessboard metrics. At the end of the loop, the center of gravity of all points closest to each of the K points is recalculated and the next iteration is started. The iteration stops when the allocation of pixels to their cluster is stable.

In the KM clustering method, the allocation of pixels to their class is either 0 or 1, but in other schemes, such as fuzzy C-means (FCM) clustering [19], it is possible to use degrees of association in the [0,1] interval for each pixel to each of the K clusters. Clustering methods are used extensively, for example, in the area of tissue analysis, as the linear mixing assumption holds only approximately for absorbance measurements [20].

6.7 EXAMPLES

6.7.1 Tablet Inspection

Spectral imaging can be used for controlling the quality of pharmaceutical tablets. It can reveal whether the constituent concentrations within a tablet match the intended formulation, whether the constituents are uniformly distributed within the tablet, and whether contaminants are present.

Typically, the ingredients used to manufacture pharmaceutical tablets are not fluorescent. In this example, we use reflectance spectroscopy to measure the amount of light that is reflected by the sample at each wavelength, as opposed to the amount of light that is fluorescently emitted at each wavelength. Every substance possesses a reflectance spectrum, but not every substance possesses a nontrivial fluorescence spectrum.

Here, we analyze 25 tablets consisting of seven known main constituents, with varying degrees of contamination by other materials, which when we carried out our analyses were unknown to us. The data were measured using an ASD (Analytical Spectral Devices, Boulder, CO) spectrometer. A library containing the spectra of the seven pure constituents in powder form was first acquired using the ASD spectrometer. Reflectance was measured every 1 nm in the range [350, 2500] nm. Both sides of the tablets were imaged. A pseudocolor image of side 1 (produced by treating the images at 650, 550, and 450 nm as the red, green, and blue components, respectively) is shown in Figure 6.2*a*. It has a spatial resolution of 72 × 72 pixels. Each tablet consisted of only about 100 spectra.

Fifteen of the tablets were uncontaminated and had the following formulation: chondroitin sulfate, 33%; glucosamine hydrochloride, 33%; microcrystalline cellulose, 25%; crospovidone, 4%; povidone, 3%; magnesium stearate, 1%; silicon dioxide, 1%. A sixteenth tablet contained no chondroitin sulfate but had the same *relative* proportions of the remaining six constituents. Another tablet (tablet 5, the second from right in the top row in Figure 6.2*a*) was 100% contaminated. The remaining eight tablets (numbers 2, 6, 9, 11, 13, 18, 21, and 24) contained between 1 and 10% contaminant

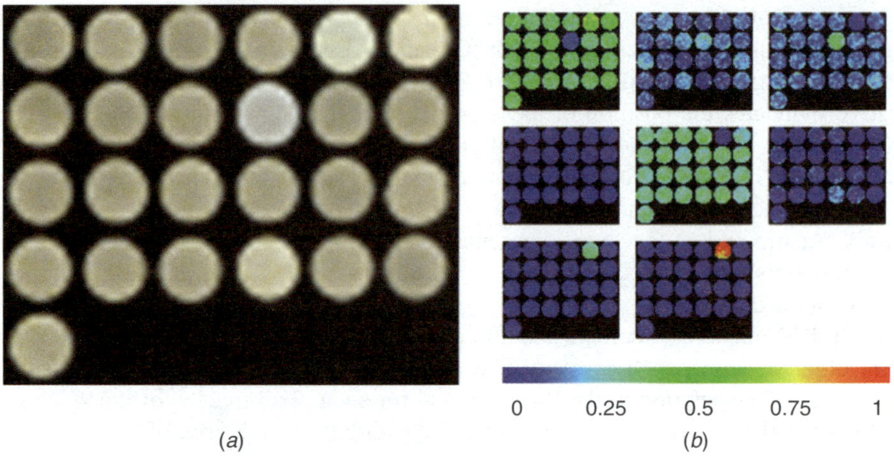

Figure 6.2 (*a*) Pseudocolor image of one side of (*b*) the 25 tablets. Estimated proportion maps for the seven pure constituents in the pharmaceutical tablets and RMS map (bottom right).

(either paracetamol or lactose) and the seven known constituents in the same relative proportions as given above.

Because there are only seven constituents, no subset selection was carried out by the Spectral Assistant software. A penalized estimate of $\mathbf{\Sigma}$ was used and the background was modeled using a low-frequency spline with two knots at 1500 and 2000 nm [21]. We have restricted the analysis to the range 1000–2500 nm, where most of the distinctive absorption features occur. Reflectance spectra were converted to absorbance spectra [absorbance = − log(reflectance)].

Figure 6.2*b* shows the estimated proportion maps for each of the seven constituents, as well as the residual mean-square (RMS) error map. Pixels which were not analyzed are shown in black, while proportions are indicated using a "heat" colormap, with the corresponding scale bar shown at the bottom of the figure.

The last map in Figure 6.2*b* (the second map in the bottom row) is the RMS map, which measures the mismatch between the observed and fitted spectra. As expected, tablet 5 has very high RMS values because it does not contain any of the seven pure materials. The estimated proportions within each tablet did not vary strikingly, indicating that in this case they were well mixed.

The RMS can also be used to identify the presence of relatively small amounts of contaminant. Figure 6.3 plots the percentage contamination of both sides 1 and 2 of 24 of the tablets (tablet 5 has been excluded) against the worst fitting (i.e., largest) RMS of the (approximately 100) pixels on that side of the tablet. It is clear that tablets with 5% contamination or more have a noticeably higher worst-fitting RMS than do tablets with smaller amounts of contamination. Instruments with higher spatial resolution than the one used in this study are likely to be able to detect even smaller contamination levels.

Based on the data in Figure 6.2, concentrations can be estimated on a per-tablet basis by averaging the proportions for all pixels in the tablet. Figures 6.4*a* to 6.4*f* show the estimated proportions for side 1 (in red) and side 2 (in blue) against the true relative proportion (in black) of six of the constituents. For the seventh constituent, magnesium stearate, whose true percentage was 1% in most of the tablets, the estimated percentage

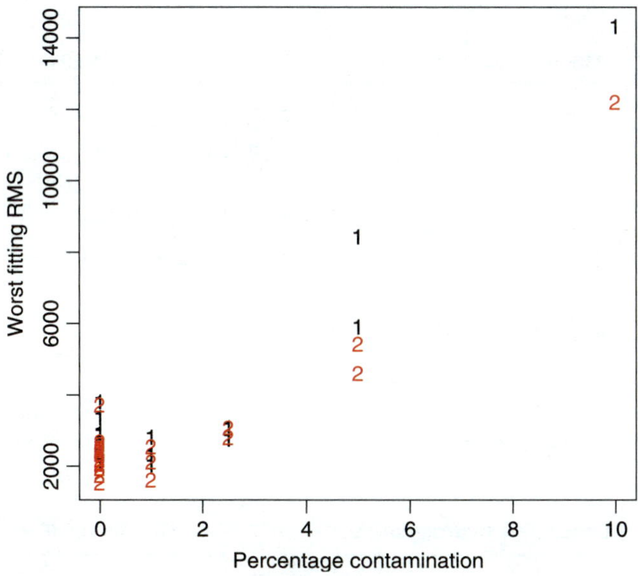

Figure 6.3 Worst-fitting RMS pixel for sides 1 and 2 for 24 tablets (tablet 5 excluded) versus percentage contamination in tablets. Poor fitting indicates contamination.

was never more than 0.4%. Therefore, the corresponding plot for this constituent is not shown. Results for both tablet sides indicate that, for uncontaminated tablets, the proportions for all constituents can be estimated to within 5% of their true values for the major constituents, and even more accurately for the minor constituents.

Apart from the 100% contaminated tablet and one tablet that contained 50% of a constituent, all tablets contained at most 33% of any constituent. It is not possible to apply successfully unsupervised unmixing to a data set where all maximum proportions are so far from 100%. In such cases, supervised unmixing should always be preferred to blind unmixing.

6.7.2 Fluorescent Microspheres

Most substances are not fluorescent. Therefore, under fluorescent microscopy, most of the signal collected from a sample containing a fluorescent probe comes from that probe. This makes fluorescence microscopy an exquisitely sensitive technique that allows focusing on those elements of the sample that are of interest, even in complex samples, such as biological cells.

Polystyrene fluorescent microspheres are useful as fluorescent tracers, as calibration standards, or as functionalized probes in many applications. For example, in tracer applications, cell lineages can be determined from a cell initially injected with microspheres and undergoing successive divisions. Subresolution limit microspheres can also be used to measure the point spread function of a microscope, the knowledge of which can be used to greatly improve image quality.

Here, a mixture of spectrally different fluorescent beads has been imaged using an Olympus FluoView™ FV1000 confocal microscope (Tokyo, Japan). Images were 512×512 pixels in size, with spectra measured at 102 equally spaced wavelengths

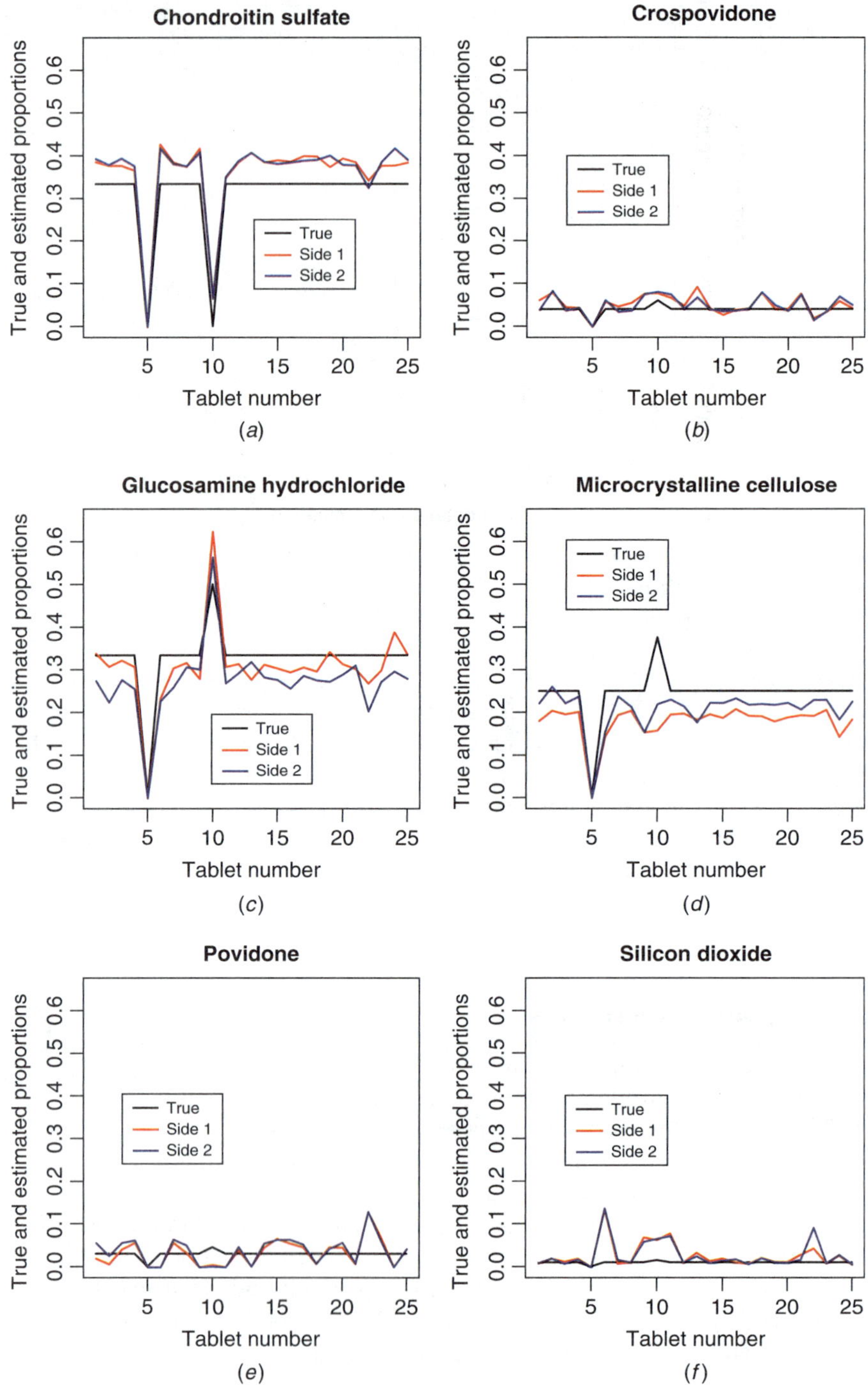

Figure 6.4 Average estimated proportions (side1 in red, side 2 in blue) of pure constituents in tablets compared to true relative proportion (in black) for six of the seven constituents.

in the visible and near-infrared range, from 490 to 794 nm. There are six types of beads, each labeled with a different dye, with 28 beads in total in the field of view. This is a somewhat contrived example, as the end members can be obtained directly by examining spectra at the center of every bead. However, the example is instructive as it illustrates well the mechanics of the blind unmixing process.

Figure 6.5 shows two images from the stack of 102 images measured at 517 and 604 nm, respectively. The set of beads that can be seen is different in both images because the beads emit in different wavelength regions. Figure 6.6 displays a few spectra, obtained at the center of a few beads, as well as in the background (at the bottom). Notice that most of them present a shoulder on their right-hand side very likely caused by Raman scattering. The Raman signal is usually very small compared to the fluorescence signal. However, here, fluorescent intensities were limited: In order to excite all bead types, the excitation wavelength was far from the maximum absorption of the beads.

Data preprocessing, including normalization, is an important step in unmixing. It is a common practice to divide each spectrum at each pixel by its mean across the wavelength range in order to reduce the variability between different spectra belonging to the same class. However, in this case, this would magnify the importance of the background (which has low SNR) in the data analysis. Thus, in this example, we calculate the MNF transform via Eq. 6.6 without preprocessing.

Figure 6.7 shows the first 9 (out of 102) MNF images. Each MNF band has been individually stretched to enhance the contrast. As expected, the successive MNF images contain decreasing amounts of visual information.

In Figure 6.8, we show pairwise plots of the first six MNF bands. Each point corresponds to a pixel from the original data set, and two-dimensional (2D) projections of the data are used because it is difficult to represent data graphically in higher dimensions. In this figure the points form straight lines, indicating pairwise linear mixing between different end members. Probably the most informative of these plots is MNF band 3 versus. MNF band 4 (or MNF band 5). This plot clearly shows six lines emanating from a central "blob". The central blob represents the background pixels, while the ends of the lines represent the centers of beads of the six types. Pixels lying

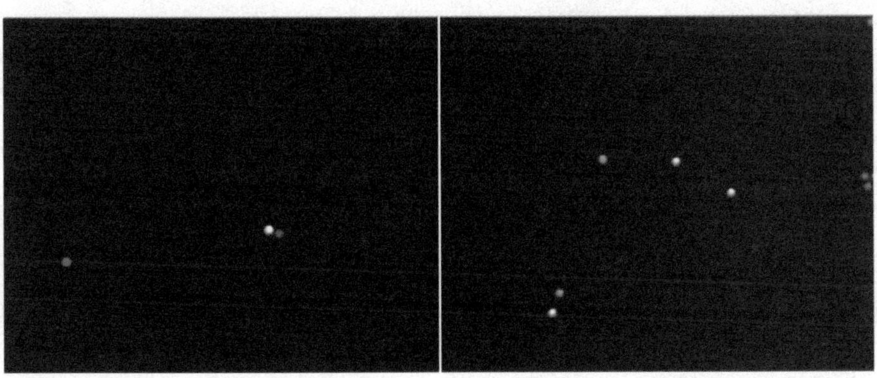

Figure 6.5 Two images from stack of 102 images of fluorescent polystyrene beads: (*a*) 517 nm, (*b*) 604 nm. The set of beads that can be seen is different in both images because the beads emit in different wavelength regions.

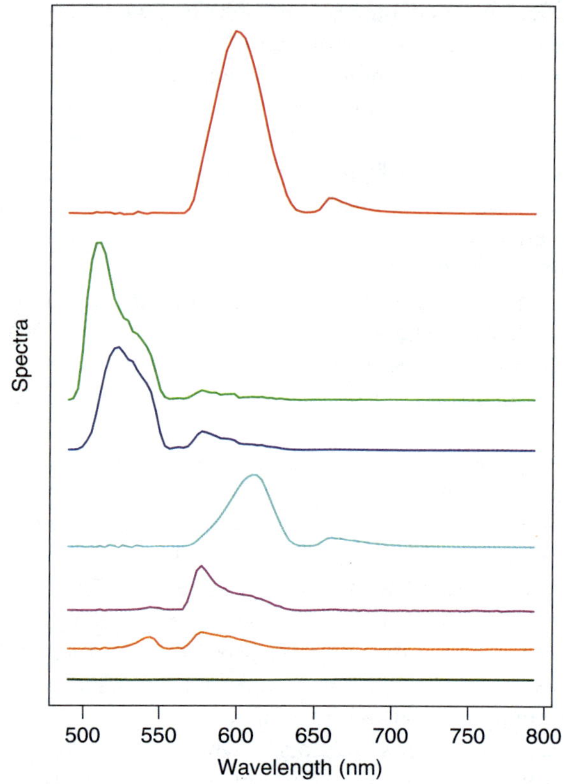

Figure 6.6 Spectra obtained at center of a few beads as well as in the background (bottom). Notice that most spectra present a shoulder on their right-hand side, likely caused by Raman scattering.

along the lines represent mixed pixels, which at first sight is surprising given that each bead contains a single fluorophore species.

In carrying out the ICE algorithm, we have to specify D, the number of end members, and M, the number of MNF bands (and hence the dimensionality of the MNF subspace) in which to carry out the end-member inference. Plots such as those in Figures 6.7 and 6.8 provide useful clues as to what values of M and D ought to be used.

We show results obtained by the ICE algorithm using seven end members in 10 MNF bands. Figure 6.9 shows the seven estimated end-member spectra on the left and their corresponding "purest" versions actually found in the image on the right. The purest version for an end member is defined as the spectrum in the data which contains the highest proportion of that end member, and this proportion is called its "purity." From top to bottom, the purities are 1, 1, 1, 0.97, 0.90, 0.84, and 0.20. As can be expected, the purest spectra with high purities are very similar to their associated end member.

Figure 6.10 shows the proportion maps and the RMS map obtained by the ICE algorithm. In such an example, we would a priori expect every fluorescent bead to display proportions equal to 100% throughout their section. However, these proportions

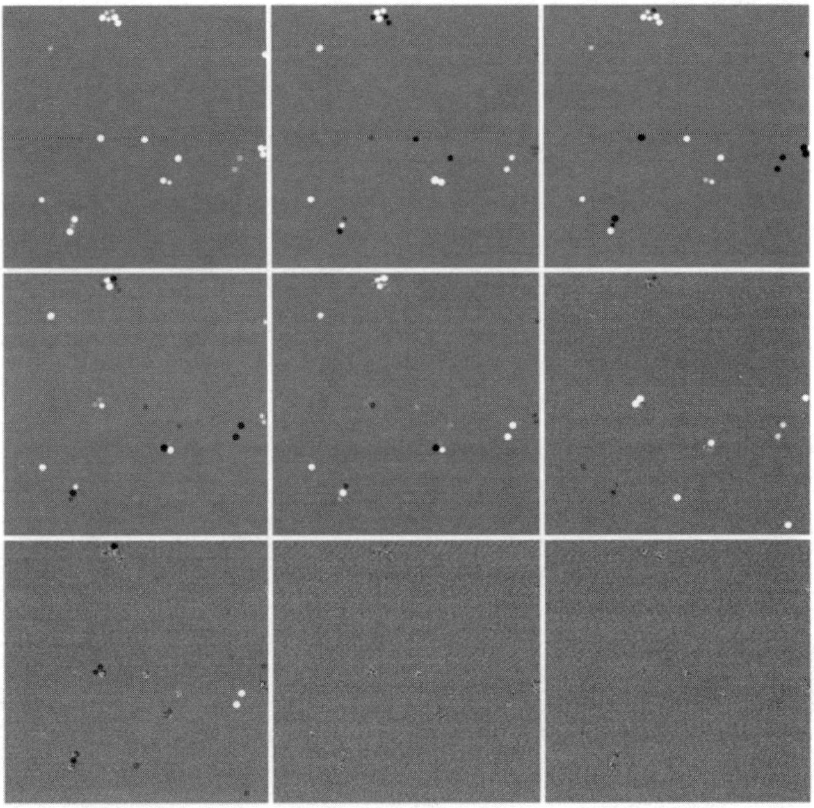

Figure 6.7 First 9 (of 102) MNF images of fluorescent beads. Each MNF band has been individually stretched to enhance the contrast. Successive MNF images contain decreasing amounts of visual information, a property ensured by the MNF transform.

are seen to decrease from the center of the beads to their periphery, with an increasing proportion of background mixed in the signal. The reason is that under the convex geometry model mixing with the background is the *only* mechanism available to model the decrease in fluorescence intensity observed from the center of the beads to their periphery.

6.7.3 Induced Mouse Lung Tumor

The last data set we consider is from a mouse in which a lung tumor has been induced and tagged using GFP (22). The image is of size 512 × 384. Fluorescence was excited with blue light (450–490 nm) and the hyperspectral data were collected every 10 nm from 500 to 650 nm using an early version of CRI's Maestro™ small animal fluorescence imaging system (Woburn, MA). The 16 images that make up the hyperspectral stack are shown in Figure 6.11. Each image has been individually stretched to enhance contrast.

The first eight MNF images are shown in Figure 6.12, and as before, they have been separately stretched to enhance contrast. Note that most of the information is contained in the first five MNF bands. So in this example we set $M = 5$.

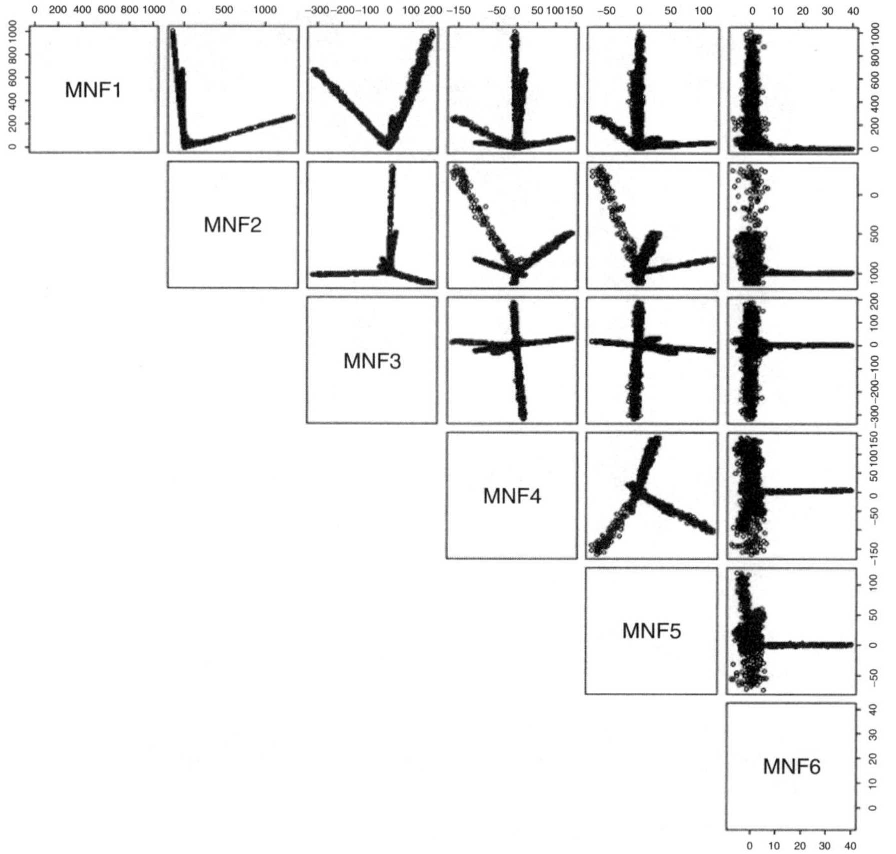

Figure 6.8 Pairwise plot of first six MNF bands for set of fluorescent microspheres. Each point corresponds to a pixel from the original data set. Lines in the plot indicate linear mixing between pure components.

Figures 6.13*a, b*, and *c* show pairwise MNF scatterplots of all 196,608 points for the first three MNF bands. If there are four end members in this image, then the convex geometry model implies that the data should be well modeled by a tetrahedron. The tetrahedron fitted by ICE in the space of the first five MNF bands is overlaid on the scatterplots in Figure 6.13, and each of the six edges is shown in a different color, although the same color is used for each edge in the different plots. In contrast to the previous example, where there was largely only pairwise mixing of the background with each end member, there is a much greater fraction of mixed pixels here, and hence the data form a cloud in MNF space. Some edges of this data cloud are curved, indicating that a linear mixture model is only an approximation in this instance. These nonlinearities could be instrumental or they could be due to absorption of the fluorescence by the tissue. However, Figure 6.13 shows that ICE is relatively resistant to noisy data and outlying observations because the fitted tetrahedron appears to fit tightly around the main part of the data cloud.

It turns out that four end members are not quite sufficient to capture all the information in the image, and in Figure 6.14 we show the results of fitting five end members

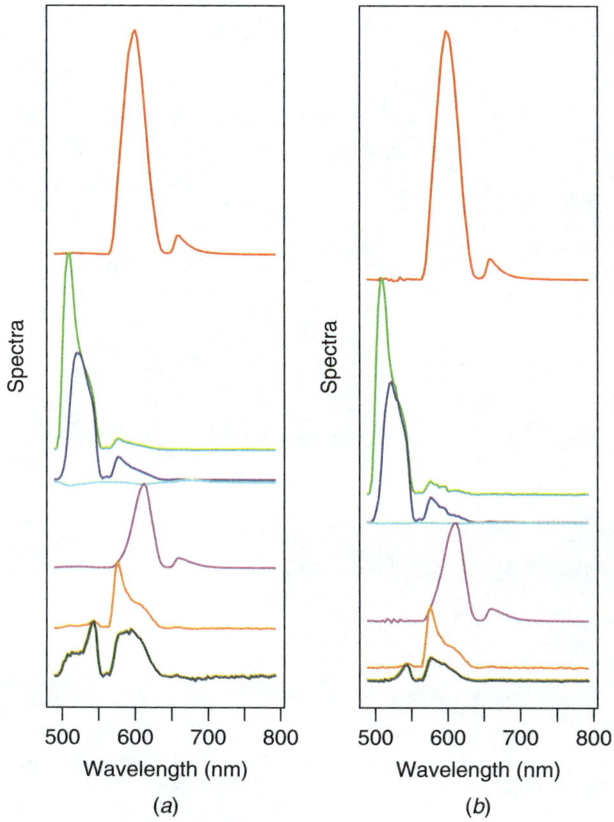

Figure 6.9 (*a*) Seven estimated end-member spectra and (*b*) their corresponding purest versions actually found in the image for a set of fluorescent microspheres. From top to bottom, the purities are 1, 1, 1, 0.97, 0.90, 0.84, and 0.20.

in five MNF bands. Figure 6.14*a* shows the estimated end-member spectra and their corresponding purest spectra. Figure 6.14*b* shows the proportion maps and RMS map. From top to bottom in Figure 6.14*a*, the purities are 1, 1, 0.93, 0.89, and 0.86, which are all quite high. The tumor is clearly identified by the fourth end member, but it is important to note that, although its spectrum contains the characteristic peak of GFP, it is actually a mixture of the tumor (GFP) spectrum *and* skin, which is given by the fifth end member. This is because we only ever see the tumor *through* the skin of the mouse. The first end member likely indicates fungal growth on the surface of the skin, and the third end member is the dark-image background. The proportion map corresponding to the second end member is very sparse. There are only 14 pixels (out of 196,608) where the proportion of this end member is greater than 0.5. All are in a connected cluster, which is just visible about halfway between the center and the top left-hand corner of the image. These may be dust particles, and although they are of no biological interest, they still represent an end member that has to be contended with.

The RMS image is stretched to enhance contrasts. Most of the red and yellow pixels are in the region outside the mouse body, which is of no interest.

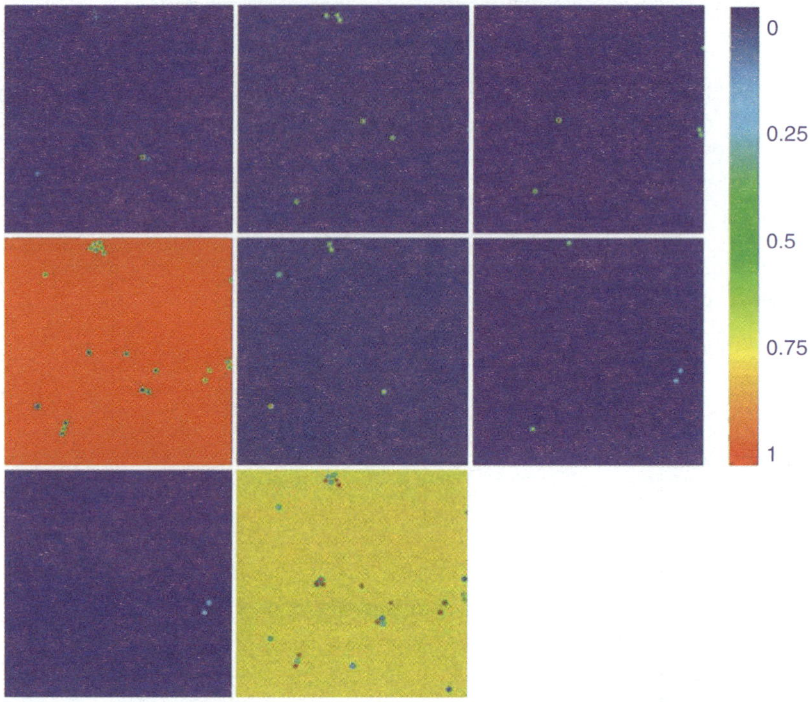

Figure 6.10 Proportion maps and RMS map obtained by ICE algorithm for images of fluorescent microspheres. The maps are arranged in order from left to right and top to bottom. The eighth map is the RMS map.

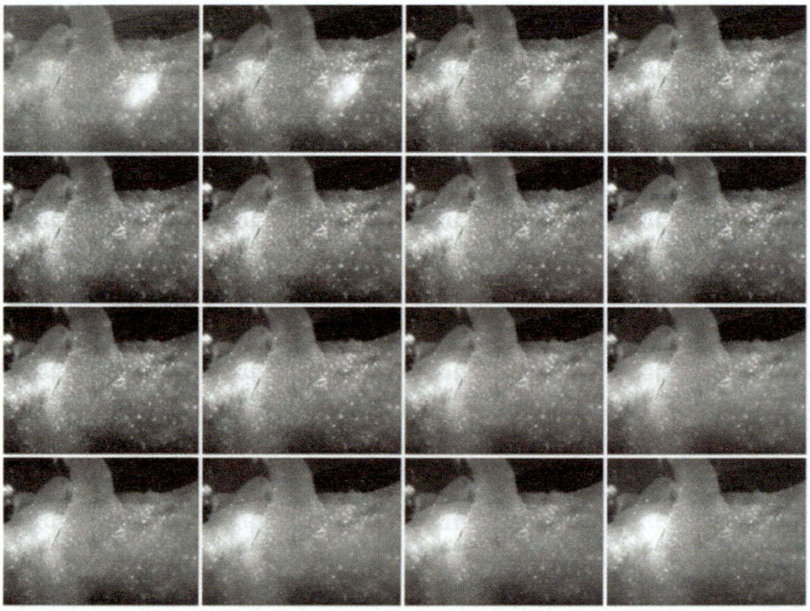

Figure 6.11 Sixteen images measured from 500–650 nm of mouse lung with GFP-labeled tumor. The sequence of images is from left to right, top to bottom. Each image has been individually stretched to enhance contrasts.

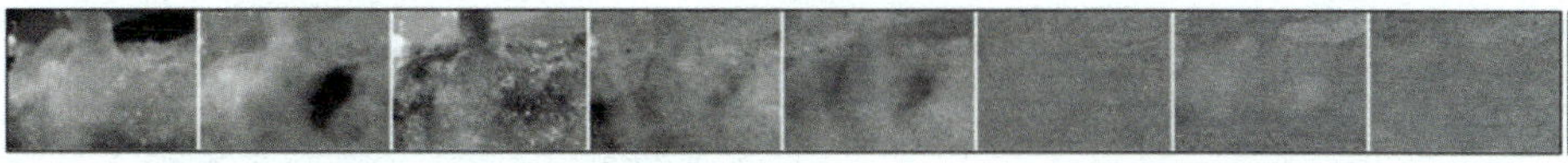

Figure 6.12 First eight MNF images of mouse lung hyperspectral image.

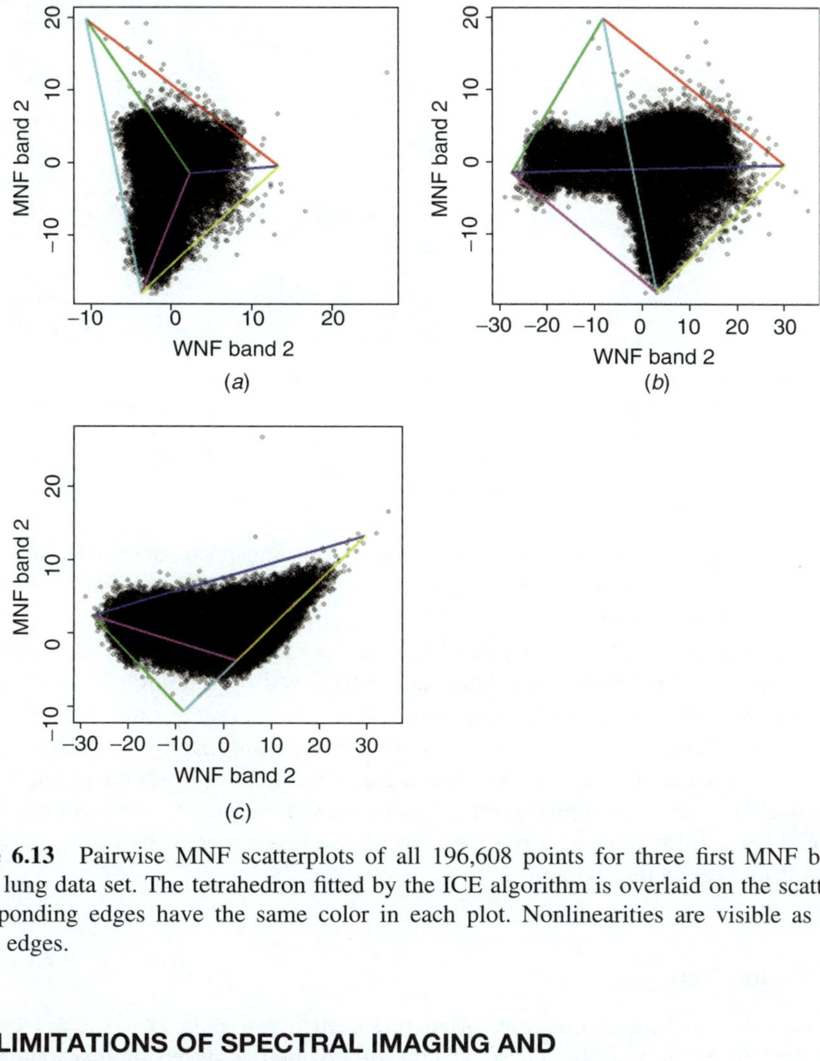

Figure 6.13 Pairwise MNF scatterplots of all 196,608 points for three first MNF bands of mouse lung data set. The tetrahedron fitted by the ICE algorithm is overlaid on the scatterplots. Corresponding edges have the same color in each plot. Nonlinearities are visible as slightly curved edges.

6.8 LIMITATIONS OF SPECTRAL IMAGING AND EXPERIMENTAL CONSIDERATIONS

6.8.1 Fast Biological Processes

Spectral imaging requires vast amounts of data to be collected, much more than when using conventional fluorescence microscopy. In the case of fixed samples, the main downside is the amount of storage space required to save and analyze these data. For fast processes, however, data acquisition must occur within the time it takes for the process to evolve significantly. This is not always possible given current limitations

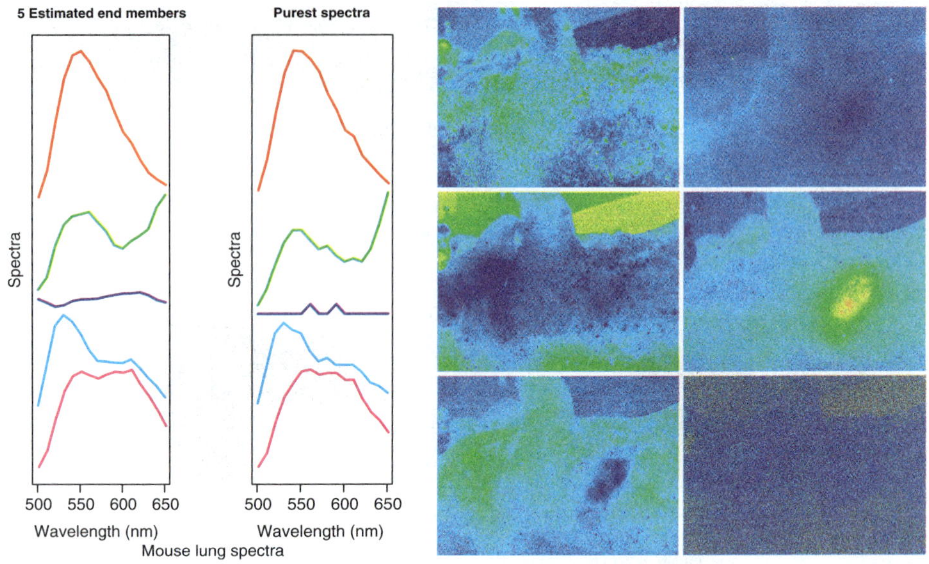

Figure 6.14 Results of fitting five end members in five MNF bands for mouse lung data set: (*a*) Estimated end-member spectra and corresponding purest spectra; (*b*) proportion maps and RMS map.

of hardware in terms of data throughput. Thus, observing processes such as cytosolic calcium waves or motile behavior represents a significant challenge that will continue to drive innovation forward.

In many instruments, the spatial resolution of spectral data can be compromised in order to limit the acquisition time. This can be achieved by reading only a fraction of the imaging sensor or by grouping pixels into 4 or 16 and reading the total sum (pixel binning). Sometimes, a line-scanning (point-scanning) approach can be used, where the sample is measured only along a fixed line (point) as a function of time. If the process itself is very well reproducible, it is possible to aggregate the results obtained for successive manifestations of the process line by line, or point by point, in order to gain a full picture of the dynamics.

6.8.2 Calibration

In supervised linear unmixing, one often relies on a set of known spectra for each species present in the sample. These spectra are deemed acquired on an "ideal instrument" and are available from libraries of spectra [23] maintained by, for example, fluorescent probe manufacturers (www.probes.com). They are valuable for experimental planning and for instrument calibration. Calibration is very important because the unmixing procedure is very sensitive to shifts and other distortions of the actual spectra measured on one's own instruments compared to library reference spectra. Instrument calibration entails measuring a set of known reference probes on one's instrument and determining correction factors at each wavelength. These factors will then be systematically and automatically applied in all subsequent measurements.

Because calibration may not be stable enough, the best experimental practice is to measure the spectra of the pure species for a specific experiment on one's own instrument. This is usually accomplished by staining and imaging the sample, one probe at a time, in the absence of all other probes. This strategy also mitigates problems associated with the sensitivity of most fluorescent probes to their immediate surroundings, as described in the next paragraph.

6.8.3 Environmental Sensitivity

Fluorescence spectra may depend considerably on the local probe environment. As a result, the actual fluorescence spectrum of a probe in a sample may be markedly different from its spectrum measured in standard conditions. In this case the process of supervised linear unmixing will deliver strongly biased results. Blind unmixing methods, which do not rely on a priori information about spectral shapes but rather infer them from the data, are particularly appropriate for dealing with this situation. However, as was mentioned in the tablet inspection example, blind unmixing works best when there are pure or almost pure representatives of all the constituents in the data set, which may not always be the case.

The sensitivity of most fluorescence probes to their local environment is not just a liability. Some of the most exciting applications of spectral imaging rely on this property. When the effects are understood and modeled appropriately, they allow precise measurements of the local acidity; the concentration of calcium and other ions; the polarity, temperature, and exciplex formation; and the proximity to another probe involved in fluorescence resonant energy transfer (FRET) [24].

6.8.4 Background Fluorescence

In linear unmixing, one assumes that the fluorescence signal can be expressed as a sum of contributions from pure components with varying fractional contributions throughout the image. The background signal poses special challenges in this model. Ideally, one would like to deal with background fluorescence as with any other pure species. However, the heterogeneity of cellular media means that one cannot expect the background to present a single spectral profile across the sample. For example, nicotinamide adenine dinucleotide (NADH), one among a host of molecules contributing to cell autofluorescence, is present in greater concentration in mitochondria [25]. Thus, several components may be required to satisfactorily model the background. In the worst cases, there may be too much heterogeneity in the background to obtain informative results with linear unmixing.

If it is possible to bleach the sample fluorescence completely, the background can be simply measured as the signal remaining after the bleaching and its contribution may be subtracted at every pixel prior to the unmixing. However, this assumes that background fluorescence is not affected by the bleaching process, an assumption that may or may not be correct and must be verified experimentally.

6.9 CONCLUSIONS

We have presented a few tools for making the best use of the wealth of information contained in spectral data sets. We have also given a few examples of the use of these tools. Many other applications are emerging across spectral ranges and imaging modalities. In some instances, such as imaging quantum dots, it is mainly the instrumentation itself that is opening new possibilities, due to its ability to measure signals at a large number of independent wavelengths. In some others, such as estimating FRET efficiency precisely, the instrumentation must be supported by the appropriate mathematical apparatus in order to perform unmixing precisely. Generally, the complexity of these algorithms tends to increase with the level of uncertainty in the experiment.

Spectral imaging not only is opening new possibilities but also simplifies existing protocols considerably. For example, we have seen that virtually any fluorescence probe combination can be used, meaning considerable savings in terms of experimental planning and engineering of fluorescent probes. Increasingly, microscopes come equipped with hyperspectral capabilities by default, including intuitive software for unmixing. Spectral imaging it seems is here to stay.

ACKNOWLEDGMENTS

We are grateful to Dennis Donley (Olympus) for the fluorescent microsphere images, to Richard Levenson (CRI) for the mouse lung images, and to a pharmaceutical company wishing to preserve anonymity for the powder and tablet samples. We thank Phil Connor for "imaging" them using CSIRO Exploration and Mining's HyChips™ system. We also thank Ryan Lagerstrom for helpful comments.

REFERENCES

1. E. Schrock, S. du Manoir, T. Veldman, B. Schoell, J. Wienberg, M. A. Ferguson-Smith, Y. Ning, D. H. Ledbetter, I. Bar-Am, D. Soenksen, et al., "Multicolor spectral karyotyping of human chromosomes," *Science* **273**(5274), 494–497 (1996).
2. C. Thaler and S. S. Vogel, "Quantitative linear unmixing of CFP and YFP from spectral images acquired with two-photon excitation," *Cytometry A* **69**(8), 904–911 (2006).
3. Y. Hiraoka, T. Shimi, and T. Haraguchi, "Multispectral imaging fluorescence microscopy for living cells," *Cell Struct. Funct.* **27**(5), 367–374 (2002).
4. B. Saleh and M. Teich, *Fundamentals of Photonics,* Wiley, New York, 1991.
5. N. Keshava, J. Kerekes, D. Manolakis, and G. Shaw, "An algorithm taxonomy for hyperspectral unmixing," *Algorithms for Multispectral, Hyperspectral and Ultraspectral Imagery, Proc. SPIE* **4049**, 42–63 (2000).
6. J. Jiang, Y. Liang, and Y. Ozaki, "Principles and methodologies in self-modeling curve resolution," *Chem. Intel. Lab. Syst.* **71**, 1–12 (2004).
7. B. Hapke, *Theory of Reflectance and Emittance Spectroscopy,* Cambridge University Press, Cambridge, 2005.
8. J. Nocedal and S. Wright, *Numerical Optimization,* Springer, New York, 1999.
9. G. Seber, *Multivariate Observations,* Wiley, New York, 1984.
10. T. Hastie, A. Buja, and R. Tibshirani, "Penalized discriminant analysis," *Ann. Stat.* **23**, 73–102 (1995).
11. A. Miller, *Subset Selection in Regression,* Chapman and Hall, London, 2002.
12. M. Berman, L. Bischof, and J. Huntington, "Algorithms and software for the automated identification of minerals using field spectra or hyperspectral imagery," *Proc. 13th Int. Conf. Applied Geol. Remote Sensing* **1**, 222–232 (1999).

13. M. Berman, H. Kiiveri, R. Lagerstrom, A. Ernst, R. Dunne, and J. Huntington, "ICE: A statistical approach to identifying endmembers," *IEEE Trans. Geosci. Remote* **42**, 2085–2095 (2004).
14. M. Berman, A. Phatak, and R. Lagerstrom, "ICE: A statistical approach to identifying endmembers in biomedical hyperspectral images," *Proc. SPIE,* **5694**, 62–73 (2005).
15. M. Berman, A. Phatak, R. Lagerstrom, and B. Wood, "ICE: A new method for the multivariate curve resolution of hyperspectral images," *J. Chemometrics,* **231**(2), 101–116 (2009).
16. A. A. Green, M. Berman, P. Switzer, and M. D. Craig, "A transformation for ordering multispectral data in terms of image quality with implications for noise removal," *IEEE T. Geosci. Remote* **26**(1), 65–74 (1998).
17. A. A. Nielsen, "An extension to a filter implementation of a local quadratic surface for image noise estimation," *Proc. Int. Conf. Image Analysis and Processing,* **199**, 119–124 (1999).
18. J. MacQueen, *Some Methods for Classification and Analysis of Multivariate Observations*, University of California Press, Berkeley, CA, 1967, pp. 281–297.
19. J. C. Bezdek, L. O. Hall, M. C. Clark, D. B. Goldgof, and L. P. Clarke, "Medical image analysis with fuzzy models," *Stat. Meth. Med. Res.* **6**(3), 191–214 (1997).
20. P. Lasch, W. Haensch, D. Naumann, and M. Diem, "Imaging of colorectal adenocarcinoma using FT-IR microspectroscopy and cluster analysis," *Biochem. Biophys. Acta.* **1688**(2), 176–186 (2004).
21. G. Wahba, *Spline Models for Observational Data*, SIAM, Philadelphia, 1990.
22. T. Yuying and C. Takashi, "Metastasis models using green fluorescent protein (GFP) as a marker," Anticancer, Inc., U.S. patent 6232523, 2001.
23. G. McNamara, A. Gupta, J. Reynaert, T. D. Coates, and C. Boswell, "Spectral imaging microscopy web sites and data," *Cytometry A* **69**(8), 863–871 (2006).
24. P. Vallotton, R. Hovius, H. Pick, and H. Vogel, "In vitro and in vivo ligand binding to the 5HT(3) serotonin receptor characterised by time-resolved fluorescence spectroscopy," *Chembiochem.* **2**(3), 205–211 (2001).
25. H. Andersson, T. Baechi, M. Hoechl, and C. Richter, "Autofluorescence of living cells," *J. Microsc.* **191**(1), 1–7 (1998).

CHAPTER 7

Correlation of Light with Electron Microscopy: A Correlative Microscopy Platform

MARKO NYKÄNEN

Research and Development Office, The Kids Research Institute at the Children's Hospital at Westmead, Locked Bag 4001, NSW 2145, Australia

7.1 INTRODUCTION

Advances in cellular and molecular imaging are bringing about a rapid reevaluation of ways to visualize dynamic processes such as intracellular protein trafficking, outcomes of medical interventions, and progress of diseases especially at subcellular and molecular levels. To achieve this, fundamental ultrastructural information needs to be supplemented by functional data collected from living specimens. Fluorescent proteins and various chemical tags and probes are providing novel insights into processes such as compound-induced responses in drug discovery. Increasing emphasis is placed on real-time analysis and investigations of living cellular and organ systems [6].

Light microscopy (LM) has been extensively used for localization studies of intracellular proteins in space and time [9, 17]. LM provides the advantage of noninvasive visualization of proteins, and it has the capacity to examine optical sections, which is especially important in living cells and tissues [22]. However, LM can only display a limited number of stained objects within the optical resolution limit, where, generally, objects smaller than 100 nm cannot be distinguished. On the other hand, electron microscopy (EM) easily extends into the subnanometer resolution limit. For either labeled or unlabeled cellular structures to be detected by EM, they must be of high enough molecular weight to effectively scatter electrons, that is, be electron dense. This is achieved by labeling of ultrastructural cellular components with electron-dense tags attached to appropriate target molecules. With such tags in place, the EM is able to provide detailed insights into subcellular architecture, in principle also in three dimensions. Moreover, EM can provide accurate quantitative information about the labeled proteins. Such quantitative EM is an essential tool in molecular morphometry. In this approach targeted molecules are labeled with ultrafine gold nanoparticles and their amount in subcellular compartments such as intracellular organelles is quantified by counting the nanoparticles observed in the image. However, EM requires cell

Fluorescence Applications in Biotechnology and Life Sciences, Edited by Ewa M. Goldys

TABLE 7.1 Summary of General Advantages and Drawbacks of LM and EM

Parameter	Confocal Scanning LM	Transmission EM
Specimen type	Live and fixed	Only fixed
Size of specimen	Up to several centimeters	Maximum few millimeters
Sample fixation and dehydration	Simple	Critical for success, needs to be optimized
Sample sectioning	Strictly optical, rapid, noninvasive	By ultramicrotomy, requires advanced skills and equipment, prone to artefacts
Postcontrasting	Not needed	Required, needs optimization
Two-dimensional (2D) resolution	Low (>100 nm)	High (<0.1 nm)
Use of microscope	High content, low throughput	High content, throughput even lower than LM
In vivo four-dimensional (4D) studies	Possible	Impossible
Label quantification	Complicated	Undemanding, e.g., immunogold labeling
Full automation	Yes	Only semiautomated
Possible Z-axis resolution	Low (>200 nm)	High (2 nm)

fixation and physical ultrathin sectioning of specimens usually down to 40 nm thick (by ultramicrotomy) [7] or even down to 8 nm thick by using the special water-soluble melamine resin Nanoplast FB101 (van Loenen Instruments), which rules out in vivo LM imaging with fluorescent proteins. It should also be noted that electron micrographs cannot provide certain important pieces of information, for example, the directionality of the visualized biological membranes. Therefore, efforts continue to bridge the gap between live cell imaging by LM and high-resolution imaging of fixed cells by EM. A successful combination of the two methodologies LM and EM offers new avenues for more detailed subcellular studies into molecular dynamics, including protein interactions and trafficking. The relative merits of both LM and EM are summarized in Table 7.1.

7.2 OVERVIEW OF TECHNIQUES USED IN CORRELATIVE MICROSCOPY

A variety of biological labeling techniques for microscopy have been developed in order to obtain specific molecular and spatial information in cells and tissues. Broadly speaking, these can be classified as labeling by molecular biology techniques (localization of genetically modified target proteins, e.g., fluorescent proteins), cytochemistry (chemical labeling of intracellular molecules), immunocytochemistry (labeling of subcellular molecular targets by antibodies), and in situ hybridization (monitoring intracellular messenger RNA by specific labeled probes suitable for LM and EM). In general, correlative microscopy (CM) refers to the circumstances in which a single specimen is examined by two or more imaging techniques or when two or more labeling probes are applied to the same sample. In the most challenging type of CM combining LM and EM, the same subcellular characteristics are correlated across different length scales.

Such integration of the EM and fluorescence images provides an additional perspective to cellular ultrastructures.

Modern advanced microscopy is prone to technical artefacts, inexperienced use, and misinterpretations of image data [2]. The CM aims to provide structural and functional molecular cell biology information by correlating the LM and EM images at exactly corresponding subcellular coordinates within the investigated cells. This is challenging since intracellular structures differ considerably even within the same specimen, and judgments by a simple analogy between the shapes observed in LM and EM may be misleading. The quantitative CM technique helps avoid such misinterpretations.

The CM utilizes diverse combinations of various LM and EM techniques which, when taken together, provide a more complete picture of real cellular structures, mechanisms, and interactions within the biological object or phenomenon under scrutiny. In addition to the LM and EM instrumentation, the CM requires a full repertoire of various optimized LM and EM specimen preparation methods in association with, for example, atomic force microscopy, scanning EM, cryoEM, and electron tomography [2, 10]. High-quality specimen preparation techniques [10, 19] are the foundation of success in CM. They should ensure specific, sensitive, and artefact-free LM and EM imaging. In this chapter we describe the experimental steps necessary for appropriate specimen preparation. We concentrate here on typical problems under investigation, for example, localization of proteins in (ultra)thin sections using antibodies coupled with fluorescent gold probes, visualization of fluorescent proteins in both living and fixed cells also by electron tomography, or staining of tissue samples for LM (histological stains) and EM (uranium salts). In such cases the frozen and chemically fixed specimens are cut into ultrathin sections and labeled with antibodies that specifically recognize the target molecules coupled with fluorescent stains (providing visibility in LM) and electron-dense stains containing atoms/molecules visible in EM such as uranium, lead, vanadate, and gold.

Figure 7.1 presents a sequence of experiments carried out in CM starting from the LM studies (Figure 7.1, top) of either living or fixed cells and proceeding toward EM ultrastructural studies by LM (Figure 7.1, bottom). The arrows indicate the various CM approaches which take us from the LM stage either directly to EM visualization (EM cathodoluminescence) or through the demanding EM sample preparation procedures such as those for cryoEM, TEM, or freeze fracture.

Highly electron-dense probes such as nanogold are necessary to trace the labeled molecular targets by EM. Once the EM labels have been put in place, they can be made visible in LM by photoconversion. Alternatively, electron-dense but fluorescent labels attached to molecules can be used, including quantum dots (QDs) attached to biomolecules [5, 14]. Electron-dense staining reagents such as lead and uranium salts are also used to visualize the subcellular structures.

The EM specimen preparation usually involves chemical fixation of the sample prior to freezing the sample at high pressure or embedding the specimen into a supporting plastic material without the freezing step. Embedding is essential for making ultrathin specimen sections by ultramicrotomy procedures. It is recommended to remove water by solvents at extremely low temperatures prior to embedding into plastic. It should be emphasized that the study of frozen samples directly by EM (cryoEM) without plastic embedding, ultramicrotomy, and postcontrasting is highly recommended whenever possible. A good alternative choice is to prepare ultrathin cryosections from frozen samples and thaw those sections for immunolabeling of target molecules at

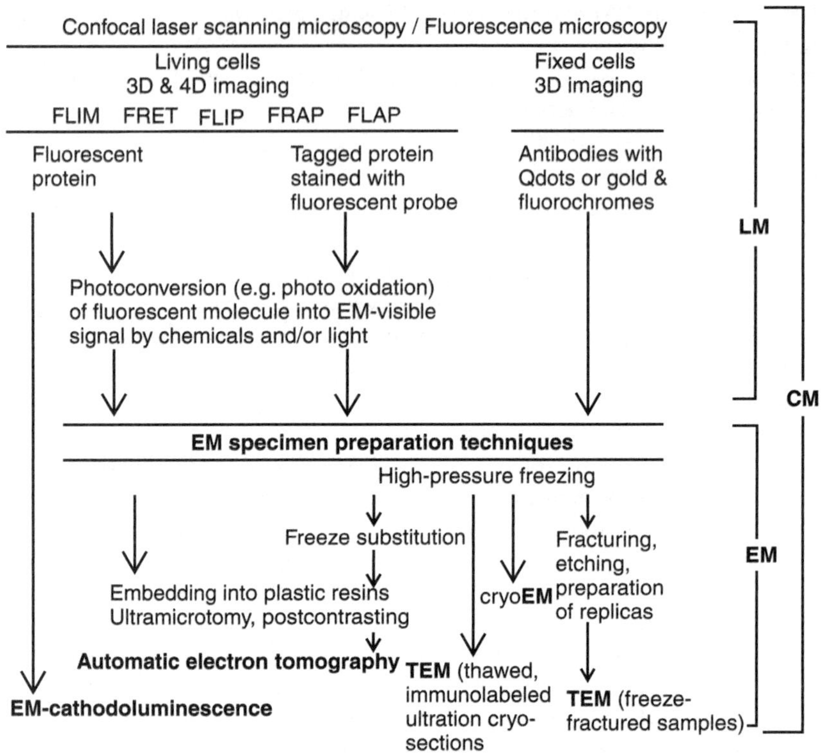

Figure 7.1 Schematic of integrated CM platform: FLIM, fluorescence lifetime imaging microscopy; FRET, fluorescence resonance energy transfer; FLIP, fluorescence loss in photobleaching, FRAP, fluorescence recovery after photobleaching; FLAP, fluorescence loss after photobleaching; TEM, transmission electron microscopy.

room temperature. The frozen EM samples can be fractured by knife at extremely low temperatures (freeze fracture). The fractured surface of membranes is often able to reveal novel unique sites with targets for labeling and visualization that are not accessible otherwise (e.g., by making thin sections). For the purpose of EM studies, these fractured specimen surfaces are replicated in metal, as described further in this chapter.

Ultimately, the success of CM depends also on numerous factors such as quality of the examined specimens (in comparison with living and fixed cells), targeted molecule(s), available labeling methods, and approaches used for ultrastructural analysis such as using specimens embedded in plastic versus cryospecimens frozen at high pressure. These issues will be discussed in more detail later.

A key feature that should be taken into initial consideration when preparing specimens for CM studies is the quality of the label or probe, such as fluorescent protein or fluorochrome or gold attached to antibody [21]. The users need to be aware of their ability to bind, life span, and sensitivity to pH changes inside cells or tissues. It is also important to note the possible toxicity of probes/labels which can interfere with vital functions of cells as well as the ability of probes to reach their molecular targets, especially in living cells and tissue. The choice of a fixation method in cells/tissues is also important, and one can use either chemical fixation or cryofixation, for example, by high-pressure freezing. The sample dehydration needs to be done with caution too. It involves removal of water from cells and tissues with solvents like acetone at extremely low temperatures in a procedure called freeze substitution. Microtomy and ultramicrotomy (thin sectioning of plastic embedded samples) and cryotomy (thin sectioning of frozen samples) also present challenges. Here numerous technical factors such as the quality of the cutting blade and cutting speed affect the results of sectioning. Deficiencies in sample preparation reduce the quality of the final results; for example, specimen artefacts can be caused by sectioning or staining, including the application of postprocessing contrast with lead and uranium. Finally, the specificity and efficiency of producing electron-dense contrast within ultrathin sections are critical in order to reveal ultrastructural architecture associated with the labeled target molecules.

7.3 CORRELATIVE MICROSCOPY OF CHEMICALLY FIXED, IMMUNOLABELED ULTRATHIN CRYOSECTIONS EMPLOYING ANTIBODIES COUPLED WITH FLUORESCENT GOLD CONJUGATES

As discussed in Section 7.1, LM uses fluorescent probes to visualize proteins of interest, as they normally have very limited or no native fluorescence. The probes could be used alone in either direct labeling (e.g., when the proteins themselves are fluorescent; Figure 7.2*e*) or indirect visualization (e.g., by using antibodies and their parts; Figures 7.2*a* and 7.2*c*). In both the direct and indirect labeling, the term *probe* is also used by referring to antibody and electron-dense metal (Figure 7.2*b*), fluorochrome, or other chemical product (Figures 7.2*f* and 7.2*g*) linked with the antibody or its fragments. The antibody is a protein that recognizes specific amino acids or other motifs in the target proteins or molecules. Simultaneous visualization of intracellular molecular targets (antigens) by LM and EM using their specific antibodies or their fragments (Fab′ or Fab_2; Figures 7.2*b* and 7.2*c*, respectively) requires probes that can be detected in both LM and EM [14].

The most frequently used probes include fluorochromes, metallic elements/ inorganic compounds (gold, QDs; Figure 7.2*d*), and enzymes. A common example of the latter is a peroxidase enzyme in cellular organelles (lysosomes) that converts the molecule with which it interacts in the cell (i.e., substrate) into a visible reaction product.

The recognition of antigen binding in the chemically fixed and liquid nitrogen frozen cells/tissues can be direct by using primary antibodies coupled directly with probes consisting of fluorochrome molecules and nanogold particles (size 1.4 nm; Nanoprobes) or ultrasmall gold (approximate size 1 nm; Aurion). Alternatively, when it is not possible to label the primary antibodies with gold or fluorochromes, indirect labeling is utilized [19, 23]. In this approach, unlabeled primary antibodies react with secondary antibodies labeled with fluorochromes and/or gold tracers. In many cases, the indirect labeling technique is the only available option to visualize molecular interactions. The availability of variously labeled probes makes it possible to carry out multiple staining. In this approach the target molecules can be localized directly with primary probes, such as fluorochromes and gold-labeled probes, whereas other target molecules are traced by probes with different labels. The optimal choice of the labeling technique depends on the repertoire of the best available probes and the existence and availability of specific antibodies tagged with various fluorochromes as well as optimal sizes of metal

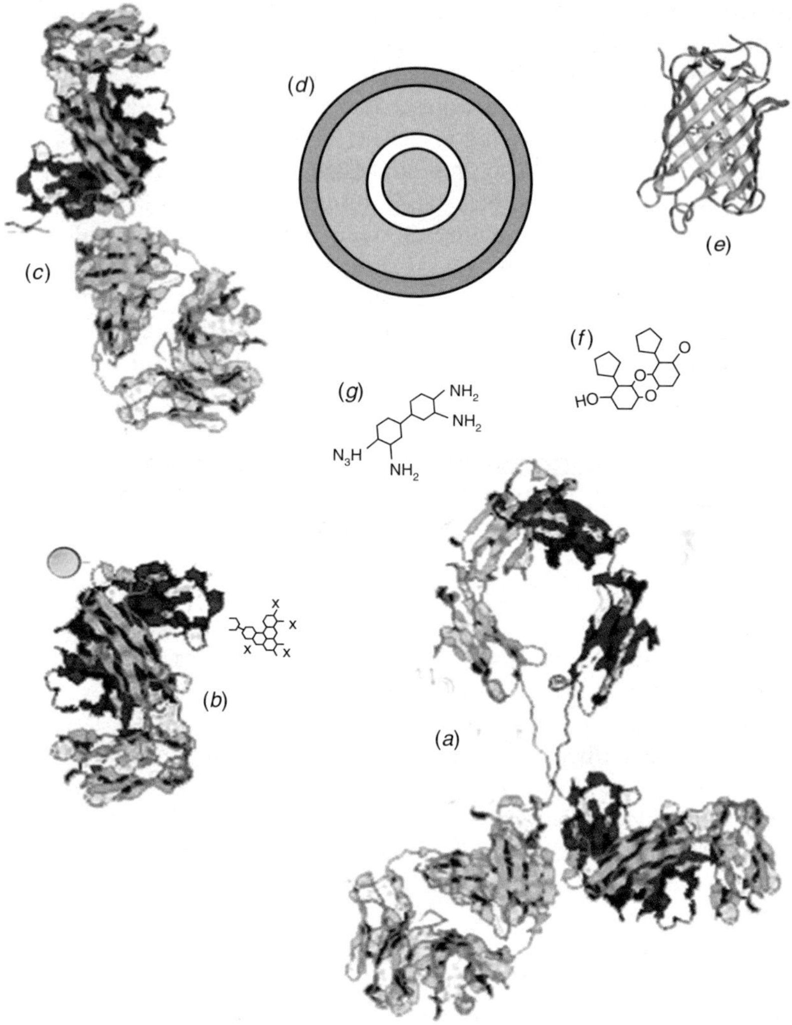

Figure 7.2 Schematic of labeling probes used in CM techniques (not to scale): (*a*) immunoglobulin molecule (antibody); (*b*) antibody fragment (Fab′) linked with nanogold and fluorochrome; (*c*) antibody fragment (Fab_2); (*d*) quantum dot; (*e*) green fluorescent protein (GFP); (*f*) bis-arsenyl fluorescent chromophore; (*g*) 3,3′-diaminobenzidine.

particles. Last but not least, one should keep in mind the optimization of specificity and sensitivity of labeling antibodies. The quality and properties of fluorochromes or other tags in the probe also affect the results of imaging in both LM and EM. Correlative microscopy demands the probes which produce as little as possible of the unspecific binding by attaching as accurately as possible only to the targeted regions of the specimen.

Examination of tissues using multiphoton laser scanning microscopy, although convenient with its large penetration depth and noninvasive optical sectioning capability, suffers from limited resolution of optical microscopy—thus the need for CM. Having discussed the CM of individual cells, we will now focus on CM tissue imaging, which presents a new and different set of complications. In CM we cross over from fluorescence microscopy to EM by using immunolabeled thin sections, and label/probe penetration inside tissue needs to be optimized to achieve good results. Tissue imaging presents problems due to large sample size—the size of a single tissue biopsy is usually from several millimeters to 1 cm—and complex multicellular architecture. In addition to the main cellular components, tissues contain numerous extracellular filamentous matrix elements such as collagen, elastin, and microfibers and other various macromolecular substances (e.g., glycoproteins). The size of typical biopsies presents a significant challenge for microscopy, whether LM or EM. With multiphoton laser scanning microscopy we can usually image only to a depth of 100 μm from the tissue surface, which is approximately 5–20 cell layers depending on the tissue and cell type. The major problem in tissue imaging is however the fact that various larger probes for localization of targets such as antibody fragments or QDs as well as gold particle diameter over 1 nm (see Figure 7.2) are unable to reach deeper regions of living or fixed tissues. In fact, they can hardly penetrate beyond the first cell layer even in the fixed tissue permeabilized by a detergent. Such a detergent (e.g., Tween) makes small "pores" in the cell membranes where the probes can traverse into the cell. It is impossible to directly deliver the antibody fragments directly into living unfixed tissue without special lipid vehicles (e.g., commercially available protein transfection methods developed for cells). The use of these vehicles in the transfection is challenging, and their delivery is generally very restricted to the outer cell layer of tissue. Thus the key approach for correlative microscopy of antibody-labeled tissue samples involves the use of (ultra)microtomy and immunolabeling and subsequent imaging of thin sections.

The important role of correlative microscopy applied to tissues emerges from the fact that accurate localization of antigen can be carried out without too much difficulty by immunoelectron (EM) microscopy, since ultrathin sections can be easily prepared from the tissue samples. However, precise localization of antigens by immunofluorescence microscopy is more complicated. Semithin (5–15-μm) (cryo)sections of tissues are relatively easy to prepare, but localization of immunofluorescence is negatively affected by out-of-focus fluorescence which limits contrast and the observed resolution. This problem is at least partially resolved by using confocal laser scanning microscopy (CLSM), which provides the optical sectioning capability. CLSM imaging removes most out-of-focus fluorescence and offers better resolution, down to a few hundred nanometers, compared to traditional fluorescence microscopy. Fortunately, ultrathin cryosections (in the average range of 70–100 nm) obtained by ultramicrotomy can also be examined by immunofluorescence, as intense enough fluorescence signals can be observed. Such ultrathin cryosections remove the problem of out-of-focus fluorescence limiting optical resolution since the sections are considerably thinner than the z dimension of an optical section (range of 200–500 nm) in CLSM. The semithin sections are not the best candidates for immunolabeling due to the inefficient penetration of probes mentioned earlier. In semithin sections (>500 nm) (just as in confocal optical sections), false colocalization (i.e., apparent localization of two different fluorochromes in the same spot but at different heights) may take place. The reason for such false colocalization is that the thickness of such sections is larger than the size of cellular organelles (50–200 nm). On the other hand, the use of ultrathin sections (70–150 nm) makes such false colocalization of molecular targets very unlikely.

Hence, the best solution to the tissue-imaging problems and to achieve the finest possible resolution in CM is to avoid using semithin sections. On the contrary, ultrathin sections are well suited for imaging by immunofluorescence, CLSM, and TEM.

The ultrathin sections can be prepared by either cryotomy where sections are taken from frozen tissue samples or ultramicrotomy, which uses tissue specimens embedded in plastic. The thin sections thus obtained are transferred on metallic, usually nickel, grids that support the film. The next step is immunolabeling by using antibodies linked with gold particles. The procedure begins with labeling the ultrathin cryosections using fluoronanogold. Such samples mounted on the specimen grid are then imaged by immunofluorescence microscopy in a standard way on a glass slide and covered with a coverslip. The coverslip and slide are subsequently removed and the specimen grid is exposed to the silver (or gold) enhancement procedure. The enhancement is carried out with the aid of chemical catalyzers that increase the size of metal particles by using a special commercially prepared solution. The enhancement reaction is controlled by the initiator and termination solutions. Typically, silver (or gold) enhancement is used to enlarge either ultrasmall gold or nanogold particles used as tags. Afterward, the sections are "postcontrasted" (i.e., negatively stained with heavy metals such as uranium salts) for visualization by TEM. The TEM examination is done with the aid of a special locator (or finder) grid which contains various numeric and geometric signs to ease navigation; this grid makes it more convenient to identify the corresponding locations in the LM and EM images [10, 23].

It is also worth noting that EM can provide information on the three-dimensional organization within cells by examining series of ultrathin cryosections (thickness of >40 nm) intersecting the region of interest and equivalent to the z stack in LM. Such measurements are labor intensive as the sections have to be individually loaded to the microscope. This approach is prone to some artefacts arising from imperfect ultracryotomy (or ultramicrotomy) and its resolution in the z-axis direction is comparable to the section thickness. An automated electron tomography (discussed below) provides a much better z-axis resolution of 2 nm or less. Despite these challenges, the CM procedure which uses ultrathin cryosections makes it possible to combine the advantages of LM and EM. The technique thus provides highly specific information on both the cellular ultrastructure and molecular dynamics in the same location.

The 3D imaging, which has traditionally been applied in biomedicine, is now increasingly applied in various areas of biology [2, 13, 14]. It is therefore important to be aware that the 2D immunoelectron microscopy images can be taken in a special way and combined to produce a 3D image. This approach, called automatic electron tomography, relies on computerized modeling of 2D images (Figure 7.3). The resolution and quality of the reconstruction depend primarily upon two TEM measurement parameters, the tilt angle and range. The resolution of tilt angle which can be achieved between each successive image has a major influence upon reconstruction quality, with smaller tilt angles producing better reconstruction. In addition, the total tilt range determines the amount of 3D data which can be obtained. For larger total tilt angles, more data will be visualized in the reconstruction. Generally, images are acquired at tilt angles of $1^\circ - 2^\circ$ between successive images and over a total tilt range of about $\pm 60^\circ - 70^\circ$. A charge-coupled device (CCD) camera is frequently used for image acquisition. Radiation injury sets a limit to the effective resolution in frozen-hydrated samples because the samples are heated and thawed in the radiation beam over time.

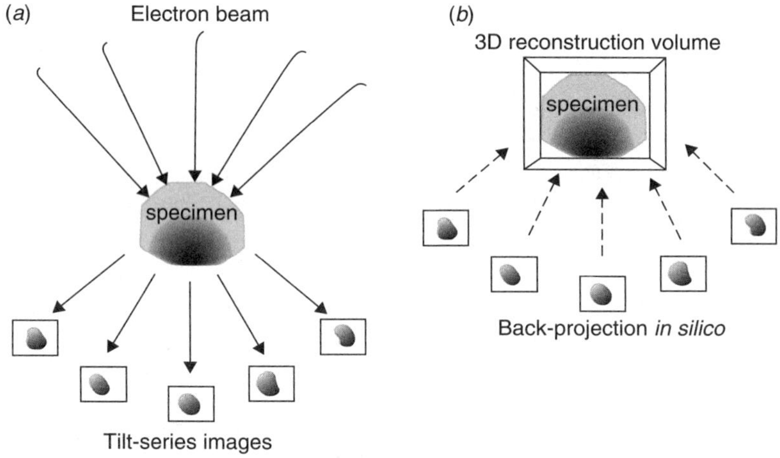

Figure 7.3 Electron tomography is based on producing a 3D reconstruction of an object from a series of TEM projection micrographs. A series of single-axis tilted images is taken. During data collection the specimen is tilted in the electron beam to generate what is known as a tilt series (*a*). The back-projection algorithms project back the mass of the specimen into the 3D reconstruction volume (*b*). When repeated for a series of projection images from different angles, the back-projected rays intersect and indicate the points where mass is found in the original structure.

It has been predicted that the resolution limit is around 2–3 nm for thick, frozen specimens.

The multidimensional data thus collected forming a tomogram provide information on actual intracellular positions of molecules of interest and their topographic relationship with subcellular ultrastructures. Such a tomogram contains quantitative insights into molecular interactions in three dimensions against the background of subcellular architecture. The automatic 3D electron tomography combined with multidimensional CLSM (with three spatial dimensions as well as temporal and wavelength of light) presents the ultimate development for the advanced CM platform.

Fluorescent proteins have provided the foundation for real-time visualization of the architecture of living cells. These proteins are effective instruments for cellular and molecular biologists since they provide high sensitivity and great versatility while minimally disturbing the examined cell, in contrast to chemical labeling. The first fluorescent protein was a GFP (Figure 7.2*e*), but presently many other variants have been identified and further engineered. Their fluorescent colors now span the entire visible range.

To trace cellular processes such as trafficking of various intracellular molecular targets, genetic engineering has to be utilized to create fusion proteins consisting of a target and a probe protein which is fluorescent. This ability of genetic targeting of protein of interest has revolutionized real-time LM and made it possible to track various cellular events. Genetically tailored reporter molecules are now frequently used; these act as active molecular indicators for monitoring of more complex cellular processes such as small-molecule messenger dynamics, enzyme activation, and protein–protein interactions. The genetically encoded fluorescent proteins can be used for labeling genes and proteins as well as, for example, drug targets of interest or in drug discovery based on live cell visualization [4]. Their broader use has now been made easier as a result of comprehensive databases obtained through cloning and more detailed characterization and optimization of such proteins.

Fluorescent proteins in living cells are well suited for applications in CM since they can be visualized without fixing cells. After fixation and further specimen preparation treatments (e.g., incorporation of an electron-dense material), they can be visualized also at an ultrastructural level, as will be explained later in this chapter. While their most significant use is in living cells, the fluorescent proteins can also be used in chemically fixed tissue specimens. This is because GFP expressed in tissues can be imaged by immunofluorescence microscopy even after fixation at mild conditions followed by dehydration and embedding into a special low-fluorescence plastic resin and after additional treatment by immunoEM.

The CM is carried out by using plastic thin sections that are first imaged by CLSM, and the selected regions can be visualized by EM in a way described earlier. As a control the specimen block surface also needs to be imaged by CLSM prior to ultrathin sectioning, as the resins can show undesired fluorescence background.

The CM approach applied to the chemically fixed tissues expressing fluorescent proteins is very powerful since even primary GFP antibodies linked with gold can be utilized for straightforward protein localization [15]. Alternatively, when the primary antibodies linked with gold are not available, the secondary antibodies (e.g., antimouse immunoglobulin antibody against the primary anti-GFP) linked with gold can be used. As mentioned earlier, GFP is able to maintain its fluorescent properties after being embedded into plastic resin. This unique characteristic is very useful for CM, and it makes it possible to analyze immunolabeled ultrathin plastic sections by CLSM and EM. The identity of subcellular coordinates is confirmed by using similar locator grids as for ultrathin cryosections.

The difficulties in the CM approach include the practical challenge of finding the same cell and/or part of a cell that has been illuminated, which is not easy in ultrathin sections. In addition, chemical fixation with dehydration and embedding into plastic resins can perturb the CM analysis since such harsh specimen preparation steps frequently reduce the specificity and sensitivity of immunolabeling. Dehydration and plastic embedding are comparatively less compatible with immunoEM than the freezing method used for making the ultrathin cryosections in cryoimmunoEM.

An illumination-based CM circumvents the above difficulties and also avoids the use of antibodies. This method is based on photoconversion, a physical process whereby a fluorescent probe within a cell or tissue is indirectly transformed (chemically and/or with light) into an electron-dense probe. Such an approach makes it possible to observe fluorescent targets or structures of interest at the EM level. An example is photo-oxidation of 3,3′-diaminobenzidine (DAB; Figure 7.2*g*). The photo-oxidation of DAB utilizes free oxygen radicals that are created upon photobleaching of a fluorescent protein (e.g., GFP) [8]. Special electron-dense probes such as gold attached to GFP are not needed since the illumination of GFP and its chromophores results in polymerization of DAB (adjacent to GFP). This produces an electron-dense precipitate which can be visualized by transmission EM, as, following precipitation, the reaction product remains in its original location. The technique delivers quantitative correlation of GFP fluorescence with the corresponding protein localization (represented by the DAB precipitate) at the EM level. The illumination-based CM technique can be performed also with thick plastic resin embedded sections, which enables 3D characterization of the target by electron tomography. This is in contrast to immunoEM, which relies on exposed antigens in thin sections. Another benefit of photo-oxidation is that DAB penetrates membranes much more easily as it is smaller in size than, for example, antibodies and their fragments. Hence, DAB performs better than other techniques in closed and very small membranous structures such as cellular junctions and transport vesicles where antigens are hard to reach by immunogold techniques.

Another technique suitable for CM is cathodoluminescence (CL), which relies on light commonly emitted by materials irradiated by an electron beam. CL imaging can be performed in parallel with scanning and transmission electron microscopies as the CL imaging system is integrated with the EM imaging unit [12, 16]. By using this approach, fluorescent proteins in the EM sample can, in principle, be directly imaged at high magnification (×10,000 and more). While the method is still under development, CL will be a valuable addition to the repertoire of CM techniques with its ability to visualize fluorescent targets by LM and EM without antibodies or photoconversion. A promising option of a novel CM methodology could involve detecting a fluorescent protein (e.g., by EM–CM) and, after that, using antibody–gold and/or photoconversion for quantitative analysis.

7.4 SPECIAL TECHNIQUES USED IN SAMPLE PREPARATION FOR CORRELATIVE MICROSCOPY: HIGH-PRESSURE FREEZING, FREEZE FRACTURING, AND FREEZE SUBSTITUTION

The EM-assisted imaging of labeled membranous structures is frequently required. This is because intracellular protein trafficking occurs within membranous vesicles that originate from several subcellular organelles (e.g., Golgi apparatus). The dynamics of the vesicular membranes plays a central role in the delivery of protein cargo from one intracellular compartment to another subcellular partition. A precise association of proteins with particular intracellular membranous structures by using conventionally prepared EM samples is very difficult. An alternative approach to ultrathin sectioning is the freeze-fracture technique, which allows fracturing at various depths of the EM specimens frozen under high pressure. The freeze-fracture technique exposes unique intracellular membranous ultrastructures because it splits the membranes along the hydrophobic internal planes (Figure 7.4). After fracturing, a metallic copy (replica) of the freeze-fractured and immunolabeled biological specimen is made (Figure 7.5). The EM imaging of such labeled metal replicas remains one of the more important CM techniques. Other specimen preparation methods for the CM studies include chemical and immunological labeling in vivo prior to high-pressure freezing (i.e., fixation of the specimen under high-pressure conditions instead of chemical fixation with aldehydes at room temperature) and freeze substitution (i.e., completely removing water from the frozen samples prior to thawing them for further processing).

The high-pressure freezing (HPF) method takes advantage of the suppression of ice nucleation and growth in water rapidly frozen at high pressures. This produces a completely vitrified but otherwise intact specimen. First, a sample is placed into a special cap (or holder) at room temperature. The cap (holder) is then transferred inside the HPF equipment where it is filled with liquid nitrogen under high-pressure conditions. The technique is well suited to various cellular samples since it provides

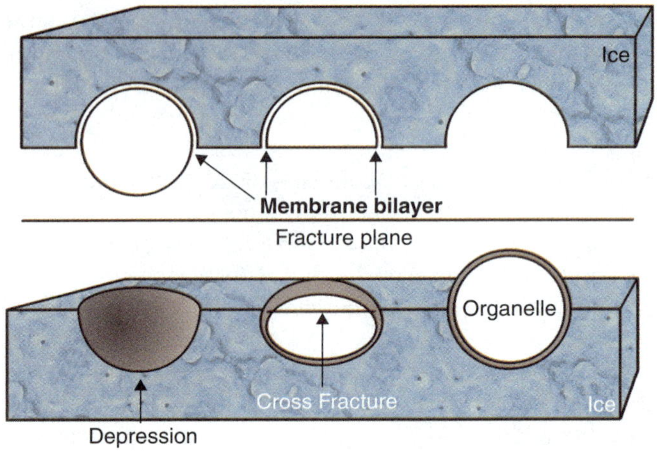

Figure 7.4 Schematic of freeze-fractured bilayer membranes of cellular organelles (e.g., membrane of nucleus).

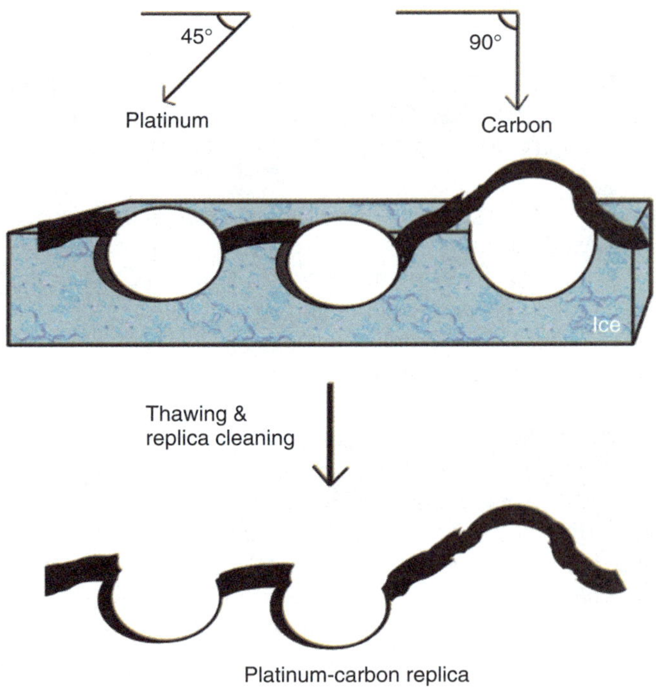

Figure 7.5 Preparation of replicas with Pt/C shadowing from freeze-fractured surfaces.

the most authentic ultrastructural landscape and can be used for preserving cells within 50–100 μm from the frozen specimen surface. The HPF technique is necessary to avoid the artefacts characteristic of conventional plunge freezing with liquid nitrogen or helium where crystallized ice tends to destroy cellular ultrastructures. The HPF has been used to capture ultrastructural details in cells grown on sapphire coverslips [18], which is important for CM since sapphire is a tissue culture substrate highly suitable for optical studies. HPF methods have also been used for correlative LM and EM on the same specimen [20] where CLSM was utilized for simultaneous fluorescence as well as transmitted and backscattered light images. Fluorescence data from a whole sample or from thin sections can also be used to merge with the TEM micrographs and the integrated image displayed by using different colors.

Following HPF, the samples undergoing freeze fracturing are transferred onto the cold table (123 K, or −150°C) of the freeze-fracturing apparatus. The selected specimen plane is exposed with successive fracturing cycles. After fracturing, samples are deep etched by sublimating the excess ice that coats fractured specimens. The next step is the preparation of a metal replica of the fractured specimen, which is performed by coating the sample with platinum (a 1–2-nm layer at an angle of 45°). The replica is further stabilized with a 10-nm layer of carbon (Figure 7.5). Finally, the samples are brought to room temperature and biological material is digested from the replicas destined for further TEM analysis.

Since EM operates under high vacuum, the specimens prepared for EM must be entirely dehydrated. In conventional chemical fixation techniques, water is removed by rinsing the sample through a series of increasing concentrations of ethanol or other appropriate solvents. Such dehydration techniques expose the sample to extraction, shrinkage, and other perturbing factors which can induce artefacts. Freeze substitution is a technique where frozen water within a sample is replaced by a solvent, usually acetone, while the sample is kept at a very low temperature. This method of dehydration preserves cellular ultrastructure reasonably faithfully, since it does not include multiple solvent changes. Freeze substitution occurs at a temperature where the sample remains frozen while the water is removed. Furthermore, since fixative agents (such as osmium) can be added to the solvent, freeze substitution can be used to simultaneously postfix and dehydrate the sample. To summarize, freeze substitution in combination with low-temperature embedding into plastic resins is a superior approach to minimize the loss of soluble cell constituents. The damage of subcellular organelles and loss of molecules is less likely to occur in rapidly frozen and properly freeze-substituted specimens.

7.5 CORRELATIVE MICROSCOPY OF FIXED TISSUE SPECIMENS USING FREEZE SUBSTITUTION

The application of various LM and EM sample preparation methods to obtain correlated image data remains difficult, especially when, for example, a tissue sample has to be cut into several pieces for different specimen preparation techniques. Hence, the EM ad LM micrographs do not always represent precisely the same region but can be considered as merely analogous. An optimal solution to the challenge could be imaging of the same tissue samples prepared for EM and LM. We have earlier described a CM technique based on a series of ultrathin sections. Unfortunately, this technique is vulnerable to several artefacts, especially during ultramicrotomy. A novel approach to visualization of tissue samples includes employing various histochemical colors. These small-molecule dyes can diffuse and thoroughly stain tissues, and the most effective include acridine orange, $DiOC_6$, Nile blue sulfate, nonyl acridine orange, and safranine T. The electron-dense uranyl acetate can also be infiltrated during freeze substitution. Prior to the staining procedure, the samples are fixed with high-pressure freezing. After freeze substitution, the tissue samples are embedded into plastic resins and polymerized and, as such, can be imaged by CSLM, also along the z axis [1]. In this approach the dyes penetrate into deeper layers of the tissue, which provides additional points of reference, and, consequently, the LM and EM can be correlated much more easily. Macroscopic characterization is carried out first by CLSM prior to preparation of ultrathin sections, then postcontrasting with electron-dense stains, and subsequently EM analysis. The CM method is also able to analyze multiply stained tissue. In this case measurements are made first by LM, and it is also possible to carry out subsequent electron tomography using thicker tissue sections.

7.6 FUTURE TRENDS: CORRELATIVE MICROSCOPY AND HIGH-CONTENT CELLULAR SCREENING

The models for complex biological systems in systems biology require integrated information from diverse experimental sources and CM brings here important insights. Large amounts of cellular localization data have already been obtained by high content cellular screening (HCS). HCS is an efficient drug discovery method that examines large numbers of living cells cultured in microtiter plates which are subjected to experiments aimed at cellular and molecular discovery [11]. HCS benefits from the use of spatially resolved techniques which reveal more in an individual experiment that just one single data point. HSC takes advantage of many tools of modern cell biology, including automated microscopy and robotic handling. Unlike in other areas of life sciences, in HCS the data collection is completely automated. The automated image-based screening allows the analysis of the effects of chemical compounds which modify cellular phenotypes. These are of interest for the development of novel pharmaceuticals and new discoveries in cell biology.

Currently HCS provides only crude information on how the acquired signals relate to cellular functions. The best resolution achievable in the HCS systems has only been on the order of 1 μm, which is satisfactory for coarse cellular target protein localization. The CM platform with its high resolution is well suited for advancing HCS and automated microcopy approaches. Optimized specimen preparation techniques are always a necessary complement to automation in microscopy and data collection and analysis.

Althought the described CM platform has not yet been fully implemented, academic research would be the first to profit from such a CM platform with its high resolution. It will be of high interest also for the biotechnology and pharmaceutical industries in the context of drug discovery and production of industrial enzymes and pharmaceuticals. The CM approach facilitates high-fidelity protein quantitation and thus a comparative analysis of cells and molecules of interest.

7.7 FUTURE TRENDS: CORRELATIVE MICROSCOPY OF FLUORESCENT IMAGES ACQUIRED BY CONFOCAL LASER SCANNING MICROSCOPY

The presented outline for an advanced CM platform (Figure 7.1) is compatible with many existing and emerging imaging technologies which are used in the studies addressing precise localization of proteins and protein–protein interactions with respect to their ultrastructural surroundings. In living cells, the kinetics of protein trafficking and molecular interactions are revealed with CLSM by employing various fluorescence detection methods (e.g., FRAP, FLIP, FLAP, FRET, and FLIM, as described elsewhere in this volume). The collected fluorescence signal can also be localized ultrastructurally by EM [4]. This chapter has provided an elementary repertoire of sample preparation methods in fluorescence and electron microscopies. Currently, biological studies comprise mostly genome and proteome approaches. However, an increasing motivation exists to elevate these studies to the cellular and subcellular levels and such a transition is well supported by CM. The CM utilizing fluorescent imaging of living organisms and the highest resolution electron microscopy will continue to assist in the discovery of new biological reactions in space and time with the highest possible accuracy.

The microscopy specialist attempting CM should be familiar with the challenges in sample preparation, imaging methodologies, and signal processing of micrographs. Last but not least, cutting-edge advanced microcopy expertise should be supplemented with outstanding knowledge about the specimen's biology [2].

REFERENCES

1. S. S. Biel, K. Kawaschinski, K. P. Wittern, U. Hinze, and R. Wepf, "From tissue to cellular ultrastructure: Closing the gap between micro- and nanostructural imaging," *J. Microsc.* **212**, 91–99 (2003).
2. F. Braet and K. Ratinac, "Creating next generation microscopists: Structural and molecular biology at the crossroads," *J. Cell. Mol. Med.* **11**, 1–5 (2007).
3. F. Braet, E. Wisse, P. Bomans, P. Frederik, W. Geerts, A. Koster, L. Soon, and S. Ringer, "Contribution of high-resolution correlative imaging techniques in the study of the liver sieve in three-dimensions," *Microsc. Res. Tech.* **70**, 230–242 (2007).
4. G. M. Gaietta, B. N. G. Giepmans, T. J. Deerinck, B. W. Smith, L. Ngan, J. Llopis, S. R. Adams, R. Y. Tsien, and M. H. Ellisman, "Golgi twins in late mitosis revealed by genetically encoded tags for live cell imaging and correlated electron microscopy," *PNAS* **103**, 17777–17782 (2006).
5. B. N. G. Giepmans, T. J. Deerinck, B. L. Smarr, Y. Z. Jones, and M. H. Ellisman, "Correlated light and electron microscopic imaging of multiple endogenous proteins using quantum dots," *Nature Methods* **2**, 743–749 (2005).
6. B. N. Giepmans, "The fluorescent toolbox for assessing protein location and function," *Science* **312**, 217–224 (2006).
7. J. M. Gillis and M. Wibo, "Accurate measurement of the thickness of ultrathin sections by interference microscopy," *J. Cell Biol.* **49**, 947–949 (1971).
8. M. Grabenbauer, "Correlative microscopy and electron tomography of GFP through photooxidation," *Nature Methods* **2**, 857–862 (2005).
9. S. L. Hanton and F. Brandizzi, "Fluorescent proteins as markers in the plant secretory pathway," *Microsc. Res. Tech.* **69**, 152–159 (2006).
10. K. Jahn, D. Barton, and F. Braet, "Correlative fluorescence—and scanning, transmission electron microscopy for biomolecular investigation," in *Modern Research and Educational Topics in Microscopy,* A. Mendes-Villas and M. Diaz (Eds.), Formatex, Spain, 2007, pp. 204–211.
11. P. Lang, K. Yeow, A. Nichols, and A. Scheer, "Cellular imaging in drug discovery," *Nature Rev. Drug Discov.* **5**, 343–356 (2006).

12. E. Kimura, T. Sekiguchi, H. Oikawa, J. Niitsuma, Y. Nakayama, H. Suzuki, M. Kimura, K. Fujii, and T. Ushiki, "Cathodoluminescence imaging for identifying uptaken fluorescence materials in Kupffer cells using scanning electron microscopy," *Arch. Histol. Cytol.* **67**, 263–270 (2004).
13. B. Koster and J. Klumpermann, "Electron microscopy in cell biology: Integrating structure and function," *Nature Rev. Mol. Cell Biol.* **4** (Suppl.), 6–9 (2003).
14. R. D. Leapman, "Novel techniques in electron microscopy," *Curr. Opin. Neurobiol.* **14**, 591–598 (2004).
15. K. Luby-Phelps, N. Gang, J. Fogerty, and J. C. Besharse, "Visualization of identified GFP-expressing cells by light and electron microscopy," *J. Histochem. Cytol.* **51**, 271–274 (2003).
16. D. Nakaji, V. Grillo, N. Yamamoto, and T. Mukai, "Contrast analysis of dislocation images in TEM-cathodoluminescence technique," *J. Electron Microsc. (Tokyo)* **54**, 223–230 (2005).
17. J. F. Presley, "Imaging the secretory pathway: The past and future impact of live cell optical techniques," *Biochim. Biophys. Acta* **1744**, 259–272 (2005).
18. R. Reipert, I. Fischer, and G. Wische, "High-pressure freezing of epithelial cells on the sapphire coverslips," **213**, 81–85 (2004).
19. H. Schwarz and M. B. Humbel, "Correlative light and electron microscopy using immunolabeled resin sections," *Methods Mol. Biol.* **369**, 229–256 (2007).
20. P. A. Sims and J. D. Hardin, "Fluorescence-integrated transmission electron microscopy images: Integrating fluorescence microscopy with transmission electron microscopy," *Methods Mol. Biol.* **369**, 291–308 (2007).
21. N. C. Shaner, P. A. Steinbach, and R. Y. Tsien, "A guide to choosing fluorescent proteins," *Nature Methods* **2**, 905–909 (2005).
22. J. Stephens and V. J. Allan, "Light microscopy techniques for live cell imaging," *Imag. Sci.* **300**, 82–86 (2003).
23. T. Takizawa and J. M. Robinson, "Correlative microscopy of ultrathin cryosections in placental research," *Methods Mol. Med.* **121**, 351–369 (2003).
24. B. A. Azfelius and A. B. Maunsbach, "Biological ultrastructure research; the first 50 years," *Tissue and Cell* **36**, 83–94 (2004).
25. G. Griffiths, *Fine Structure Immunocytochemistry,* 1st ed., Springer, Berlin, 1996.
26. M. A. Hayat, *Principles and Techniques of Electron Microscopy: Biological Applications,* 4th ed., Cambridge University Press, Cambridge, 2000.
27. A. B. Maunsbach and B. A. Afzelius, *Biomedical Electron Microscopy: Illustrated Methods and Interpretations,* 1st ed., Academic, New York, 1999.
28. C. Stolinski, *Freeze-Fracture Replication of Biological Tissues: Techniques, Interpretation, and Applications,* Academic, New York, 1975.

CHAPTER 8

Fluorescence Resonance Energy Transfer and Applications

ANDREW CLAYTON

Cell Biophysics Laboratory, Ludwig Institute for Cancer Research, Victoria 3050, Australia

8.1 WHAT IS FRET?

Förster (or fluorescence) resonance energy transfer (FRET)* is defined as the transfer of electronic excitation from an initially excited donor fluorophore to a proximal acceptor chromophore via a nonradiative (dark) process (see Figure 8.1). FRET has wide application in biological sciences and biotechnology for measuring structure, conformation, and associations between fluorescently tagged biological macromolecules on the length scale of 1–10 nm. This chapter will describe the technique of FRET and its applications in microscopy and spectroscopy.

8.1.1 Theory of FRET

In what follows we present the key equations of FRET that are standard in the biochemical literature. More generalized treatments using radiationless transition theory and quantum electrodynamics are beyond the scope of this chapter. The interested reader is directed to excellent recent reviews of these advanced topics.

The theory of FRET, first successfully described by Förster, treats the process as a nonradiative transfer of energy between two fluorescent molecules referred to as the donor and acceptor. A classical and relatively simple physical analogue is the behavior of coupled oscillators, such as a pair of tuning forks vibrating at the same frequency one of which can stimulate the other to vibrate and produce sound. FRET is a nonradiative phenomenon with no light energy exchanged between the two molecules. The most important features of FRET are the length scale of operation (1–10 nm) and the distance dependence of the phenomenon. According to FRET theory, the rate of energy transfer is given by the equation

$$K_{\mathrm{FRET}} = \left(\frac{1}{\tau_D}\right)\left(\frac{R_0}{R}\right)^6 \tag{8.1}$$

*Also referred to as RET (resonance energy transfer) and EET (electronic energy transfer).

Fluorescence Applications in Biotechnology and Life Sciences, Edited by Ewa M. Goldys

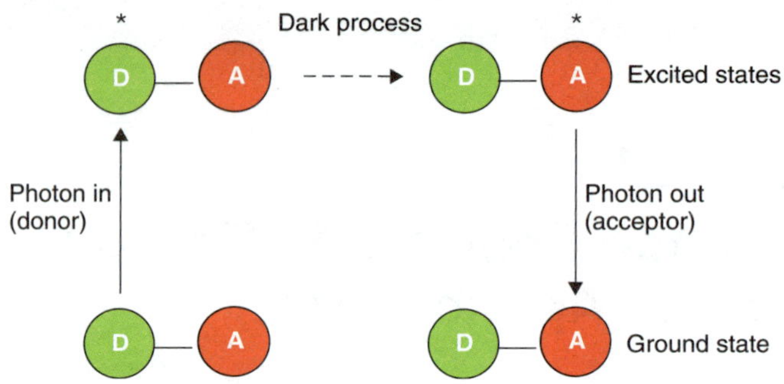

Figure 8.1 FRET between donor (D) and acceptor (A).

where R_0 is the Förster critical transfer distance (a constant for a given donor–acceptor pair), τ_D is the excited-state lifetime of the donor in the absence of acceptor (a constant for a given donor), and R is the distance separating the donor and acceptor molecules (this is a variable depending on how far away they happen to be). In practice the donor–acceptor separation R is approximated as separation between the donor–acceptor chromophores. The Förster critical transfer distance is defined as the donor–acceptor separation for which the FRET efficiency is 50% or the rate of FRET is equal to the rate of donor decay in the absence of acceptor. The Förster critical transfer distance essentially provides the length scale over which FRET can be reliably measured and, for most donor–acceptor pairs used in FRET studies, the range is between 2 and 7 nm.

The Förster critical transfer distance can be calculated for any given donor–acceptor pair and depends on their certain fluorescence properties and their relationship to one another (such as the degree of spectral overlap of donor emission and acceptor absorption spectra, the quantum yield of the donor, and the relative orientation of the donor and acceptor transition moments). Given these quantities, the magnitude of R_0 can be calculated by the expression

$$R_0 \text{ (nm)} = 0.0211\left[\kappa^2 J(\lambda) n^{-4} Q_d\right]^{1/6} \tag{8.2}$$

where $J(\lambda)$ is the overlap integral in the region of donor emission and acceptor absorption (expressed in nanometers), n is the refractive index of the medium (for water, $n = 1.333$), Q_d is the fluorescence quantum yield of the donor (range 0–1), and κ^2 is the so-called orientation factor, which describes the relative orientation between the dipoles on the donor and acceptor (range 0–4).

Of the three parameters in Eq. 8.2 the value of $J(\lambda)$ can be calculated on the basis of tabulated or directly measured fluorescence properties; the refractive index and quantum yield can also be found in resource books. The orientation factor is the most difficult to estimate precisely since its value cannot be determined in a simple way by direct measurement. Instead, workers either assume a particular value (usually $\frac{2}{3}$) or use measurements of fluorescence polarization to narrow down the range of possible orientation factors. If we make certain simplifying assumptions about the random motion of molecules, certain approximations of this factor can be obtained. In the limit that donors and acceptors rotate rapidly on the timescale of FRET, a value for κ^2 of $\frac{2}{3}$ is used (the dynamic orientation averaging limit). This value is a good approximation if the donor and acceptor can undergo significant and unrestricted rotational motion or if the acceptor chromophore has multiple polarized absorption bands in the overlap region with the donor emission. Because the orientation factor is largely an unknown, absolute measurements of distance are difficult to make with high precision. It is important to bear this in mind when designing any experiment based on FRET. It is safer to compare relative distances (using the same donor and acceptor probes) or changes in distance (from the same donor/acceptor probe). Choosing dyes that are able to rotate freely at their point of attachment or donor acceptor pairs with multiple polarized absorption transitions can narrow the uncertainty posed by the orientation factor.

On the basis of measured optical properties of the donor and acceptor the spectral overlap integral is calculated in the following manner:

1. Record the absorption spectrum of the acceptor and present the vertical axis in extinction coefficient units [$\varepsilon(\lambda)$, M^{-1} cm^{-1}] and the horizontal axis in units of wavelength (λ, nanometers). Store the $x-y$ pairs (λ, $\varepsilon(\lambda)$).
2. Record the donor emission spectrum in the absence of acceptor and normalize the area under the spectrum to be equal to unity. Store the $x-y$ pairs (λ, $F(\lambda)$)
3. Compute the overlap integral. For each λ raise it to the fifth power and then multiply by the corresponding λ, $\varepsilon(\lambda)$ and λ, $F(\lambda)$ [i.e., compute $\lambda^5\lambda\varepsilon(\lambda)F(\lambda)$]. Now compute the sum $\sum\lambda^5(\lambda)F(\lambda)$. These operations can be written into a simple computer program or even more simply they can be carried on a spreadsheet (using column multiplication followed by row summation).

The Förster critical transfer distance for various commonly used donor–acceptor pairs can be found on various websites, reviews, and publications. It is important to note that solvent, temperature, pH, ionic strength, and fluororophore–macromolecule interactions can all influence the spectral overlap integral. For these reasons it is prudent to measure the spectral overlap integral on the actual samples of interest.

8.2 WHY FRET CAN BE USEFUL

The strong distance dependence of the FRET phenomenon means that its biggest use by far in the biosciences is in measuring distances or proximity relationships between labeled sites of macromolecules or macromolecular complexes. To appreciate its use and limitations as a "spectroscopic ruler," it is useful to express the energy transfer rate in terms of energy transfer efficiency.

The efficiency of energy transfer (or quantum yield of energy transfer) is defined in the same way as any other excited-state process. The efficiency is given by the rate of energy transfer k_{FRET} divided by the sum of rates of all the processes leading to depletion of the donor excited state, $\sum k$:

$$E = \frac{k_{\text{FRET}}}{k_{\text{FRET}} + \sum k} \tag{8.3}$$

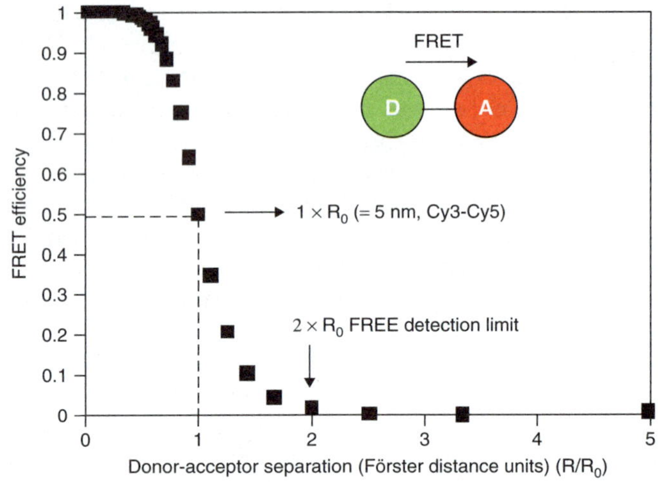

Figure 8.2 Plot of FRET efficiency as function of separation of donor and acceptor chromophores. The efficiency is represented in fraction units ($0 = 0\%$, $1 = 100\%$). The donor–acceptor separation is represented in units of Förster distance (R_0 units). For typically used donor–acceptor pairs R_0 is in the 5-nm (± 2 nm) range.

Using the definition for the lifetime of the donor $\sum k = 1/\tau_D$ and Eq. 8.1, the distance dependence of this quantity can finally be obtained as

$$E(R) = \frac{(R_0/R)^6}{(R_0/R)^6 + 1} \tag{8.4}$$

Figure 8.2 illustrates a plot of the energy transfer efficiency versus the distance as predicted from a FRET mechanism. The efficiency of transfer is greater than 90% at distances much shorter than the Förster distance (i.e., $R/R_0 < \frac{2}{3}$) and less than 10% at distances greater than 1.5 times the Förster distance and undergoes a rapid transition about the Förster distance (i.e., $R/R_0 = 1$).

The strong distance dependence in the energy transfer efficiency makes it especially useful to biologists for measuring the following:

Average distances between specifically labelled sites (with intrinsic or extrinsic probes).

Changes in proximity between donor and acceptor due to conformational changes or association/dissociation (especially sensitive near $R = R_0$).

Interactions inside cells between donor and acceptor tagged biological macromolecules. Any measurable FRET implies the two probes are less than 10 nm apart and thus the molecules are interacting.

8.3 HOW FRET CAN BE MEASURED

The occurrence of FRET perturbs the fluorescence properties of the donor molecule and the acceptor molecule. These perturbations are listed in Table 8.1 and form the basis of the methods which are employed to detect or measure FRET.

TABLE 8.1 Photophysical Consequences of FRET

Fluorescence Property	Donor Emission	Acceptor Emission	Sensitized Acceptor Emission
Quantum yield or Intensity	Decreases	Unchanged	Increases
Lifetime	Shortened	Unchanged	Lengthened
Anisotropy	Increases	Unchanged	Decreases
Photobleaching	Rate decreases	Unchanged	Either

FRET depletes the donor excited state and competes with donor excited-state deactivation processes. FRET decreases donor fluorescence quantum yield and decreases the magnitude of the donor excited-state lifetime. FRET from a donor to acceptor fluorophore populates or sensitizes the acceptor excited state. If the acceptor is fluorescent, the acceptor fluorescence will increase in the presence of FRET.

While the various effects of FRET imply the existence of multiple universal measurement strategies, in practice it is useful to separate FRET measurements according to whether they are performed in a cuvette (spectroscopy) or in the microscope.

8.3.1 Applications of FRET in Spectroscopy

Careful measurements of FRET in the cuvette can provide valuable information on the conformation and associations of appropriately labeled biological macromolecules in solution. Figure 8.3 provides a visual summary of the four main spectroscopic approaches. Brief experimental protocols and applications of the formulas are given below.

In Table 8.2 we have summarized the main measurement strategies and the appropriate formulas used to compute FRET efficiencies from spectral data.

FRET Efficiency Measured from Donor Emission Spectrum FRET decreases the fluorescence quantum yield of the donor. Instead of directly measuring the quantum yield of donor fluorescence, in practice one normally compares the magnitude of donor emission in the absence and presence of acceptor. This situation is illustrated in Figure 8.3*a*.

Requirements: Donor-conjugated sample, acceptor-conjugated sample, donor–acceptor-conjugated sample, ultraviolet–visible (UV–Vis) spectrometer, fluorometer.

- *Step 1* Make up solutions of the donor-conjugated sample and the donor–acceptor-conjugated sample to identical absorbance (<0.05) at the long-wavelength absorption maximum of the donor. There should be no acceptor absorbance at this wavelength.
- *Step 2* Measure the fluorescence spectrum of the donor-conjugated sample and the donor–acceptor-conjugated sample exciting at the donor wavelength used in step 1.
- *Step 3* Measure the fluorescence spectrum of a dilute solution of the acceptor-conjugated sample.
- *Step 4* If the donor fluorescence spectrum and the acceptor fluorescence spectrum are well separated, then choose a fluorescence wavelength of the donor

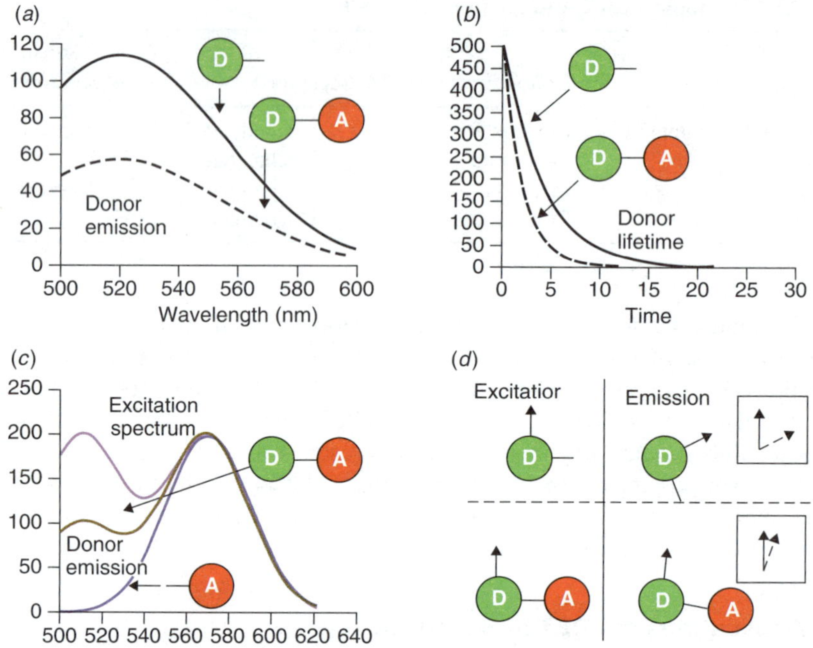

Figure 8.3 FRET measured by spectroscopy. (*a*) FRET decreases intensity of fluorescence from donor. (*b*) FRET shortens fluorescence lifetime of donor chromophore. (*c*) FRET increases amount of acceptor fluorescence that originates from donor excitation. Blue curve: acceptor excitation spectrum normalized to acceptor absorption. Purple curve: absorbance spectrum of donor–acceptor conjugate. Brown curve: acceptor fluorescence excitation spectrum of donor–acceptor conjugate. (*d*) FRET increases polarization anisotropy of fluorescence. Photoselection by polarized excitation generates a highly polarized distribution of dipoles. By molecular rotation during the excitation state lifetime the emitted light becomes depolarized. FRET shortens the time delay between photoselection and donor emission and hence decreases the amount of depolarization by rotation.

TABLE 8.2 Quantifying FRET by Spectroscopy

Fluorescence Property	Donor Measurement	Sensitized Acceptor Measurement
Quantum yield or intensity	$E_{FRET} = 1 - (I_{d-a}/I_d)$	$E_{FRET} = (I_{da}/I_d)(\epsilon_d/\epsilon_a)$
Lifetime	$E_{FRET} = 1 - (\tau_{d-a}/\tau_d)$	
Anisotropy	$E_{FRET} = (r_{da} - r_d)/(r_0 - r_d)$	Decreases

where the acceptor does not fluoresce. Read or record the intensity value of the donor-conjugated sample (I_d) and the intensity value of the donor–acceptor conjugated sample (I_{d-a}).

- *Step 5* Compute the FRET efficiency by using

$$\text{FRET efficiency} = 1 - \frac{I_{d-a}}{I_d} \tag{8.5}$$

[*Variations:* In some instances there may be considerable overlap in the emissions of the donor and acceptor. This method relies on obtaining the fluorescence contribution from the *donor only*. To obtain the *donor*, subtract a normalized (tail-matched) fluorescence spectrum of the acceptor (step 3) from the donor–acceptor conjugate fluorescence spectrum.]

FRET Efficiency Measured from Sensitized Acceptor Fluorescence FRET from an initially excited donor fluorophore to a fluorescent acceptor results in fluorescence from the acceptor. Evidence for donor absorption in the fluorescence excitation spectrum of the acceptor provides definitive proof for FRET.

Requirements: donor-conjugated sample, acceptor-conjugated sample, donor–acceptor-conjugated sample, UV–Vis spectrometer, fluorometer.

- *Step 1* Make up dilute solutions of all three conjugated samples.
- *Step 2* Measure the absorption spectra in the region of donor and acceptor absorption for all three solutions.
- *Step 3* Measure the fluorescence excitation spectra monitoring acceptor fluorescence of the acceptor conjugate solution and of the donor–acceptor conjugate solution. Measure the fluorescence excitation spectrum of the donor conjugate solution (monitoring donor fluorescence).
- *Step 4* Compare or overlay the absorption spectrum of the donor–acceptor conjugate with the fluorescence excitation spectrum of the donor–acceptor conjugate using a plotting/graphics program. If the spectra are identical in shape, this means that acceptor emission results from donor excitation and FRET is occurring and is very efficient (if the spectra overlap *exactly*, this corresponds to 100% FRET!). If the excitation spectrum of the donor–acceptor conjugate resembles the absorption spectrum of the acceptor only, then this means that donor absorption does not result in acceptor fluorescence and the FRET efficiency is low or beyond measurable detection limits. The ratio of the acceptor emission intensities at two excitation wavelengths (corresponding to donor excitation and acceptor excitation) and the ratio of donor absorbance and acceptor absorbance derived from the donor–acceptor conjugate are sufficient to compute the energy transfer efficiency.
- *Step 5* Compute the FRET efficiency in the following fashion:

$$\text{FRET efficiency} = \frac{\text{abs(acceptor wavelength)}}{\text{abs(donor wavelength)}} \times \frac{\text{acceptor intensity (exciting donor wavelength)}}{\text{acceptor intensity (excite acceptor)}} \tag{8.6}$$

FRET Efficiency Measured from Fluorescence Lifetime of Donor FRET shortens the excited-state lifetime of the donor because it provides an extra nonradiative deactivation process. Lifetime measurements require specialized instrumentation.

Requirements: donor-conjugated sample, donor–acceptor-conjugated sample, time-resolved spectrometer (frequency or time domain).

- *Step 1* Make up dilute solutions of the donor- and donor–acceptor-conjugated samples (absorbance at exciting wavelength <0.1–0.2).

- *Step 2* Choose a wavelength of excitation to selectively excite the donor and monitor donor emission. Measure the donor fluorescence lifetime of the donor-conjugated sample (τ_d) and the donor–acceptor-conjugated sample (τ_{d-a}).
- *Step 3* Compute the FRET efficiency by using

$$\text{FRET efficiency} = 1 - \frac{\tau_{d-a}}{\tau_d} \tag{8.7}$$

[*Variations:* In many instances the time-resolved fluorescence decay of the donor and/or donor–acceptor will not be described by a single lifetime component. The energy transfer efficiency can still be evaluated provided the amplitude-weighted average lifetime is used instead. For example, for a two-component decay with amplitudes a_1 and a_2 and lifetimes 1 and 2, the average lifetime is given by $\langle\tau\rangle = (a_1 < \tau_1 > +a_2 < \tau_2 >)/(a_1 + a_2)$.]

FRET Measured from Donor Fluorescence Anisotropy The steady-state fluorescence anisotropy measures the extent of angular motion (tumbling or local fluorophore motion) during the excited-state lifetime of the molecule. A decrease in the excited-state lifetime of the donor will increase the fluorescence anisotropy. For a simple model of rotation, the spherical rotator, anisotropy measurements can be used to provide an indirect measure of fluorophore lifetime (see Chapter 1).

Requirements: donor-conjugated sample, donor–acceptor-conjugated sample, fluorometer equipped with polarizers or plate reader with polarization capability.

- *Step 1* Make up dilute solutions of the donor- and donor–acceptor-conjugated samples (absorbance at exciting wavelength <0.1–0.2).
- *Step 2* Choose a wavelength of excitation to selectively excite the donor and monitor donor emission. Measure the donor fluorescence anisotropy of the donor-conjugated sample (r_d) and the donor–acceptor-conjugated sample (r_{d-a})
- *Step 3* Compute the FRET efficiency in the following fashion:

$$\text{FRET efficiency} = 1 - \frac{r_0 - r_{d-a}}{r_0 - r_d} = \frac{r_{d-a} - r_d}{r_0 - r_d} \tag{8.8}$$

where r_0 is the anisotropy of the donor in the absence of rotation (the anisotropy measured in vitrified medium), r_d is the anisotropy of the donor fluorescence from the donor-conjugated sample, and r_{d-a} is the donor fluorescence anisotropy of the donor–acceptor-conjugated sample.

8.3.2 Applications of FRET in Microscopy

FRET microscopy is a tool that enables nanoscale proximity relationships between fluorescently tagged molecules to be examined in spatial domains down to the resolution of the light microscope (≈200–300 nm). This is particularly relevant to the study of protein–protein interactions, conformation, enzyme activity, or ion concentration inside living cells or within subcellular organelles, which require resolution of a micrometer or less.

FRET measurements in the microscope face special challenges since it is difficult to control or determine solute concentrations and intensity measurements are affected by multiple instrumental and sample-dependent factors. Standard microscopes use filters to isolate fluorescence from excitation light and hence do not provide spectral shape information. For these reasons some rather elegant methods have been introduced that circumvent these issues.

Figure 8.4 diagrammatically summarizes the new FRET approaches that are particularly applicable to the microscope including representation of FRET images and histograms.

In Table 8.3, we have summarized the main measurement strategies and the appropriate formulas used to compute FRET efficiencies from microscopic data. Brief experimental protocols and applications of the formulas are given below.

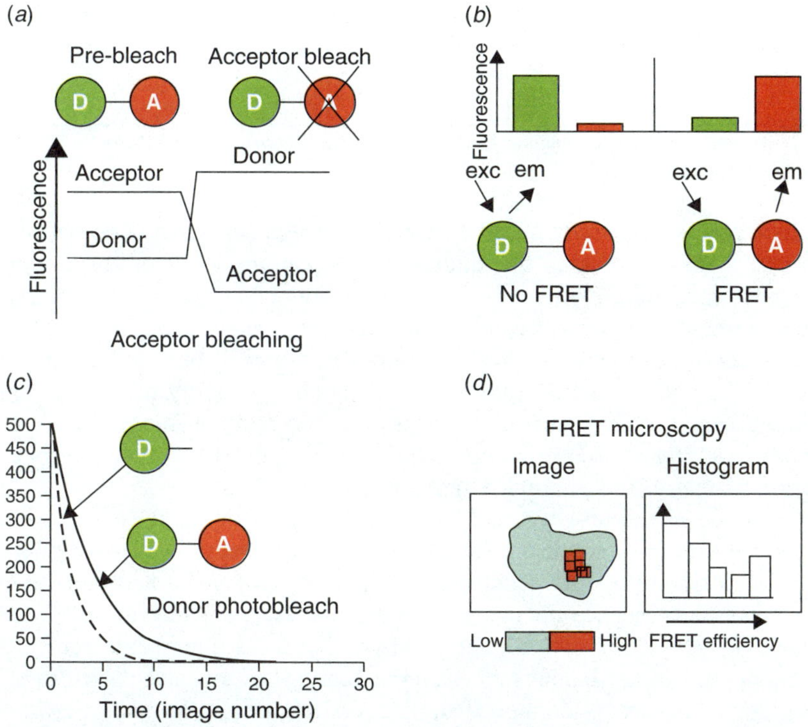

Figure 8.4 FRET measured by microscopy. (*a*) FRET from donor to acceptor decreases the intensity of fluorescence from the donor. The acceptor photobleaching method measures the increase in donor fluorescence by photochemically destroying the acceptor in a donor–acceptor pair. The prebleach donor and acceptor fluorescences are first measured, then the acceptor is bleached until it no longer fluoresces. The donor fluorescence after acceptor bleaching is then remeasured. (*b*) FRET increases the amount of acceptor fluorescence that originates from donor excitation and decreases the directly excited donor fluorescence. In the microscope normally donor and acceptor emission filters are used and the two intensity values upon donor excitation are compared (ratiometric or filter-cubed FRET). (*c*) Repetitive or continuous illumination results in fading or photobleaching of the donor chromophore. FRET from donor to acceptor lengthens the photobleaching time of the donor chromophore. (*d*) In FRET microscopy the FRET efficiency can be imaged as a function of position (e.g., in a cell) or can be represented as a frequency histogram.

TABLE 8.3 Quantifying FRET by Microscopy

Fluorescence Property	Method	Samples Required	Measurements	Energy Transfer Expression
Donor or intensity	Acceptor photobleaching	Donor + acceptor, donor, acceptor	Donor intensity before and after bleaching, acceptor	$E_{FRET} = 1 - I^{PRE}/I^{POST}$
Sensitized emission from acceptor	FRET-cubed method	Donor, acceptor, donor + acceptor	Seven different intensity measurements	$E_{APP} = [F^{DA}(i) - F^{D}(i)R_D - F^{A}(i)R_E]/F^{A}(i)$
Donor photo-bleaching	pbFRET	Donor, donor + acceptor	Photobleaching, anisotropy	$E_{FRET} = 1 - k_{d-a}/k_d$
Anisotropy	heteroFRET	Donor, donor + acceptor	Donor, anisotropy	$E_{FRET} = (r_{da} - r_d)/(r_0 - r_d)$
Lifetime	FLIM, FLI	Donor, donor + acceptor	Image, donor fluorescence lifetimes	$E_{FRET} = 1 - \tau_{d-a}/\tau_d$

Note: FLI, fluorescence lifetime imaging; FLIM, fluorescence lifetime imaging microscopy.

FRET Efficiency Measured from Donor Emission with Acceptor Photobleaching FRET decreases the fluorescence quantum yield of the donor. In the acceptor photobleaching method the intensity of donor fluorescence is measured from cells containing the donor–acceptor-conjugated molecules. Then the acceptor chromophore is continuously and selectively illuminated until it becomes completely photobleached. The photobleached acceptor cannot act as an energy transfer acceptor. The donor fluorescence is then remeasured again and the relative fluorescence before and after photobleaching is used to compute the energy transfer efficiency. This is an elegant method because the photobleached acceptor provides the required reference for the donor signal in the absence of FRET. Control measurements with acceptor-only and donor-only samples are also necessary to correct for any inadvertent photobleaching of the donor and possible occurrence of spectral spillage of acceptor fluorescence into the donor fluorescence channels. This method is applicable to any fluorescence microscope. It works best with a photostable donor and a photolabile acceptor.

Requirements: donor-conjugated sample (control), acceptor-conjugated sample (control), donor–acceptor-conjugated sample, confocal or wide-field microscope with excitation source and detector.

- *Step 1* Measure the donor emission from the donor–acceptor-conjugated sample. Store the image (=donor image prebleach, I^{pre}).
- *Step 2* Choose a laser wavelength or excitation filter to selectively excite the acceptor. Measure the acceptor fluorescence from the donor–acceptor sample. Then continuously illuminate the acceptor.
- *Step 3* Remeasure the acceptor fluorescence. If not equivalent to background levels, repeat Step 2. If equivalent to background levels, move to Step 4.
- *Step 4* Change the laser or filter set to selectively excite the donor. Remeasure the donor emission from the donor–acceptor-conjugated sample. Store the image (=donor image postbleach, I^{post}).

- *Step 5* Repeat steps 2–4 using identical conditions as the donor–acceptor-conjugated sample for the donor-conjugated control. The ratio ($= (I_D^{\text{post}}/I_D^{\text{pre}})$) between the postbleach (I_D^{post}) and prebleach donor-only (I_D^{pre}) conjugated sample corrects for any inadvertent bleaching of the donor that occurs at the acceptor excitation wavelength.
- *Step 6* Compute the energy transfer efficiency as

$$E_{\text{FRET}} = 1 - \left(\frac{I^{\text{pre}}}{I^{\text{post}}}\right)\left(\frac{I_D^{\text{post}}}{I_D^{\text{pre}}}\right) \tag{8.9}$$

[*Variations:* (a) Instead of bleaching the whole area in the field of view, it is useful to select a small region of interest to bleach. The area outside the bleach region provides an internal standard. (b) Instead of completely bleaching the acceptor, it is possible to partially bleach the acceptor and monitor the donor emission as a function of gradual bleaching of the acceptor. The energy transfer efficiency can be obtained by extrapolation to complete acceptor bleaching.].

FRET Efficiency Measured from Sensitized Acceptor Fluorescence FRET from an initially excited donor fluorophore to a fluorescent acceptor results in fluorescence from the acceptor. Evidence for donor absorption in the fluorescence excitation spectrum of the acceptor provides definitive proof for FRET. In commercially available microscopes it is not possible to directly record excitation and absorption spectra. Instead, measurements using a combination of excitation and detection filters are performed to extract the sensitized acceptor fluorescence. Donor excitation/donor detection, donor excitation/acceptor detection, and acceptor excitation/acceptor detection are the filter combinations. Donor-only and acceptor-only samples are required to provide spectral spillage correction factors. The correction factors and controls are critical and require carefully matched samples in terms of signal intensity.

These measurements can be automated and provide rapid readout suitable for live cell studies. In the authors' opinion these intensity-based measurements are best used with intramolecular FRET samples where the donor and acceptor are attached to a single macromolecular chain (fixed stoichiometry). Changes in the FRET can be ascertained as a simple intensity readout.

- *Step 1* The first correction factor is to determine the relative detection efficiencies of the donor emission through the donor and acceptor filter sets. Image a sample containing donor-only molecules. Take an image using a donor excitation and acceptor detection filter set. Store the image. Take an image using donor excitation and donor detection. Store the image. Divide the total image intensity using acceptor detection by the total image intensity using donor detection. Store this value as R_D.
- *Step 2* The second correction factor involves determining the relative extinction of the acceptor when excited at the acceptor and donor wavelengths. Image a sample containing acceptor-only molecules. Excite the sample with a donor excitation/acceptor detection filter combination, then store the image. Repeat with an acceptor excitation/acceptor detection filter combination and store the image. Divide the total acceptor intensity obtained by donor excitation by the total acceptor intensity by acceptor excitation. Store this value as R_E.

- *Step 3* Take images of the donor–acceptor sample. Image the acceptor emission upon acceptor excitation $F^{\mathrm{A}}(i)$, the donor fluorescence upon donor excitation $F^{\mathrm{D}}(i)$, and the acceptor emission upon donor excitation $F^{\mathrm{DA}}(i)$ at each pixel location i of an image.
- *Step 5* Compute the *apparent* FRET efficiency as follows:

$$\text{FRET efficiency} = \frac{F^{\mathrm{DA}}(i) - F^{\mathrm{D}}(i)R_D - F^{\mathrm{A}}(i)R_E}{F^{\mathrm{A}}(i)} \tag{8.10}$$

FRET Efficiency Measured from Donor Photobleaching Photobleaching is a photochemical process that occurs in the excited state and leads to destruction of the chromophore. An example is the gradual fading that one sees if a colored garment is left out in the sun for long periods. The rate of bleaching depends on environmental conditions (oxygen concentration), the intensity of the exciting light, and the lifetime of the excited state. All other things being equal, the longer a fluorophore remains in the excited state, the greater the chance that the fluorophore is bleached. Conversely, if the excited state is depleted by a process like FRET, then photobleaching is harder to achieve and it requires longer exposures to light to achieve the same level of photobleaching. The donor photobleaching method relies on this proportionality relationship between the fluorescence lifetime and the rate of photobleaching. It is a simple method that can be used on any microscope with a detector. It works best with a photolabile donor and a photostable acceptor.

- *Step 1* Selectively excite the donor-conjugated sample in the absorption region of the donor and measure or scan an image of the donor fluorescence. Store or record the image.
- *Step 2* Repeat Step 1 until emission is at background levels. *Hint*: Select the time lapse mode in a confocal microscope or repeat image acquisition on a wide-field microscope with the lamp left on. Save the time lapse images.
- *Step 3* Repeat steps 1 and 2 with the donor–acceptor-conjugated sample.
- *Step 4* Select a region of interest on the donor cells and donor–acceptor cells and plot the intensity versus time for the two data sets. Fit the data to an exponential function or sum of exponentials. Compute the mean photobleaching rate of the donor and the donor with acceptor.
- *Step 5* Compute the FRET efficiency as

$$\mathrm{E}_{\mathrm{FRET}} = 1 - \frac{k_{d-a}}{k_d} \tag{8.11}$$

[*Variations: Revised Step 4:* An alternative to exponential fitting is to rely on the observation (by Hirshfeld, see [1]) that the area under a photobleaching curve is a constant for a given fluorophore. The image of an unbleached donor divided by the sum of the images of the donor during complete photobleaching is a measure of the relative quantum yield of the donor. If the same analysis is carried out for the donor–acceptor-conjugated sample, then the FRET efficiency can be calculated as

$$E_{\mathrm{FRET}} = 1 - \left(\frac{I(1)_{d-a}}{I(1)_d}\right)\frac{\Sigma I_d}{\Sigma I_{d-a}} \tag{8.12}$$

where $I(1)_{d-a}$ and $I(1)_d$ are the prebleach mean intensities of the donor–acceptor and donor conjugates and ΣI_d and ΣI_{d-a} are the summed mean intensities of the time lapse images during photobleaching from first to last for the donor-conjugated sample and the donor–acceptor conjugate. This method is computationally efficient and simple.]

FRET Measured from Donor Fluorescence Anisotropy The steady-state fluorescence anisotropy measures the extent of angular motion (tumbling or local fluorophore motion) during the excited-state lifetime of the molecule. A decrease in the excited-state lifetime of the donor will increase the fluorescence anisotropy since the molecule has effectively "run out of light" before it has a chance to rotate appreciably. For a simple model of motion, the spherical rotator, anisotropy measurements can be used to provide an indirect measure of fluorophore lifetime.

Requirements: donor-conjugated sample, donor–acceptor-conjugated sample, microscope equipped with polarizers.

- *Step 1* Choose a wavelength of excitation (laser excitation) or filter set [lamp or light-emitting diode (LED) excitation] to selectively excite the donor and monitor donor emission. Measure the donor fluorescence anisotropy of the donor-conjugated sample (r_d) and the donor–acceptor-conjugated sample (r_{d-a})
- *Step 2* Compute the FRET efficiency as

$$\text{FRET efficiency} = 1 - \frac{r_0 - r_{d-a}}{r_0 - r_d} = \frac{r_{d-a} - r_d}{r_0 - r_d} \quad (8.13)$$

Where r_0 is the anisotropy of the donor in the absence of rotation (the anisotropy measured in vitrified medium), r_d is the anisotropy of the donor fluorescence from the donor-conjugated sample, and r_{d-a} is the donor fluorescence anisotropy of the donor–acceptor-conjugated sample.

8.4 EMERGING APPLICATIONS INCLUDING NOVEL FRET PROBES

In discussing applications of FRET to the biosciences it is useful to distinguish two idealized types of FRET experiment, intramolecular FRET and intermolecular FRET.

8.4.1 Intramolecular FRET

In this type of FRET donor and acceptor fluorophores are attached to two different regions on a single monomeric biomacromolecular chain. Changes in the separation of the two probes can be conveniently inferred by measuring the change in donor and/or acceptor intensities.

Intramolecular FRET has been used in the development of assays to measure ion concentration, enzyme activity, and phosphorylation reactions and to study folding of biological macromolecules (Figure 8.5).

In assays designed to measure protease activity, the biosensor consists of a FRET donor and a FRET acceptor linked via an amino acid sequence that contains the recognition and cleavage site of the protease (Figure 8.5*a*). When no enzyme is present, the donor–linker–acceptor biosensor is intact and FRET occurs from the donor to

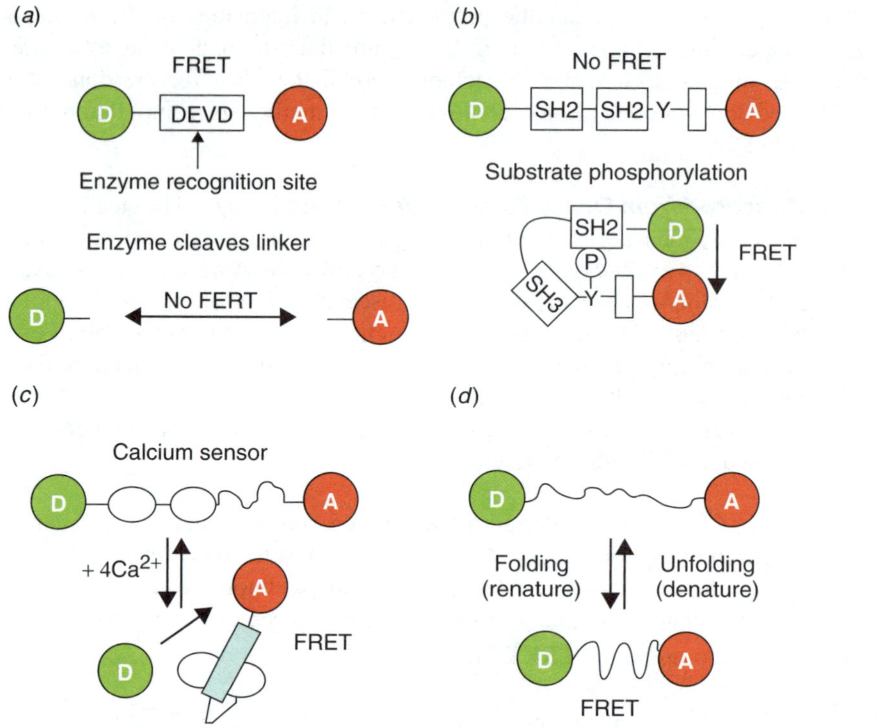

Figure 8.5 Intramolecular FRET biosensors: (*a*) enzyme activity; (*b*) phosphorylation; (*c*) calcium sensor; (*d*) macromolecular folding/unfolding.

the acceptor. When enzyme is present, it cleaves the linker holding the donor and acceptor at close proximity and the donor and acceptor diffuse apart. The onset of enzyme activity is measured by a decrease in the FRET between the donor and acceptor.

Phosphorylation/dephosphorylation is a key chemical modification in the signal transduction processes of proteins in living cells. An intramolecular FRET sensor has been designed that is based on a change in donor–acceptor distance upon phosphorylation of a specific tyrosine within a donor–Sh2–Sh3–Y–Sh3–acceptor system. In the tyrosine phosphorylated form the Sh2 module binds to the phosphotyrosine and causes a conformational change that brings the donor and acceptor moities closer together. In this example the increase in FRET indicates that the tyrosine residue has been phosphorylated by its target kinase (Figure 8.5*b*).

Calcium sensors based on intramolecular FRET have employed the calcium-binding protein, calmodulin, as their substrate. When calmodulin binds four calcium ions, it undergoes a large conformational change that brings the N- and C-termini into FRET proximity (Figure 8.5*c*).

A significant problem in biochemistry and biophysics is an understanding of the folding of proteins, DNA, and RNA. FRET-based assays that take advantage of the different donor–acceptor distances in the folded compared to the unfolded state are finding widespread use in characterizing the thermodynamics, kinetics, and single-molecule behavior of the folding process (Figure 8.5*d*).

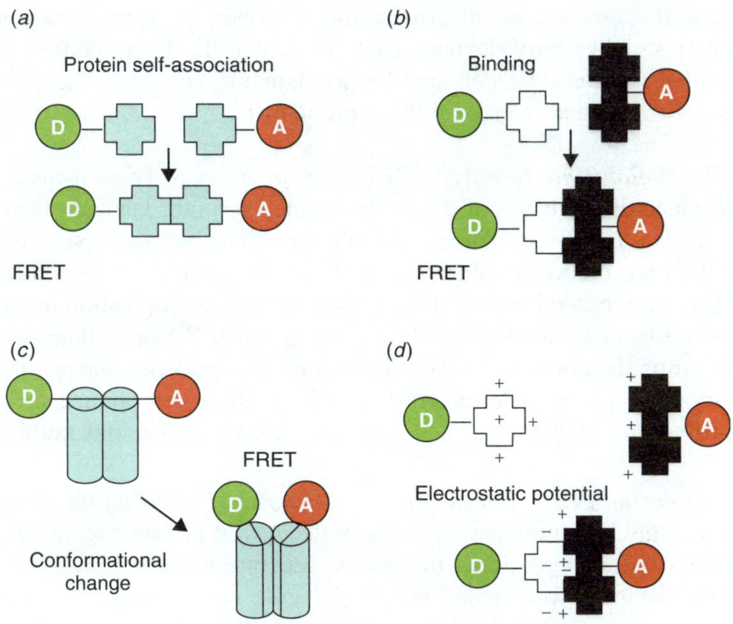

Figure 8.6 Intermolecular FRET biosensors: (*a*) self-association; (*b*) binding; (*c*) conformational change within macromolecular complex; (*d*) Electrostatic potential.

8.4.2 Intermolecular FRET

In this configuration donor and acceptor fluorophores are attached to separate biomacromolecules (Figure 8.6).

A major feature of biochemical reactions and intracellular pathways is the noncovalent association or binding between two (or more) biological macromolecules. When such macromolecules are attached to appropriate fluorophores acting as donors and acceptors, the binding interactions between them can be studied by FRET. FRET occurs in the bound complex when the donor and acceptor are in nanoscale proximity but not when the two binding partners are unbound and separated by distances outside the FRET range. In the test tube, FRET-based binding assays can also be used to obtain quantitative information about the thermodynamics and kinetics of the binding interaction. In the cell, FRET microscopy can be used to detect for the presence and spatial location of the binding interaction. High-throughput FRET assays can also be devised to conduct screens for inhibitors. When the molecules in question are identical, then FRET provides a measure of the self-association, dimerization, or more generally oligomerization of the molecule. FRET can also be used to examine conformational changes within a macromolecular complex. FRET between judiciously placed donor and acceptor tags can reveal conformational changes that are important to biological function.

8.5 ADVANCED FRET METHODS

The measurement of a FRET efficiency can be used to obtain an average donor–acceptor distance provided there is a single donor and a single acceptor in the

FRET process. If there is a broad distribution of donor–acceptor distances or if the donor–acceptor stoichiometry deviates from 1 : 1, then the interpretation of FRET in terms of detailed structural models can be problematic. However, there are methods "for experts only" that can overcome these problems:

1. *High-Resolution Time-Resolved FRET Measurements* These measurements can determine distance distributions of donor–molecule–acceptor labeled macromolecules in solution. For a unique or narrow distribution of donor–acceptor distances the time-resolved decay of donor fluorescence should be a single exponential function. However, if in the ensemble the macromolecule has a population distribution of donor–acceptor distances, then this will give rise to a distribution of donor excited-state lifetimes. By fitting the time-resolved decay of donor fluorescence, the parameters of the distance distribution can be determined. Examples include determining the end-to-end distance distributions of peptides, DNA, RNA, carbohydrates, and multimeric complexes.

2. *Single-Molecule FRET Measurements* Instead of inferring the distance distribution from a single measurement on many molecules, it is now becoming possible to measure FRET from a single donor to a single acceptor and determine the population distribution of distances from many single-molecule measurements. Single-molecule techniques require no synchronization of the population. This is especially important for complex macromolecules and living biological systems where it is difficult to synchronize conformations and biological states. Single-molecule measurements can detect rare events that would otherwise be lost or averaged out in an ensemble measurement. Moreover, dynamic information can be obtained, for example, the average time it takes to switch between two conformational states. Single-molecule measurements require specialized instrumentation and software.

3. *Determining Stoichiometry of FRET Interactions* The occurrence of intermolecular FRET between donor-labeled macromolecule and a separately labeled acceptor–macromolecule is often interpreted as due to a 1 : 1 interaction, in other words, due to formation of a hetero- or homodimer. Measurements of the FRET signal at varying ratios of donor-labeled and acceptor-labeled macromolecule can be analyzed in terms of simple oligomeric forms—dimer, trimers, tetramers, or high-order species. An understanding of stoichiometry is particularly important when interpreting changes in FRET from multimeric complexes. A change in FRET could result from a conformational change at constant stoichiometry or to association–dissociation of the complex or both.

REFERENCES

1. E. A. Jares-Erijman and T. M. Jovin, "FRET imaging," *Nat. Biotechnol.* **21**(11), 1387–1395 (2003).
2. G. D. Scholes, "Long-range resonance energy transfer in molecular systems," *Annu. Rev. Phys. Chem.* **54**, 57–87 (2003).

3. G. Bunt G and F. S. Wouters, "Visualization of molecular activities inside living cells with fluorescent labels," *Int. Rev. Cytol.* **237**, 205–277 (2004).
4. M. Sugawa, Y. Arai, A. H. Iwane, Y. Ishii, and T. Yanagida, "Single molecule FRET for the study on structural dynamics of biomolecules," *Biosystems*, **88**(3), 243–250 (2006).
5. P. Wu and L. Brand, "Resonance energy transfer: Methods and applications," *Anal. Biochem.* **218**(1), 1–13 (1994).

CHAPTER 9

Monitoring Molecular Dynamics in Live Cells Using Fluorescence Photobleaching

NECTARIOS KLONIS and LEANN TILLEY
Department of Biochemistry, La Trobe University, Melbourne, Victoria 3086, Australia

9.1 INTRODUCTION

Photobleaching is the irreversible loss of fluorescence from a sample exposed to light. It is the reason fluorescent dyes (either as solids or in solution) and samples used for fluorescence microscopy need to be protected from exposure to light unless they are in the process of being measured or imaged. In cuvette-based measurements the fluorescence intensity of the photobleached sample can often be partially restored by simply mixing the contents of the cuvette. This is because only a small proportion of the total cuvette contents are in the light path and hence subject to illumination, and thus mixing the contents replenishes the unbleached molecules in the illuminated area. Unlike the situation in a cuvette, the fluorescent molecules in fixed samples used for immunofluorescence microscopy are immobile whereas those present in live cell samples are typically confined to a small organelle or structure. Thus, when subjected to Kohler illumination in an epifluorescence microscope (which evenly illuminates the whole field of view), the same fluorescent molecules are continuously illuminated and there is no opportunity for "fresh" unbleached molecules to replenish the bleached molecules. Thus photobleaching or fluorescence fading is often a serious problem in fluorescence microscopy and a range of measures are usually employed to limit the degree of bleaching. However, the ability to selectively bleach some molecules in a sample provides the basis for a number of photobleaching techniques that are widely employed in microscopy and can provide a great deal of information about molecular and cellular dynamics.

Photobleaching methods are increasingly being utilized in cell biology to investigate many aspects of macromolecular and cellular dynamics in live cell preparations. This is due to two major technological advances, the first being the development of green fluorescent protein (GFP) fusion technology which has permitted fluorescently tagged proteins to be targeted to various intracellular compartments and to be studied in an almost native state in the living cell. Major progress has also been made in the "user friendliness" of commercial confocal microscopes with software that makes it possible

Fluorescence Applications in Biotechnology and Life Sciences, Edited by Ewa M. Goldys

to design photobleaching measurements much more easily. Together, these technologies help to obtain significantly more information from a cell expressing a GFP fusion protein than just its location and relative intensity within a particular compartment.

This chapter describes the theoretical basis for performing photobleaching measurements using a laser scanning confocal microscope. We begin with a quick description of the photobleaching process and explain how photobleaching permits the determination of molecular dynamics. This is followed by a discussion of the basic principles of confocal microscopy and the components of confocal microscopes that can be manipulated to perform a photobleaching measurement. Finally, a number of examples are provided to illustrate the type of information that can be obtained using such approaches. This chapter is aimed at the beginner, and it is designed to be descriptive with the mathematics kept to a minimum.

9.2 PHOTOBLEACHING THEORY

At room temperature, essentially all the molecules are present in the ground state. Upon illumination with light of an appropriate energy/wavelength, an electron can jump to a high vibrational level of the first excited state, a process that typically takes about 10^{-15} s. The molecule rapidly ($\sim 10^{-12}$ s) relaxes to the lowest vibrational energy level of the excited state in a process known as internal conversion. The now-excited molecule can persist in this state for a period on the order of nanoseconds (10^{-9} s) before it relaxes back to its ground state. The excess energy in the transition from the excited to the ground state can be released via radiative or nonradiative means—the former case results in the emission of fluorescence which has a lower energy (longer wavelength) compared to the excitation light. The time that the molecule spends in the excited state is relatively long on the atomic/molecular timescale. During this time other interactions and processes may take place that form the basis for a number of fluorescence techniques, including polarity sensing (solvent relaxation), assessment of molecular mobility (anisotropy), fluorescence quenching, and resonance energy transfer.

Only a small proportion of the total population of fluorophores is excited by the relatively low light intensities typically used in fluorescence measurements. The individual molecules can undergo consecutive excitation/emission cycles since they are effectively regenerated in the ground state following emission. Indeed, in the simplest case the fluorescence intensity should be proportional to the light intensity because increasing the light intensity increases the population of excited molecules. In addition, illumination of molecules with a constant light intensity might be expected to produce a constant "steady-state" fluorescence emission. While this is generally true at low illumination levels and at short illumination times, this breaks down at high illumination levels or even at low illumination levels continued for a long time. This gradual loss of fluorescence is termed *photobleaching*.

Photobleaching is a consequence of the generally increased reactivity of molecules in the excited state. In the excited state, molecules can undergo chemical reactions or rearrangements which produce a new chemical entity that is no longer fluorescent (the photobleached species). However, the time a typical fluorophore spends in the excited state (about 1 ns) means that most of the excited molecules do not have sufficient time to produce the nonfluorescent species before they return to the ground state. But some of them do, and once they have reacted, they are removed from the pool of the fluorescent molecules. The remaining fluorescent molecules continue cycling between the ground and excited states and they continue to be vulnerable to the same excited-state reactions, which will eventually take away their ability to fluoresce. The net result is a reduction in the concentration of unbleached molecules and hence a reduction in the steady-state fluorescence intensity. In the end all fluorescent molecules will bleach—it is simply a question of how many excitation/emission cycles they undergo before photobleaching. Thus, the rate/extent of bleaching can be increased by increasing the illumination intensity or by increasing the duration of the illumination. It is important to appreciate that photobleaching is the consequence of a photochemical reaction and that the products of such reactions (including free-radical species) may perturb the system being investigated. This is particularly so for live cell imaging where prolonged illumination and bleaching might lead to cell damage or even death. It is therefore prudent to minimize illumination intensity and duration in such applications. Similarly, even where photobleaching is the desired result, it is prudent to only illuminate for the minimum time required and to be aware there is always the possibility that the bleaching event itself might affect the cell.

9.3 DYNAMICS OF MACROMOLECULES

9.3.1 Macromolecular Mobilities

Photobleaching measurements can provide information on the rates of movement of macromolecules. Even if this is not the question that is being addressed in a particular measurement, a qualitative understanding of macromolecular dynamics is required in order to properly design a measurement and to interpret the results.

The biomolecules in a living cell (with relatively few exceptions) do not occupy fixed positions and usually undergo some Brownian motion. The molecules undergo random translational (sideways) and rotational (tumbling) movements. Photobleaching experiments provide information of the lateral movements while tumbling can be measured using other techniques such as fluorescence anisotropy, not discussed here. A small biomolecule such as a protein in solution exhibits isotropic diffusion (i.e., its motion is similar in all three dimensions; Figure 9.1*a*). Its rate of translational movement is described by its translational diffusion coefficient (D_t), which has units of

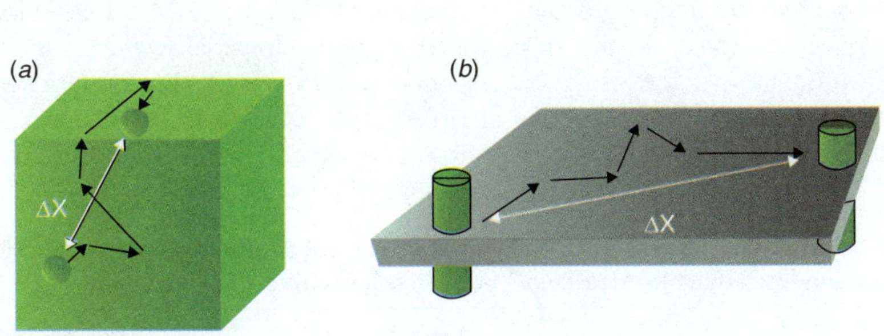

Figure 9.1 Translational diffusion of a macromolecule in (*a*) solution and (*b*) a membrane. The black arrows represent the position of a soluble molecule (sphere, *a*) or a membrane-embedded molecule (cylinder, *b*) at different times. The diffusion of the sphere is isotropic (uniform) in three dimensions, whereas that of the cylinder is isotropic only in two dimensions in the plane of the membrane. In both cases, a measure of mobility is given by the translational diffusion coefficient, which is the mean-square displacement over time ($\Delta x^2/4\ \Delta t$) and depends on the size of the diffusing species and the viscocity of the medium.

micrometers squared per second and can be thought of as the typical cross-sectional area a molecule will visit in its random motion per unit time. The magnitude of D_t is influenced by a number of factors, including the viscosity of the medium, but most critical from our point of view is its dependence on size: For a spherical molecule, D_t is inversely proportional to the radius (r). For a nonspherical molecule, the precise value of D_t is a more complex function of both the shape and size of the molecule. However, the general relationship holds whereby large molecules exhibit slower diffusion than smaller molecules.

For molecules located in a membrane translational diffusion out of the plane of the membrane is prevented because the hydrophobic regions of these molecules need to remain associated with the acyl chain region of the membrane bilayer. Thus the translational diffusion of phospholipids and membrane proteins is limited to lateral motions in the plane of the membrane which is largely isotropic (uniform) in two dimensions. For example, transmembrane proteins can be considered as cylinders embedded within the viscous medium of the membrane that are capable of diffusing in the plane of the membrane (Figure 9.1*b*). The general relationship between the D_t value for a transmembrane protein and its size still holds, so that larger membrane proteins exhibit smaller values of D_t. However, D_t is much less sensitive to size compared to soluble molecules (which are able to move freely in space) so that much larger changes in size are required to produce equivalent changes in D_t.

The diffusion coefficients of a number of biological molecules are summarized in Table 9.1. In order to get a feeling for what these numbers represent, we will now consider these D_t values in the context of a spherical cell with a diameter of 10 μm. These dimensions are similar to those of a typical mammalian cell nucleus or a red blood cell, both of which are discussed later. Small solutes and typically sized soluble monomeric proteins can diffuse freely within the internal volume of this simple cell. Within a time period of 1 s, an individual molecule will move fast enough to sample the whole-cell volume. In contrast, the movement of phospholipids and membrane proteins is restricted to the surface of the cell. Such molecules are expected to diffuse about 100-fold more slowly due to the increased viscosity of the membrane and will sample only ~0.1% of the total membrane surface area on a 1 s timescale. In practice, phospholipids, glycophosphatidylinositol (GPI)–linked proteins, and transmembrane proteins that are associated with the internal membranes of cells display close to the diffusion rates predicted on the basis of their dimensions. However, many integral membrane proteins, particularly those associated with the plasma membrane, diffuse much more slowly than predicted and are effectively motionless on a timescale of 1 s. This is due to interactions with other proteins or cellular elements or to steric restrictions

TABLE 9.1 Diffusion Coefficients of Typical Biological Macromolecules and Their Expected Recovery Times in Idealized Spot Photobleaching Measurement

Solute	D (μm²/s)	Recovery Time ($\tau_{1/2}$)[a]
Protein in solution	10–100	0.1 ms
Phospholipid in membrane	0.1–1	1 s
Protein in membrane		
Theoretical	0.1–1	1 s
Measured	0.01–0.1	5 min

[a]Assuming an instantaneous spot bleach with a Gaussian radius of ≈1 μm (see text).

on mobility imposed by the underlying cytoskeleton. Some membrane proteins exhibit no lateral movement on much larger timescales approaching minutes. This is believed to reflect very tight interactions with the underlying cytoskeleton.

9.3.2 Fluorescence Recovery After Photobleaching

Fluorence recovery after photobleaching (FRAP) was developed to measure the dynamics of fluorescently labeled membrane-associated proteins. The general design of a FRAP experiment is shown in Figure 9.2. The fluorescence intensity within a small region of the membrane is monitored using a low-intensity beam that causes little bleaching. A short pulse of high-intensity laser light is then used to bleach molecules within the illuminated region. This results in a decrease in intensity when the region is assessed again with low-intensity illumination. As bleached molecules diffuse out of the illuminated area and unbleached molecules diffuse into the area, the fluorescence is observed to increase or recover over time. Since the recovery of fluorescence is a direct result of the lateral movement of the fluorescently labeled molecules, an analysis of the kinetics of fluorescence recovery can provide the diffusion coefficient of the molecule and thus its molecular dimensions.

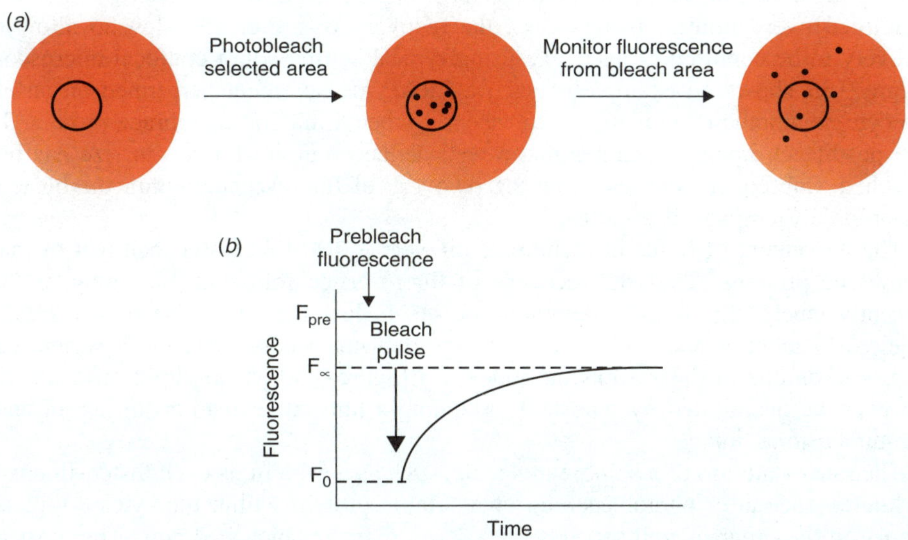

Figure 9.2 Design of "classical" FRAP experiment to measure the dynamics of membrane-embedded protein. (*a*) Surface view of fluorescently labeled protein molecules (yellow dots) within a membrane (red). The fluorophores attached to the molecules within the illuminated region (black circle) are bleached by high-intensity illumination and become nonfluorescent (black dots). Over time, these molecules diffuse out of the illuminated area while unbleached molecules diffuse in. (*b*) Changes in fluorescence intensity within bleached region during FRAP measurement. The illumination level is kept low during the monitoring phases to limit bleaching so that a constant prebleach fluorescence (F_{pre}) is observed. The fluorescence decreases to F_0 immediately after the bleach event and recovers to a value of F_∞ over time. In this example, the postbleach fluorescence does not reach the prebleach fluorescence due to the presence of an immobile population (see text). The proportion of the population which is immobile can be calculated as $(F_\infty - F_o)/(F_{pre} - F_o)$.

In practice, the recovery kinetics are also dependent on other instrumental/experimental factors, such as the size of the area bleached, the precise geometric relationship between the bleaching beam and the region bleached, and indeed the degree of bleaching. Thus relating the diffusion time to the molecular size of the integral membrane protein can be complex. It also means that care has to be taken when comparing the recovery kinetics of different samples. In order to keep things simple, for the purpose of this review we will use the half-time of recovery ($\tau_{1/2}$) as an empirical measure of the recovery kinetics. The value of $\tau_{1/2}$ is inversely proportional to the value of D_t if the conditions of measurement are kept the same (e.g., a similar sized area is bleached in a similar region of the cell).

The intensity profile of the laser beam that is used to illuminate or bleach a specimen is typically described by a Gaussian distribution (i.e., the intensity is brightest at the center of the beam and decays with distance from the center). For a Gaussian beam of radius ω impinging on a flat surface, the following relationship holds: $\tau_{1/2} \propto \omega^2/4D_t$. Table 9.1 illustrates typical recovery times for various biomolecules assuming a 1 μm bleach spot. An appreciation of the likely magnitude of the recovery time is important in the design of an experiment and in the interpretation of the results. Ideally, the bleach time should be much shorter than $\tau_{1/2}$ and the kinetics should be monitored over times much longer than $\tau_{1/2}$. In the case of a plasma membrane protein, bleach times can be on the order of hundreds of milliseconds and the recovery should be monitored over minutes. In this case, the recovery is sufficiently slow to allow the recovery to be captured as an image using typical settings on a confocal microscope. Figure 9.3*a* shows an example of such a FRAP measurement performed on an erythrocyte membrane containing a fluorescently labeled integral membrane protein. The first postbleach image illustrates that a well-defined region of 1 μm in size has been bleached. Subsequent images show the recovery of fluorescence within the bleached region on a timescale of minutes.

The movement of lipids in membrane bilayers is 100-fold faster than that of many membrane proteins. Thus the recovery of fluorescence following bleaching of fluorescently labeled lipids in a membrane occurs in less than 1 s. The time resolution required to monitor such a fast recovery is often not accessible using a typical confocal microscope in the *xy* imaging mode. As Figure 9.3*b* shows, lipid diffusion can, however, be quantitated by repeatedly scanning a line rather than acquiring an entire two-dimensional image.

The rate of motion of a soluble molecule, such as a protein, is even faster. Recovery of fluorescence after photobleaching of a soluble protein within the cytosol typically occurs on the order of milliseconds for a 1 μm diameter bleached area. The measurements of such fast processes are not feasible using most confocal microscopes since they require submillisecond bleach times and millisecond time resolution. Figure 9.3*c* shows the fluorescence profile obtained upon application of a bleach pulse to an erythrocyte containing a fluorescent protein. Bleaching is observed, but there is no defined bleach spot in the illuminated region (indicated by the arrow). Instead, there is even bleaching throughout the entire cytoplasm of the cell. This is because a significant fraction of the total population of labeled proteins pass through the beam path during the 20-ms bleach time and are bleached. The bleached and the unbleached molecules are evenly distributed throughout the entire compartment of this small-sized cell by the time the first line of the postbleach image is acquired.

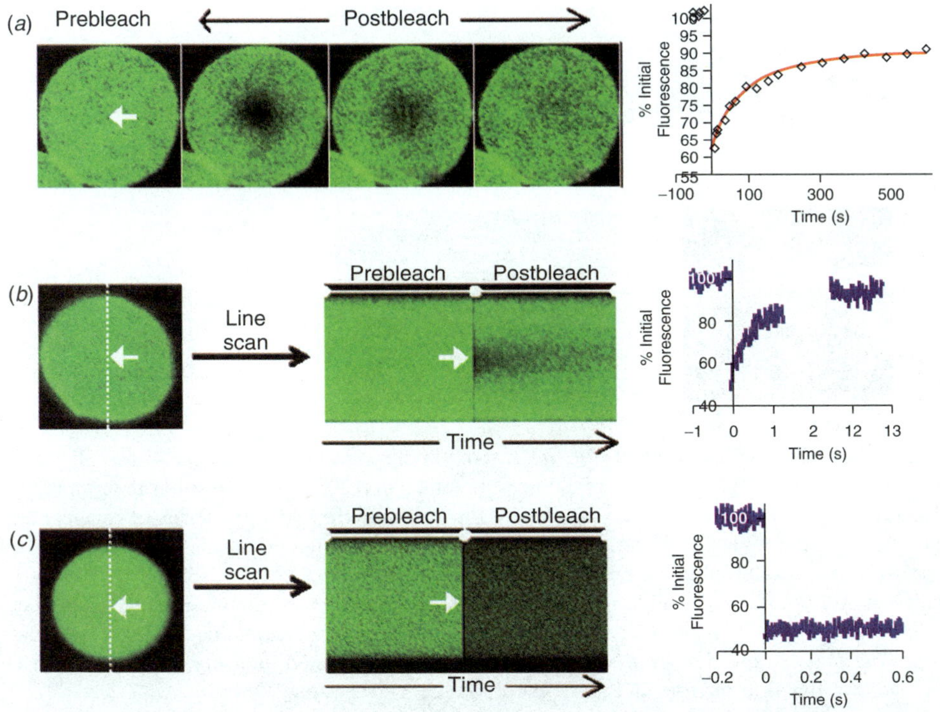

Figure 9.3 Fluorescecne recovery profiles of different macromolecule classes in erythrocyte: (*a*) single transmembrane helix plasma membrane protein, glycophorin A, labeled with fluorescein; (*b*) lipid probe, DiI, incorporated into erythrocyte membrane; (*c*) carboxyfluorescein–albumin incorporated into cytoplasm of resealed erythrocyte. The cells were subjected to spot bleaching in the regions indicated by the white arrows for 200, 100, and 20 ms, respectively. In (*b*) and (*c*), a line scan at the section indicated by the dotted line was used rather than a two-dimensional image to improve the time resolution. The data represent the fluorescence recorded in continuous line scans over a period of time. The fluorescence intensity in the bleached region is presented in the graphs at the right.

The above discussion does not mean it is impossible to measure protein diffusion in larger cells using a confocal microscope. In this case, by increasing the bleached area, it is possible to use the dependence of $\tau_{1/2}$ on ω^2 to bring the recovery time into the experimentally accessible range. Figure 9.4*a* shows a recovery profile of carboxyfluorescein-labeled albumin in solution following a 2-s bleach. The recovery is slow enough to be followed using two-dimensional image acquisition because of the large bleach area. This large area is achieved not because of a larger beam illumination profile—the same optics were used as in the previous examples that show micrometer-sized bleached regions. The larger bleached region is instead a consequence of diffusion of the fluorescein–albumin that occurred *during the bleaching event* and *during the acquisition* of the first postbleach image. The black dot in this figure corresponds to a structure of the same dimensions as the erythrocytes shown on the previous figure and illustrates the difficulty of performing these measurements within small compartments.

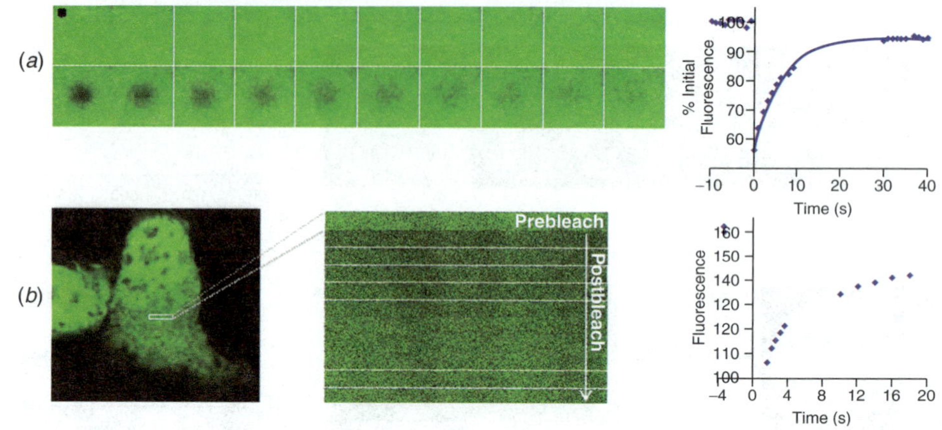

Figure 9.4 FRAP measurements of (*a*) carboxyfluorescein-labeled bovine serum albumin in solution and (*b*) GFP in cytoplasm of cultured mammalian (COS) cell. The solution of fluorescent albumin (*a*) was imaged before (top series of images) and after (bottom series of images) a 2-s spot bleach in the center of the field of view using a 100 × 1.4 numerical aperture (NA) objective lens. The time resolution is 1 s per image. The black circle in (*a*) has a diameter of 10 μm. For the COS cell (*b*), the rectangular region was bleached by repeated imaging using unattenuated laser power. Pre- and postbleach series of images of this region were obtained using an attenuated laser. The plots on the right of the images represent the integrated intensity within the bleached regions as a function of time and show the fluorescence recovery .

Figure 9.4*b* shows that using this approach it is also feasible to quantitate the diffusion of a small molecule within a relatively large-sized cell. In this case a rectangular "slice" within the cytoplasm of a cultured mammalian (COS) cell was imaged and bleached. As shown in the recovery profile, the bleached area is sufficiently large for there to be sufficient recovery to be analyzed. In principle, similar measurements performed in different cells could be used to identify differences in the diffusion coefficient.

In a FRAP measurement where only a small proportion of the total pool of fluorescent molecules are bleached and where all the labeled molecules are mobile, the fluorescence in the bleached region will recover to a value very close to its value prior to the bleach event. Such behavior is usually observed with lipids in membranes (Figure 9.3*b*). However, for many plasma membrane proteins the fluorescence often does not recover to its prebleach value (Figure 9.3*a*). This is thought to be due to the presence of a second, immobile population of proteins. The degree to which the fluorescence signal recovers can be used to calculate another useful parameter, f_{mob}, which is the fraction of the population that is mobile on the timescale of the measurement (Figure 9.2*b*). However, one should be aware that there can also be incomplete recovery due to overbleaching of the sample, as illustrated in the examples in Figures 9.3*c* and 9.4*b*. In these cases, the recovery does not approach its initial value because a significant fraction of the total population has been bleached. This can occur when the labeled species is moving very rapidly and molecules move in and out of the beam during the bleach phase. An inspection of the fluorescence profile in the first postbleach image will reveal whether this is occurring as the intensity in regions at some distance from the illuminated area will decrease in intensity.

9.4 PHOTOBLEACHING MEASUREMENTS WITH CONFOCAL MICROSCOPE

The wide availability of the laser scanning confocal microscope has led to increased interest in photobleaching measurements for various research applications. The hardware/software of most modern commercial confocal microscopes allows the user to design and perform a range of photobleaching measurements to address a wide variety of questions. A general understanding of the principles behind the confocal microscope and its associated components is necessary to optimize the design of photobleaching measurements and to properly interpret the data that are generated. In this section we explore the general principles of confocal imaging and examine the various components of the instrument that are important in performing photobleaching measurements. Photobleaching measurements can be performed on all currently available confocal microscopes, though some types of measurements are easier to perform on some instruments than on others.

Confocal microscopes are used to obtain images of thin optical sections of cells without the need for physically sectioning the cells. They are therefore particularly useful for live cell imaging. A laser is focused by the objective lens of the microscope to a diffraction-limited point within the sample. The fluorescence emitted from the illuminated region is collected back through the objective and focused through a pinhole prior to reaching the detector. The pinhole is positioned at the confocal position so that only light from the focal plane and not from the out-of-focus regions is detected. The size of the pinhole can be altered to control the level of out-of-focus light entering the detector and to set the "thickness" of the optical section. A fluorescence image of the optical section is built up pixel by pixel by scanning the focused illumination beam across the sample and reading the fluorescence intensity at each pixel position.

A number of features of the confocal microscope can be exploited to optimize the design of photobleaching measurements. These are described below:

1. *Acousto-Optical Tunable Filter (AOTF)* Commercial confocal microscopes are equipped with an AOTF that can be used to rapidly adjust the intensity of the laser. This affects not only the intensity of the detected fluorescence but also the degree of bleaching. The AOTF setting is usually adjusted to a relatively low value leading to low laser intensity during the imaging phase of the measurement to limit the degree of bleaching. Monitoring several successive images gives an indication of whether the AOTF setting is sufficiently low to keep bleaching during the imaging phase to an acceptable level. In contrast, an unattenuated laser is used during the bleaching phase to minimize the bleach time.

2. *Photomultipier Tube (PMT) Gain* The intensity of the fluorescence signal measured by the PMT can be increased by adjusting (increasing) its voltage. Although this increases the signal, it also amplifies background and noise, especially at very high gain settings. Except for very weakly fluorescent samples, a trade-off can usually be found between a high gain setting and a minimum AOTF setting to optimize image quality while minimizing bleaching during the imaging phase of an experiment.

3. *Confocal Pinhole* The size of the pinhole affects the "thickness" of the optical section examined in an image. This size can be adjusted by the user and it primarily affects optical spatial resolution. There is a trade-off between the "thinness" of the optical section and the intensity of light that reaches the detector with smaller pinholes

leading to lower levels of detected light, and this lowers the quality of the resulting fluorescence image. In many cases it may be acceptable to sacrifice spatial resolution in photobleaching measurments by opening the pinhole in order to increase the measured fluorescence intensity. It is important to note that increasing the pinhole size increases the intensity of light reaching the detector by a less stringent rejection of the out-of-focus fluorescence. The procedure does not increase or affect in any way the actual intensity of illumination and hence the degree of bleaching.

4. *Scan Speed* Most confocal microscopes offer the option of performing slow, medium, or fast scans, which is a useful way of adjusting the time resolution of a measurement. However, the scan speed affects the pixel dwell time. Increasing the scan speed will decrease the time spent collecting the signal at each pixel and increase the noise of the measured signal. Although decreasing the scan speed will improve the signal-to-noise ratio of the fluorescence signal, it may also increase the degree of bleaching during the imaging phase of the experiment.

5. *Uni- or Bidirectional Line Scanning* The confocal image is built up pixel by pixel and horizontal line by horizontal line. The default setting on most instruments is for unidirectional scanning, which means that each line in the image is scanned in the same direction (e.g., left to right). This means that time is wasted repositioning the laser on the left-hand side before the next line is imaged. In the bidirectional scanning mode, a raster-type scan is used which increases image acquisition speed twofold. In this mode, every second line is scanned in the same direction but adjacent lines are scanned in opposite directions. This can cause problems with the precise registration of adjacent lines in the image, but these problems can usually be overcome using the methods for phase correction that are supplied with the instrument software

6. *Image Averaging* The quality of an image can be improved by averaging a number of images. The averaging can be performed on a frame-by-frame or line-by-line basis. Frame averaging involves averaging a number of successive two-dimensional images. Movements of cells or subcellular components during the image acquisition time will produce blurriness or "trailing" effects depending on the degree of movement. In the line-averaging mode a single line is repeatedly imaged and averaged before moving to the next line. This approach is preferable in live cell measurements, in particular when examining structures that may exhibit a degree of movement during the course of an image scan. Although both types of image averaging increase the quality of data in an image, they decrease the time resolution. Averaging can also significantly increase the level of bleaching during the image acquisition phase of the measurement since the sample is subjected to a greater dose of illumination.

7. *Pixel Resolution* A "standard" two-dimensional confocal image may be made up of 512×512 pixels and typically take $\sim$1 s to acquire. Lowering the pixel resolution (e.g., to 256 x 256 or 64 x 64) can have advantages. For example, a decrease in the number of pixels scanned will increase the speed of image acquisition (improve time resolution). This will also substantially decrease the degree of bleaching during image acquisition. For example, decreasing the resolution from 512 x 512 to 256 x 256 without adjusting the zoom factor will decrease the total illumination dose in the scanned field (and hence the bleaching) by a factor of 4. This may be useful in situations when bleaching is very fast.

8. *Zoom* A major advantage of the confocal microscope is its ability to zoom into a region of interest within a field of view. However, it is important to be aware that

increasing the zoom without adjusting the pixel resolution will substantially increase the degree of bleaching. For example, zooming into a feature of interest by a factor of 4 while maintaining the pixel resolution at 512 x 512 means that the total illumination intensity that was used to generate the unzoomed image is now concentrated in an area one-sixteenth of the original size. Hence the degree of bleaching will similarly increase by a factor of 16. For this reason, it is often advisable to adjust the pixel resolution when zooming in on features. In fact, the simplest photobleaching measurement that can be performed on all instruments is to zoom in on a defined region of a sample and use high pixel resolution and an unattenuated laser to rapidly bleach a region and then to zoom out.

9. *Types of Scans* Different types of scans can be performed on many confocal microscopes. A "typical" scan may involve an xy scan to produce a two-dimensional image. As mentioned earlier, such a scan can take on the order of 1 s to acquire, which may be too slow to capture many processes. A substantial increase in time resolution can be obtained by scanning a single line. Such xt scans, as shown in Figures 9.3*b* and *c*, can be used to obtain a time resolution on the order of milliseconds. Further improvements in time resolution can be obtained by simply parking the laser over a region of the sample and repeatedly measuring the intensity. In principle, such an approach can lead to submillisecond time resolution, though this application is not available on many commercial confocal microscopes.

Overall Methodology of Photobleaching Measurements A general photobleaching measurement involves three phases: (i) the acquisition of prebleach images, (ii) the bleach event, and (iii) the acquisition of postbleach images. When designing a measurement, two important considerations are to minimize the time of the bleach event and to limit the degree of bleaching occurring during the image acquisition phase. It is important to use the lowest feasible laser power during image acquisition. The resultant low-fluorescence signals can be partly compensated for by opening the pinhole or increasing the PMT gain. Other ways of minimizing bleaching include using fewer averages, decreasing the zoom factor and/or pixel resolution, or simply acquiring fewer images. A small degree of bleaching is often unavoidable, especially in weakly fluorescent samples which require a higher laser power for imaging. An "internal" control in the field of view, such as another cell that is not subjected to the bleaching event, can be used to correct for unavoidable bleaching. Alternatively, the prebleach series of images can be used to determine the amount of bleaching per image and an exponential correction factor can be used to correct the fluorescence intensity in the postbeach series of images. The bleaching phase of the experiment can be performed in a number of ways:

1. *Zoom Bleach* The simplest bleaching experiment involves zooming into a region of interest with high pixel resolution and laser power and repeatedly imaging the region until significant bleaching is obtained. Zooming out to a larger field of view can be used to visualize the recovery process. This approach can be used on any confocal microscope. It has limited time resolution but is useful for slowly diffusing species or in applications where large-sized bleach areas are employed.
2. *Line or Rectangular Bleaching* An unattenuated laser scanning in the xt mode can be used to bleach diffraction-limited lines across the scanned field of view.

Rectangular areas can also be defined and bleached, as illustrated in Figure 9.4*b*. The advantage of using line and rectangular bleach profiles is that methods for quantitative analysis of these experiments have been developed.

3. *Region-of-Interest (ROI) Bleaching* ROIs of almost any size and shape can be defined on a prebleach image and the defined regions on the sample subjected to increased laser power to selectively bleach the ROI. The advantage of ROI bleaching is that irregularly shaped subcellular structures such as Golgi can be selectively bleached. The disadvantage of this method is the loss of time resolution. In bleaching the ROI, the instrument still scans a rectangular selection incorporating the defined ROI but only switches the AOTF to the unattenuated laser power when in the ROI. It typically takes much longer to bleach ROI-defined structures compared to other bleaching modes because of the time wasted scanning the region which is not subjected to high-intensity illumination.
4. *Spot Bleaching* For situations requiring increased time resolution, a spot bleach approach can be used. This involves defining a point (or multiple points) on the prebleach image of a sample. The unattenuated laser is parked over this point for a defined period of time to produce localized illumination of the sample. The bleach "spot" is actually a diffraction-limited point whose dimensions are defined by the optics of the system, in particular the objective lens used. A 100 × oil objective with a 1.4 NA will produce a beam with a Gaussian radius of ~0.2 μm in the *xy* image plane and ~0.6 μm in the *z* direction. The dimension of the bleached spot will appear larger in the scanned image because of the point spread function of the lens used for imaging. In addition, as is evident in Figure 9.4*a*, any diffusion that occurs during the time it takes to perform the bleaching and acquire the first postbleach image will spread the bleached molecules, which will affect the apparent size of the bleached area observed in the first postbleach image.

It is important to appreciate the different spatial bleaching profiles obtained using a spot bleach and other bleach modes such as the "zoom" bleach. As illustrated in Figure 9.5, utilizing a parked beam (spot bleach) largely restricts the bleached area

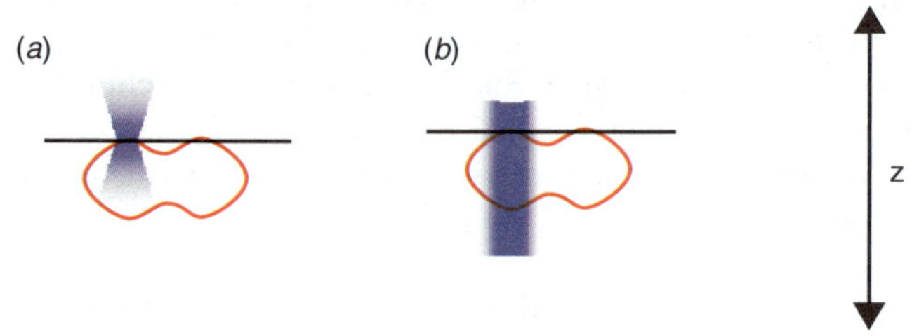

Figure 9.5 Comparison of (*a*) spot bleaching and (*b*) zoom bleaching. The sample is shown in red and the black line corresponds to the focal plane in the *xy* direction. In (*a*), the laser is parked in a position at the top of the cell for the bleaching event. The illumination (blue) and thus the region of bleaching are essentially confined to this region. There is relatively little illumination and bleaching at the bottom of the cell. In (*b*), a small region of the surface is selected and scanned with high-intensity illumination using the zoom function. In this case, the levels of illumination and bleaching are similar at different points along the *z* direction and there is significant bleaching at the bottom of the cell.

to the point of focus, although there is some illumination and bleaching in regions above and below the plane of focus that may not be visualized, especially if a closed pinhole is utilized. In contrast, when a region is subjected to an xy scan, the integrated intensity at, above, and below the plane of focus is approximately equal. Hence all regions above and below the focal plane that is scanned are bleached to a similar extent. It should be pointed out that the situation is different when using multiphoton excitation—in this case illumination and bleaching are both confined to the plane that is imaged (i.e., what you see is what you bleach!).

The time employed for the bleach event depends on a variety of factors, including the properties of the fluorophore, the laser power, the objective lens, the type of bleach being employed, the diffusion coefficient of the molecule being examined, and the size and shape of the structure through which it diffuses. With a 20-mW laser, we find that fluorophores such as fluorescein are readily bleached with an unattenuated laser in tens of milliseconds, whereas GFP typically requires bleach times 10 times greater. Ideally, the bleach time should be much less than the half time for recovery, but it is not always feasible to achieve bleaching on a millisecond timescale. This imposes limitations on the types of processes that can be measured. Note that in the case of GFP, which typically requires bleach times of a few hundred milliseconds, monitoring the recovery over a similar timescale may not be particularly accurate and care has to be taken in interpreting results.

9.5 PHOTOBLEACHING APPLICATIONS

In this section we present examples illustrating the types of information that can be obtained from different photobleaching measurements. Many of the examples are measurements obtained using erythrocytes infected with the malaria parasite, *Plasmodium falciparum*. To appreciate the subsequent examples, a brief introduction into the cell biology of the malaria parasite–infected erythrocyte is necessary.

Figure 9.6 shows a schematic representation of an infected erythrocyte. The parasite is enclosed in the erythrocyte within a parasitophorous vacuole that is formed during parasite invasion. A number of changes occur to the infected erythrocyte during parasite growth. Extensions of the parasitophorous vacuolar membrane develop; sometimes these seem to be continuous and sometimes they seem to break off to form distinct entities. These structures are referred to as the tubulovesicular network. Other membrane-bound structures called Maurer's clefts are found just under the host membrane and electron-dense structures called knobs appear in the host membrane. As it grows, the parasite exports a number of proteins to these external structures in the host cell. It is still not entirely clear how these structures are generated and how parasite proteins are trafficked to these compartments. Many of the examples presented describe our approach of using GFP fusion proteins targeted to these compartments to gain a greater insight into these novel trafficking mechanisms and into the changes that occur during parasite growth.

9.5.1 Macromolecular Organization

FRAP measurements provide information on factors that affect the diffusivity of molecules. Although viscosity can be one of these factors, it is usually the size of

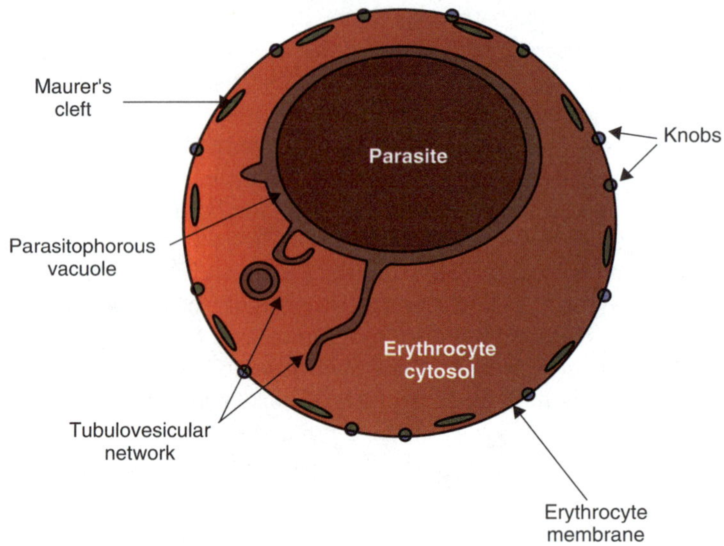

Figure 9.6 Compartments within an erythrocyte infected with malaria parasite.

the molecular complex that is measured. FRAP is a good technique for looking at properties such as molecular size and degree of immobilization of macromolecules. Figure 9.7*a* shows an experiment examining control and parasite-infected erythrocytes in which a host membrane protein, called band 3, has been selectively labeled with the fluorophore eosin. A region of the erythrocyte membrane is bleached using spot illumination. In uninfected erythrocytes ~50% of the band 3 molecules are mobile on a timescale of minutes. This is because some of the band 3 molecules are linked through to the underlying membrane skeleton. In contrast, almost all the band 3 molecules in the infected erythrocyte membrane are immobile on this timescale. This is due to alterations to the organization of the host cell membrane induced by the parasite. The FRAP measurements combined with biochemical analyses indicate that parasite-induced oxidative stress causes aggregation and crosslinking of the band 3 protein [5].

Figures 9.7*b* and *c* show examples of FRAP measurements performed on an infected erythrocyte in which a GFP fusion protein is targeted to the space between the parasite plasma membrane and the parasitophorous vacuole membrane. In the first example, the image reveals a smooth rim of fluorescence surrounding the parasite (at least within the resolution limits of light microscopy) whereas in the second example the fluorescing compartment resembles a necklace of beads. Spot bleaching produces a localized loss of fluorescence which recovers with a $\tau_{1/2} \sim 15\,\mathrm{s}$ (Figure 9.7*b* and data not shown). In both cases the rate of recovery is slower than expected for a freely diffusing protein in an unrestricted compartment. As illustrated in Figure 9.3*c*, application of a bleach pulse to a compartment containing a freely mobile protein produces even bleaching throughout the entire compartment. That is, the recovery is faster than can be measured ($\tau_{1/2} < 0.1\,\mathrm{s}$). An increased viscosity within the vacuole or the incorporation of the protein into a large supramolecular complex could explain the slower diffusion of the GFP fusion proteins in the malaria parasite. Another possibility is that the slow diffusion results from the constricted geometry of the compartment. Electron micrographs show that the parasitophorous vacuole is narrow and closely

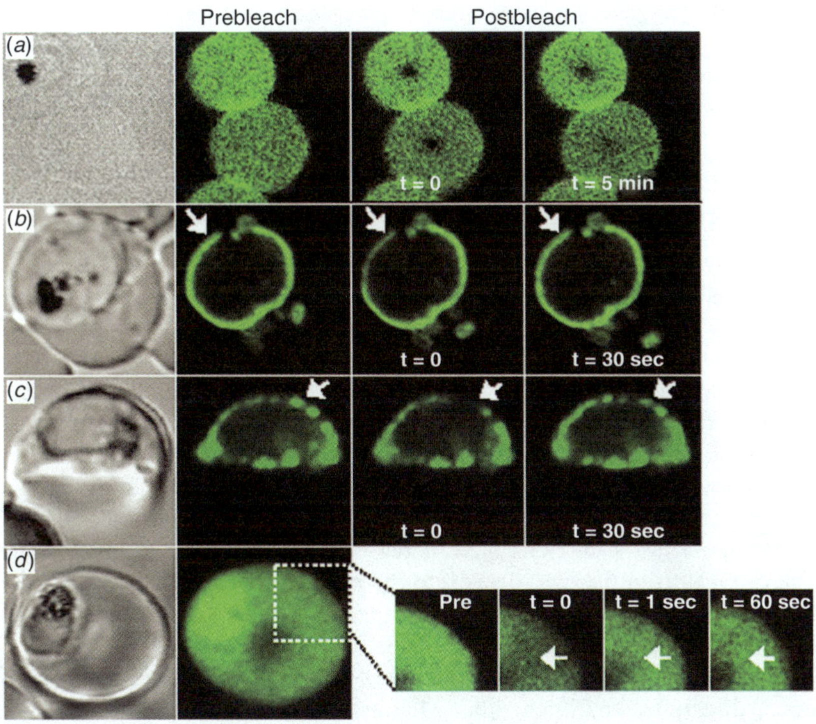

Figure 9.7 FRAP measurements in erythrocytes infected with malaria parasites. Each panel of images shows a differential interference contrast image (grey scale) and pre- and postbleach fluorescence images (green) of the infected erythrocytes. The arrows point to the regions bleached and the times at which the images are collected after the bleach event are indicated. (*d*) Zoom function was used to image a region of the cell for the FRAP measurement. (*a*) Uninfected erythrocyte (bottom cell) and infected erythrocyte (top cell) with malaria parasite clearly visible in differential interference contrast image. The host membrane protein, band 3, has been labeled with the fluorescent probe eosin. The two cells were spot bleached in rapid succession in the middle of each cell. Partial recovery of fluorescence is observed in the uninfected erythrocyte but no recovery in the infected erythrocyte. This indicates complete restriction of the movement of band 3 in infected erythrocytes. (*b*, *c*) Parasites are transfectants expressing a GFP fusion protein targeted to the parasitophorous vacuole. Bleaching is followed by recovery, but the recovery rate is slower than expected theoretically, possibly due to the constricted nature of the compartment. (*d*) GFP fusion protein is located in the host cytoplasm (another pool of GFP is also evident within the parasite). Again the recovery rate is slower than expected theoretically; this may be due to the formation of large complexes.

apposed to the parasite membrane. This may restrict the diffusion of molecules within the compartment [2].

Figure 9.7*d* shows a FRAP analysis of a GFP-tagged parasite protein that is targeted to the erythrocyte cytoplasm. In this measurement we have zoomed in on a particular region of the cytoplasm with low pixel resolution (64×64) and line averaging in order to obtain high-quality spatial information while attempting to improve temporal resolution. Application of a laser pulse induces limited localized bleaching and the recovery is complete by the time the second postbleach image is acquired. Again this recovery profile is slower than expected for free diffusion of a protein monomer. In this case the data suggest that the protein is part of a much larger complex within the erythrocyte cytoplasm and hence diffuses more slowly [4]. Overall, although the rapid recovery characteristics preclude an accurate determination of the size of this complex, it is still possible to get some qualitative information on relatively fast diffusive processes.

9.5.2 Monitoring Movement between Different Compartments

Not all recovery observed in a FRAP measurement reflects the simple translational diffusion of a molecule. In order to interpret a particular experiment, some knowledge of the expected diffusional behavior of the molecule of interest may be required. Figure 9.8*a* shows an example of a FRAP analysis of GFP expressed in the cytoplasm of a cultured mammalian cell. GFP is also present in the cell nucleus as it can move into this compartment through the nuclear pores. Application of a laser pulse to the nuclear region results in even bleaching throughout the entire nucleus because GFP diffuses fast enough to sample the entire nuclear compartment during the bleach pulse. The depleted nuclear compartment is clearly delineated in the postbleach image. The fluorescence signal in the nucleus then increases over time. This recovery reflects the movement of GFP from the cytoplasm into the nucleus through the nuclear pores. This approach has been used to investigate the sequence signals and metabolic factors that influence the transport of proteins through the nuclear pores.

Figure 9.8*b* illustrates an example where recovery is due to association–dissociation interactions. In this experiment the Maurer's clefts structures (submicrometer–micrometer size compartments) within the infected erythrocyte cytosol are targeted

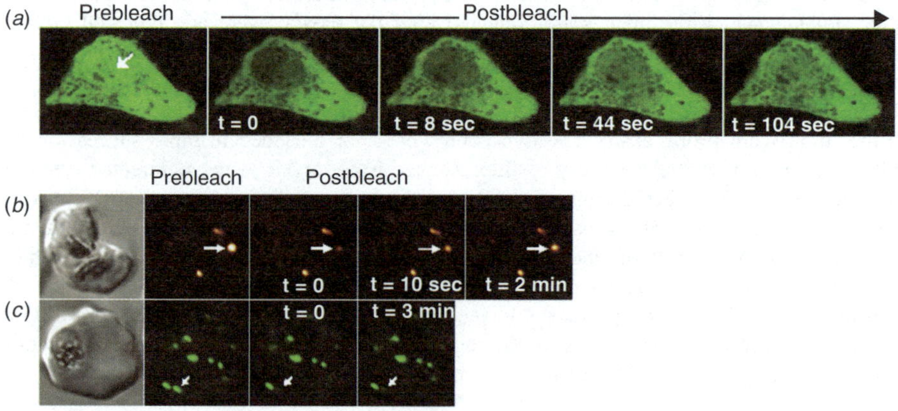

Figure 9.8 FRAP measurements showing recovery due to different cellular processes. Differential interference contrast images are shown in grey scale and fluorescence images in green. Cells were bleached in the regions indicated by the white arrow using spot illumination and postbleach images were recorded at the times indicated. (*a*) Cultured mammalian cell (COS) expressing GFP in cytoplasm. Some GFP is also present in the nucleus and it is this pool that was subjected to bleaching (indicated by arrow). (*b*, *c*) Erythrocytes infected with malaria parasite transfectants expressing GFP fusion proteins that are associated with Maurer's clefts. The transfectant in (*b*) is expressing a peripheral protein that is exchanging with a cytoplasmic pool. The transfectant in (*c*) is expressing an integral membrane protein. The lack of fluorescence recovery indicates that this compartment has no connections to adjacent compartments.

by a soluble GFP fusion protein that transiently associates with these structures. Spot bleaching of an individual Maurer's cleft results in the selective loss of fluorescence of the targeted structure, with some recovery of fluorescence over time [3]. The observed recovery in this case reflects the interchange between cytoplasmic and Maurer's cleft–associated pools of this molecule. In contrast, a different GFP-tagged parasite protein targeted to the same structure exhibits no recovery on a similar timescale (Figure 9.8*c*), suggesting that it is more tightly associated with the Maurer's clefts [6]. This approach helps judge which proteins are tightly associated with a given structure and which are not.

FRAP measurements have also been utilized to examine the organization and reorganization of organelles and to examine the connectivities between different subcellular compartments. For example, the entire Golgi network of a cell can be bleached using a ROI scan. In such live cell measurements, fluorescence recovery can occur on a timescale of tens of minutes due to trafficking of proteins from the endoplasmic reticulum (ER) to the Golgi.

9.5.3 Fluorescence Loss in Photobleaching

In FRAP measurements, a small proportion of the total population of fluorophores is bleached and recovery of fluorescence due to the movement of unbleached molecules into that region is measured. In a related method, fluorescence loss in photobleaching (FLIP), a defined area of the cell is bleached and other regions of the cell are monitored to see if they undergo a loss of fluorescence. Such a loss indicates that the two regions of the cell must be interconnected. FLIP usually involves repeatedly subjecting a region of the cell to short laser pulses. Ideally, the pulses are spaced at time intervals similar to the recovery time to allow unbleached molecules time to diffuse into the illuminated area. Given enough time and a sufficient illumination dose, all molecules that are in regions connected to the illuminated area will eventually be bleached.

Examples of FLIP measurements performed on fusion GFPs targeted to the parasitophorous vacuole of an infected erythrocyte are shown in Figure 9.9. In Figure 9.9*a* repeated bleaching of a localized region of the parasitophorous vacuole causes loss of fluorescence throughout the entire rim. This demonstrates that the GFP fusion molecules can freely diffuse throughout this compartment. However, the fluorescence in some structures that appear superficially close to the parasitophorous vacuole is not affected. This is more clearly seen in Figure 9.9*b*, where the fluorescence of the structure indicated by the blue arrowhead is unaffected by the bleach events. This indicates that molecules are not free to diffuse between the two regions of the cell; that is, they are distinct compartments.

Parasites expressing GFP in the necklace of bead structures within the parasitophorous vacuole exhibit interesting behavior in a FLIP experiment. Only the regions subjected to the laser beam are bleached (Figure 9.9*c*). Thus, the GFP fusion must be restricted to discrete subcompartments surrounding the parasite. Together, the FLIP and FRAP measurements provide a picture of the parasitophorous vacuole as a complex structure that is divided into subcompartments. Sometimes these compartments are connected, allowing the free diffusion of molecules between them; at other times connectivity is lost. FRAP and FLIP measurements provide complementary information, and it is often advantageous to perform both analyses, preferably on the same cell. The former provides information about the diffusion of molecules and the latter about the connectivity of compartments.

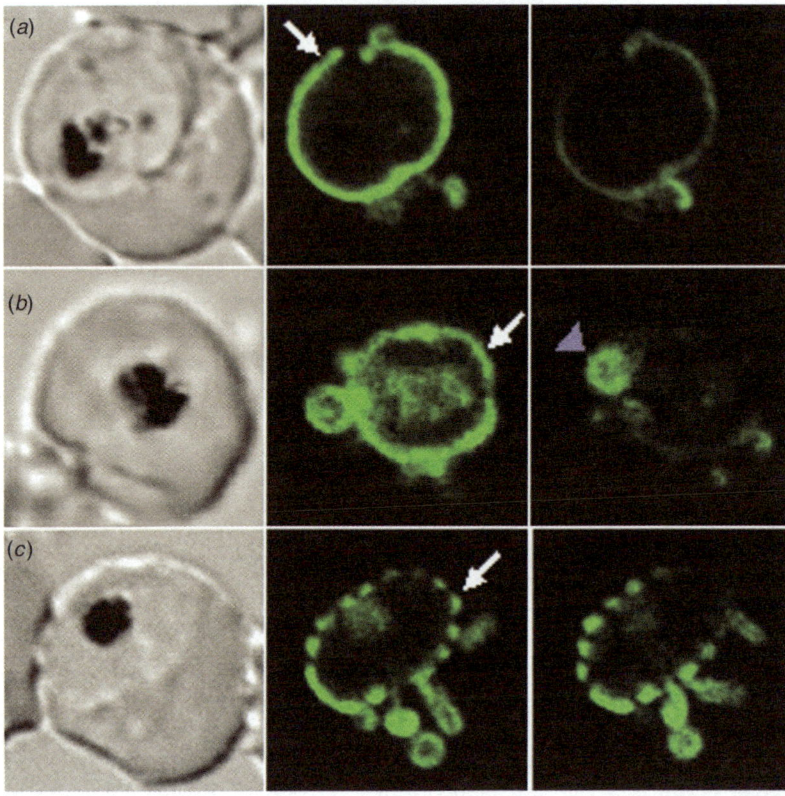

Figure 9.9 FLIP measurements in malaria parasite transfectants expressing GFP fusion protein targeted to parasitophorous vacuole. Shown are differential interference contrast images in grey scale and fluorescence images in green. The fluorescence images on the left correspond to the images obtained prior to the bleaching events. The cells were repeatedly bleached using spot illumination in the regions indicated by the white arrows. The fluorescence images on the right represent the fluorescence images obtained after bleaching.

9.5.4 Fluorescence Resonance Energy Transfer

Fluorescence resonance energy transfer (FRET) helps to determine whether two fluorescently labeled components are part of single macromolecular complex. FRET relies on the nonradiative transfer of energy from one probe in the excited state (the donor) to another probe in the ground state (the acceptor) when the two are in close proximity (typically within 5 nm). As a result of FRET the excited-state donor decays to the ground state without emitting light in the expected wavelength range. This means that a donor fluorophore undergoing FRET will exhibit both a decrease in the rate of radiative decay (which can be measured as a decrease in its fluorescence lifetime) and a decrease in the intensity of fluorescence emission.

A change in fluorescence lifetime affects the rate at which a molecule is bleached because it affects the length of time the molecule spends in the excited state and hence the probability of undergoing a chemical reaction prior to returning to the ground state. A consequence of this is that any process, such as FRET, that decreases the fluorescence lifetime will also decrease the observed rate of bleaching of the molecule.

Thus a simple way of identifying FRET is to measure the rate of bleaching of the donor in the absence and presence of the acceptor fluorophore.

The photobleaching rate can be determined relatively easily using a epifluorescence or confocal microscope. In the former case, the sample is repeatedly imaged as a means of bleaching the sample. Under Kohler illumination all parts of the cell receive essentially the same total illumination dose so changes in the rate of bleaching should in most cases reflect changes in the underlying lifetime. A similar approach can be utilized with a confocal microscope though care has to be applied to ensure that all samples being compared are imaged using the same laser power, pixel resolution, zoom setting, and averaging. All regions above and below the plane of focus should receive the same total dose of illumination (see Figure 9.5*b*).

The photobleaching rate is determined from the bleach series on defined ROIs within the cell by fitting an exponential decay function to the loss of fluorescence intensity. A similar analysis can be performed on a pixel-by-pixel basis if the appropriate software is available to provide detailed spatial information on FRET throughout the cell.

Another very simple way to identify FRET is by selectively bleaching the acceptor. As the acceptor is destroyed, FRET is prevented and the fluorescence intensity of the donor increases. This approach is illustrated in Figure 9.10. The prebleach images show fluorescence micrographs of a fixed erythrocyte probed with a primary antibody against the cytoskeletal component spectrin and subsequently labeled with red and green fluorescent secondary antibodies. The region of the cell indicated by the arrow was subjected to high-intensity spot illumination to selectively bleach the red (acceptor) fluorophore. As is evident in the fluorescence images, but particularly in the difference images, the loss of red fluorescence is associated with increasing intensity of the green fluorescence. This indicates that the secondary antibodies are in close proximity, as would be expected if they were binding to the same primary antibodies, which in turn should be binding to the repetitive spectrin element in the erythrocyte cytoskeleton.

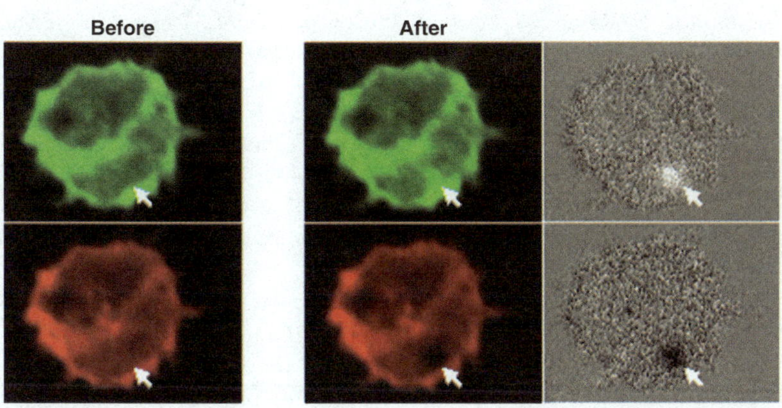

Figure 9.10 FRET analysis by acceptor photobleaching. Fixed erythrocyte samples were probed with a primary antibody against the cytoskeletal protein spectrin, and secondary antibodies labelled with green and red fluorophores. The red fluorophores were bleached by spot illumination at the position indicated by the white arrow; the loss of red fluorescence is associated with an increase in green fluorescence. This is particularly evident in the difference images shown in greyscale on the right where increases in fluorescence are represented as white and decreases as black.

Photobleaching-based FRET measurements suffer the major disadvantage that they require significant loss of fluorescence from the cell for accurate quantitation. Thus they are not suitable for long-term imaging of live cells. However, they have the advantage that they are relatively straightforward and can be performed on any epifluorescence or confocal microscope and can answer the basic question: Are these two molecules of interest part of the same complex within the cell.

9.6 CONCLUSIONS

Photobleaching methods can be utilized in a wide variety of ways to provide insights into macromolecular interactions and cellular dynamics. Almost all the approaches described here can be performed by novice users on standard confocal microscopes. Thus, rather than simply generating information on the spatial location of a fluorescent species, the user can obtain a more detailed picture of dynamic events in living cells. Further advances in instrumentation that will allow ever more detailed analysis of cellular processes are becoming available. For example, the technique of fluorescence correlation spectroscopy provides information about fast diffusive processes that is not available using photobleaching methods. Similarly, advances in the availability and utility of photoactivatable probes that change their color upon illumination provide whole new approaches to studying cellular dynamics. These will surely keep both the cell biologist and the microscopist busy for many years to come.

For a more detailed and technical account of photobleaching, see [1].

REFERENCES

1. N. Klonis, M. Rug, I. Harper, M. Wickham, A. Cowman, and L. Tilley, "Fluorescence photobleaching analysis for the study of cellular dynamics," *Eur Biophys J.* **31**, 36–51 (2002).
2. A. Adisa, M. Rug, N. Klonis, M. Foley, A. F. Cowman, and L. Tilley, "The signal sequence of exported protein-1 directs the green fluorescent protein to the parasitophorous vacuole of transfected malaria parasites," *J Biol Chem.* **278**, 6532–6542 (2003).
3. M. E. Wickham, M. Rug, S. A. Ralph, N. Klonis, G. I. McFadden, L. Tilley, and A. F. Cowman, "Trafficking and assembly of the cytoadherence complex in *Plasmodium falciparum*-infected human erythrocytes," *EMBO J.* **20**, 5636–5649 (2001).
4. E. Knuepfer, M. Rug, N. Klonis, L. Tilley, and A. F. Cowman, "Trafficking of the major virulence factor to the surface of transfected *P. falciparum*-infected erythrocytes," *Blood* **105**, 4078–4087 (2005).
5. P. D. Parker, L. Tilley, and N. Klonis, "*Plasmodium falciparum* induces reorganization of host membrane proteins during intraerythrocytic growth," *Blood* **103**, 2404–2406 (2004).
6. C. Spycher, M. Rug, N. Klonis, A. F. Cowman, H.-P. Beck, and L. Tilley, "Genesis of and trafficking to the Maurer's cleft secretory compartment of malaria parasite-infected erythrocytes," *Mol. Cell. Biol.* **6**, 4074–4085 (2006).

CHAPTER 10

Time-Resolved Fluorescence in Microscopy

TREVOR A. SMITH, CRAIG N. LINCOLN, and DAMIAN K. BIRD

Ultrafast and Microspectroscopy Laboratories, School of Chemistry, University of Melbourne, Victoria 3010, Australia

10.1 INTRODUCTION

Fluorescence-based detection is among the most sensitive characterization techniques available, capable of achieving single-photon and single-molecule detection levels. Moreover, it can be used to probe the three spatial dimensions with high resolution through a variety of fluorescence microscopy techniques. As discussed elsewhere in this volume, emission intensity is dependent on a variety of physical and environmental variables, such as fluorescence quantum yield; temperature; pH; solvent properties such as viscosity and polarity; the concentration of oxygen, impurities, heavy atoms, and ions; fluorophore concentration; excitation and emission wavelength; polarization; excitation intensity; and time after excitation. Due to the many phenomena that can affect fluorescence intensity, resolving the fluorescence signal in time relative to the excitation event potentially provides far more additional information, particularly through discriminating between time-dependent and time-independent processes. In this chapter we will concentrate on this attractive advantage of fluorescence-based techniques. This will be discussed in a general sense initially, and then the application of various time-resolved fluorescence techniques will be discussed with particular emphasis on methods appropriate for time-resolved fluorescence imaging on the micrometer and submicrometer scale. Time-resolved fluorescence imaging has developed into a mature science and is being used in an increasingly wide range of disciplines, including biology, chemistry, forensics, [1] physics, and even the arts, such as in the studies of Michelangelo's statue of David. [2]

10.2 PHOTOPHYSICS AND DEACTIVATION OF EXCITED STATE

The fundamentals of photochemistry, photophysics, and photobiology are well documented in numerous textbooks and in Chapter 1 of this book. Excellent overviews

Fluorescence Applications in Biotechnology and Life Sciences, Edited by Ewa M. Goldys

of the principles of fluorescence spectroscopy have also been published [3, 4], so we provide here only a brief summary of the points salient to fluorescence microscopy. Once formed, the excited electronic state of a molecule will survive for only a limited time, characteristic of the particular molecule and the specific state involved. The molecule will lose its excess energy to return to a preferred lower energy state, which it can do through a number of radiative and nonradiative pathways, each with its own characteristic rate of deactivation, as discussed in Chapter 1. In most, but not all cases, the deactivation of the excited state is a random, spontaneous process, occurring with a first-order rate constant, with the rate constant for each process usually designated k_{ij}. Since the concentrations of the various excited states can be dealt with just as any other concentrations in chemical reactions, the rate of change in the population of a given energy level can be considered by combining the terms of all the deactivation pathways contributing to the overall photophysical properties and dynamics of the molecule. If the concentration of an excited state, such as the first excited singlet state, is designated $[M^*]$, the rate of change of this concentration can be defined as:

$$\frac{d[M^*]}{dt} = -(k_{\text{ISC}} + k_{\text{IC}} + k_R + k_{\text{VR}})[M^*] = -k[M^*] \qquad (10.1)$$

The fluorescence lifetime τ_f represents the lifetime of the excited state of the molecule, which is related to the various rate constants for deactivation of the excited state, that is:

$$\tau_f = \frac{1}{k_{\text{ISC}} + k_{\text{IC}} + k_R + k_{\text{VR}}} \qquad (10.2)$$

Integration of Eq. 10.1 gives the familiar exponential decay of the population of the excited state (Eq. 10.4, in which A is the amplitude parameter), and relates the intensity of fluorescence emanating from M^* as a function of time after excitation, $I(t)$, to the fluorescence lifetime of the emitting species, M^*, as depicted in Figure 10.1a:

$$[M^*] = [M^*]_0 e^{-kt} \qquad (10.3)$$

$$I(t) = Ae^{-t/\tau_f} \qquad (10.4)$$

The fluorescence lifetime is also related to the fluorescence quantum yield ϕ_f as:

$$\phi_f = \frac{k_R}{k_{\text{ISC}} + k_{\text{IC}} + k_R + k_{\text{VR}}} = k_R \tau_f \qquad (10.5)$$

The timescales over which the various photophysical processes occur are summarized in Figure 10.2. Internal conversion, intersystem crossing, and vibrational relaxation typically occur over picosecond and subpicosecond timescales. Typical fluorescence lifetimes (i.e., lifetime of the excited state, such as S_1, Figure 10.2) are of picosecond to nanosecond durations. Phosphorescence, on the other hand, occurs on significantly longer timescales and therefore is less likely, under normal experimental conditions, to be competitive with fluorescence or other radiative or nonradiative deactivation pathways.

In addition to the processes discussed above, the intensity of emission from a fluorophore may be reduced through various, often nonradiative, processes competing with fluorescence. These may include energy transfer from a higher energy donor to a lower energy acceptor, static and dynamic excited-state quenching processes (e.g., due to the presence of oxygen), and excited-state aggregation formation at high chromophore concentrations. Due to the similarities of the timescales of the various processes involved, fluorescence can be used to report on these processes and others, including chromophore rotation. In the presence of these additional pathways through which the excited state might be deactivated, additional rate constants must be included in the expression for the quantum yield (and therefore the fluorescence lifetime). Thus, any additional excited-state deactivation mechanisms will result in a reduced fluorescence quantum yield ϕ'_f (Eq. 10.6) reflected in a concomitant reduction in the fluorescence lifetime τ'_f (cf. Eq. 10.5). This reduction in fluorescence lifetime is illustrated in Figure 10.1*b*, in which the *intensity* of the decay has been normalized to that of the decay in Figure 10.1*a*. This highlights the ability, through the process of resolving the emission temporally, to discriminate between reductions in quantum yield due to time-dependent and time-independent mechanisms (e.g., between static and dynamic quenching or between losses due to collection efficiency variations and dynamic quenching processes):

$$\phi'_f = \frac{k_R}{k_{\text{ISC}} + k_{\text{IC}} + k_R + k_{\text{ET}} + k_Q + \cdots} = k_R \tau'_f \tag{10.6}$$

10.3 TIME-RESOLVED FLUORESCENCE MEASUREMENTS

We have just noted that time-resolved measurements provide additional information about molecular fluorescence, which may be difficult to gain from fluorescence intensity or its spectral characteristics. A fluorophore's spectral characteristics may provide

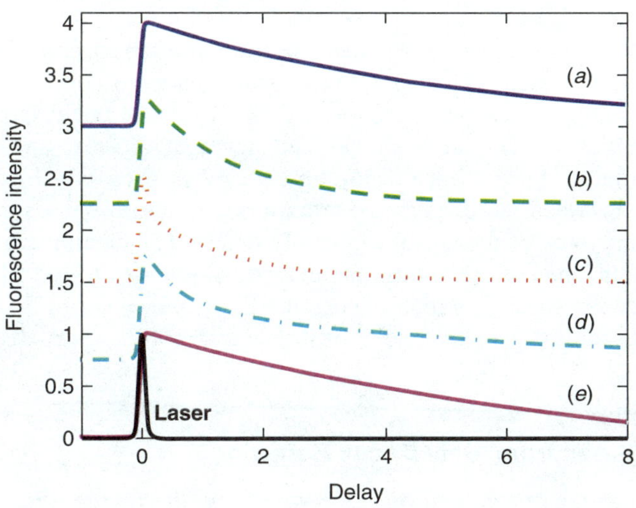

Figure 10.1 Time-resolved fluorescence decay profiles of (*a*) fluorophore exhibiting simple (exponential) excited-state decay, (*b*) the same fluorophore experiencing additional excited-state decay processes, (*c*) fluorescence decay corrupted by scattered light, (*d*) multiexponential decay profile, and (*e*) influence of instrument response function.

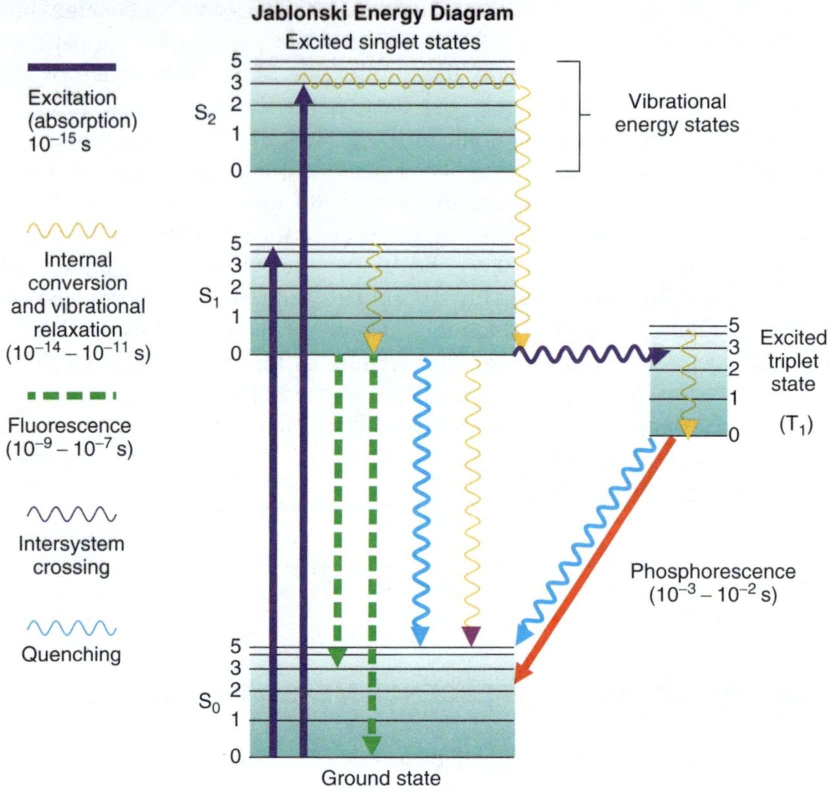

Figure 10.2 Jablonski diagram showing energy levels and approximate timescales for various photophysical processes.

a certain degree of discrimination between species, but often spectral shifts can be subtle, for example, members of the porphyrin family undergo concentration-dependent aggregation, resulting in very modest spectral shifts in both the absorption and emission spectra [5]. However, the monomer and aggregate species are known to have significantly different fluorescence decay time characteristics, which can be exploited to discriminate between these species. Furthermore, due to the many phenomena that can affect the *intensity* of the signal ultimately detected (including scattered light and the collection efficiency of the optical and detection systems), the added degree of discrimination between species available when the fluorescence signal is resolved in time relative to the excitation event can help overcome some of the shortfalls of steady-state methods.

10.3.1 Deviations from Ideal Decay Behavior

The discussion above concerning the case where the fluorescence decay is described by a single, defined decay constant (or fluorescence lifetime) is valid if the emission emanates from only one fluorescing species within a homogeneous environment. This is, however, an ideal case, and many processes, in particular, molecular aggregation, species heterogeneity, and concentration quenching, may be prevalent in the conditions experienced in many common microscopy situations and can be identified and quantified using decay functions that deviate markedly from the simple exponential model that predicts a single fluorescence lifetime.

Under circumstances such as molecular aggregation or species heterogeneity, the concept of a single, defined fluorescence lifetime is invalid, and the emission decay may be better described by a linear combination of n contributing components, as in the equation (Figure 10.1d):

$$I(t) = \sum_{i=1}^{n} a_i \ \exp^{-t/\tau_i} \tag{10.7}$$

Often the identity of these individual components cannot be clarified, and this fitting method may not lead to a meaningful interpretation. We should be aware that a variable chemical environment may give rise to a large variety of excited states that can have very similar, yet different, fluorescence lifetimes [6]. In such a case, detection of individual discrete states, as discussed above, is not feasible, and a *distribution* of components may be more appropriate to describe the time dependence of the emission. Distributions of decay times can be analyzed in terms of a predetermined or assumed functional form, such as a Gaussian distribution. Alternative methods, including the exponential series (ESM) [7] or maximum-entropy methods (MEMs) [8, 9], assume nothing about the form of the distribution and report back on the shape and center of the distribution based on a large set of fixed lifetime values. The adjustable variables are the amplitudes (preexponential factors) corresponding to each fluorescence decay time. Unfortunately, in most time-resolved fluorescence imaging situations, it is not possible to record an adequately high number of counts per pixel in a realistic time period to justify ESM or MEM approaches.

In Förster resonance energy transfer measurements, where a distribution of energy transfer distances may be appropriate, decay functions of the form given by Eq. 10.8 may be applicable:

$$I(t) = I_0 \int P(r) \ \exp\left[-\frac{t}{\tau_D} - \frac{t}{\tau_D}\left(\frac{R_0^6}{r^6}\right)\right] \ dr \tag{10.8}$$

where r is the donor–acceptor distance, τ_D is the donor fluorescence lifetime, and the distance distribution $P(r)$ can be of any form; however, it is often assumed Gaussian in shape, for example:

$$\mathrm{P(r)} = \frac{\alpha_n}{Z} \exp\left[-\frac{1}{2}\left(\frac{r - r_{\mathrm{av}}}{\sigma}\right)^2\right] \ [10]$$

In some cases, nonexponential decay functions may be applicable, such as the general form given by Eq. 10.9, which is valid for the emission decay profile of an energy donor molecule undergoing s-dimensional Förster energy transfer to a distribution of an excess of acceptor molecules [11, 12]:

$$I(t) = A \ \exp\left(-b_1 t - b_2 t^{\frac{s}{6}}\right) \tag{10.9}$$

Due to the complex (e.g., multi- or nonexponential) nature of many fluorescence decay profiles, the term "average fluorescence lifetime" is often used. The correct use of the term "average" in this context has been discussed elsewhere [13]. When measuring fluorescence lifetimes, it is possible to calculate different average lifetimes, the two most commonly used being the "intensity average" and the "amplitude average" lifetime.

The intensity average lifetime is based on the observation that the fluorescence intensity contribution of a component, i, is proportional to the product $a_i\tau_i$. The intensity average lifetime is the average amount of time a fluorophore spends in the excited state and is given by:

$$\langle\tau\rangle_f = \frac{\sum a_i\tau_i^2}{\sum a_i\tau_i} \tag{10.10}$$

The amplitude average lifetime is defined by Eq. 10.11 and can be interpreted as the lifetime a fluorophore would have if it had the same steady-state fluorescence as the fluorophore with several lifetimes. The same definitions of average lifetimes apply when the time-dependent fluorescence profile is described by a *distribution* of lifetime components:

$$\langle\tau\rangle_a = \frac{\sum a_i\tau_i}{\sum a_i} \tag{10.11}$$

10.3.2 Time-Resolved Fluorescence Techniques

A number of experimental approaches exist by which the emission may be resolved in time. Broadly speaking these time-resolved fluorescence methods can be categorized as operating in either the time or frequency domain. In the time domain, there are numerous techniques that can be further categorized as discussed below. The choice of the most appropriate method depends on a number of factors that will be outlined in this section.

Frequency Domain Methods Frequency domain methods exhibit many attractive features and have gained popularity over many years, particularly among the biological community. For more detailed discussion the reader is referred to [3, 14, 15]. The early development and subsequent popularity of this approach largely stem from the influence of one of the fathers of fluorescence science, Gregorio Weber [16]. Frequency domain methods rely on the delay in the emission following photoexcitation, resulting from the finite lifetime of the intervening excited singlet state. The light source is modulated at some frequency and so the emitted light will also be modulated at this same frequency, only with some phase lag δ and some loss in the depth of the modulation relative to the (promptly) scattered excitation light, as depicted in Figure 10.3.

Both the phase shift δ and the relative demodulation D are related to the fluorescence lifetime τ_f and the modulation frequency (in hertz) f through Eqs. 10.12 and 10.13:

$$D = \text{relative demodulation} = \frac{D_f}{D_s} = \frac{1}{\sqrt{1 + 4\pi^2 f^2\tau_f^2}} \tag{10.12}$$

where D_s and D_f relate the maximum and minimum intensities of scattered light and the fluorescence, respectively; that is, $D_s = (S_{\max} - S_{\min})/(S_{\max} + S_{\min})$ and $D_f = (F_{\max} - F_{\min})/(F_{\max} + F_{\min})$:

$$\tan\,\delta = 2\pi f\tau_f \tag{10.13}$$

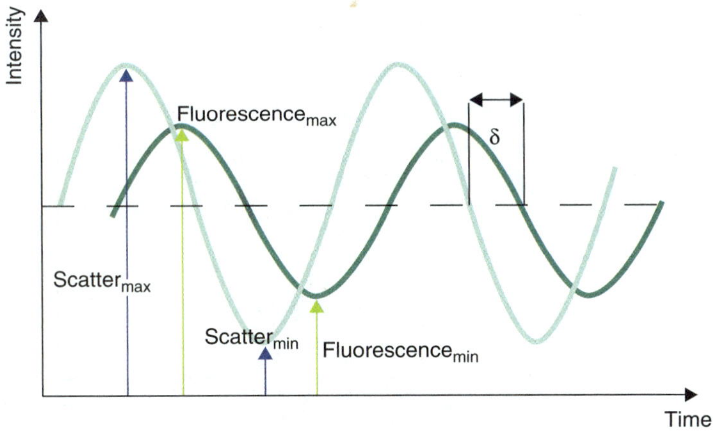

Figure 10.3 Schematic of concept of frequency domain time-resolved measurements.

The gain of the detector is modulated at the same (homodyne) or at a slightly different (heterodyne) frequency [17]. For the most precise measurements, both the phase and demodulation can be recorded and analyzed simultaneously to extract the fluorescence lifetime τ_f. The optimum modulation frequency for a given experiment depends on the fluorescence lifetime of the given sample and can be chosen using the equation:

$$f = \frac{1}{2\pi\tau_f} \qquad (10.14)$$

Since fluorescence lifetimes are usually of the order of nanoseconds or picoseconds, modulation frequencies of hundreds of megahertz are commonly used, although frequency domain instruments operating up to several gigahertz using the high-frequency components inherent in high-repetition-rate, short-duration pulse light sources (e.g., mode-locked lasers or synchrotrons) [18] and high-bandwidth detectors have also been reported [19].

To resolve the components of more complex (e.g., multiexponential) decay functions, phase and demodulation measurements performed over a range of frequencies are necessary [20, 21]. In many cases the phase and demodulation are analyzed as a function of a range of frequencies and plots of the type shown in Figure 10.4 analyzed globally [22].

A number of advantages of frequency domain methods over time domain equivalents have been discussed elsewhere [23], which perhaps partially accounts for the popularity of this approach. One of the main advantages of the frequency domain approach is that the influence of the finite pulse width, substructure, and jitter associated with the detector and electronics need not be taken into account. Compare this with time domain measurements in which the convolution of the instrument response function (IRF; Figure 10.1*e*) with the actual decay model function [24], as discussed below, is necessary. This also circumvents the problems associated with determining a suitable IRF at the appropriate wavelength, which is also a recognized problem in time domain techniques. In frequency domain measurements, very high accuracy in the phase and in the modulation frequency determination is achieved relatively easily, meaning that fewer photons are required to achieve a desired accuracy in the recovered parameters

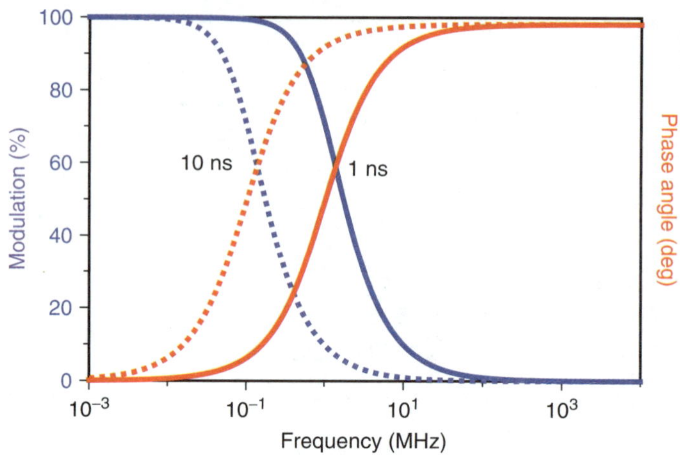

Figure 10.4 Modulation (blue) and phase angle (red) as function of modulation frequency for fluorescence decay times of 1 ns (solid line) and 10 ns (dashed line).

[23]. Also frequency domain methods are often regarded as having superior ability to resolve lifetimes that are not significantly different from one another.

Time Domain Methods In the time domain approach the examined quantity is the time decay of the fluorescence intensity, produced in response to an excitation pulse, as shown in Figure 10.1. Although simple in principle, in this method a serious challenge to be overcome is related to the low intensity of emitted light throughout the $I(t)$ decay profile. The different methods used in the time domain approach attempt to handle the extremely low time-dependent signal in different ways. Low-pulse-repetition-rate laser sources may deliver enough energy within a short (e.g., nanosecond) pulse to create a sufficiently large population of excited-state molecules that the entire time-dependent fluorescence signal has enough intensity to be measured for each individual laser pulse. The detected emission intensity is then recorded on a digital oscilloscope or other form of transient digitizer, through which several pulse events can be averaged to improve signal-to-noise (S/N). This approach, which can be referred to as "impulse response," requires detectors such as a photomultiplier tube or photodiode with suitably rapid temporal characteristics while maintaining adequate detection sensitivity. This often requires a compromise between the required gain and the desired temporal response since the time response of the oscilloscope is proportional to the product of the resistance R and capacitance C of the input, and the gain (or voltage deflection) is proportional to the product of the current I produced by the photodetector and the termination resistance R. Usually, 50 Ω termination is used rather than the common value of input impedance in many oscilloscopes of 1 MΩ. These time response signals can suffer from S/N problems and are inherently restricted in time resolution principally by the detector rise and fall time and the bandwidth of the electronics. In order to increase the S/N, it is tempting to increase the input pulse energy, which has severe consequences relating to sample damage. High-repetition-rate pulsed sources, such as a mode-locked laser, synchrotron, nanosecond light-emitting diode (LED), or picosecond laser diode, rarely provide enough energy per pulse to generate sufficient emission signal to be resolved using "impulse response" detection methods. Under

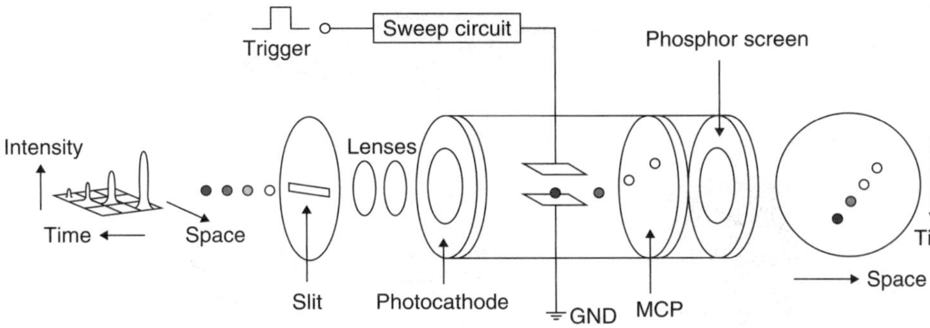

Figure 10.5 Schematic of space and time information provided by streak camera.

such circumstances, other time domain approaches implemented in specialised devices are required. These are described below.

Streak Cameras A streak camera is a device capable of resolving fluorescence down to subpicosecond timescales. These devices can be operated in an impulse response mode or synchronized to a high-repetition-rate light source [25, 26]. A schematic diagram of a streak camera is shown in Figure 10.5. In such devices, the emission is converted to an electric signal beginning with the generation of an electron beam by the focused light impinging on a photocathode in the streak tube. The number of photoelectrons generated at the photocathode is proportional to the intensity of the incident light. In the streak tube these electrons are accelerated and directed toward a phosphor screen. A high-speed voltage ramp, which is synchronized to the arrival of the incident light, is applied across the electron beam. This sweep voltage deflects the electrons producing an intensity image with a time-dependent position on a phosphor screen. This so-called streak image shows the intensity distribution of the incident light, by which the positions of the electrons can be determined in one direction over the passage of time. The emission from the phosphor streak image is then detected with a sensitive array detector such as a charge-coupled device (CCD) camera. Using this method, the temporal intensity distribution of the light being measured can be displayed as the spatial intensity distribution on the phosphor screen.

Streak cameras are capable of providing excellent time resolution, in some cases down to hundreds of femtoseconds, but are an expensive option and their applicability is somewhat limited, particularly since it is often the case in synchroscan systems that the device is designed for a quite specific pulse repetition rate. Signal-to-noise issues can also be problematic in some cases.

Gated Optical Intensifiers Another sensitive light detection device capable of fast time resolution is the gated optical intensifier (GOI) or intensified charge-coupled device (ICCD) camera. Light incident on the photocathode of the detector is converted to photoelectrons, which are amplified through the channels of a microchannel plate (MCP; Figure 10.6) before impinging on a phosphor, the emission of which is integrated within the CCD camera.

The intensifier can be thought of as a very fast shutter in the context of conventional photography, and its gain is triggered in synchrony with the excitation pulse, and through accurate digital delay electronics, the width and delay of the amplification

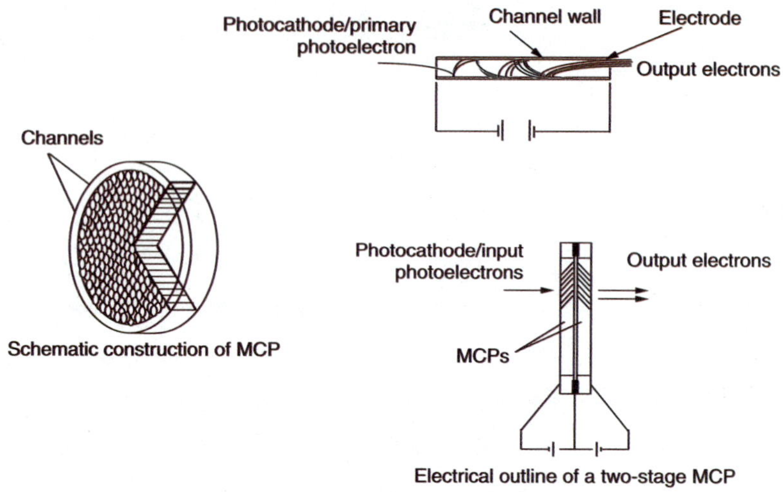

Figure 10.6 Schematic of principle behind microchannel plate photomultiplier tubes.

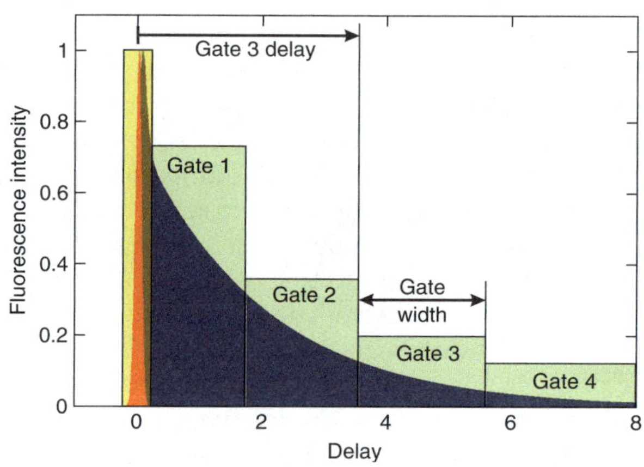

Figure 10.7 Schematic of gated or boxcar description of time-resolved fluorescence measurements.

(gain) period can be adjusted. The intensity at a given delay is integrated in the pixels of the CCD over a given number of excitation pulses, and the intensity decay profile is built up on an image-by-image basis by incrementing the delay between excitation and triggering of the intensifier. This is the so-called boxcar mode depicted in Figure 10.7, taking its name from the similar configuration established using boxcar integrators. Devices capable of being triggered at high (megahertz) repetition rates and with gate widths as short as <100 ps are available [27]. Other devices operate at lower repetition rates (~10 s of Hz) and with gate widths of a few nanoseconds [28, 29].

Photon Counting As discussed, one of the most attractive advantages of fluorescence detection is that it is essentially a background-free technique and can be implemented with extreme sensitivity since light can be detected and resolved in time at the single-photon level using a variety of devices. Some CCD cameras can operate at close to single-photon levels, and the single photons can be integrated in each pixel (as discussed above for GOIs). Alternatively, the individual photons in each pixel can simply be counted using a single-element photon-counting detector such as a photomultiplier tube (PMT), MCP, or single-photon avalanche photodiode (SPAD). Single-photon counting on its own is, however, incapable of providing temporal resolution and additional provisions need to be made to extract the desired time-dependence of the fluorescence. The most common of these is time-correlated single-photon counting (TCSPC), or single-photon timing [3, 24, 30]. TCSPC is an extremely sensitive technique with time resolution down to a few picoseconds, limited essentially by the transit time spread induced by the time response of the photodetector and electronics. TCSPC is a flexible method that can be applied to a wide variety of experimental configurations, including microscopy. It relies on the ability to accurately time the arrival of single photons of fluorescence relative to the time of photo-excitation of the sample. Under these conditions, the probability of each excitation pulse generating a single photon emission event is significantly less than unity (typically 1% probability). Thus each excitation/single-photon detection event provides one count. A fast electronic ramp [time-to-amplitude converter (TAC)] is activated upon excitation of the sample and stopped upon detection of the single photon of emission. An electrical pulse with a voltage that is proportional to the time between the start and stop events is sent to a multichannel analyzer which associates one count in the appropriate channel corresponding to the voltage of the pulse from the TAC (Figure 10.8). The electronics are reset and the excitation, timing, and channel allocation process is repeated over a large number of excitation events until a sufficient number of counts in each channel has been acquired. The resulting data represent a histogram of the number of counts versus channel number (which is proportional to the voltage of the input pulses, and hence the time after excitation that photon detection events have occurred). Since the probability of an emission event occurring is highest immediately after the excited state is formed and decreases with time thereafter, this histogram reflects the decay of the fluorescence intensity, from which the fluorescence decay parameters, such as the fluorescence decay time, can be recovered through curve-fitting analysis. Since this is a highly statistical process, the S/N can be improved simply by increasing the number of excitation events (i.e., counting for longer periods). The use of high-repetition-rate light sources is exploited to great advantage allowing high rates of excitation and single-photon detection. The time resolution of this method is limited by the transit

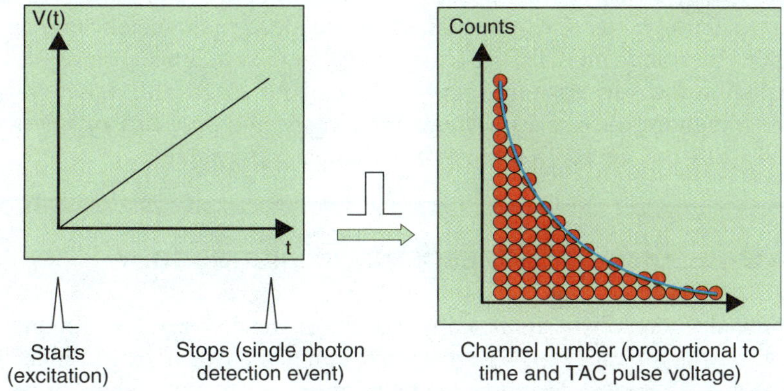

Figure 10.8 Schematic of principle of time-correlated single-photon counting

time spread of the detection system, which is itself a convolution of the detector timing characteristics (not its actual rise or fall time), and the jitter associated with the various electronics components. Following appropriate data analysis and through use of the best MCP or SPAD detector, decay time components down to a few picoseconds are achievable.

In modern TCSPC electronics [31, 32], the collected photon counts can be tagged with a variety of additional information, including the detector from which they originate. Coupled with multielement detectors [33], a series of fluorescence decay profiles recorded at, for example, a series of emission wavelengths can be collected simultaneously. This potentially increases dramatically the rigor with which several decays can be analyzed simultaneously and globally [22].

One advantage of time domain methods such as TCSPC over frequency domain measurements is that data are, to some, more intuitive to interpret since they are represented as the fluorescence intensity decay as a function of time from which nonexponentialities might be more readily identified. As mentioned above, one important distinction between the frequency domain and all time domain methods is that the timing response of the detection system must be taken into account in the latter (Figure 10.1*e*). That is, the fluorescence decay will be corrupted by the finite width and substructure of the IRF. In such cases the measured decay profile $I(t)$ is actually a "convolution" of the IRF, $P(t)$, with the true fluorescence decay $F(t)$:

$$I(t) = P(t) \otimes F(t) = \int_0^t P(t')F(t - t')\,dt' \tag{10.15}$$

where $\otimes$ indicates a convolution and t' is a "dummy" time variable.

To derive the true decay profile $F(t)$, the effect of $P(t)$ must be removed, or deconvolved from $I(t)$, which adds complexity to the analysis of the decay curve. Several methods by which Eq. 10.15 can be solved to extract the decay parameters have been developed, with varying degrees of success, versatility, and computational complexity, and are dealt with in detail elsewhere [24, 30]. Generally the method of choice is *nonlinear least squares iterative reconvolution* (NLLSIR) whereby a model function is selected (e.g., a single exponential; Eq. 10.4) and initial guesses made for each parameter to be determined (e.g., fluorescence lifetime τ_f and amplitude). This function is then convoluted with the IRF and the resulting profile compared to the experimental decay. The deviation between the convoluted and experimental curves is minimized through iterative adjustment of the decay parameters until a selected convergence criterion is met. This process can be applied to a wide range of functional forms, including the various nonexponential functions discussed above. With use of appropriate weighting factors to account for the specific statistics of the acquisition method, NLLSIR can be applied to any time domain technique.

10.4 TIME-RESOLVED FLUORESCENCE IN MICROSCOPY

In conventional fluorescence microscopy, the fluorescence *intensity* is monitored as a function of location of a focused light source over a given region of a sample. This may be achieved in a range of experimental configurations, employing lamps or lasers as the excitation source, combined with far-field, near-field, confocal, and even multiphoton detection techniques. In these fluorescence microscopy methods, the emission intensity recorded at each spatial location is produced by the integration of all photons emitted within the duration of the excitation and over the entire emission period (given by the fluorescence lifetime) of the excited state. Another way of expressing this is that the fluorescence quantum yield of a fluorophore is proportional to the integrated area under the fluorescence decay profile, which from integration of Eq. 10.4 over all times gives a value of $A\tau$. These imaging modes are therefore described as "steady-state" methods.

If the temporal information contained in the fluorescence decay can be recorded as a function of spatial location in a sample, fluorescence images can be acquired that correspond to different times after photo-excitation. This *time-resolved fluorescence microscopy* (TRFM) mode has developed substantially in recent years into a mature form of imaging, available commercially using a range of both wide-field, multifocal [34] and laser scanning methods. These latter methods can be applied to scanning single- and multiphoton excitation as well as methods exceeding the diffraction limit of spatial resolution by use of techniques such as scanning near-field optical microscopy (SNOM) [35]. TRFM methods have also been applied to the rapidly developing "superresolution" techniques based on structured illumination [36].

The discussion in Section 10.3.1 serves to highlight both the advantages and potential difficulties in applying time-resolved fluorescence concepts to fluorescence imaging. It is worth noting that TRFM is more commonly termed *fluorescence lifetime imaging microscopy* (FLIM), but as discussed, it is not uncommon, especially in situations common in microscopy, that a single fluorescence "lifetime" is not observed, and so the term "fluorescence lifetime imaging" is somewhat of a misnomer and so should be treated with some caution. For this reason, the term *time-resolved fluorescence imaging* is preferred and used by the authors.

A variety of methods exist for achieving the time-resolved fluorescence mode of imaging, based on the methods of time-resolved fluorescence detection discussed above. The main methods of TRFM are discussed below. It is important to recognize that all the various methods available for TRFM have their advantages and shortcomings, thus making no single method ideal for all circumstances or sample types. Ultimately, each method relies on its ability to collect enough fluorescence signal in each location on the sample from which the required temporal detail can be extracted. In all cases this is fundamentally limited by the number of photons being emitted by the sample within the dwell time of the excitation source on each specific spatial location in the sample. An excellent review of the various TRFM techniques is available elsewhere [37].

Frequency domain detection can be adapted to TRFM applications whereby the analysis of the phase shift (and/or relative demodulation) is performed at each specific location of the focused excitation source. Frequency domain TRFM instruments have been developed that employ either single- or multichannel (ICCD) detection. Single-channel detection using, for example, PMTs can be implemented by scanning the excitation source over the sample (e.g., using x,y galvo scanners) or scanning the sample (e.g., using a three-dimensional piezoelectric scanner unit) and the signal analyzed as a function of the pixel location [17]. Alternatively, MCP [19] or ICCD [27] devices may be operated up to the gigahertz regime in wide-field microscopy configurations [38]. Some low-cost alternative frequency domain devices for TRFM applications have also been reported recently [39, 40] which promise to bring this mode of TRFM into increasingly wide use.

A large range of time domain TRFM methods exist based on the various concepts discussed above. Impulse response methods have been used for TRFM [41] as well as phosphorescence imaging, as discussed elsewhere [14], but are generally limited in time resolution (specifically by the detector used), the S/N achievable, and instrumental artefacts. Streak cameras are reasonably widely used for bulk fluorescence decay measurements but can also be used for TRFM whereby an optical image is generated by recording a streak image, providing the intensity, location, and time information, at every pixel. TRFM applications using a streak camera with 20-ps resolution have been reported [25], but this mode is not in wide use, possibly related to the expense and complexity of correct operation of such devices.

The "gated" or "boxcar" concept of time-resolved fluorescence illustrated in Figure 10.7 can be applied to fluorescence imaging applications using a variety of detection modes. If fluorophores with different fluorescence lifetimes are present in different locations, then it can be envisaged that an image generated from photons emitted at long times after excitation might look significantly different to one generated from photons emitted immediately after excitation since the fluorescence of the short-lived species will have decayed and therefore will not be present at late times. In addition, if scattered light, be it Raman or Rayleigh scatter, is prevalent, then this time-gated approach can be used to gate short-timescale information (dominated by scatter; Figure 10.1c) from fluorescence (longer timescale signal) as illustrated by the yellow and blue portions shown in Figure 10.7.

Gated emission can be implemented in the impulse response approach by integrating the intensity of emission within a period using a boxcar averaging unit or the capabilities of modern digital oscilloscopes. GOIs [42] operating at low repetition rates ($\sim$10 s of Hz) and with gate widths of a few nanoseconds [28, 29] or at high (kilohertz-to-megahertz) repetition rates and with gate widths as short as $<$100 ps [27] are attractive devices for time-resolved fluorescence imaging [36]. In such devices a series of images is acquired sequentially by incrementally increasing the delay of the triggering of the intensifier relative to the excitation event. Each individual gated image can be acquired in a short time depending on the integration time required to generate adequate S/N. The generation of a complete series of gated images can be achieved in a matter of seconds to minutes. Alternatively, just one early and one late gated image may be acquired and a "lifetime" image generated assuming a simple decay relationship between the intensities at the two time gates in each pixel of the image. GOI (ICCD) devices are not suitable for conventional scanning confocal imaging; however, they can be used for nondescanned multiphoton imaging or multifocal [34] confocal (or multiphoton) imaging. The other mode of confocal imaging appropriate for such devices is Nipkow disk scanning confocal imaging [43], whereby the emission is distributed over the ICCD element and an image is generated rapidly.

An example of a time-resolved fluorescence image of an onion skin stained with ethidium bromide and Nile red and collected using such an ICCD system operated in the time domain is shown in Figure 10.9. The excitation source used was the visible output of a femtosecond optical parametric amplifier (Coherent RegA/OPA 9400). The intensifier was synchronized to the operating laser pulse repetition rate of 250 kHz and a series of images was collected with sequential acquisition using a gate width of $\sim$200 ps and steps in the delay of 100 ps. Upon intercalation, ethidium bromide locates within the cell nuclei and exhibits a small emission spectral shift (610–595 nm), which restricts the ability to spectrally isolate the emission. However, the bound form

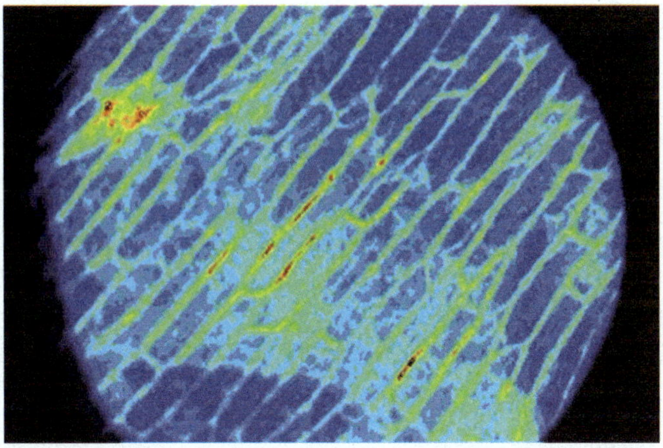

Figure 10.9 Time-resolved fluorescence imaging of onion skin stained with fluorescent probes ethidium bromide and Nile red.

undergoes an enhancement in ϕ_f of ~20 times and an increase in fluorescence lifetime τ_f from 1.8 to ~23 ns compared to the unbound form. Nile red is a lipid environment probe that exhibits enhanced emission in low-polarity regions (τ_f ~ 1.8 compared with 4.2 ns). The different emission decay times represented on a false-color scale from blue (short, ~2 ns) to red (long, ~20 ns) are clearly discernible in the figure.

Photon-counting modes can be exploited in a range of remarkably sensitive TRFM methods. De Grauw and Gerritsen [44] have developed a gated method that exploits the sensitivity of photon counting coupled with fast switching and accurate digital delay chips. This method enables the recording of time-resolved fluorescence information on the subnanosecond to microsecond timescales, on a pixel-by-pixel basis at high count rates, and with a high detection efficiency. This method is therefore applicable to single-channel detection in microscopy modes in which the focused spot or sample is scanned, such as confocal or multiphoton fluorescence imaging. Typically four images, corresponding to four time gates of Figure 10.7, are collected simultaneously, from which a "lifetime image" can be generated using the four intensity values corresponding to each pixel. This concept, illustrated in Figure 10.10, is now marketed commercially as the LIMO system by Nikon [45].

The advantage of this approach is that all single-photon counts are used and the four images are generated simultaneously, in contrast to the sequential gating approach commonly used for GOIs. Sample exposure is thereby reduced compared to many other methods, making this approach attractive for photolabile or moving samples. An example of where this gated technique of TRFM has proved effective in this respect is in the study of a chlorinated merino wool fiber excited at 280 nm and emission collected between 300 and 600 nm (Figure 10.11). Figures 10.11*a*, *b*, and *c* are images corresponding to increasing delays of 1.2 ns after excitation, and Figure 10.11*d* is the lifetime merged images generated from Figures 10.11*a*, *b* and *c*. This illustrates how scattered excitation light can be filtered through temporal discrimination. The image in the second channel is somewhat sharper than the first, which is corrupted by scattered light. Scattered light is especially prevalent in the current example, which was collected using a new "deep UV" confocal microscope operating at 280 nm. The high photon

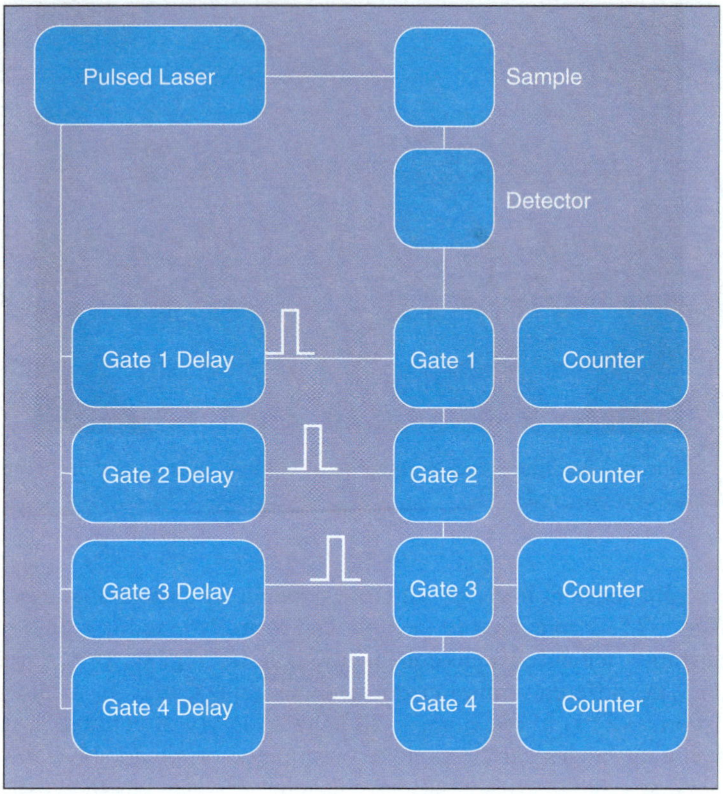

Figure 10.10 Schematic of gated photon counting technique (LIMO).

energy involved in UV confocal microscopy necessarily limits the exposure that each pixel can withstand without photodegradation, yet this TRFM approach proved effective in acquiring images of adequate S/N using the endogenous emission of the components of the wool. That is, no artificial fluorescence labeling was required.

Limitations of the method result from the relatively long gate duration currently achievable with the digital delay circuitry and from the limited number of gate and counter channels. The limited number of time elements restricts the rigor with which decay functions more complex than a simple exponential decay (as discussed in Section 10.3.1) can be analyzed. TCSPC, on the other hand, records many more time elements. Single PC-based cards based on TCSPC detection are marketed [31, 32] that are capable of recording a complete fluorescence decay profile of typically several hundred to a few thousand time channels for every pixel of a scanned array (e.g., 256×256 pixels). This enables time-gated images at any chosen delay and gate width to be generated post data collection. Due to the high level of temporal information recorded by TCSPC, this method also represents the best opportunity to analyze data on the basis of the complex decay functions discussed earlier that can result from (or be used to model) processes such as energy transfer. In order to implement accurate NLLSIR analysis (especially for the more complex model functions), a minimum of several hundreds or thousands of counts per time channel must be acquired. If the

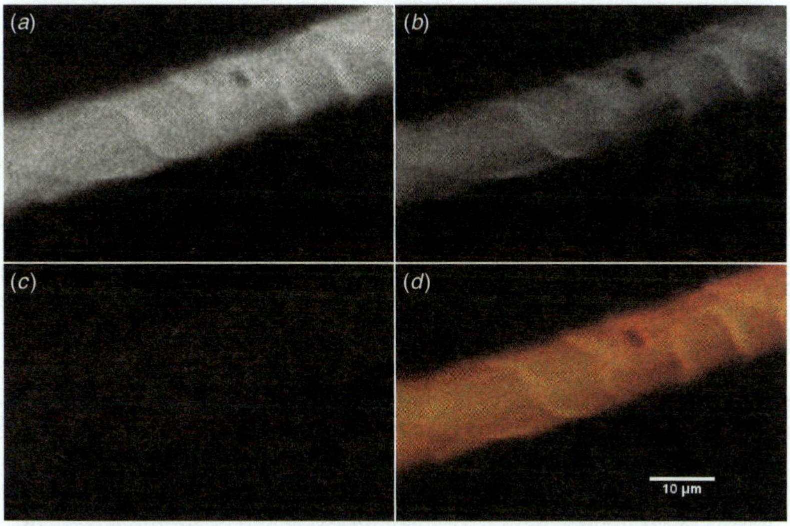

Figure 10.11 TRFM image of wool fiber recorded using LIMO method: (*a*–*c*) increased delays of 1.2 ns; (*d*) lifetime merge of (*a*)–(*c*).

decay is collected into several hundred time channels and over a reasonable number of pixels, photon count rates must be quite high—something that is not readily achievable in many samples. This highlights one major disadvantage of the TCSPC approach, namely that, in order to acquire a sufficient S/N ratio in each pixel, in the absence of high photon count rates, long data acquisition times or multiple scans are often required (depending on the sample's emission and detection efficiency), which can limit this method's applicability in photolabile or rapidly moving samples.

This approach has been used in a diverse range of fields following scanning single- and multiphoton fluorescence studies. Examples of such images are given in Figure 10.12 generated following two-photon excitation of the endogenous fluorescence of full-thickness dermatomed sections of human abdominal skin. This was achieved using a TCSPC card [31] in conjunction with a mode-locked

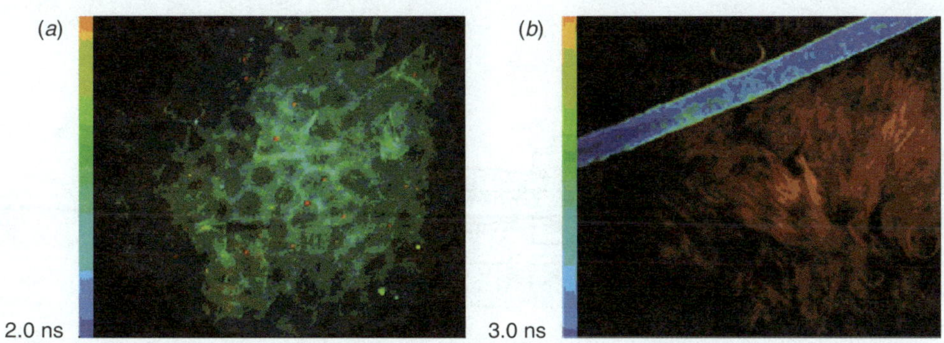

Figure 10.12 Time resolved fluorescence images: (*a*) reconstructed from autofluorescence present in stratum corneum of human abdominal skin; (*b*) of single human hair over collagen fibers.

Ti–sapphire laser operating at 780 nm [46]. Figure 10.12*a* was acquired at a depth of 2 μm relative to the skin surface. The pseudocolor mapping represents that of the weighted average τ_m of the short, τ_1, and the long, τ_2, exponential decay components. Individual corneocytes are clearly visualized in the stratum corneum, as are small scattering contaminants on the skin surface. Figure 10.12*b* shows a time-resolved fluorescence image of a single human hair over collagen fibers. The blue line (longer lifetime) is due to endogenous emission from human hair, which is easily distinguished from the second-harmonic generated (SHG) signal produced by the collagen fibers (orange, very short time scale) or any light scattering (instantaneous).

A related method of TRFM based on TCSPC using a position-sensitive picosecond MCP detector has been developed [47–49] and is available commercially [50]. Spatial information along the x,y directions can be obtained by replacing the usual disk anode of a conventional MCP with a quadrant anode. The incident photon produces a cone-shaped cloud of electrons at the output face of the second MCP. The center of this cone hits the four segments of the quadrant anode at a spatial position corresponding to that of the photon (Figure 10.13). The quadrant anode splits the electric pulse into four portions whose individual magnitudes depend on the x,y coordinate of the incident photon. The four charge packets are amplified, discriminated, and fed to an analogue circuit for calculation of the x,y coordinates from the ratio of the four charge signals.

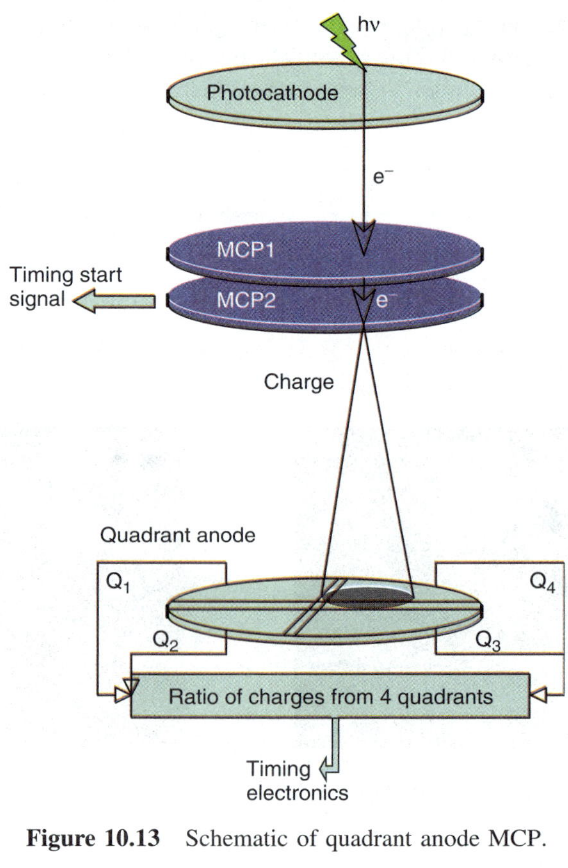

Figure 10.13 Schematic of quadrant anode MCP.

The timing information is derived from an auxiliary pulse from the second MCP that is used to start the TAC together with a stop pulse as in conventional TCSPC.

Such instruments are capable of producing an IRF with full width at half maximum (FWHM) of ~120 ps, providing a time resolution of <15 ps after convolution of the IRF is accounted for. They can also provide spatial resolution of <100 μm on the photocathode, that is, ~400 × 400 channels over an active diameter of 22 mm. Such a system has been employed in a study using wide-field photon-counting FLIM to study Förster resonance energy transfer (FRET) in fixed mammalian cells expressing either cyan fluorescent protein (CFP) or a fusion of CFP and yellow fluorescent protein (YFP) and living fungal cells expressing either Cerulean or a Cerulean–Venus fusion protein [51]. In these measurements, the high-precision FLIM data were able to reproducibly resolve multiple fluorescence decays, thereby revealing new information about the fraction of the protein population that undergoes FRET and reducing error in the measurement of donor–acceptor distances. Besides the wide-field configuration, this quadrant anode system can be implemented in a confocal mode when coupled with a Nipkow disk scanning system [43] or in picosecond fluorescence anisotropy imaging [50].

It should be noted that a conventional (steady-state) fluorescence image can still be generated through the spatial variation of the time-integrated emission intensity of any of these TRFM methods, that is, opening the gate width to cover the entire decay profile.

10.4.1 Factors That Influence Choice of TRFM Method

Important factors that influence the most appropriate choice of technique for a particular application are the required time information and resolution, the light source and detector that are available, and the photochemical/photophysical properties and stability of the sample. Another major factor is cost.

Time Resolution The required time resolution is largely dictated by the dynamics of the processes to be investigated and the emission characteristics of the sample. For example, fluorescence decay times are typically on the order of a few nanoseconds and so time resolution of a nanosecond or so may be adequate for many routine measurements. On the other hand, some emitting species can be substantially longer lived. For example, quantum dots (nanocrystals) can exhibit emission lifetimes extending to several tens of nanoseconds. It is worth mentioning in passing that the time-resolved emission imaging techniques discussed here can also be adopted to other emission regimes such as phosphorescence, which can occur on the microsecond or millisecond timescales, with an associated relaxation in the required specifications in terms of pulse width or detector temporal response. Despite nanosecond resolution being adequate for resolving emission in time for many situations, sometimes it is the purpose of the measurement to resolve the dynamics of a given process, for example, FRET, which can occur on substantially faster timescales than the typical "lifetime" of the excited state. For such purposes, ultrashort light pulses (high-frequency components) and ultrafast (broad-bandwidth) detection techniques are required.

TCSPC or frequency domain methods can generally provide the highest degree of time information at the expense of long data acquisition times. Gated methods such as the use of ICCD imaging can be configured to provide many time channels, but the overall time resolution may not be as high as that achievable with the best detectors in TCSPC or frequency domain methods. The LIMO gated method provides very few time-gated images, but it is sufficient to generate informative time-resolved fluorescence images in many cases [44] and has other benefits.

Light Source The available light source largely dictates the form of TRFM that is achievable. If a nonpulsed [i.e., continuous wave (CW)] light source, such as an LED, CW laser, or lamp, is all that is available, time-resolved fluorescence imaging can be achieved using the frequency domain methods discussed briefly above. The minimized expense and complexity of the light source and the breadth and ease of selection of excitation wavelengths of such devices are key advantages of these methods over those that operate in the time domain. The ultimate limitation in time resolution achievable is then the stability and upper frequency at which the light source and detector can be modulated, but instruments operating in the megahertz-to-gigahertz (corresponding to the nanosecond-to-picosecond) range are available.

In the time domain, other factors are important regarding the light source. The pulse duration is one such factor. Devices are now available that can produce nanosecond, picosecond, and femtosecond duration pulses at high pulse repetition rates over a range of excitation wavelengths. Among these are nanosecond flash lamps [52], nanosecond LEDs [53], picosecond laser diodes [54], mode-locked lasers, and synchrotrons. The selection of excitation wavelength can be achieved by a range of heads in the case of nanosecond LEDs or picosecond diode lasers or through tunable sources such as picosecond dye lasers, titanium–sapphire lasers, or synchrotrons. The high peak power of these latter sources affords the possibility to further convert the excitation wavelengths through nonlinear frequency conversion devices such as frequency doubling/tripling units, devices based on optical parametric processes, and continuum generation in photonic crystal fibers (PCFs) [55]. The use of these PCF devices in TRFM applications is in its infancy, but they show great promise in opening up the available excitation range available to these and other modes of microscopy.

The laser pulse repetition rate is also an important factor. This can largely dictate the specific method of time domain fluorescence imaging that is adopted. Intensified CCD cameras can sometimes be synchronised at megahertz repetition rates, although these devices are more commonly restricted to much lower repetition rates. Time domain techniques based on single-photon timing benefit from high (megahertz) repetition rate sources in order to gain sufficient photon statistics. Nanosecond LEDs can operate at pulse repetition rates of megahertz. Laser diodes, mode-locked lasers, and synchrotrons typically operate at somewhat higher pulse repetition rates (tens of megahertz). These high pulse repetition rates correspond to time intervals between the pulses of ~10 ns. Consider the fluorescence decay of a typical fluorophore and recall that while the "fluorescence lifetime" of many common fluorophores used in fluorescence microscopy may be on the order of several nanoseconds, this corresponds to the time it takes for the emission to decay to $1/e$ of its initial intensity. The emission continues for several "lifetimes" after excitation, which means that the fluorescence intensity may not have decayed completely before the next laser pulse arrives to reexcite the sample. Therefore, if a subsequent excitation pulse arrives before the emission intensity arising from the initial pulse has decayed completely, the temporal fluorescence response will be additionally complex, resulting in a so-called "sawtooth decay" (Figure 10.14). The analysis of the decay profile (and hence the fluorescence image) is then additionally complex due to the corruption of the emission decay caused by the residual

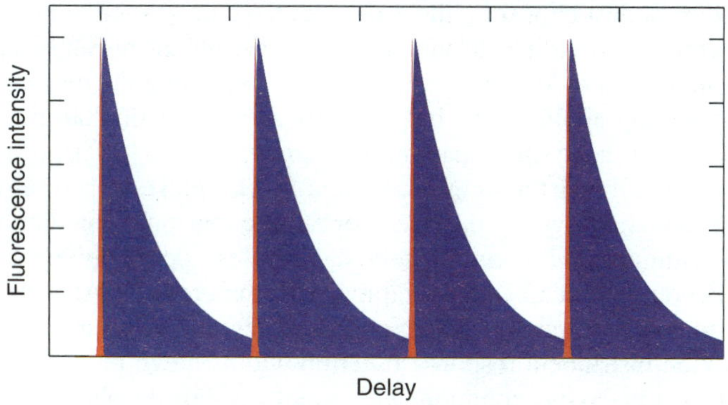

Figure 10.14 "Sawtooth" fluorescence decay resulting from interpulse separation being insufficient to allow complete decay of emission from preceding pulse.

emission from the preceding pulse. This is particularly troublesome in time-resolved fluorescence studies in which the information associated with the early times of the decay is specifically required, as is often the case in FRET experiments. Techniques of accounting for this have been reported in the literature [56], but their use is not widely adopted.

The other related problem associated with the use of high-repetition-rate pulse sources is that of saturation (or bleaching) of the ground state. This can result from a buildup of population of long-lived, "dark" intermediate species, including triplet states, radical cations, and photochemical products, and so fewer molecules will have returned to the ground state ready for absorption of another photon, and the observed emission signal intensity will therefore decrease over time.

These issues associated with pulse repetition rate are often neglected in time-resolved fluorescence microscopy and other techniques relying on the use of mode-locked lasers (including multiphoton fluorescence microscopy). Despite statements to the contrary [37], we consider it better practice to remove the problem in the first place by reducing the laser pulse repetition rate. The pulse repetition rate can be variably selected on many picosecond laser diodes or nanosecond LEDs or pulses can be selected from the pulse train with a Pockel Cell, Bragg cell pulse picker, intracavity dumper [57], or similar pulse selection device in the case of mode-locked lasers. Another attractive alternative is the use of a high-repetition-rate (100 s of kilohertz) laser amplifier that not only reduces the laser repetition rate but also overcomes losses associated with the usual pulse repetition rate reduction devices by amplifying the energy of the selected pulses.

Detector Various devices are available for the detection and ultimately the resolution of the emission in time. The choice of detector is often a compromise between the desired sensitivity, active detection area, time resolution, and the funds available. It is also related to whether time or frequency domain techniques are chosen. Intensified CCD cameras are an attractive, yet often expensive option with high-sensitivity, large active areas conducive to direct imaging applications and reasonably good time resolution (down to ~80 ps dependent on repetition rate) [27]. Photomultiplier tubes capable of time resolution in the nanosecond to ~200-ps scales are routinely available. For improved time resolution, the MCP photomultiplier is often preferred; however, these devices are expensive and are susceptible to damage by excessive exposure to light. Even under modest exposure, these devices have only a limited lifespan. Suitable devices are marketed providing, in the best case, instrument response function widths of ~25 ps. Avalanche photodiodes are increasingly becoming the detectors of choice in many photon-counting applications, but they still have their limitations. These devices are reasonably robust, have high quantum efficiency, require lower power supply voltages, and produce a transistor–transistor logic (TTL) pulse in response to a photon being detected, which alleviates the need for subsequent pulse modification (e.g., the need for a discriminator). For time-resolved purposes, single-photon avalanche photodiodes are becoming increasingly common. Commercial SPADs have impressive specifications in terms of photon detection efficiency and, with active quenching circuitry, can provide instrument response function widths down to ~10 s of picoseconds FWHM [58–60]. One issue common with many avalanche photodiodes is the size of their active area. This is especially important in time-resolved applications since the temporal response is generally inversely related to the device's active area. For example, the active area of the highest time resolution SPADs is only tens of micrometres. This has implications on the efficiency with which the fluorescence photons may be presented to the detector; however, they are ideally suited to applications where the emission is in the form of a point source, such as single-molecule imaging and when the emission is confined to an optical fiber. Another problem reported with these devices is a long, count rate–dependent diffusion tail in the IRF which cannot be readily accounted for in the convolution process [61].

Properties of Sample A number of issues relating to the nature of the sample are also worthy of consideration. The photophysical and photochemical properties of the sample and the intensity of the light source also influence the success or otherwise of the TRFM experiment. This primarily relates to the photostability of the sample. The quantum yield and absorption cross section of the sample can also influence the selection of the most appropriate technique. A sample that moves, degrades, or otherwise changes within the time frame of the imaging experiment dictates that a rapid collection technique be employed and that multiple scans cannot be carried out. In many cases this may make the TCSPC method less effective than the LIMO or ICCD approaches. On the other hand, if a high degree of rigor is required in the analysis of the time decay of the sample, TCSPC or frequency domain imaging methods might be a more appropriate choice.

Cost Despite the indisputable power of TRFM, most methods discussed above involve a high level of instrumentation and expertise, making this a reasonably expensive mode of microscopy in terms of equipment. However, this is a rapidly developing area and the costs are expected to reduce with the advancements made. Most methods require short pulse light sources, but the range of such sources is increasing and the cost decreasing. The frequency domain approach, which does not necessarily require ultrashort pulsed sources, is perhaps the most promising area in which significant cost savings can be made, in terms of both the light source and the mode of detection [39, 40]. Multiphoton microscopes are becoming increasingly common in biotechnology laboratories, and the required mode-locked laser is one of the major expenses of this mode of microscopy; however, the size, cost, and complexity of these systems are

TABLE 10.1 Summary of Advantages and Disadvantages of Various Methods of TRFM

TRFM Method	Light Source	Sample Properties[a]	Temporal Resolution	Imaging Modes	Cost
Frequency domain	Wide choice of tunable CV or mode locked[b]	—[b]	Picosecond resolution with GHz detection[b]	Wide-field or scanning confocal or multiphoton[b]	Moderate for MHz, expensive for GHz, potentially very reasonable [39, 40]
Impulse response methods	Low repetition rate, high energy per pulse (μJ–mJ)	Potential for sample damage, high concentrations	Time response limited by detector (typically to ns)	Low spatial resolution	Reasonable[b]
Streak camera	Low repetition rate, intense, or high repetition rate, synchroscan	—	Typically ps but about 200 fs possible[b]		Expensive ($100 s of thousands), difficult to use properly
Gated optical imaging	Low repetition rate, ns mJ systems High repetition rate (kHz to MHz), nJ systems	Minimized sample exposure possible	Nanosecond or $\sim$100 ps (depends on repetition rate)[b]	Wide-field or spinning disk or multifocal confocal/multiphoton	Expensive ($10 s–100 s of thousands)
Gated photon counting	High repetition rate, low energy, single channel	Minimized sample exposure[b]	Subnanosecond few time channels	Confocal, multiphoton, near field	Moderate ($10 s–100 s of thousands)
TCSPC	High repetition rate, low energy, single-channel detection	Potential for sample damage, by long/multiple exposure	10 s–100 s of picoseconds[b]	Confocal, multiphoton, near field	Moderate ($10 s of thousands)
Quadrant anode MCP	High repetition rate, low energy	—	100 s of picoseconds	Wide field	($100 s of thousands), relatively undeveloped

[a] Signifies a clear benefit.
[b] Affected by quantum yield, absorption cross section, photostability, aggregation, motion (live cell), acquisition time, and penetration depth/opacity.

reducing rapidly. The short pulses can be exploited more fully through the implementation of TRFM for a relatively modest additional investment. The cost of expertise and personnel is also an important consideration since the analysis of time-resolved fluorescence data can be inherently complex, especially when performed rigorously. Skill must be acquired in the generation and interpretation of time-resolved fluorescence images.

The various criteria discussed illustrate why no single method of TRFM is ideal for all imaging situations, but usually one method will exhibit distinct advantages over others. In light of the discussion above, Table 10.1 summarizes which methods are most beneficial in addressing each of the factors to be considered when selecting the most appropriate method of TRFM.

10.5 CONCLUSIONS

Time-resolved fluorescence imaging is a mature, yet still rapidly developing microscopy modality. It is applicable to and becoming more widely employed in many disciplines including the biomolecular sciences. As excitation sources and detection instrumentation develop further and costs are reduced, the popularity of the mode will only increase due to the additional information and discrimination provided compared to conventional (steady-state) fluorescence imaging. Although more commonly termed fluorescence lifetime imaging (FLIM), it has been illustrated that there are several phenomena that can complicate the temporal decay of the emission beyond a simple, single fluorescence lifetime. The term FLIM might therefore be considered as an oversimplification or misnomer, although it has been generally adopted throughout the fluorescence imaging community. There are numerous techniques operating in either the frequency or time domain that can be implemented. It is most common that one particular mode is adopted within a given laboratory (with a few exceptions). However, it is stressed that each method has its intrinsic advantages and disadvantages, and therefore no single technique is ideally suitable to every TRFM application or scenario. Ultimately, the limiting factor is the number of fluorescence photons that can be generated within each pixel of the image. There are numerous factors that influence the most appropriate method for a given situation, which influence the collection of these photons, and these have been discussed.

REFERENCES

1. D. K. Bird, K. M. Agg, N. W. Barnett, and T. A. Smith, "Time-resolved fluoresence microscopy of gunshot residue: An application to forensic science," *J. Microsc.* **226**, 18 (2007).
2. L. Toniolo, A. Sansonetti, R. Cubeddu, G. Valentini, and D. Comelli, "FLIM—fluorescence lifetime imaging," in *Exploring David. Diagnostic Tests and State of Conservation*, S. Bracci, F. Falletti, M. Matteini, and R. Scopigno (Eds.), Giunti Editore S.p.A., Florence-Milan, 2004, p. 154.
3. J. R. Lakowicz, *Principles of Fluorescence Spectroscopy*, 3rd ed., Springer, Singapore, 2006.
4. B. Valeur, *Molecular Fluorescence*, Wiley-VCH, Brisbane, 2002.

5. L. E. Bennett, K. P. Ghiggino, and R. W. Henderson, "Singlet oxygen formation in monomeric and aggregated prophyrin c," *J. Photochem. Photobiol. B: Biol.* **3**, 81 (1989).
6. D. R. James, Y.-S. Jiu, P. De Mayo, and W. R. Ware, "Distributions of fluorescence lifetimes: Consequences for the photophysics of molecules adsorbed on surfaces," *Chem. Phys. Lett.* **120**, 460 (1985).
7. B. D. Wagner, D. R. James, and W. R. Ware, "Fluorescence lifetime distributions in homotry-tophan derivatives," *Chem. Phys. Lett.* **138**, 181 (1987).
8. A. K. Livesey and J. C. Bochon, "Analyzing the distribution of decay constants in pulse-fluorimetry using the maximum entropy method," *Biophys. J.* **52**, 693 (1987).
9. A. Siemiarczuk, B. D. Wagner, and W. R. Ware, "Comparison of the maximum entropy and exponential series methods for recovery of distributions of lifetimes from fluorescence lifetime data," *J. Phys. Chem.* **94**, 1661 (1990).
10. D. Klostermerier and D. P. Millar, "Time-resolved fluorescence resonance energy transfer: A versatile tool for the analysis of nucleic acids," *Biopolymers* **61**, 159 (2002).
11. M. Hauser, U. Klein, and U. Gösele, "Extension of Förster's theory of long-range energy-transfer to donor-acceptor pairs in systems of molecular dimensions," *Z. Phys. Chem.* **101**, 255 (1976).
12. M. Yokota and O. Tanimoto, "Effects of diffusion on energy transfer by resonance," *J. Phys. Soc. Jpn.* **22**, 779 (1967).
13. A. Sillen and Y. Engelborghs, "The correct use of 'average' fluorescence parameters," *Photochem. Photobiol.* **67**, 475 (1998).
14. T. W. J. Gadella, T. M. Jovin, and R. M. Clegg, "Fluorescence lifetime imaging microscopy (FLIM): Spatial resolution of microstructures on the nanosecond time scale," *Biophys. Chem.* **48**, 221 (1993).
15. X. F. Wang and B. Herman, *Fluorescence Imaging Spectroscopy and Microscopy*, Wiley-Interscience, New York, 1996.
16. R. D. Spencer and G. Weber, "Measurements of subnanosecond fluorescence lifetimes with a cross-correlation phase fluorometer," *Ann. N.Y. Acad. Sci.* **158**, 361 (1969).
17. P. T. C. So, T. French, W. M. Yu, K. M. Berland, C. Y. Dong, and E. Gratton, "Two-photon fluorescence microscopy: Time-resolved and intensity imaging," in *Fluorescence Imaging Spectroscopy and Microscopy*, X. F. Wang and B. Herman (Eds.), Wiley, New York, 1996, p. 351.
18. J. R. Alcala and E. Gratton, "A multifrequency phase fluorometer using the harmonic content of a mode-locked laser," *Anal. Inst.* **14**, 225 (1985).
19. G. Laczko, I. Gryczynski, Z. Gryczynski, W. Wiczk, H. Malak, and J. R. Lakowicz, "A 10 GHz frequency domain fluorometer," *Rev. Sci. Instrum.* **61**, 2331 (1990).
20. G. Weber, "Resolution of the fluorescence lifetimes in a heterogeneous system by phase and modulation microscopy," *J. Phys. Chem.* **85**, 949 (1981).
21. A. Squire, P. J. Verveer, and P. I. H. Bastiens, "Multiple frequency fluorescence lifetime imaging microscopy," *J. Microsc.* **197**, 136 (1997).
22. E. Gratton, "Globals for spectroscopy," http://www.lfd.uci.edu/globals/unlimited/.
23. E. Gratton, "Time resolved fluorescence spectroscopy," in *Workshop on Fluorescence Spectroscopy in the Biosciences*, W. Sawyer (Ed.), University of Melbourne, Melbourne, Australia, 1997.
24. D. V. O'Connor and D. Phillips, *Time-Correlated Single Photon Counting*, Academic, London, 1984.
25. M. Fujiwara and W. Cieslik, "Fluorescence lifetime imaging microscopy: Two dimensional distribution measurement of fluorescence lifetime," *Meth. Enzymol.* **414**, 633 (2006).

26. R. V. Krishnan, H. Saitoh, H. Terada, V. E. Centonze, and B. Herman, "Development of a multiphoton fluorescence lifetime imaging microscopy system using a streak camera," *Rev. Sci. Instrum.* **74**, 2714 (2003).
27. La Vision, PicoStar HR ICCD, http://www.lavision.de/products/cameras/ultrafast_gated cameras.php.
28. Andor, ICCD, http://www.andor.com/products/cameras/?app = 208.
29. Roper, ICCD, http://www.roperscientific.de/pimax.html.
30. W. Becker, *Advanced Time-Correlated Single Photon Counting Techniques*, Springer, Heidelberg, 2005.
31. Becker and Hickl GmbH, "SPM830 single photon counting module," http://www.becker-hickl.de/tcspc.htm#spc830.
32. Picoquant GmbH, "TimeHarp Single photon counting module," http://www.picoquant.com/getfs.htm?products/timeharp200/timeharp200.htm.
33. Becker and Hickl GmbH, "PML-16 16 channel photomultiplier head," http://www.becker-hickl.de/spectral.htm#pml16.
34. M. Straub and S. W. Hell, "Fluorescence lifetime three-dimensional microscopy with picosecond precision using a multifocal multiphoton microscope," *Appl. Phys. Lett.* **73**, 1769 (1998).
35. N. Yamamoto, H. Muramatsu, L. M. Do, E. M. Han, T. Kato, and M. Fujihira, "Study of energy transfer from excited TPD to Alq in organic electroluminescent devices by time-resolved fluorescence spectroscopy using a scaning near-field optical atomic force microscope," *J. Microsc.* **202**, 395 (2001).
36. S. E. D. Webb, Y. Gu, S. Lévêque-Fort, J. Siegel, M. J. Cole, K. Dowling, R. Jones, and P. M. W. French, "A wide-field time-domain fluorescence lifetime imaging microscope with optical sectioning," *Rev. Sci. Instrum.* **73**, 1898 (2002).
37. W. Becker and A. Bergmann, "Lifetime imaging techniques for optical microscopy," www.becker-hickl.de/pdf/tcvgbh1.pdf.
38. Lambert Instruments, "Fluorescence lifetime imaging—FLIM," http://www.lambert-instruments.com/product_details/1_english/2_products/9_fluorescence_lifetime_imaging/29_lifa_system.
39. E. Gratton, "FLIM box," http://www.lfd.uci.edu/research/.
40. M. J. Booth and T. Wilson, "Low-cost, frequency-domain, fluorescence lifetime confocal microscopy," *J. Microsc.* **214**, 36 (2004).
41. E. P. Buurman, R. Sanders, A. Draauer, H. C. Gerritsen, J. J. F. van Deen, P. M. Houpt, and Y. K. Levine, "Fluorescence lifetime imaging using a confocal laser scanning microscope," *Scanning* **14**, 155 (1992).
42. K. Dowling, M. J. Dayel, M. J. Lever, P. W. French, J. D. Hares, and A. K. L. Dymooke-Bradshaw, "Fluorescence lifetime imaging with picosecond resolution for biomedical applications," *Opt. Lett.* **23**, 810 (1998).
43. Yokogawa, "CSU10 Nipkow disk scanner," http://www.yokogawa.co.jp/SCANNER/english/products/csu10e.html.
44. C. J. de Grauw and H. C. Gerritsen, "Multiple time-gate module for fluorescence lifetime imaging," *Appl. Spectrosc.* **55**, 670 (2001).
45. Nikon, "LIMO," http://www.nikoninstruments.com/.
46. D. K. Bird, A. L. Schneider, A. C. Watkinson, B. Finnin, and T. A. Smith, "Navigating transdermal diffusion with multiphoton fluorescence lifetime imaging," *J. Microsc.*, **230**, 61 (2008).
47. I. Gautier, M. Tramier, C. Durieux, J. Coppey, R. B. Pansu, J. C. Nicolas, K. Kemnitz, and M. Coppey-Moisan, "Homo-FRET microscopy in living cells to measure monometer-dimer transition of GFP-tagged proteins," *Biophys. J.* **80**, 3000 (2001).

48. K. Kemnitz, L. Pfeifer, and M. R. Ainbund, "Detector of multichannel spectroscopy and fluorescence lifetime imaging on the picosecond timescale," *Nucl. Instrum. Meth. Phys. Res. A.* **387**, 86 (1997).
49. M. Tramier, T. Piolot, I. Gautier, V. Mignotte, J. Coppey, K. Kemnitz, C. Durieux, and M. Coppey-Moisan, "Homo-FRET versus hetero-FRET to probe homodimer in living cells," *Methods Enzymol.* **360**, 580 (2003).
50. Europhoton GmbH, "MCP FLIM," http://www.europhoton.de/.
51. M. Millington, G. J. Grindlay, K. Altenbach, R. K. Neely, W. Kolch, M. Benčina, N. D. Read, A. C. Jones, D. T. F. Dryden, and S. W. Magennis, "High-precision FLIM-FRET in fixed and living cells reveals heterogeneity in a simple CFP-YFP fusion protein," *Biophys. Chem.* **127**, 155 (2007).
52. D. J. S. Birch and R. E. Imhof, "Coaxial nanosecond flashlamp," *Rev. Sci. Instrum.* **52**, 1206 (1981).
53. C. D. McGuinness, K. Sagoo, D. McLoskey, and D. J. S. Birch, "A new sub-nanosecond LED at 280 nm: Application to protein fluorescence," *Meas. Sci. Technol.* **15**, L19 (2007).
54. Picoquant GmbH, "Picosecond diode lasers," http://www.picoquant.com/_lightsources.htm.
55. Crystal Fibre Femtowhite, "Continuum generation in photonic crystal fibres," http://www.crystal-fibre.com/products/femtowhite.shtm.
56. Y. Sakai and S. Hirayama, *J. Lumin.* **39**, 145 (1988).
57. APE GmbH, "PulseSwitch," http://www.ape-berlin.de/gb/products/pulseswitch.html.
58. S. Cova, "Single photon avalanche photodiodes," http://intranet.dei.polimi.it/res/spad/.
59. Picoquant GmbH, "Single photon avalanche photodiodes," http://www.picoquant.de/_instrumentation.htm.
60. Becker and Hickl GmbH, "Single photon avalanche photodiodes," http://www.becker-hickl.de/detectors_new.htm.
61. Becker and Hickl GmbH, "Single photon avalanche photodiodes," http://www.idquantique.com/products/files/id100-becker.pdf.

CHAPTER 11

Fluorescence Correlation Spectroscopy

THOMAS DERTINGER

Department of Chemistry and Biochemistry, University of California Los Angeles, Los Angeles, California 90095, USA

IRIS VON DER HOCHT

Max-Planck-Institute of Biophysics, D-60438 Frankfurt, Germany

ANASTASIA LOMAN, INGO GREGOR, and JÖRG ENDERLEIN

Institute of Physics, Georg-August University, D-37077 Göttingen, Germany

11.1 INTRODUCTION

Thermally induced random movement called diffusion is one of the fundamental properties exhibited by molecules in solution. It is characterized by the diffusion coefficient D, which reflects the average speed at which individual particles move. It is directly related to the size of the molecules via the Stokes–Einstein relation

$$D = \frac{k_B T}{6\pi \eta r_H} \tag{11.1}$$

where k_B denotes the Boltzmann constant, T the temperature, η the viscosity of the solution, and r_H the radius of a sphere that represents the size of the molecule. It becomes clear that any change of the size (and therefore r_H) will change the diffusion coefficient of the molecules. Such changes occur to most biomolecules—in particular proteins, RNA, and DNA—when they interact with their environment (e.g., bind ions or other biomolecules), perform biologically important functions (e.g., enzymatic catalysis), or react to changes in environmental parameters such as pH, temperature, or chemical composition (e.g., protein unfolding). Therefore, the ability to precisely measure diffusion coefficients is significant for a range of applications, for example, monitoring important conformational changes in proteins upon ion binding or unfolding. However, many biologically relevant conformational changes produce rather small changes in molecular size on the order of angstroms (see, e.g., [1]). To monitor such small changes, it is necessary to measure the diffusion coefficient with an accuracy of better than a few percent. Such measurements can be done using a technique of fluorescence correlation spectroscopy.

Fluorescence Applications in Biotechnology and Life Sciences, Edited by Ewa M. Goldys

Fluorescence correlation spectroscopy (FCS) is a technique originally introduced by Elson, Magde, and Webb in the early seventies [2–4]. In its original form it was invented for measuring diffusion, concentration, and chemical/biochemical interactions/reactions of fluorescent or fluorescently labeled molecules at nanomolar concentrations in solution. There are numerous excellent reviews and overviews of FCS [5–7] and there is even a complete book devoted to it [8]. The present chapter gives a very general introduction to the philosophy of FCS, trying to be self-contained, developing the fundamental principles of FCS but describing also recent methodological advances which are not well covered by previous reviews.

Qualitatively, the core idea of the method can be understood quite easily. Let us assume that one has a measurement system capable of exciting and detecting the fluorescence of solved molecules in solution within a very small volume (for a moment, let us postpone all the technical details). The system is characterized by this so-called volume of detection, a region in solution where fluorescence excitation and detection take place.

Due to their random motion, molecules will enter and leave the detection volume over time. In response the measured fluorescence signal (which can be considered to be proportional to the number of molecules in the detection volume) will fluctuate strongly (see Figure 11.1).

In FCS, the detected time-varying fluorescence signal is correlated with a time-shifted replica of itself) for different values of time shift τ (lag time). The result is the so-called autocorrelation function (second-order correlation function, in short

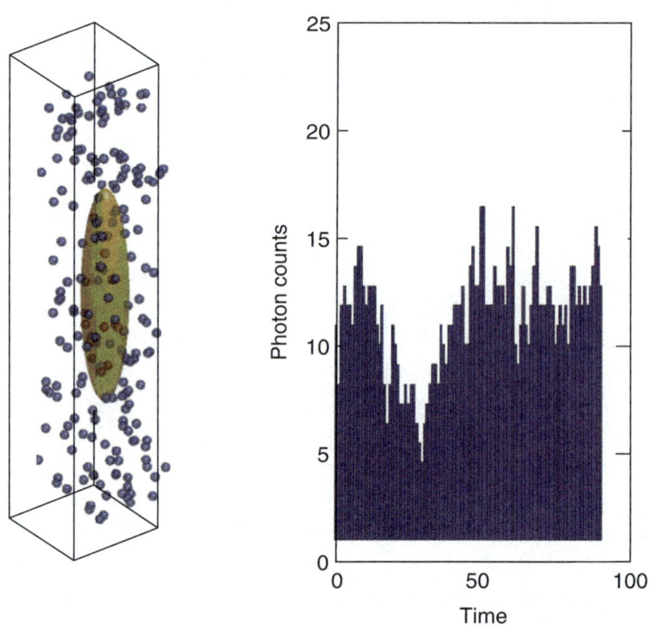

Figure 11.1 Left: schematic of detection region (yellow) where effective fluorescence detection takes place. When molecules (blue spheres) diffuse in and out of this region, they generate a highly fluctuating fluorescence signal (right) due to the continuously changing numbers of fluorescent molecules within the detection region.

ACF), which is calculated as

$$g(\tau) = \langle I(t)I(t+\tau)\rangle_t \tag{11.2}$$

where $I(t)$ is the fluorescence signal at time t, $I(t+\tau)$ is the time-shifted replica, τ is the time shift, and the triangular brackets denote averaging over all time values t. The physical meaning of the autocorrelation is that it is directly proportional to the probability to detect the present signal after the time period τ again. From the definition of the ACF it follows that its value for $\tau = 0$ equals the second moment of the measured signals: $g(0) = \langle I(t)I(t)\rangle_t = \langle I^2(t)\rangle_t$. The limit for infinite lag time τ is $g(\infty) = \langle I(t)\rangle_t^2$, the square of the mean fluorescence signal. Therefore, the amplitude of the ACF equals the variance of the signal distribution:

$$g(0) - g(\infty) = \langle I^2(t)\rangle_t - \langle I(t)\rangle_t^2 = \sigma^2 \tag{11.3}$$

In the case of our experiment we can identify the "signal" with the number of particles in the detection volume. In general, the probability to find N particles that enter and leave the volume randomly obeys a Poissonian distribution. This distribution is characterized by the fact that mean and variance are the same. From this it follows that the amplitude of the ACF is proportional to N upon a constant offset proportional to N^2. Here N stands for the average number of particles in the detection volume. Traditionally in FCS one works with a normalized ACF defined as

$$G(\tau) = \frac{g(\tau)}{g(\infty)} - 1 \tag{11.4}$$

This function has zero offset and its amplitude is proportional to N^{-1}.

In the following we assume that the concentration of fluorescent molecules in solution is so small that on average only one molecule is present within the detection volume. So the autocorrelation will give us the probability to find a molecule in the detection volume after the time τ if there is one now. This probability is composed of two basically different terms. The fluorescence signals detected at time zero and at time τ can originate from unintentional fluorescence background or from different fluorescing molecules and therefore do not have any physical correlation (provided there is no interaction of the different fluorescing molecules).

These events will contribute to a constant offset of $g(\tau)$ that is completely independent on τ (the joint probability to detect two physically uncorrelated signals is completely independent on the time distance between their detection). Alternatively, the two signals can originate from one and the same molecule and are then physically correlated (see Figure 11.2).

Let us start with some very simple qualitative considerations concerning the lag time dependence of $g(\tau)$. Suppose a molecule is close to the center of the detection volume. Then there will be a high probability to detect a high-fluorescence signal over a certain period from this molecule. This means that the fluorescence signal will be *highly correlated* in time within that period. When the molecule in its random motion due to diffusion approaches the boundary of the detection volume, this correlation will progressively decrease, that is, the probability to see the fluorescence signal will decrease in time, until the molecule has completely diffused away from the observation

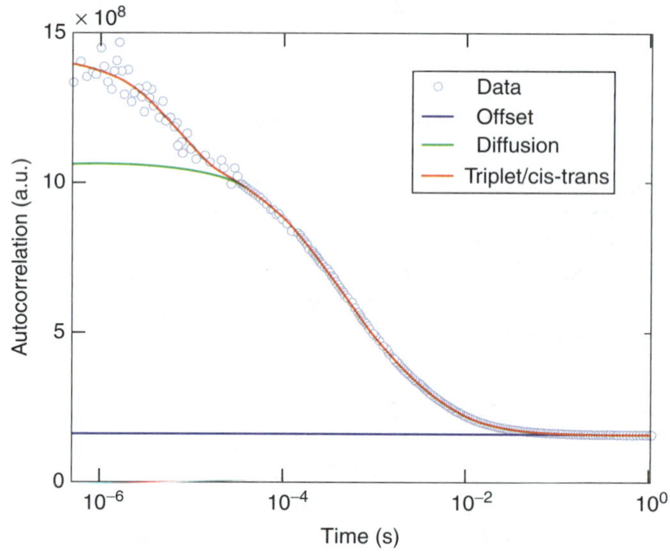

Figure 11.2 Anatomy of typical autocorrelation curve. On the microsecond timescale, fast photophysical processes such transitions into the triplet state lead to a partial loss of the fluorescence autocorrelation. On the millisecond timescale, autocorrelation becomes smaller due to the diffusion of molecules out of the detection region (green). The long-time constant offset (blue) is due to the completely uncorrelated signals. Open circles: measured data (aqueous solution of the dye Alexa633).

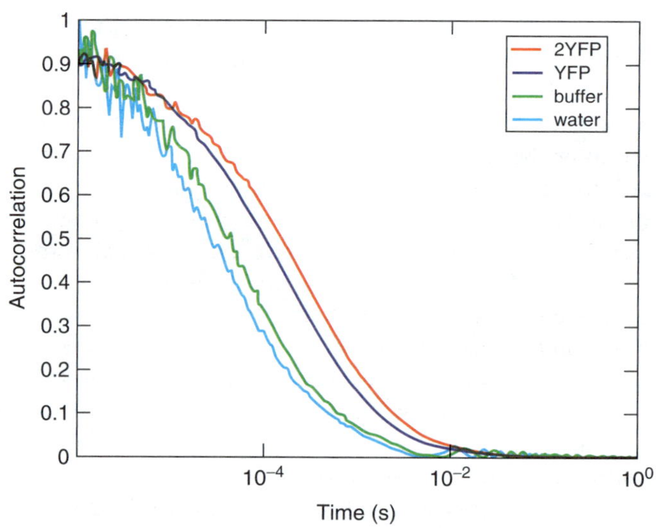

Figure 11.3 Effect of values of diffusion coefficients on shape of autocorrelation curves. Four measurements are shown: purified water (light blue) and salt buffer solution (green) that contain rapidly diffusing fluorescent contaminations, aqueous solution of yellow fluorescent protein (YFP, blue) showing much slower diffusion, and aqueous solution of two coupled YFPs bound together by a short amino linker, displaying even slower diffusion.

volume and the correlation is completely lost. It is important that the temporal decay of the correlation, that is, the temporal decay of $g(\tau)$ with increasing lag time τ, is proportional to the diffusion speed of the molecule: The larger the diffusion coefficient, the faster the fluorescence correlation decays (see Figure 11.3).

A second important property of the autocorrelation function is its dependence on the concentration of fluorescing molecules. It is rather obvious that the fluorescence intensity fluctuations will be larger for smaller molecule concentrations. Indeed, if one has, on average, only a signal molecule within the detection volume, then the diffusion of this molecule out of this volume or the diffusion of another molecule into this volume will cause a significant change of the measured fluorescence intensity. Conversely, if the average number of fluorescing molecules within the detection volume is rather large (e.g., several hundred), then the departure or arrival of a single additional molecule causes only small signal variations. Intuitively, one may expect a direct connection between the average number of molecules within the detection volume (i.e., concentration) and the amplitude of the fluorescence signal fluctuations. And indeed, as will be discussed below, there is a direct connection between the inverse concentration of fluorescing molecules and the amplitude of the autocorrelation function.

Thus, FCS measurements can provide information about diffusion and concentration of fluorescing molecules. Any process that alters one (or both) of these quantities can also be measured by FCS. The binding of two proteins in solution is a good example: By labelling one of the binding partners with a fluorescence label and monitoring with FCS the changing value of the diffusion coefficient of the labeled molecules upon binding of their binding partner, one can directly measure binding affinities and kinetics.

11.2 OPTICS OF FLUORESCENCE CORRELATION SPECTROSCOPY

From the beginning of FCS in the 1970s it took nearly two decades until the technique experienced a renaissance in biophysics. The realization of stable and reliable setups required lasers with high beam quality and temporal stability, low-noise single-photon detectors, and high-quality microscope objectives with nearly perfect imaging quality at high numerical aperture. Achieving small, few-cubic-micrometer detection volumes made it possible to study samples at reasonably high concentrations and reduced measurement times.

The standard optical setup for performing FCS measurements is based on a confocal epifluorescence microscope, as schematically shown in Figure 11.4 [9]. Fluorescent molecules are dissolved in an aqueous solution that is placed on top of a microscope slide housing a small chamber to hold the liquid with a coverslip to minimize evaporation. For inverted microscopes one has to put the sample upside down because the microscope objective always has to look through the coverslip. A collimated high-quality laser beam is coupled via a dichroic mirror into an objective with high numerical aperture. The dichroic mirror is reflective at the laser's wavelength and transmissive at the wavelengths of the fluorescence emission. It is important to minimize the detection volume to achieve the tightest possible focusing of light. Fluorescence light generated in the sample is collected by the same objective (so-called epifluorescence collection) transmitted through the dichroic mirror and focused onto a circular confocal aperture. The confocal aperture effectively rejects fluorescence light that is

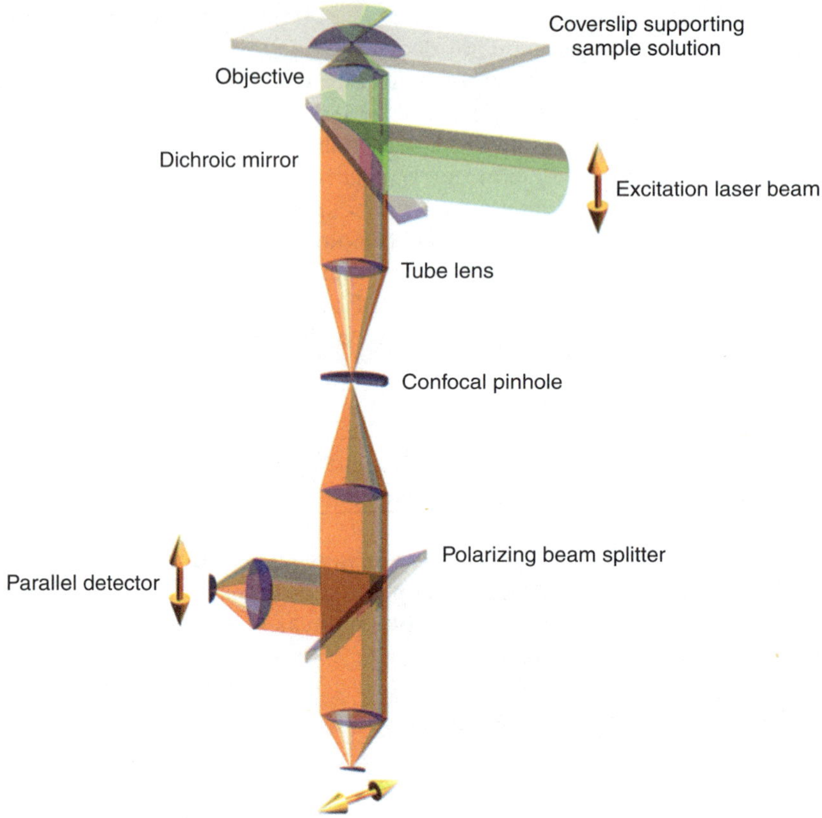

Figure 11.4 Schematic diagram of confocal laser epi-fluorescence microscope typically used in FCS. Shown is a setup with a linearly polarized excitation laser. Detection is carried out by using two detection channels following the splitting of light with a polarizing beamsplitter. The detectors are usually SPADs photomultiplier tubes. The vertical position of the objective can be accurately adjusted using a piezoactuator (not shown).

generated outside the focal plane. Behind the aperture, the fluorescence light is refocused onto a sensitive light detector, usually a single-photon avalanche diode (SPAD) or a specially configured photomultiplier. The combination of near-perfect focusing of excitation light and confocal detection of fluorescence generates an effective detection volume of approximately 0.5 μm in diameter in the focal plane and a few micrometers along the optical axis.

The exact shape and size of the detection volume determine the shape and temporal decay of the autocorrelation function. For example, the smaller the detection volume, the faster molecules diffuse out of it and the faster is the decay of the autocorrelation function, and vice versa. Thus, the features of the detection volume are weaved into the shape autocorrelation function. As we will see below, knowing the exact shape of the detection volume makes it possible to calculate the shape of the autocorrelation function. The autocorrelation function can then be used to fit experimental data and to obtain the diffusion constants and/or concentration values of the fluorescent molecules.

It is one of the central features of FCS that the accuracy of these values critically depends on the exact knowledge of the detection volume. We will discuss this topic in more detail in Section 11.4.

11.3 PRACTICAL ASPECTS OF FCS EXPERIMENTS

In what follows we discuss some experimental points of FCS measurements that the user can control in order to obtain reliable results. FCS provides information about molecular diffusion, sample concentration (especially changes and relative values), brightness, aggregation, and chemical and conformational kinetics requiring minute amounts of sample. Any particles can be the subject of investigation as long as they are soluble. If the size of the particle reaches the dimensions of the detection volume, one has to modify the data evaluation, but in most cases this is not a problem. Necessarily the particles or molecules of interest have to carry a fluorescent group. For example, nucleic acids can be site specifically labeled with fluorescent probes with minimal effect on their hybridization. Green fluorescent protein (GFP) and many of its mutants can be fused genetically to proteins of interest providing highly specific in vivo labeling. FCS used in combination with fluorescent proteins is a powerful tool for protein studies. If the fluorophore is introduced by a labeling reaction, great care has to be taken in order to get rid of all excess fluorophore molecules that have not bound to the target molecule. Another concern during labeling is the possibility that a fluorescent label might influence the interaction of the labeled particle with other molecules. This can usually be resolved by choosing an appropriate fluorescent dye bound at a minimally disruptive labeling site.

FCS performs at its best if the average number (over time and space) of target molecules in the detection volume is around 1. Lower numbers also work well but will increase measurement time (due to lower fluorescence signal) as well as the amount of background signal. Higher numbers will work also, but the amplitude of the ACF will be decreased. It is not recommended to work with more than 10 molecules at a time in the detection volume. For an estimation of a proper concentration one can assume the size of the detection volume to be $\sim$1 fL. The concentration of one particle per femtoliter corresponds to the concentration $c \approx 1.7$ nmol/L. One also needs to be cautious about adsorption as adsorption processes can easily happen on glass–water interfaces. Since the total amount of sample is usually on the order of a few tenths of microliters, adsorption can dramatically and uncontrollably decrease the concentration, especially in the case of proteins. This should be avoided as much as possible because it is essential to know exactly the concentration of all involved molecules for determination of binding coefficients of rate constants. The low concentrations required for FCS can also be a limiting factor if the K_D for the interaction of interest is much higher. One can overcome these limitations by enclosing the substances in vesicles or other compartments where the local concentration in the interior can be much higher.

For most measurements the examined particles or molecules are diluted not in pure water but in a proper buffer to control pH and concentrations of ions and other substances that are essential. However, each ingredient in the buffer can contain impurities that can increase dramatically the signal background. It is crucial to check the working buffer in the instrument before preparing the sample. In particular, if the excitation wavelength is below 550 nm, one should try to keep the number of ingredients and their concentration as low as possible. The presence of signal background due to fluorescence or scatter affects the amplitude of the correlation curve but usually not its decay parameters.

Before one starts to run an experiment with rare and valuable samples, one should check the performance of the instrument using a standard sample solution. This standard typically is a solution of the pure dye that you have used to label your sample. When exciting below 500 nm, one should also consider Raman scattering. Water has a strong and broad Raman band with wavenumber ν_{Ra} between 3100 and 3600 cm^{-1}. The wavelength of the Raman signal can be calculated as $1/\lambda_{\mathrm{Ra}} = 1/\lambda_{\mathrm{exc}} - \nu_{\mathrm{Ra}}$. One should use emission filters that efficiently cut off the Raman emission. In this sense bandpass filters are favurable over long-pass filters. Some instruments offer the possibility to select the size of the confocal aperture. Do not be tempted to choose diameters larger than 150 μm. A larger diameter would unreasonably extend the long axis of the detection volume. The highly opened microscope objectives work optimal near the surface of the coverslip. One should also avoid focusing too far in the solution. The influence of the surface does not usually extend further than 10 μm. Measuring between 15 and 30 μm away from the interface should give best results. To improve reproducibility and comparability, one should always measure at the same distance from the surface.

During measurement it is worth monitoring the mean count rate. It should usually stay constant during the measurement. A decrease or increase may in some cases be expected, for example, if one wants to monitor the progress of a reaction. In general, it is likely to be an indication of problems, for example, aggregation, photobleaching, evaporation, and instrument drift.

11.4 QUANTITATIVE EVALUATION OF FCS MEASUREMENTS TO OBTAIN DIFFUSION CONSTANTS AND CONCENTRATION

The qualitative behavior of the autocorrelation function in an FCS measurement and its connection with the diffusion coefficient and concentration of the solved fluorescent molecules were explained in the introductory section. We will now deal with the problem of how to obtain quantitative values for these variables. We will start by considering the standard measurement setup as described in Section 11.2 (one-focus setup), next extensively discuss the pitfalls and problems of one-focus FCS, and finally describe and analyze a recently developed modification of standard FCS, the so-called two-focus FCS, that has much improved measurement performance in terms of precision and reproducibility.

11.4.1 One-Focus FCS

For quantitatively evaluating an FCS measurement, we have to find a suitable model of the autocorrelation function as a function of the diffusion coefficient and concentration. Following Eq. 11.2, the autocorrelation function is the correlation of the fluorescence intensity with a time-shifted replica of itself calculated for all possible lag times τ. The measured signal $I(t)$ comes from the fluorescence of all the molecules within the sample plus uncorrelated background I_{bg} (light scattering, electronic noise, etc.):

$$I(t) = I_{\mathrm{bg}} + \sum_j I_j(t) \tag{11.5}$$

where the index j refers to the jth molecule and the summation runs over all molecules in the sample. Thus, the autocorrelation function $g(\tau)$ is given by

$$g(\tau) = \left\langle \left(I_{bg}(t) + \sum_j I_j(t) \right) \left(I_{bg}(t+\tau) + \sum_k I_k(t+\tau) \right) \right\rangle$$
$$= \sum_j \left\langle I_j(t) I_j(t+\tau) \right\rangle + \sum_{j \neq k} \overline{I}_j \overline{I}_k + \sum_j \overline{I}_j \overline{I}_{bg} + \overline{I}_{bg}^2 \tag{11.6}$$

where the triangular brackets and bars again denote averaging over all possible time values t. In the last line, we took into account that fluorescence signals coming from different molecules are completely uncorrelated (provided there is no intermolecular interaction). Because all molecules in solution are indistinguishable, the last equation can be simplified further to

$$g(\tau) = N\langle i(t)i(t+\tau)\rangle + N(N-1)\langle i(t)\rangle^2 \tag{11.7}$$

where i is the measured fluorescence signal of any molecule and N is the total number of molecules present in the sample. Thus, the task of modeling the function $g(\tau)$ reduces to calculating $\langle i(t)i(t+\tau)\rangle$, the correlation function of the fluorescence signal from one and the same molecule, and $\langle i \rangle$, the average fluorescence signal contribution of a single molecule.

The correlation $\langle i(t)i(t+\tau)\rangle$ of the fluorescence signal from one and the same molecule can be easily derived when remembering its physical meaning: It is proportional to the chance of detecting a fluorescence signal from one and the same molecule at time $t+\tau$ after it was detected at time t. The probability to find a molecule within an infinitely small volume dV anywhere in the sample is equal to dV/V, where V is the total sample volume. At this point we have to mathematically express the chance of detecting a fluorescence signal from a molecule at a given position $\mathbf{r}$ in the sample. For this purpose we introduce a probability function $U(\mathbf{r})$, that tellingly is called the molecule detection function (MDF). So, the value of the MDF at a position $\mathbf{r}$; that is, $U(\mathbf{r})$ is proportional to the probability to detect a fluorescence signal from a molecule at this position. The MDF depends on many experimental conditions, but generally has its maximum in the focal plane and on the optical axis and rapidly falls off to zero if one moves away from the molecule.

Furthermore, the chance that the molecule diffuses from position $\mathbf{r}$ to position $\mathbf{r}+\boldsymbol{\rho}$ within time τ is given by the solution of the diffusion equation for the given initial (molecule at position $\mathbf{r}$) and boundary conditions. For a sample with far removed boundaries this solution has the simple form

$$G(\boldsymbol{\rho}, \tau) = \frac{1}{(4\pi D\tau)^{3/2}} \exp\left(-\frac{|\boldsymbol{\rho}|^2}{4D\tau}\right) \tag{11.8}$$

where D is the diffusion coefficient of the molecule. Finally, the chance to detect a photon from the molecule at the new position $\mathbf{r}+\boldsymbol{\rho}$ is again proportional to the value of the MDF at this position, that is, to $U(\mathbf{r}+\boldsymbol{\rho})$. Thus, the autocorrelation $\langle i(t)i(t+\tau)\rangle$ is calculated as the product of all these individual contributions and averaging over all possible initial and final positions of the molecule, that is, integrating over $\mathbf{r}$ and $\boldsymbol{\rho}$.

Before the final calculation can be carried out, the MDF $U(\mathbf{r})$ has to be specified. A very simple approximation of the MDF is usually adopted, that of a three-dimensional Gaussian distribution, that is,

$$U(\mathbf{r}) = \kappa \exp\left[-\frac{2}{a^2}(x^2+y^2) - \frac{2}{b^2}z^2\right] \tag{11.9}$$

where κ is a constant, (x, y, z) are Cartesian coordinates centerd at the intersection of the focal plane and optical axis and with z being the optical axis, and a and b are the characteristic half axes of the cylindrically symmetric, Gaussian-shaped detection volume. This corresponds to the lowest order polynomial expansion of ln $U(\mathbf{r})$ (due to symmetry axial and mirror symmetry, the terms linear in x, y, z are absent). The characteristic parameters a and b are not known a priori and are usually determined by reference measurements on a sample with known diffusion coefficient.

Using the expression of Eq. 11.9, the single-molecule autocorrelation $\langle i(t)i(t+\tau)\rangle$ can now be explicitly calculated as

$$\begin{aligned}\langle i(t)i(t+\tau)\rangle &= \frac{\varepsilon^2}{(4\pi Dt)^{3/2}}\int_V d\mathbf{r}\int_V d\boldsymbol{\rho}\; U(\mathbf{r}+\boldsymbol{\rho})\,\exp\left(-\frac{|\boldsymbol{\rho}|^2}{4Dt}\right)U(\mathbf{r})\\ &= \left(\frac{\pi^{3/2}}{8}\right)\frac{\varepsilon^2a^2b}{(1+4Dt/a^2)\sqrt{1+4Dt/b^2}}\end{aligned} \tag{11.10}$$

where ε is an constant factor which takes into account the overall detection efficiency of the measurement system and absolute fluorescence brightness of the molecules (defined by absorption cross section and fluorescence quantum yield). In a similar way, the average fluorescence signal coming from one molecule is given by

$$\langle i(t)\rangle = \varepsilon\int_V d\mathbf{r}\; U(\mathbf{r}) = \left(\frac{\pi^3}{8}\right)^{1/2}\varepsilon a^2 b \tag{11.11}$$

Thus, the final result for the total autocorrelation reads

$$\begin{aligned}g(\tau) &= \frac{N}{V}\frac{\varepsilon^2}{(4\pi Dt)^{3/2}}\int_V d\mathbf{r}\int_V d\boldsymbol{\rho}\; U(\mathbf{r}+\boldsymbol{\rho})\,\exp\left(-\frac{|\boldsymbol{\rho}|^2}{4Dt}\right)U(\mathbf{r})\\ &\quad+\left[I_{\text{bg}}+\frac{N\varepsilon}{V}\int_V d\mathbf{r}\;U(\mathbf{r})\right]^2\\ &=\left(\frac{\pi^{3/2}}{8}\right)\frac{c\varepsilon^2a^2b}{(1+4Dt/a^2)\sqrt{1+4Dt/b^2}}+\left[I_{\text{bg}}+\left(\frac{\pi^3}{8}\right)^{1/2}c\varepsilon a^2b\right]^2\end{aligned} \tag{11.12}$$

where c denotes the concentration of fluorescent molecules (numbers per volume) and we used the fact that in the limit of large sample volume $N/V \to c$ and $N(N-1)/V^2 \to c^2$. An important property of the autocorrelation function is that in case of negligible background the concentration of the fluorescent species can be derived from Eq. 11.12 via

$$\frac{g(\infty)}{g(0)-g(\infty)} = c\frac{\left[\int d\mathbf{r}\;U(\mathbf{r})\right]^2}{\int d\mathbf{r}\;U^2(\mathbf{r})} \tag{11.13}$$

where we have taken into account that $G(\boldsymbol{\rho}, \tau)$ in Eq. 11.8 approaches a δ function for $\tau \to 0$. Using Eq. 11.13, we can define the *effective detection volume* V_{eff} as

$$V_{\mathrm{eff}} = \frac{\left[\int d\mathbf{r}\, U(\mathbf{r})\right]^2}{\int d\mathbf{r}\, U^2(\mathbf{r})} \tag{11.14}$$

so that the left-hand side of Eq. 11.13 equals cV_{eff}, that is, the mean particle number within V_{eff}, directly connecting the autocorrelation function amplitude with concentration. One can use the analytical model of Eq. 11.12 to fit it to the experimental data. A proper model function would be

$$\begin{aligned} g(\tau) &= \frac{A}{(1+\alpha t)\sqrt{1+\beta t}} + B \\ A &= \frac{\sqrt{\pi^3}}{8} c\varepsilon^2 a^2 b \quad B = \left[\frac{\sqrt{\pi^3}}{2\sqrt{2}} c\varepsilon a^2 b + I_{\mathrm{bg}}\right]^2 \\ \alpha &= \frac{4D}{a^2} \qquad \beta = \frac{4D}{b^2} \end{aligned} \tag{11.15}$$

By measuring a sample of known concentration and diffusion constant, one can calibrate the detection volume and determine the parameters a, b, and ε:

$$a^2 = \frac{4D}{\alpha} \qquad b = \sqrt{\frac{4D}{\beta}} \qquad \varepsilon^2 = \frac{8A\alpha\sqrt{\beta}}{c\sqrt{(4\pi D)^3}} \tag{11.16}$$

Although this may seem a proper way of analyzing FCS data, it is rather unproductive to try to obtain reliable results from this approach. At first, one commonly has to take into account a decrease in molecular brightness, causing an additional decay of the ACF in the microsecond time regime. This can be approximated by introducing a multiplicative exponential decay term. This way one ends up with six parameters for fitting a rather unstructured data curve. Second, one can only roughly estimate the real concentration of the sample due to adsorption effects. Also the diffusion constants of possible standards are known to have errors about 50%. These facts explain why this approach is disadvantageous, even disregarding the fact that the assumption of a three-dimensional Gaussian-shaped MDF (Eq. 11.9) is rather inappropriate too. Accordingly, the physical meaning of the parameters a and b is rather dubious. The best way of doing FCS measurements are *relative* measurements, where, for example, the unknown diffusion coefficient of a sample is measured relative to a reference. The question of how good the MDF model is may be unimportant as long as it yields sufficiently good-quality fit of the autocorrelation function. As can be directly seen by inspecting the first line in Eq. 11.12, the diffusion coefficient enters all expressions only as a multiplying factor of the time t. Under identical optical conditions, two autocorrelation functions $g(t) - g(\infty)$ of two different molecular species are connected by stretching or compressing the vertical and horizontal axes. The transformation factor of the time axes is then equal to the ratio of the diffusion coefficients of the two species, and the ratio of the amplitudes of the ACFs is equal to the ratio of the products of concentration and fluorescence brightness. This is of course strictly correct only if the autocorrelation functions are exclusively determined by diffusion. In most real situations, there are several other contributions to an autocorrelation function coming from fast photophysical processes or other dynamic processes that affect the molecule's fluorescence. However, the above statement always remains valid for the *diffusion-related* part of an autocorrelation function. Under strictly identical experimental conditions, FCS is remarkably successful for making conclusions concerning the diffusion constant changes by a certain factor or the concentration changes by a certain amount.

Let us take a closer look at why it is so difficult to obtain absolute values from FCS experiments and why sometimes relative changes are prone to errors. First, one always has to measure against a reference, that is, a sample of fluorescing molecules with an a priori known diffusion coefficient. This is unsatisfactory in the sense that such a standard does not exist yet. The values found in the literature are often inaccurate, with errors of 50% or more. Second and much more problematic is the need to maintain *identical optical conditions in both sample and reference measurements, which is extremely difficult*. In recent years, it has become clear that the actual shape of the MDF is extremely sensitive to many optical and photophysical factors and can easily change from one measurement to another. The most severe will be briefly discussed here (for more details, see [10]).

The first common problem is that most water immersion objectives used in FCS setups are designed to image through a coverslip of specific thickness. In this sense, the coverslip acts as the last optical element of an objective, and the optical quality of imaging (and laser focusing) critically depends on the exact matching between the coverslip thickness, the objective to which it is adjusted, and its actual thickness. Figure 11.5 illustrates what happens when the actual coverslip thickness is different

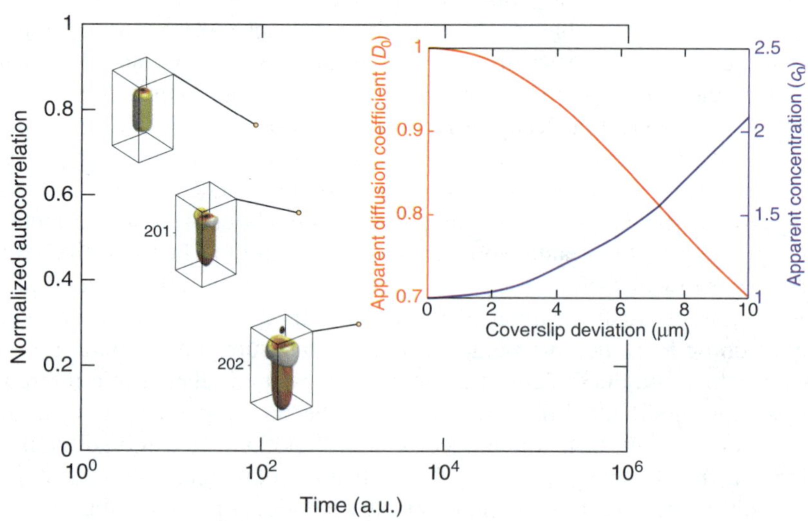

Figure 11.5 Left to right: MDF and autocorrelation function for three increasing values of coverslip thickness difference of 0, 5, and 10 μm compared to design value. Box size of MDF displays is $1 \times 1 \times 2$ μm^3; the number next to the box gives the center position along the optical axis in micrometers. Note the shift of the center of the MDF along the optical axis for increasing values of thickness difference. Inset: dependence of apparent diffusion coefficient and concentration on thickness difference.

from the design value by only a few micrometers, and in such a case severe optical aberrations are introduced. The autocorrelation function is then deformed and shifts toward longer lag times. The increased volume and the MDF produce increased diffusion times, that is, apparently lower diffusion coefficients and apparently increased concentration (there are more molecules present in the detection volume because the latter has become larger). In general, any aberration results in an increased detection volume and thus leads to the same trend of an apparently lower diffusion coefficient and higher concentration with increasing aberration. The impact on the apparent concentration is much stronger than on the apparent diffusion, resulting, for example, for a coverslip thickness difference of 10 μm to an error of over 100% for the diffusion coefficient and of roughly 30% for the concentration. It should be noted that the errors shown here are largely unaffected when the position of the focus is varied.

This is in stark contrast to the second problem considered here, the effect of refractive index mismatch. An optical microscope using a water immersion objective is optimally corrected for imaging in water. However, in many biophysical applications buffer solutions are used with slightly different refractive indices, typically in the range between 1.333 and 1.360. Figure 11.6 shows the impact of refractive index mismatch on the MDF and autocorrelation function and, subsequently, on the apparent diffusion coefficient and concentration. In contrast to the coverslip thickness, the aberrations introduced by refractive index mismatch accumulate with increasing distance of the focus from the coverslip surface because an increasingly thicker layer of solution

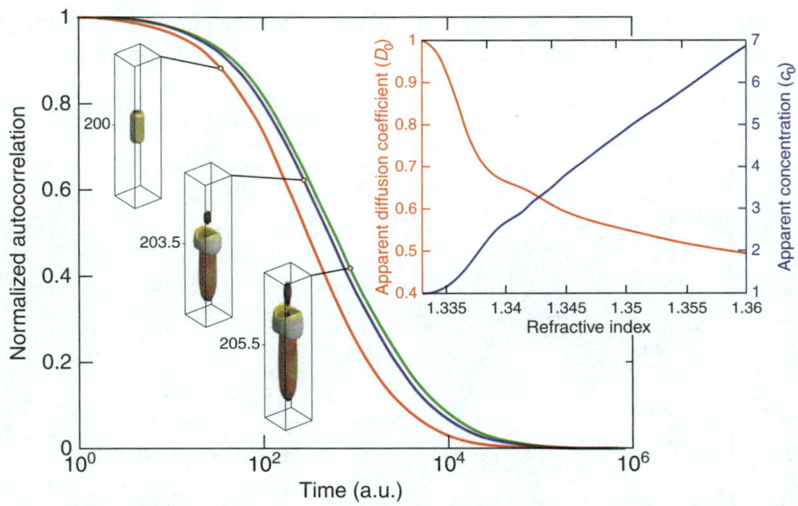

Figure 11.6 Left to right: MDF and ACF for three increasing values of refractive index of the sample solution of 1.333, 1.346, and 1.360. Box size of the MDF displays is 1 × 1 × 5 μm^3. Note again the shift of the center of the MDF along the optical axis for increasing values of refractive index. Inset: dependence of apparent diffusion coefficient and concentration on refractive index. The impact of even slight refractive index mismatch is much more dramatic than that of coverslip thickness. This is mostly due to the large distance of the focus position from the coverslip surface (200 μm, the default value of the commercial instrument, Confocor I by Carl Zeiss).

with mismatched refractive index lies between the optics and the detection volume. The effect of refractive index mismatch can be greatly reduced when positioning the detection volume closer to the surface.

A third and particularly intriguing problem in FCS measurements is the dependence of the autocorrelation function on excitation intensity due to optical saturation. Optical saturation occurs when the excitation intensity becomes so large that a molecule spends more and more time in a nonexcitable state, so that increasing the excitation intensity does not lead to a proportional increase in emitted fluorescence intensity. The most common sources of optical saturation are (i) excited-state saturation, that is, the molecule is still in the excited state when the next photon arrives; (ii) triplet state saturation, that is, the molecule undergoes intersystem crossing from the excited to the triplet state so that it can no longer become excited until it returns back to the ground state; and (iii) other photoinduced transitions into a nonfluorescing state, such as the photoinduced cis–trans isomerization in cyanine dyes, or the optically induced dark states in quantum dots. The detailed relationship between fluorescence emission intensity and excitation intensity can be very complex [11] and even be dependent on the excitation mode (pulsed or continuous wave) [12], but a sufficiently good approximation of the dependence of fluorescence intensity on excitation intensity is given by the simple relation

$$I_{\text{fluo}} \propto \frac{I_{\text{exc}}}{1 + I_{\text{exc}}/I_{\text{sat}}} \tag{11.17}$$

where I_{fluo} and I_{exc} are the fluorescence and excitation intensity, respectively, and I_{sat} is a parameter called the saturation intensity, which describes the saturation behavior of a given dye. Figure 11.7 shows how optical saturation changes the shape of the MDF and autocorrelation function and the apparent diffusion coefficient and concentration. An important special feature of optical saturation is the behavior of apparent diffusion and

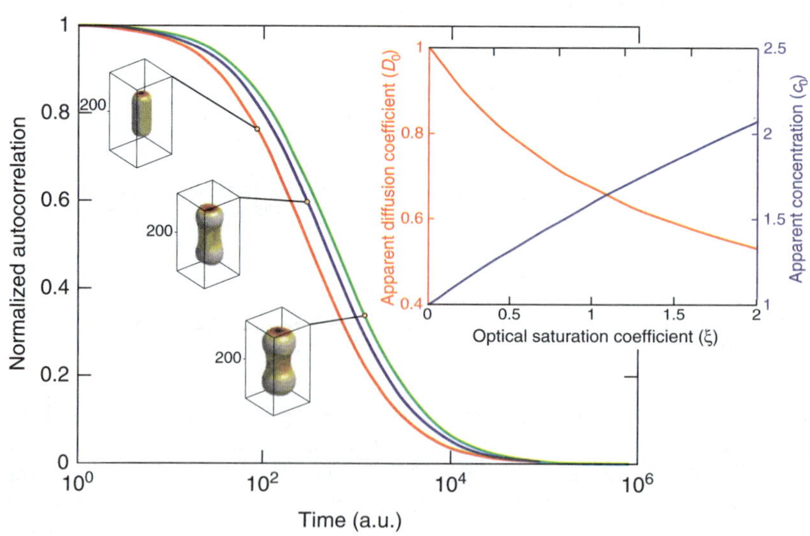

Figure 11.7 Left to right: MDF and ACF for three increasing values of optical saturation. Box size of the MDF displays is 1 × 1 × 2 μm^3. Inset: dependence of apparent diffusion coefficient and concentration on optical saturation, that is, excitation intensity.

concentration in the limit of vanishing excitation intensity: The slopes of the apparent diffusion and concentration curves have their largest absolute value at zero saturation, whereas for coverslip thickness difference or refractive index mismatch the slope of the curves tends to zero for vanishing aberration.

To better understand the reason for such behavior, we need to consider an ideal Gaussian excitation profile $I = I_0 \exp(-x^2/2)$. To simulate saturation we transform this distribution using $I^* = I/(1 + I/I_{sat})$ for different values of I_{sat}. A measure of the width of the distribution is its mean-square deviation. Figure 11.8 shows the widening of such a profile due to saturation. As can be seen, the relative change in profile is largest in the limit of zero intensity $I_0 \to 0$, explaining why one sees the biggest change of an autocorrelation function at low saturation levels.

All these effects make a quantitative evaluation of standard FCS measurements rather unreliable. The core problem is the absence of an *extrinsic and fixed-length scale* in the experiment. Even relative measurements are problematic due to the strong dependence of an FCS result on optical saturation, which is itself determined, in a complex manner, by the photophysics of a particular dye. Even more, the photophysical parameter of one and the same dye can change upon binding to a protein or other target molecule! The next section describes a recent modification of the standard FCS measurement that seems to solve this long-standing problem and makes it possible to perform reproducible, quantitative, and absolute measurements of diffusion coefficients.

11.4.2 Two-Focus FCS

Several modifications of FCS have been proposed to obtain a better defined detection volume, that is, a better defined MDF, by introducing an external ruler into the measurement which is lacking in standard FCS. A relatively easy way to do that is

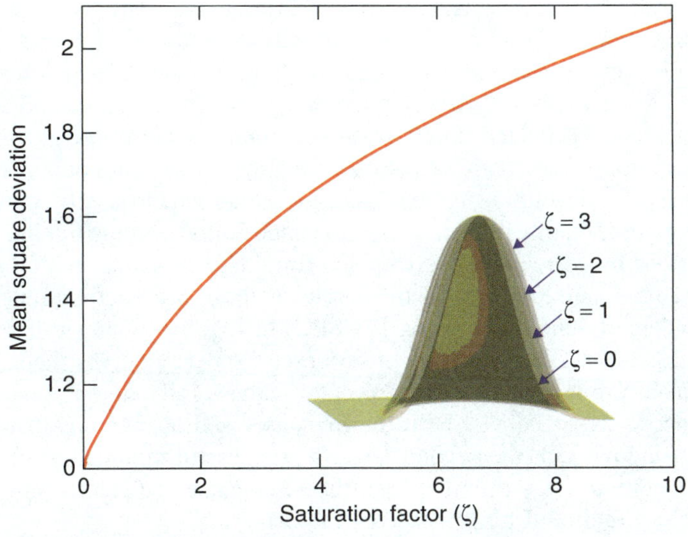

Figure 11.8 Change of mean-square deviation of distribution $I/(1 + I/I_{sat})$ with increasing optical saturation.

two-focus FCS (2fFCS)* [13]. This technique satisfies two requirements: (i) It introduces an external ruler into the measurement by generating two overlapping laser foci of precisely known and fixed distance and (ii) it generates the two foci and corresponding detection regions in such a way that the corresponding MDFs are sufficiently well described by a simple two-parameter model yielding accurate diffusion coefficients when applied to 2fFCS data analysis. Both these properties enable the measurements of absolute values of the diffusion coefficient with an accuracy of a few percent. Moreover, the new technique is robust against all the above-mentioned optical problems that are interfering in standard FCS measurements.

The 2fFCS setup, as shown in Figure 11.9, is based on the same standard confocal epi-fluorescence microscope as was shown in Figure 11.4. However, instead of using a single excitation laser, the light of two identical, linearly polarized pulsed diode lasers is combined by a polarizing beamsplitter. Both lasers are pulsed *alternately* with a high repetition rate (~40–80 MHz), an excitation scheme which is called pulsed interleaved excitation (PIE) [14]. Both beams are then coupled into a polarization-maintaining single-mode fiber. At the output, the light is again collimated. Thus, the combined light consists of a train of laser pulses with alternating orthogonal polarization. The beam is then reflected by a dichroic mirror toward the microscope's water immersion objective, but before entering the objective, the light beam is passed through a Nomarski prism that is normally used in differential interference contrast (DIC) microscopy [15]. The Nomarski prism is an optical element that deflects the laser pulses into two different directions according to their corresponding polarization. Thus, after focusing the light through the objective, two overlapping excitation foci are generated with a small lateral shift between them. The distance between the beams is uniquely defined by the chosen Nomarski prism and is independent of the sample's refractive index, coverslip thickness, or optical saturation, because all these effects introduce aberrations but will not change the distance between the axes of propagation of both focused laser beams.

As in one-focus FCS, the generated fluorescence is collected by the same objective, passed through the Nomarski prism and the dichroic mirror, and focused onto a single circular aperture which is positioned symmetrically with respect to both focus positions and chosen to be large enough to easily transmit light from both foci. After the pinhole, the light is collimated, split by a nonpolarizing beamsplitter cube, and focused onto two light detectors. Dedicated single-photon counting electronics is used to record the detected photons from both detectors with picosecond temporal resolution. The picosecond temporal resolution is now used to decide which laser has excited which fluorescence photon, that is, in which laser focus/detection volume the light was generated. This is done by correlating the detection time of each photon with the time of the last preceding laser pulse. A typical histogram of these time correlations, a so-called time-correlated single-photon counting (TCSPC) histogram, is shown in Figure 11.10.

In Figure 11.10, we see two different fluorescence decay curves that correspond to the two alternately pulsing lasers. In the data analysis, all photons that fall into the first time window are associated with the first laser and all photons that fall into the second time window with the second laser. A successful application of this method requires, of course, that the time between the laser pulses be significantly larger than the fluorescence lifetime of the fluorescent molecules.

*A commercial version of this technique is available from PicoQuant GmbH in Berlin (Germany).

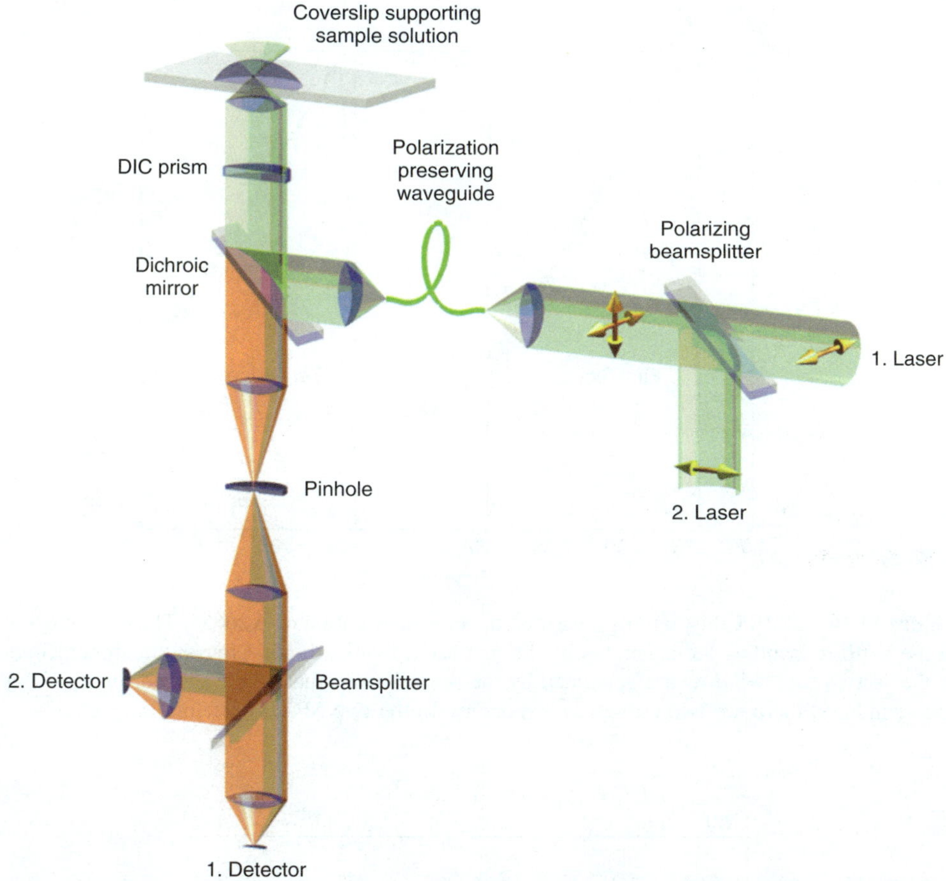

Figure 11.9 Schematic of 2fFCS setup. Excitation is provided by two interleaved pulsed lasers of the same wavelength. The polarization of each laser is linear but orthogonal to each other. Light is then combined by a polarizing beamsplitter and coupled into a polarization maintaining optical single-mode fiber. After leaving the fiber, the laser light is collimated by an appropriate lens and reflected by a dichroic beamsplitter through a DIC prism. The DIC prism deflects the laser light into two beams according to the polarization of the incoming laser pulses. The microscope objective focuses the two beams into two laterally shifted foci. Fluorescence is collected by the same objective. A lens focuses the detected fluorescence from both excitation foci on a single pinhole. Subsequently, the fluorescence light is split by a 50/50 beamsplitter and detected by two SPADs.

Once we establish which photon was generated in which detection volume, the autocorrelation functions for each detection volume as well as the cross-correlation function between the two detection volumes can be calculated. The cross-correlation function is calculated in a similar way as the autocorrelation function but correlating photons only from different detection volumes. The cross-correlation function at lag time τ is thus proportional to the likelihood to see a photon from the second detection volume at time $t + \tau$ if there was a detection event from the first detection volume at time t and vice versa. A typical 2fFCS measurement is presented in Figure 11.11.

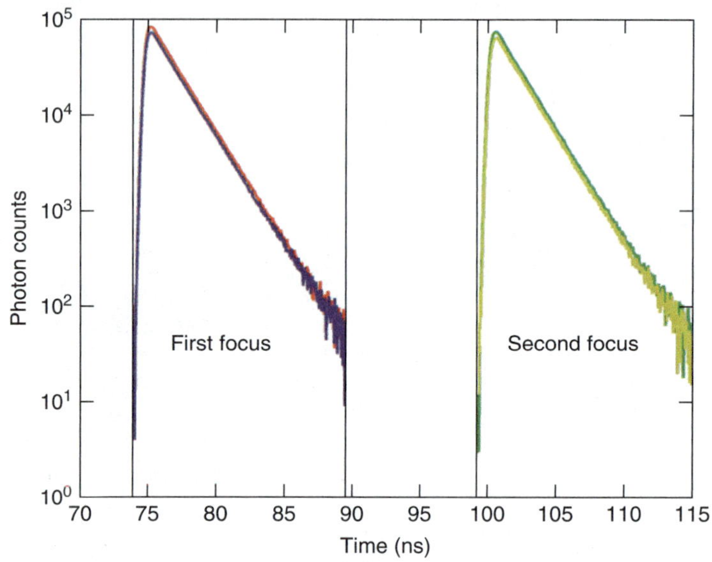

Figure 11.10 TCSPC histograms measured on aqueous solution of Atto655. The photon counts in the left time window are generated by the first laser, that is, the first focus; the photon counts in the second time window are generated by the second laser, that is, the second focus. In both time windows, there are two curves corresponding to the two SPAD detectors, respectively.

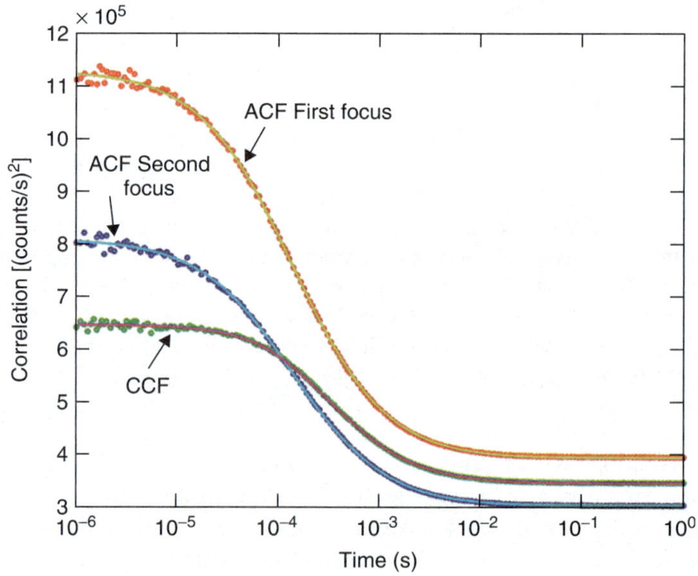

Figure 11.11 2fFCS measurement of nanomolar aqueous solution of Atto655. Shown are the autocorrelation functions for the first focus, the second focus, and the cross-correlation between both foci (CCF). The *shape* of both ACFs is virtually identical. Circles are experimental values; solid lines are global fits as described in the text.

A crucial point for a successful 2fFCS data analysis is to have an appropriate model function for the MDF. A suitable expression is given by

$$U(\mathbf{r}) = \frac{\kappa(z)}{w^2(z)} \exp\left[-\frac{2}{w^2(z)}(x^2 + y^2)\right] \tag{11.18}$$

where $\kappa(z)$ and $w(z)$ are functions of the axial coordinate z (optical axis) defined by

$$w(z) = w_0 \left[1 + \left(\frac{\lambda_{\mathrm{ex}} z}{\pi w_0^2 n}\right)^2\right]^{1/2} \tag{11.19}$$

and

$$\kappa(z) = 2\int_0^a \frac{d\rho\, \rho}{R^2(z)} \exp\left(-\frac{2\rho^2}{R^2(z)}\right) = 1 - \exp\left(-\frac{2a^2}{R^2(z)}\right) \tag{11.20}$$

where $R(z)$ is defined by an expression similar to Eq. 11.19:

$$R(z) = R_0 \left[1 + \left(\frac{\lambda_{\mathrm{em}}}{\pi R_0^2 n}\right)^2\right]^{1/2} \tag{11.21}$$

In the above equations, λ_{ex} is the excitation wavelength and λ_{em} the center emission wavelength, n is the refractive index of the immersion medium (water), a is the radius of the confocal aperture divided by the magnification, and w_0 and R_0 are two (generally unknown) model parameters. Equation 11.6 is nothing else than the scalar approximation for the radius of a diverging laser beam with beam waist radius w_0. Equation 11.18 is a modification of the three-dimensional Gaussian we have already come across when discussing one-focus FCS. It says that in each plane perpendicular to the optical axis the MDF is approximated by a Gaussian distribution having width $w(z)$ and amplitude $\kappa(z)/w^2(z)$. Using the parameterization of the MDF as given by Eqs. 11.18–11.21, the auto- and cross-correlation curves of the two-focus setup can be calculated as

$$g(t,\delta) = g_\infty(\delta) + \frac{\varepsilon_1\varepsilon_2 c}{4}\sqrt{\frac{\pi}{Dt}} \int_{-\infty}^{\infty} dz_1 \int_{-\infty}^{\infty} dz_2$$
$$\frac{\kappa(z_1)\kappa(z_2)}{8Dt + w^2(z_1) + w^2(z_2)} \exp\left[-\frac{(z_2 - z_1)^2}{4Dt} - \frac{2\delta^2}{8Dt + w^2(z_1) + w^2(z_2)}\right] \tag{11.22}$$

Here, we have taken into account that the MDFs of both detection volumes are identical but shifted by a distance δ along the x axis (along unit vector $\hat{\mathbf{x}}$) and having potentially two different overall detection efficiencies ε_1 and ε_2. Equation 11.22 is certainly more complicated than the simple expression of the second line in Eq. 11.12 but not much harder to handle numerically on a PC.

Data fitting is performed with least-square fitting of the model curve (Eq. 11.22) against the measured autocorrelation functions ($\delta = 0$, $\varepsilon_1\varepsilon_2$ replaced by either ε_1^2 or ε_2^2) and cross-correlation functions *simultaneously* in a global fit. As fitting parameters we need to use $\varepsilon_1 c^{1/2}$, $\varepsilon_2 c^{1/2}$, D, w_0, and R_0 as well as three offset values g_∞.

The distance δ between the detection regions is determined by the properties of the Nomarski prism and has to be exactly known a priori, thus introducing an external length scale into data evaluation. It is important to notice that a crucial criterion of fit quality is required not only to simultaneously reproduce the temporal shape of both autocorrelation functions and the cross-correlation function but also to reproduce their three amplitudes $g_{t\to 0} - g_\infty$ using only the two parameters $\varepsilon_1 c^{1/2}$ and $\varepsilon_2 c^{1/2}$. The relation between the amplitudes of the CCF and the amplitudes of the autocorrelation functions is determined by the overlap between the two MDFs and thus by the shape parameters w_0 and R_0. Thus, achieving good fit quality for the relative amplitudes of the autocorrelation functions and the cross-correlation function makes it easier to find the correct values of these parameters.

Due to the presence of an external length scale determined by the distance δ between the detection volumes and a reasonably accurate model of the MDF, 2fFCS gives superior accuracy and stability when measuring diffusion. An optimal distance between the two foci is ~400 nm, giving a sufficiently large overlap between the detection volumes so that the amplitude of the cross-correlation function between both detection volumes is roughly one-half of the amplitude of each autocorrelation function. Larger distances will lead to significantly longer measurement times to accumulate a sufficiently good cross-correlation, while smaller distances will lead to a cross-correlation function too similar to the autocorrelation functions so that fitting becomes increasingly unstable.

The superior performance of 2fFCS is shown in Figure 11.12. Shown are the determined diffusion coefficients of the dye Atto655 in aqueous solutions of guanidine

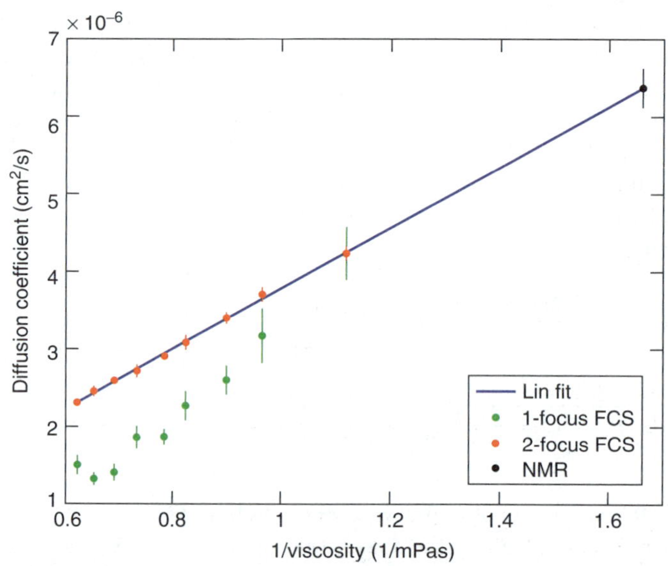

Figure 11.12 Dependence of diffusion coefficient of Atto655 in aqueous GdHCl solutions and in d_4-deuterized methanol at 25°C as function of solvent viscosity. Solid line is linear least-square fit to all data. Standard deviations are shown as error bars and are each derived from 10 repeated measurements. For comparison, the results of single-focus FCS using a standard model that assumes a three-dimensional Gaussian MDF are also shown. Because single-focus FCS can only measure relative values of diffusion coefficient, the value for pure water was used as reference value.

hydrochloride (GdHCl). The concentration of GdHCl was varied from zero to 6 M between different measurements, leading not only to a strong increase in solution viscosity but also to a significant increase in the refractive index of the solution. According to the Stokes–Einstein relation we expect to find a linear relationship between the diffusion coefficient and the inverse of the viscosity.

Indeed, 2fFCS precisely yields these results, despite increasing aberrations introduced by the refractive index mismatch. Moreover, as is also shown in Figure 11.12, the *absolute* values of the diffusion coefficient perfectly match those determined by pulsed-field gradient nuclear magnetic resonance, an independent spectroscopic method capable of measuring absolute diffusion coefficients. The achievable accuracy of 2fFCS in diffusion coefficient measurements was estimated to be smaller than 5%, opening the possibility to measure changes in the hydrodynamic radius of nanometer-sized molecules on the order of 1 Å.

11.5 CONCLUSION

We presented here a thorough introduction to FCS with strong emphasis on its application for precise diffusion measurements. We also carried out a thorough analysis of the optical performance of a confocal laser scanning microscope (CLSM) which has much wider importance for high-resolution fluorescence imaging. Of course, many other and more important applications of FCS could not be included in this chapter due to space constraints. From the description of the FCS as presented in this chapter it should be clear that any process that influences the temporal behavior of a molecule's fluorescence will have an impact on the ACF. Thus, FCS can also be used to measure, for example, fast photophysical processes [16], fast intramolecular structural dynamics [17], or stoichiometry of molecular complexes [18]. There are multiple applications of FCS and ingenious variants of FCS and FCS analysis, and the reader is referred to the excellent reviews cited in the introduction.

REFERENCES

1. A. M. Weljie, A. P. Yamniuk, H. Yoshino, Y. Izumi, and H. J. Vogel, "Protein conformational changes studied by diffusion NMR spectroscopy: Application to helix-loop–helix-calcium binding proteins," *Protein Sci.* **12**, 228–236 (2003).
2. D. Magde, E. Elson, and W. W. Webb, "Thermodynamic fluctuation in a reacting system—measurement by fluorescence correlation spectroscopy," *Phys. Rev. Lett.* **29**, 705–708 (1972).
3. E. L. Elson and D. Magde, "Fluorescence correlation spectroscopy. I. Conceptual basis and theory," *Biopolymers* **13**, 1–27 (1974).
4. D. Magde, E. Elson, and W. W. Webb, "Fluorescence correlation spectroscopy. II. An experimental realization," *Biopolymers* **13**, 29–61 (1974).
5. J. Widengren and Ü. Mets, "Conceptual basis of fluorescence correlation spectroscopy and related techniques as tools in bioscience," in *Single-Molecule Detection in Solution—Methods and Applications,* C. Zander, J. Enderlein, and R. A. Keller (Eds.), Wiley-VCH, Berlin, 2002, pp. 69–95.
6. P. Schwille, "Fluorescence correlation spectroscopy and its potential for intracellular applications," *Cell. Biochem. Biophys.* **34**, 383–408 (2001).

7. S. T. Hess, S. Huang, A. A. Heikal, and W.W. Webb, "Biological and chemical applications of fluorescence correlation spectroscopy: A review," *Biochemistry* **41**, 697–705 (2002).
8. R. Rigler and E. Elson (Eds.), *Fluorescence Correlation Spectroscopy*, Springer, Berlin, 2001.
9. M. Böhmer and J. Enderlein, "Single molecule detection on surfaces with the confocal laser scanning microscope," in *Single-Molecule Detection in Solution—Methods and Applications,* C. Zander, J. Enderlein, and R. A. Keller (Eds.), VCH-Wiley, Berlin/New York, 2002, pp. 145–183.
10. J. Enderlein, I. Gregor, D. Patra, T. Dertinger, and B. Kaupp, "Performance of fluorescence correlation spectroscopy for measuring diffusion and concentration," *Chem. Phys. Chem.* **6**, 2324–2336 (2005).
11. J. Enderlein, "Dependence of the optical saturation of fluorescence on rotational diffusion," *Chem. Phys. Lett.* **410**, 452–456 (2005).
12. I. Gregor, D. Patra, and J. Enderlein, "Optical saturation in fluorescence correlation spectroscopy under continuous-wave and pulsed excitation," *Chem. Phys. Chem* **6**, 164–170 (2005).
13. T. Dertinger, V. Pacheco, I. von der Hocht, R. Hartmann, I. Gregor, and J. Enderlein, "Two-focus fluorescence correlation spectroscopy: A new tool for accurate and absolute diffusion measurements," *J. Chem. Phys. Chem* **8**, 433–443 (2007).
14. B. K. Müller, E. Zaychikov, C. Bräuchle, and D. Lamb, "Cross talk free fluorescence cross correlation spectroscopy in live cells," *J. Biophys.* **89**, 3508–3522 (2005).
15. D. B. Murphy, S. Schwartz, E. D. Salmon, K. R. Spring, M. Parry-Hill, R. T. Sutter, and M. W. Davidson, http://www.microscopyu.com/articles/dic/dicindex.html.
16. J. Widengren, R. Rigler, and Ü. Mets, "Triplet-state monitoring by fluorescence correlation spectroscopy," *J. Fluoresc.* **4**, 255–258 (1994).
17. H. Neuweiler, A. Schulz, M. Böhmer, J. Enderlein, and M. Sauer, "Measurement of submicrosecond intramolecular contact formation in peptides at the single-molecule level," *J. Am. Chem. Soc.* **125**, 5324–5330 (2003).
18. J. Sýkora, J. K. Kaiser, I. Gregor, W. Bönigk, G. Schmalzing, and J. Enderlein, "Exploring fluorescence antibunching in solution for determining the stoichiometry of molecular complexes," *Anal. Chem.* **79**, 4040–4049 (2007).

CHAPTER 12

Flow Cytometry

RUSSELL E. CONNALLY
Macquarie University, North Ryde, New South Wales 2109, Australia

GRAHAM VESEY and CHARLOTTE MORGAN
BTF Pty., North Ryde, New South Wales 2113, Australia

12.1 WHAT IS FLOW CYTOMETRY?

Flow cytometry is a technique which enables rapid analysis of many thousands of micrometer-sized particles per second. It uses a fluid stream to transport cells through a narrow region, the excitation zone that is illuminated by an intense beam of light. The resultant scatter and fluorescence signal is highly correlated with cell physiology. As a consequence of the large number of cells analyzed, accurate statistical data can be gathered on cell populations. Specialized *sorting* flow cytometers can separate particles according to their size, surface characteristics, or fluorescence signatures. A unique feature of flow cytometry is that particles/cells are analyzed individually. This contrasts with most other fluorescence analysis methods in which measurements are made for a bulk volume of sample containing a large number of particles. Flow cytometers permit measurements to be taken a cell at a time with throughputs of around 70,000 cells per second.

Figure 12.1 illustrates the basic components of a flow cytometer, where a laser is typically used as the light source and detectors are arranged to collect scattered light in the forward direction (forward scatter) and orthogonal to the excitation beam (side scatter). The intense excitation can also excite fluorescence either from intrinsic autofluorophores within the cells or from special fluorescent labels attached to their surface. The optical signals are converted to electrical pulses for storage and analysis using a high-speed dedicated computer system. The data are often represented as a two-axis scatter plot for the identification, enumeration, and sorting of unique cell populations.

The light collected from the excitation zone may originate from two processes: *light scattering*, where a beam of light changes its direction, and *fluorescence emission*, where the excitation light is absorbed and reemitted at a longer wavelength(s) or color. The scattering and fluorescence characteristics are uniquely dependent on the physical characteristics of the cell, as shown in Figure 12.2 Therefore, by carrying out

Fluorescence Applications in Biotechnology and Life Sciences, Edited by Ewa M. Goldys

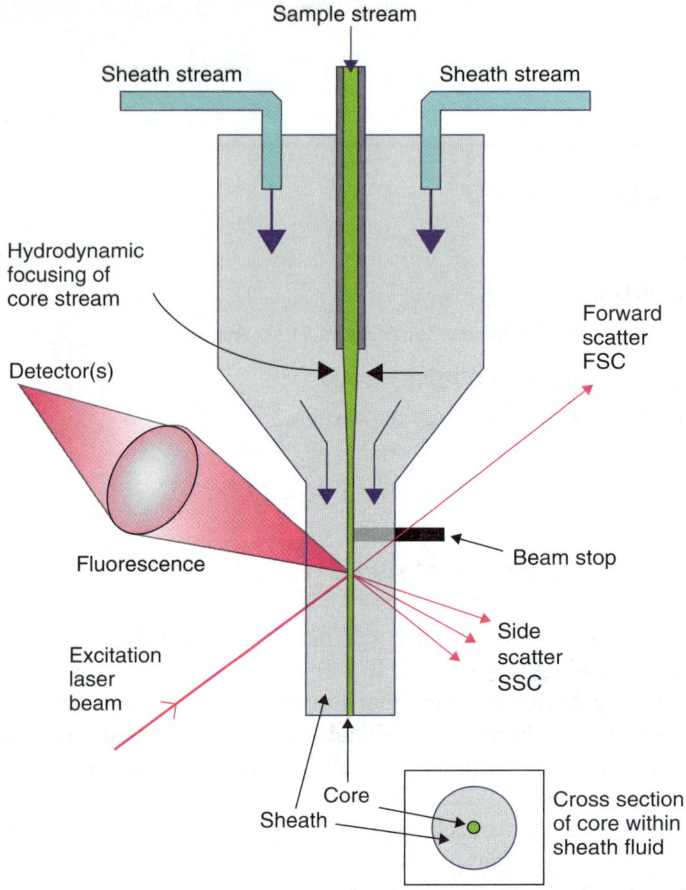

Figure 12.1 Flow cell schematic illustrating how diameter of core stream can be compressed or hydrodynamically focused as it enters excitation zone by controlling ratio of sheath and sample stream pressures. A laser beam is focused to a small elliptical region within the core stream and the forward propagation of the beam is blocked by a beam stop so that only scattered light can be detected in the forward direction (FSC). Side scatter (SSC) is detected at right angles to the beam, although at reduced intensity compared to the forward direction. Fluorescence is also collected at right angles to the incident beam using sensitive detectors to register the faint signals.

a combination of scattering and fluorescence measurements at a range of wavelengths, it is possible to measure features such as cell size and shape. Moreover, flow cytometry can probe internal cellular components or functions that can be visualized using fluorescent compounds introduced to the cells. Consequently, the applications of flow cytometry are numerous, and this has led to the widespread use of these instruments in the biological and medical fields.

12.1.1 History of Flow Cytometry

Early instrumentation of the 1940s and 1950s was mainly directed toward blood cell counting by instruments called hemocytometers. They were relatively insensitive due

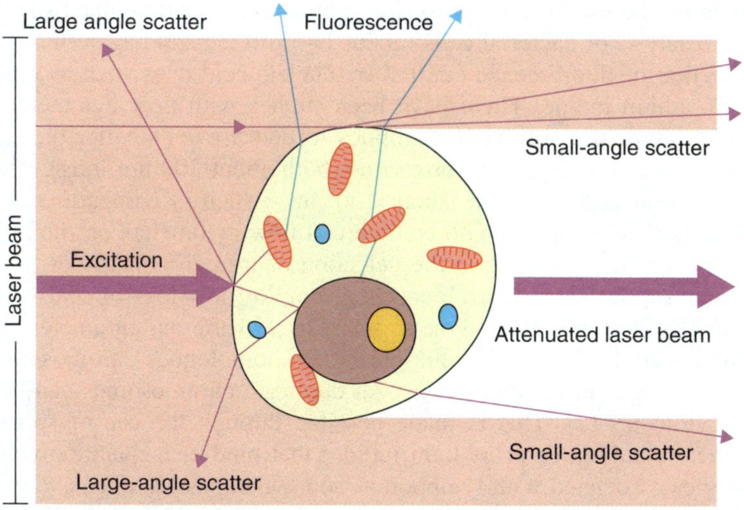

Figure 12.2 Model cell shown interrupting excitation beam to illustrate potential sources of scatter and fluorescence emission. Side-scatter signal is information rich and strongly influenced by refractive components within cells and cell surface topography. Forward scatter is frequently useful to provide an indication of particle size and can provide information about the state of the cell since dead cells refract light differently. Certain cellular components (porphyrins, proteins, etc.) will fluoresce when excited at appropriate wavelengths.

to the reliance upon side-scatter signals alone. In the 1950s Wallace Coulter introduced the concept of measuring cell volume by observing the increase in electrical impedance as cells interrupted the current path between two electrodes. In comparison to the saline core, cells represent a much higher electrical impedance. The Coulter counter could measure cell volume (size) with greater precision than SSC-based hemocytometers and was quickly adopted for this role. Following the introduction of fluorescence detection for DNA in the 1960s, optical detection became the preferred modality. Fluorescence detection became increasingly important as new protocols were introduced, and by 1979, cytometers were equipped with detectors for both small- and large-angle light scatter and two fluorescence channels.

The first reported use of a laser excitation source for flow cytometry originated from a Los Alamos group in 1969 that used an argon–ion laser to measure DNA distributions in populations of tissue culture cells and human leukocytes. Prior to analysis, the cells were exposed to dyes that intercalated within the DNA to render their nuclei fluorescent. Helium–neon lasers were also employed around 1970 by Kamenstsky in the Cytograf and Cytofluorograf; the latter instrument was also equipped with an argon–ion laser for excitation at 488 nm to better excite fluorescein-labeled cells. Large water-cooled lasers that often required industrial-level power supplies were thereafter integrated into many commercial designs and this trend continued for many years. More recently the emphasis has moved to benchtop instruments relying on solid-state lasers, air-cooled argon ion and/or helium–neon excitation that operates from conventional mains supply.

Flow cytometry has been particularly successful in the areas of microbiology and molecular biology, where particle size is most appropriate for this modality. Flow cytometers were originally designed to examine comparatively large mammalian cells such as red blood cells (5 μm diameter), but the increase in flow cytometer sensitivity brought about by the use of more powerful light sources enabled much smaller cells to be detected. Analysis of bacterial cells (about 1–5 μm in size) began in the mid-1970s through detection of fluorescence emitted by nucleic acid dyes such as ethidium bromide and propidium iodide. There have been studies with flow cytometers equipped with powerful lasers and special beam optics to detect even smaller biological particles such as T4 bacteriophage and pox virus (both about 300 nm long). The practical size detection limit appears to be about 150 nm, which is comparable to a typical virus particle; however, there are no commercial flow cytometers on the market today with sufficient sensitivity to enable the detection of free virus particles. Modern flow cytometers are sophisticated instruments that employ low-loss optical elements and multiple sensitive detectors to analyze as many as 17 different parameters from a single detection event [1]. Cells with multiple sets of homologous chromosomes (ploidy) or cells at later stages in the cell cycle with duplicate chromosomes can be identified using flow cytometry [2]. This is made possible through the use of special fluorescent molecules (ethidium or propidium iodide) that bind near quantitatively to DNA. Cell pathologies associated with lymphomas and leukemias are intensively studied for surface markers of diagnostic and prognostic value. The DNA content of tumor cells can be used to determine the proliferative activity of the cells and thereby help in determining the best form of chemotherapy to apply for cancer treatment. Alternative less expensive technologies are under development, yet at the time of this writing, flow cytometry remains the method of choice for monitoring lymphocyte levels in the blood of AIDS patients. The technology has been applied to analyze cell surface proteins for identifying a successful match for organ transplants and to separate X- and Y-chromosome sperm cells for artificial insemination of animals. Flow cytometry has such a diverse range of applications, including space travel. A small lightweight flow cytometer was recently assessed on the International Space Station (ISS) to determine whether it would give comparable data to a ground-based flow cytometer, with an aim of using this technology to diagnose astronaut illness and to conduct in-flight research into the effects of weightlessness on human physiology (Partec Cyflow; International Space Station, 2003).

12.1.2 Flow Cytometry Fundamentals

Flow cytometers direct a fluid stream containing particles for analysis through a narrow region, the excitation zone where an intense beam of light is focused. Light scattered from particles is collected at small angles ($0.5^\circ - 10^\circ$) in the forward direction (FSC) and at right angles to the beam axis (SSC). Cells or particles that range in size from submicrometer (ultramicrobacteria) to tens of micrometers (nucleated blood cells) should ideally pass through the excitation zone in single file to ensure that scatter and fluorescence signals are representative for each detection event. To achieve this aim, hydrodynamic focusing is used to compress the core stream to a diameter of 10 μm or less and distribute cells axially within the stream. It is not practicable to confine the core stream using a micrometer-sized orifice since flow blockage would be a constant problem. Instead, a small core size is achieved using a larger orifice (75–120 μm) to inject the core stream into a rapidly flowing saline sheath. The pressure and flow rate of the sheath fluid can be varied to control the core stream diameter. An appropriate core diameter can be "programmed" to ensure that cells or particles under analysis travel single file through the excitation zone. The principle of hydrodynamic focusing is illustrated in Figure 12.3.

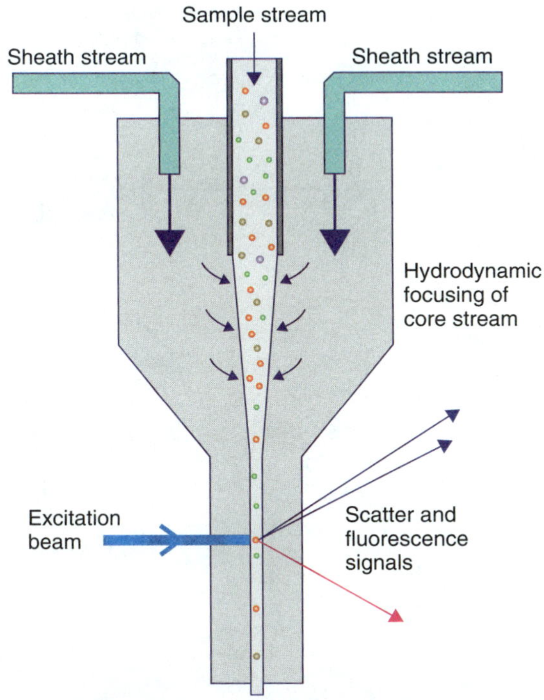

Figure 12.3 Flow of particles through excitation zone. It is important to distribute cells individually within the core stream so that scatter and fluorescence signals relate only to a single cell. This is achieved through hydrodynamic focusing of the core stream to force cells/particles to travel through the excitation zone in single file.

Forward-scatter light provides an indication of particle size; however, this is highly dependent on the refractive index of the particles and the core stream. The side-scatter detector captures light scattered at larger angles, the intensity of which is to some degree size dependent but influenced strongly by surface roughness and internal granularity of the particles detected. The side-scatter and fluorescence detectors are positioned at right angles to the beam axis. Fluorescence is typically analyzed in a number of different spectral bands through the use of a network of reflective dichroic filters (filters that only reflect certain wavelengths of light), as shown in Figure 12.4. Each detector converts the photons into electronic signals that are amplified, digitized, and processed by a microcontroller. In most instruments, there is provision to process and manipulate detector output as a logarithmic value. Both FSC and SSC signals can be useful for cell analysis. Typically the output data from a flow cytometer are in the form of a scatter plot, as shown in Figure 12.5*a*, whereby two signals are plotted against each other. The signals used most often are FSC versus SSC, SSC versus fluorescence bandwidth, or two different fluorescence bandwidths if two separate fluorochromes are used. Each dot on the scatter plot represents an event or particle passing through the light beam and creating a detectable signal. The differing signals produced form distinguishable groups or populations within the scatter plot and can help to define fundamental differences within a particle or cell suspension. For example, white blood cells can be clearly differentiated into three different classes using only the FSC and SSC signals, as shown in Figure 12.5*a*. Differentiation requires cell staining with dyes

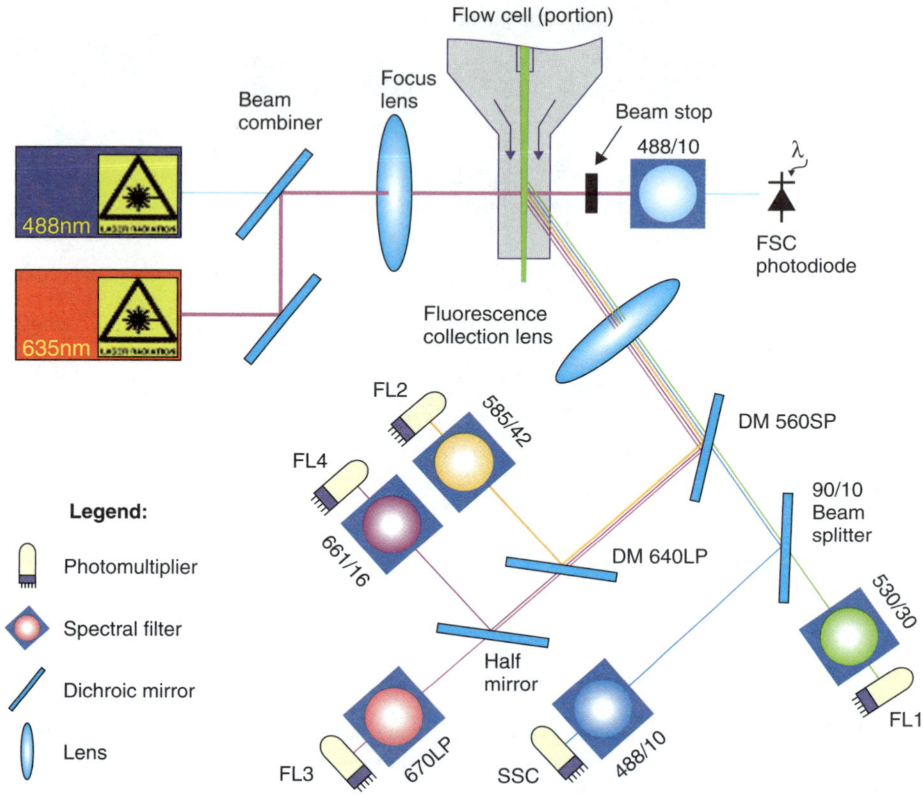

Figure 12.4 Detection optics for a typical flow cytometer such as the FACSCalibur from Becton Dickinson. The strong FSC signal is easily detected with a photodiode while the weaker SSC and fluorescence signals are registered on photomultipliers with high gain. The fluorescence signals in this instrument are captured by four channels: FL1 (green), FL2 (orange), FL3 (red), and FL4 (far red).

such as ethidium or propidium iodide (PI) which intercalate between the bases in a duplex strand of DNA and fluoresce strongly only in this configuration. Fluorescence intensity of dividing cells treated with these compounds is roughly proportional to DNA content and can be used to classify them into the G_0/G_1 phase or G_2/M postreplicative phase populations (see Figure 12.5*b*). Propidium iodide does not readily penetrate intact cell membranes to interact with the DNA and thus cells that show red nuclear fluorescence are presumed to have a disrupted membrane and can therefore be classified as dead or dying.

The three-dimensional dot-plot shown in Figure 12.5*c* shows *Pseudomonas* cells that were treated both with PI (red fluorescence) and Syto 9 (green fluorescence). The *X* axis represents the logarithmic intensity of green fluorescence signal (FL1) while the log intensity of red fluorescence (FL3) is plotted on the *Y* axis. The height (*Z* axis) is a linear representation of cells counted, in this case a count of thresholded FSC events. The dead population can clearly be discriminated from live cells using these parameters. The FSC signal is often used to trigger a sequence of operations once the signal strength exceeds a certain threshold value. The threshold value is above the "noise" level, resulting from random scatter events and corresponds to higher intensity

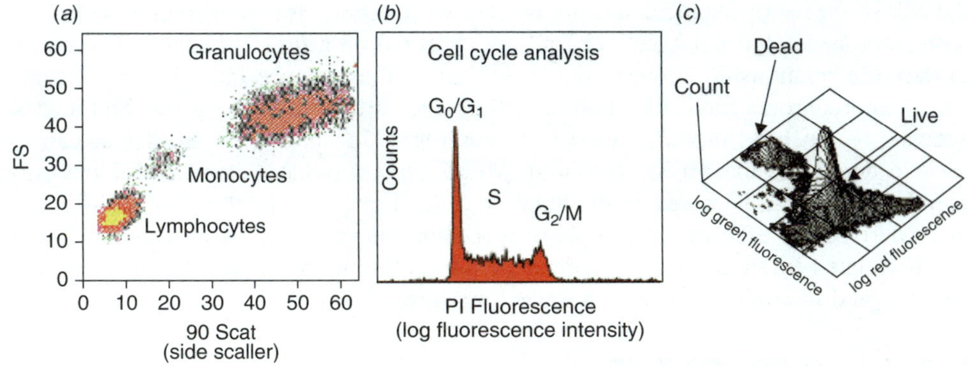

Figure 12.5 Presentation of data in flow cytometry. The application software on a flow cytometer can be configured to display cytometric data in a wide variety of formats. (*a*) Use of three parameters for label-free analysis of blood sample, relying only on unique scattering signal for each cell type. The *X* and *Y* coordinates are intensity values for the SSC and FSC signals while event frequency is color coded. (*b*) Use of flow cytometry for cell cycle analysis of population of cells. Here event frequency corresponds to the *Y* axis and fluorescence intensity of PI to the *X* axis. PI can be used to study the cell cycle since this reagent binds to DNA in a stoichiometric manner such that there is a direct relationship between DNA content and PI fluorescence. In this case the membrane was slightly damaged to allow penetration of the dye. Instead of using color, an isometric format such as that seen here for (*c*) of antibiotic-treated *Pseudomonas aeruginosa* can be used to highlight three different parameters. The cells were stained with the BacLight Live/Dead kit and the log green fluorescence arises from Syto 9 label while the log red fluorescence corresponds to PI intensity. (Courtesy of J. Paul Robinson.)

FSC signals generated when a particle enters the excitation zone. Detection of a cell would trigger processing of the FSC and SSC signals that could be used to classify the event.

Fluorescent labeling is used in flow cytometry to assist in cell recognition. Rare cells can be more readily discriminated from the total population if a specific marker exists on their surface that can be recognized by an antibody. Antibodies are proteins that can be engineered to bind to a specific macromolecule (antigen) that identifies the cell. Immunofluorescence is a technique that relies upon fluorescent labeling of the antibodies so that cells presenting the target antigen attract these antibodies, which renders them fluorescent, greatly facilitating their detection with flow cytometry. Immunofluorescent labeling became far more accessible following Kohler and Milstein's publication in 1975 describing the use of fused cells (hybridomas) for continuous production of monoclonal antibodies which are highly specific proteins for particular antigens [3]. These fused cells greatly simplified the monoclonal antibody production. The binding of fluorescently labeled antibodies to specific antigens is used as the basis for diagnostic detection of bacterial cells, protozoan cysts such as *Cryptosporidium* and *Giardia*, cancerous cells, or virus (e.g., HIV)–infected cells.

12.1.3 Sensitivity of Flow Cytometers

Flow cytometer sensitivity is often expressed in the form of molecules of equivalent soluble fluorochrome (MESF) units. The MESF threshold essentially reports the number of molecules of fluorochrome that the cytometer can detect. In order to measure the MESF, beads of identical size are labeled with varying levels of the fluorochrome, with some beads left unlabeled, and all are analyzed on a flow cytometer. The aim is to derive a relationship between the logarithm of fluorescence intensity to the number of fluorochrome molecules bound to the bead surface. Following flow cytometric analysis of the bead mixture, a least-squares regression plot is obtained that can be used to determine the MESF threshold. MESF units provide a standard for intensity correlation that can be based on the fluorochrome of interest, and thus the MESF needs to be derived for each new fluorophore type. For example, autofluorescence intensity can be related to an equivalent number of fluorochrome molecules if unstained cells are analyzed in conjunction with the bead mixture.

12.2 EXCITATION SOURCES

The cells or particles are transported rapidly through the excitation zone at a speed of 1–10 m/s. A powerful light source is required to excite strong fluorescence and scatter signals during the brief interval that a particle or cell is illuminated by the excitation beam. While early cytometers employed tungsten filament lamps, they were quickly superseded by much stronger mercury arc lamps. The broad spectral range of light emitted by arc lamp emission (Hg and Xe) conveniently provided a wide range of excitation wavelengths which could be selected or filtered by appropriate choice of the excitation filter set. It was a demanding task, however, to design an efficient optical system to provide a sufficient amount of filtered light in the excitation zone to ensure satisfactory detection sensitivity. Nevertheless, a number of impressive instruments were designed to operate using arc lamp excitation, including the first instrument designed for fluorescence detection. Fluorescence signals are much weaker than forward and orthogonal scatter signals, and this places stringent demands on instrument sensitivity when a relatively weak excitation source is used (compared to lasers). For example, a 100-W mercury arc lamp (HBO-100) delivers about 30 mW of optical power across the spectral range 365–435 nm and about 10 mW at 365 nm alone. A Hg lamp was used to excite fluorescence from cells stained with antibodies in the world's first demonstration of the fluorescence-activated cell sorting (FACS) flow cytometer. The first commercial flow cytometer (1969) available worldwide, the ICP-11 Impulscytophotometer, used a mercury arc lamp (HBO-100). This instrument sparked further design efforts from other groups since the mercury arc lamp delivered satisfactory amounts of light only in the blue and UV region of the spectrum and was poorly suited to excite strong emission from fluorescein, one of the most commonly used fluorophores [4]. Beckman Coulter currently markets a flow cytometer that employs a mercury arc lamp for excitation in conjunction with a laser source at 488 nm (Cell Lab Quanta SC). Partec also equips its advanced CyFlow ML instrument with a mercury arc lamp and an array of red, green, yellow, and blue solid-state lasers. The principal advantage of mercury arc lamps is the strong line at 365 nm (10 mW from HBO-100 lamp) that is not easily available from laser sources.

12.2.1 Laser Excitation

Lasers are near-ideal excitation sources for flow cytometry since the coherent radiation permits the beam to be focused to a very small spot size of high intensity. Laser sources are typically brighter at the beam center and weaker at the beam periphery, displaying

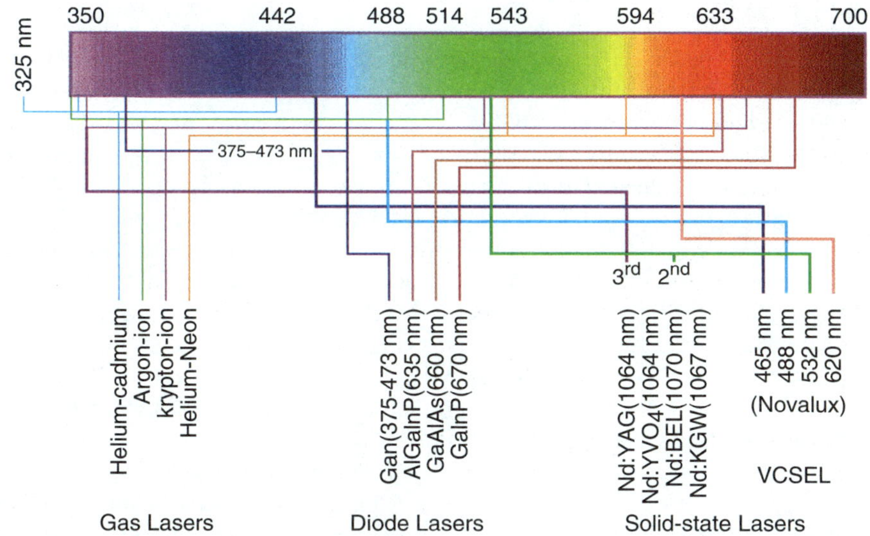

Figure 12.6 Laser excitation wavelengths cover visible spectrum and beyond. Gas lasers such as the argon–ion laser have found wide application in flow cytometry but are progressively being replaced by newer technologies. Shorter wavelengths have become more accessible with the introduction of diode lasers spanning the UVA region from 375 to 404 nm. Diode lasers are compact and relatively inexpensive, but a gap exists for the green/yellow region of the spectrum. Solid-state lasers operating in the green/yellow region have been available for years and vertical-cavity surface-emitting lasers (VCSELs) have recently been demonstrated to offer excellent beam quality at high output power over a range of important wavelengths.

what is known as a Gaussian energy distribution. If the beam were focused to a small spot encompassing the core, cells illuminated at the beam periphery would generate weaker signals than similar cells passing through the beam center. Identical particles or cells would therefore generate scatter or fluorescence signals with a large variation in their mean intensity. To avoid this problem, the laser beam is focused to an oval shape typically 70 μm across by 20 μm long to limit intensity variations across the 10-μm core stream to less than 2%.

12.2.2 Gas Laser Sources

Fluorescein is maximally excited at 494 nm, producing emission in the yellow (514 nm), and its isothiocyanate derivative was the first commercially available, practical antibody labeling reagent patented in 1960. The argon–ion laser efficiently excites fluorescein emission at 488 nm and can also deliver output in the UV (351 nm), blue (468 nm), and green (514 nm). Few commercial lasers were available in the 1960s and, among these, the argon–ion laser was clearly superior in terms of versatility, reliability, and cost. Consequently, the majority of laser-excited flow cytometers included an argon–ion laser. Flow cytometers developed since then are often equipped with a range of (gas) laser sources including krypton–ion, helium–neon, and helium–cadmium; see Figure 12.6 for details on specific emission wavelengths for these devices.

12.2.3 Diode Lasers

Gallium–indium phosphide laser diodes emitting at 670 nm were available in the early 1980s; however, most manufacturers retained their HeNe lasers at least until shorter wavelength versions operating at 635 nm reached the market in 1995. The shorter wavelengths were achieved by fabricating the diodes from aluminium–gallium–indium phosphide. Simple, dedicated instruments designed to precisely count CD4 T cells have been built using only a 635-nm diode laser as the excitation source. New diode laser sources fabricated with gallium nitride (GaN) can deliver diffraction-limited continuous-wave output at 375, 405, 440, and 473 nm with typical power levels of 18–75 mW [5]. Single-mode laser-diodes avoid the drawbacks associated with gas lasers relating to cost, size, power, thermal management, and optical noise.

Diode lasers generally require beam correction. The beam from a diode laser is typically elliptical in shape with a divergent and uneven (astigmatic) wavefront. Beam circularity can be achieved by passing the beam through a pair of anamorphic prisms and a circular aperture. A weak cylindrical lens on the output side can then be used to apply astigmatic correction to deliver a near-Gaussian, circular beam shape. Other techniques include microlensing within the diode packaging; this has the advantage of simplicity and efficiency. The placement of a microlens with a high numerical apperture (NA) immediately in front of the emitting face ensures virtually all the optical energy is captured and circularized without the need for correcting prisms.

If some coupling loss can be tolerated, the diode beam may be fiber coupled to remove astigmatism and yield a superior circular beam free of astigmatism. In this approach a flat wavefront ensures the beam can be finely focused to a diffraction-limited spot.

12.2.4 Solid-State Lasers

Coherent emission can be excited from certain glass or crystalline materials configured in a resonant cavity when pumped by an external source (e.g., flash-lamp or diode laser). While many crystalline substrates can be induced to lase under appropriate excitation, Nd–YAG (neodymium–yttrium–aluminum–garnet) is probably one of the better known materials which can be pumped with a diode laser source at around 808 nm to deliver multiwatt output at 1064 nm. This technique is suitable for pumping other lasing crystals such as Nd–YVO_4 (neodymium–yttrium–vanadate) with a higher absorbance coefficient than YAG. These can be excited to lase at 914, 1064, and 1342 nm with high efficiency. Compact design and single-longitudinal-mode output are two important benefits available from Nd–YVO_4-based systems. Other neodymium-doped crystals that can be pumped at around 809 nm include lanthanum–beryllate Nd–BEL (Nd–$La_2Be_2O_5$) and potasssium–gadolinium–tungstate Nd–KGW [Nd–$KGd(WO_4)_2$]. These crystals emit in the infrared, and generation of visible wavelengths is achieved using a nonlinear optical process to generate the second (SHG) or third harmonic (THG) of the input wavelength. The related processess of sum frequency generation (SFG) or difference frequency generation (DFG) can also be used to generate wavelengths that are otherwise not accessible using SHG or THG. Solid-state sources typically have a superior beam profile to diode lasers and deliver a circular beam with a Gaussian energy distribution and low wavefront error. Their output can however be noisy, especially when mode competition is not suppressed.

It is important to mention novel laser sources such as VCSELs. Faced with a plummeting market demand in the communications industry, a Californian manufacturer (Novalux) of VCSELs adapted its product to deliver visible wavelengths. VCSELs first emerged onto the market about 10 years ago as a low-cost, high-yield laser emitting in the infrared. Novalux modified the structure of the devices to permit introduction of a nonlinear optical material within the intracavity space to achieve highly efficient second-harmonic conversion of infrared light. Necsel (Novalux-extended cavity surface-emitting laser) products were first marketed in 2002 as the Protera 488-5 blue laser system providing 5-mW TEM00 output with $<0.2\%$ root-mean-square (rms) optical noise. In 2006 a high-brightness Necsel RGB (red/green/blue) array was demonstrated to provide enhanced color and brightness compared to a conventional TV projection source. The Necsel array emits red at 620 nm, green at 532 nm, and blue at 465 nm with output powers approaching 3 W for each beam. The entire package is reported to be smaller than a matchbox and suitable for mass production; thus economies of scale would apply. Unlike most edge-emitting diode lasers, surface-emitting lasers can deliver a near-circular beam with a Gaussian energy distribution that is optimal for coupling to lenses or optical fiber. In the authors' opinion, these are the lasers of the future for cytometry applications.

12.3 SIGNAL DETECTION AND ANALYSIS

12.3.1 Forward Scatter

Forward scatter produces the most intense signal for flow cytometry detection. The majority of light scattering is observed to occur at small angles (0.5°–5°) to the incident beam with smaller particles scattering light at larger angles. Forward-scatter signals are a reliable indicator of the presence of a cell within the excitation zone. Quantitative interpretation of signal intensity is difficult because at dimensions approaching the wavelength of light the scattering of light cannot be easily predicted. However, certain features can be tracked to features of particles. The particle size is an important factor, and forward scatter is frequently useful to provide an indication of particle size. The difference in the refractive index of the particle and core stream also has a strong influence on the scatter angle. This effect can be employed to derive insights into cell populations. For example (other factors being equal), refractive elements within a cell (blood granulocytes) will produce stronger scatter (increased amplitude of light bursts) than similar cells without such structures (e.g., blood lymphocytes). Forward scatter also provides information about the state of the cell (alive or dead). This is because cells with damaged membranes (dead cells) have a lower refractive index and smoother surface, resulting in decreased forward scatter.

12.3.2 Side Scatter

Scatter at 90° to the incident beam is termed orthogonal or side scatter, and intensive studies were conducted in the mid-1970s to determine the relative "information value" of scatter collected over a range of different angles. Scatter signals collected at angles as small as 18° from the beam axis were found to hold the same information content as scatter orthogonal to the beam axis. In terms of instrument design, it is easier to implement side-scatter detection orthogonal to the beam axis as part of the fluorescence collection optics. It was later demonstrated by Salzman et al. [6] that a combination of forward- and side-scatter signals could distinguish blood lymphocytes, monocytes, and granulocytes from each other without any chemical pretreatment (fixing or staining). We are now aware that the side-scatter signal is information rich and strongly influenced by refractive components within cells and cell surface topography. Shapiro and others have also observed a correlation between total protein content of a cell and side-scatter intensity [7]. Such signals have been used to assess nuclear morphology since condensed chromatin in the nuclei increases scatter. Other researchers have reported the use of DNA dyes in conjunction with side scatter to discriminate cells with mitotic nuclei (cells with twice the DNA content). Refractile inclusions in cells or the presence of gas vacuoles can result in strong side-scatter signals that can be used in conjunction with forward-scatter signals to distinguish different cell populations.

The intensity of side scatter is considerably reduced in comparison with forward scatter and the coefficient of variation (CV) is much higher for side scatter due to the extreme sensitivity of scatter intensity to small variations in the size of the particles/cells.

12.3.3 Fluorescence

From about the 1980s onward, most commercial flow cytometers supported at least two fluorescence channels. The popular FACScan (Becton Dickinson) supported three-color cell analysis and more recent BD instruments such as the FACSCalibur and FACSAria support four- and nine-color cell analysis, respectively. Figure 12.7 illustrates the advanced fluorescence detection arrangement used on the Becton Dickinson FACSAria.

12.3.4 Issues in Flow Cytometry Using Fluorescence: Fluorescence Compensation

Although the new commercially available cytometers on the market are supporting more and more sophisticated fluorescence detection systems, the detection of fluorescence is not straightforward. The emission spectrum of most fluorescent dyes is relatively broad; for example, fluorescein emission peaks at around 520 nm with a full width at half maximum (FWHM) of about 40 nm, but emission can be detected from 490 nm to beyond 600 nm. Fluorescence detection on a flow cytometer is designed (typically) to collect broad spectral "bands of interest" (FL1, green; FL2, orange; and FL3, red) that span more than 200 nm of the visible spectrum. Returning again to our fluorescein example, fluorescence emission will be collected primarily in FL1, but a smaller portion of the fluorescence will be detected by the FL2 detector. This can become problematic when multiple fluorophores are employed with spectral overlap on their emissions. Such overlap occurs with phycoerythrin and fluorescein with both channels receiving signal contributions from "out-of-band" emission (regions A and B in Figure 12.8), reducing the instrument capability to make quantitative determinations. To overcome this problem, the cytometer needs to be calibrated with a single fluorophore and the ratio of signal contribution to adjacent channels noted. The signal on the primary channel is then used to proportionally reduce gain on the adjacent channel according to the previously observed ratio. This is known as "one-way compensation," and for accurate measurement of our phycoerythrin signal, the process must be extended to the other channel in a similar manner to give "two-way compensation."

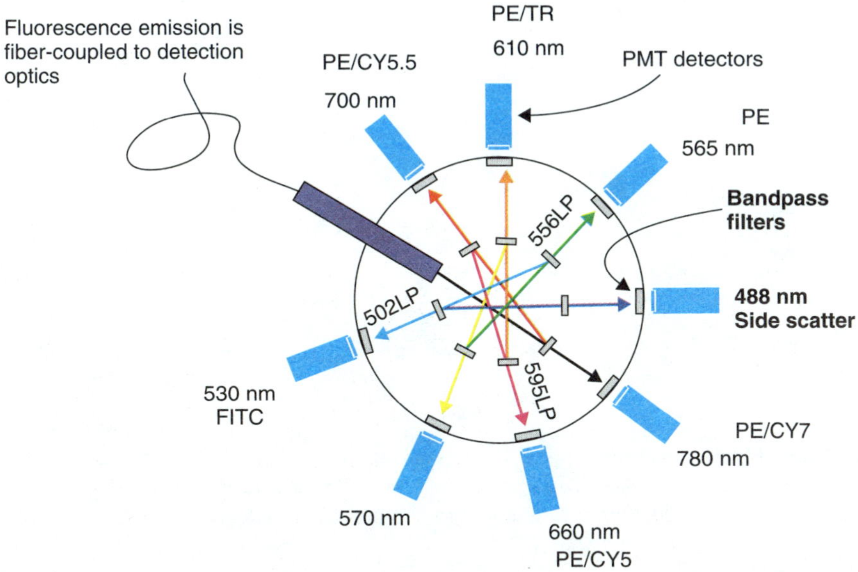

Figure 12.7 Schematic of FACSAria instrument from BD Biosciences. It departs radically from conventional detection schemes by collecting fluorescence from the excitation focal point using optical fibers and delivering the emission to a ring of detectors as shown here. Collection efficiency is optimized by transmitting the longest wavelengths to the first photomultiplier tube (PMT) and reflecting the shorter wavelengths to the next PMT through a series of long-pass dichroic mirrors. Bandpass filters in front of each PMT allow fine tuning of the collected signal. Since reflection is more efficient than transmittance, this design greatly increases the multicolor detection capabilities of the instrument.

The process becomes increasingly difficult with more spectral channels, and modern instruments provide an automated process for achieving fluorescence compensation across multiple channels.

The electronics in a flow cytometer is an important part of the system. The FSC signal is strong and can be captured with a low-cost photodiode whereas SSC and fluorescence signals are generally much weaker and require a sensitive PMT for detection. The PMT can amplify weak fluorescence signals by several orders of magnitude (2×10^7) if required. Maximum amplitude of a signal from the detection electronics is typically limited to 10 V peak to peak and dynamic range of the signals can range over five orders of magnitude. Conventionally this large range is handled by processing the signal through logarithmic amplifiers (log amps) that output the logarithm of the input voltage. Log amps that respond accurately across the required range are complex and expensive circuits that can be eliminated if the input signals are digitized. Modern instruments increasingly rely on digital signal processing and utilize high-speed analog-to-digital (A/D) conversion to sample detector signals. To accommodate a reasonable dynamic range for the instrument, the A/D conversion process must digitize the signal with 16-bit (65,536-channel) resolution or greater [the Coulter EPICS XL is reported to digitize to 20-bit (1,048,576-channel) precision]. Once in digital form, the data can be processed using a digital signal processor to perform such operations as peak detection, integration, and convolution of input signals.

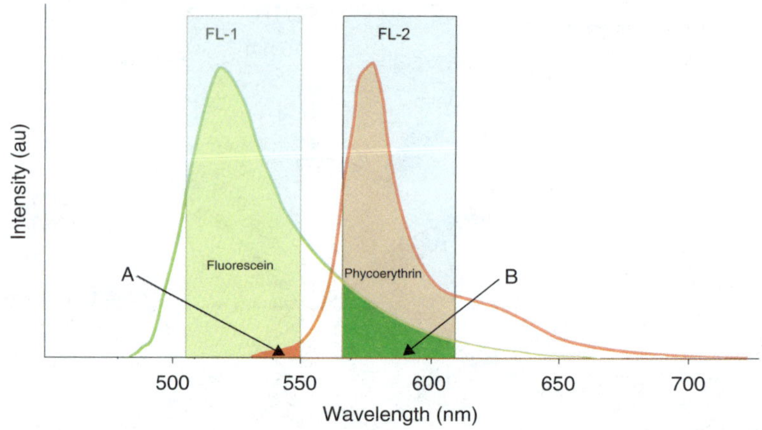

Figure 12.8 Fluorescence overlap of fluorescein and phycoerythrin. Many fluorophores emit over a broad spectral band that may span two or more fluorescence channels. Natural autofluorescence can also compete with a synthetic fluorescence label to degrade quality of the collected data.

12.3.5 Multiparameter Analysis

Modern flow cytometers such as the CyFlow ML or FACSAria are capable of 13- or 9-color analysis, respectively. An instrument would rarely need to be configured to monitor the full range of available channels; instead various scatter and color channels are used to "gate" or select a desired subset of the sample population. The sequence of events initiated by the passage of a target particle, for example, a granulocyte labeled with an immunofluorophore, through the excitation zone of the cytometer begins with the forward-scatter burst of photons. An FSC signal pulse that exceeds a programmed threshold value is registered as a positive detection event, triggering the electronics to capture SSC and fluorescence signal information. The FSC signal will diminish as the target particle exits the excitation zone, falling below threshold and terminating signal collection for that event. Modern instruments capture this sequence by slicing the event into hundreds of individual time packets for which signal intensity from all channels is digitally recorded (16–20-bit resolution). Modern multicolor flow cytometers have led to the development of complex protocols with as many as 17 colors analyzed in conjunction with scatter signals [1]. To represent these datasets, bivariate (two-axis) data plots are usually generated using two key parameters to discriminate populations that are then subjected to further two-dimensional gating using additional parameters. Information content tends to increase exponentially with the number of parameters, and identification of populations within this multidimensional space is often beyond the capacity of human operators. Analysis of such datasets using automated clustering algorithms has been shown to be useful [8].

12.4 CELL SORTING

As well as being a powerful cell analysis tool, flow cytometry can be used to physically sort cells using information from the various detectors as discriminators. Sorting enables purification of a particular cell type from a complex mixture. The most widely

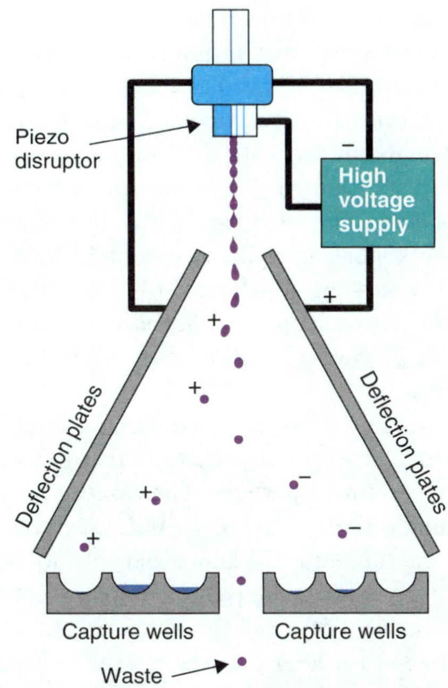

Figure 12.9 Sorting process. Collection of the desired cells following their identification was a design goal from the earliest days of flow cytometry. The system shown here can operate at high speed and is employed on most modern flow cytometers. A piezoelectric transducer within the flow cell body oscillates at frequencies from 10 to 300 kHz to induce the exiting flow stream to break up into a train of small, evenly shaped droplets. On identifying a desired cell or particle, the instrument electronics places a charge on the droplet at the moment prior to it separating from the main stream (the last attached drop). As the drop passes between the two charged plates, it experiences an attractive/repulsive force proportional to its charge and can thus be directed into individual receiving wells.

used method of sorting cells by flow cytometry is known as droplet deflection sorting. It relies on the use of a piezoelectric transducer in the flow cell to induce droplet formation in the flow stream (Figure 12.9). An alternating electrical drive is applied to the transducer, causing the flow cell pressure to oscillate in phase with transducer displacement. Oscillation of the flow cell pressure induces undulations to form in the flow stream as it exits the flow cell. Further downstream from the flow cell, the undulations become more pronounced until the stream breaks up into individual droplets. The last undulation in the stream before the stream breaks up into droplets is known as the last-attached droplet.

If a particle is to be collected, then an electric charge is placed on the sheath fluid at the exact time the particle is in the last-attached droplet. The charge is maintained for the duration of a full cycle of the piezoelectric crystal. This results in a single droplet, the one containing the particle to be sorted, being charged. Downstream from the flow cell the stream of droplets passes between two plates, one positively and one negatively charged. As the charged droplet passes between the energized plates, it is deflected from its path to permit collection. Sorting can be performed at a rate of several thousand times per second on modern instruments.

Major problems associated with droplet deflection cell-sorting technology arise from the complexity of instrument setup that requires an operator with a high degree of skill and experience and instability of the droplet stream. To calibrate the instrument, fluorescent beads are sorted onto a microscope slide using a range of different settings. The sorted droplets are then examined with a fluorescence microscope and the number of beads within each drop is counted. Once set up, the droplet stream is carefully monitored by a video camera. The position of the last-attached droplet tends to be unstable, particularly when sorting samples that contain large numbers of particles or with particles that clump. Frequent adjustment of both the frequency and amplitude of the signal applied to the piezoelectric crystal is necessary to stabilize the position of the last-attached droplet. Figure 12.9 illustrates a sorting instrument based on the last-attached-droplet process.

An alternative form of sorting is used on the Becton Dickinson FACSCalibur flow cytometer. This sorting process uses a capture tube that is mechanically moved in and out of the sample stream to capture a particle. The capture tube is positioned within the sheath stream but just outside the stream of particles. A continuous stream of sheath fluid travels through the capture tube. When a particle to be sorted is detected, the capture tube is moved slightly so that the particle enters the capture tube. This capture tube format requires less intervention from the operator and once calibrated using fluorescent beads can be left to run for long periods of time, whereas the droplet deflection sorting method requires constant monitoring. The limitation of the mechanical capture tube is the maximum speed of sorting. The capture tube is physically moved in and out of the sorting fluid stream; therefore, the tube is limited to sorting a maximum of 300 events per second.

A similar mechanical sorting mechanism is used by the sorting instrument manufactured by the German company Partec. The advantage of these mechanical sorting mechanisms is that the flow cytometer is simple to operate, is completely stable, and requires no calibration or complex setup procedure to be performed prior to sorting particles. It is simply a case of switching on the instrument, analyzing a sample, and sorting the particles of interest. There are, however, two major limitations of this mechanical sorting technology. First, the maximum sort speed is 300 cells per second as previously described for the Becton Dickinson FACSCalibur flow cytometer. Second, the constant stream of sheath fluid has to be collected along with the sorted particles, resulting in the sorted particles being contained in a large volume of fluid (typically 1–50 mL depending on the time of the collection process). The particles therefore have to be concentrated to much smaller volumes before they can be analyzed or visualized with a microscope. Smaller sort volumes are now possible; for example, Morgan et al. [9] reported a method for modifying the sorting mechanism within a FACSCalibur cytometer to enable particles to be sorted in volumes of less than 20 μL. A comparison of different cell-sorting methods is illustrated in Table 12.1.

12.5 APPLICATIONS OF FLOW CYTOMETRY

12.5.1 Calibration

Micrometer-sized beads have broad applications in flow cytometry, both as calibration reagents and as components in diagnostic and detection assays. Calibration microspheres can be designed to simultaneously establish both sensitivity and range of a flow cytometer. Cytometers are calibrated using a mixture of identically sized beads labeled at (typically) five different fluorescence levels. Beads with the least label simulate weakly labeled and autofluorescent cells, while the more strongly labeled beads provide a full range of intensities calibrated with approximate MESF values (see Section 12.1.3) to determine the relative fluorescence intensity of target cells. Calibration is a frequent practice which needs to be performed at least daily and whenever detection protocols are changed.

12.5.2 Use of Beads for Diagnostic Purposes

Although fluorescent beads are primarily used as a calibration tool for flow cytometers, there are technologies available to bind specific probes to beads. The specificity of the probe combined with the size and easy cytometer detection of the fluorescent bead enables the detection of small biomolecules which are beyond the normal detection limit of flow cytometers. Thus flow cytometry bead or microsphere assays are gaining increasing prominence as a diagnostic method, for example, to detect small biomolecules.

Free molecules of nucleic acid are too small to be detected using conventional flow cytometry. However, there is an approach for the analysis of DNA and RNA based on microspheres. Luminex (Austin, TX) supplies bead kits that are designed to be used with flow cytometry to analyze DNA or RNA molecules. Microspheres (5.5 μm in diameter) manufactured from a polystyrene polymer containing varying proportions of red and orange fluorophores are designed to permit classification (gating) of the beads based on their fluorescence signature. The beads can be divided into 100 different subsets based on their fluorescence signatures. Each subset of beads is labeled with a nucleic acid capture probe (DNA/RNA) that targets a specific DNA sequence. The target DNA or RNA is amplified using PCR (polymerase chain reaction) and subsequently labeled with a green fluorescent dye. The amplified DNA is then reacted with the labeled beads. The beads are then analyzed to determine which subsets are coated with the fluorescently labeled DNA.

This technology is a powerful tool for the analysis of PCR products. When combined with a generic PCR assay, such as one that amplifies a range of different viral or

TABLE 12.1 Comparison of Different Sorting Methods

Parameter	Droplet Deflection Sorting	Mechanical Sorting
Maximum speed of sorting	50,000 sorts per second	300 sorts per second
Volume of liquid containing sorted particle	<2 μL	1 mL
Setup time	0.5–2 h	No setup required
Stability	Poor: requires constant monitoring and frequent recalibration	Very stable: requires no calibration
Required operator skill level	High: significant experience necessary to set up and operate	Operator can be trained within a few hours
Cost	>$500,000	$100,000–$200,000

bacterial DNA sequences, it allows for the rapid detection and identification of a large range of microorganisms as well as the assessment of a viral load. This is because the level of DNA label fluorescence is directly related to the number of viral nucleic acids attached to each bead [10].

12.5.3 Water Testing

Cryptosporidiosis can be a life-threatening disease for those with damaged or suppressed immune systems. For this reason, testing is required for the presence of *Cryptosporidium* oocysts within drinking water. During the testing procedure the cysts are first isolated from most other particulate matter in the water; however, there is still some carry-over of naturally fluorescent debris/algae/mineral particles. Highly specific detection of oocysts within this matrix can be achieved using two-color immunofluorescent labeling of the pathogen followed by analysis on a FACS flow cytometer. The addition of the second parameter makes it possible to reduce false-positive detection numbers 20-fold compared to conventional single-color detection. Techniques such as these have the potential to allow on-line analysis of water samples, eliminating the requirement for complex enrichment protocols.

12.5.4 Milk Analysis

To monitor the quality and safety of milk requires enumeration of both somatic cells (any bovine cells other than the reproductive cells) and microbial cells. The detection of somatic cells by flow cytometry requires the lipid components of milk to be removed. Lipid globules can be removed by centrifugation of the milk sample at 14,000 *g* for 10 min; a detergent wash with Triton X-100 can also aid the removal of lipids. Once the lipids are removed, somatic cells can be distinguished from milk proteins by staining the cells with acridine orange. The stained cells are detected by analysis of the green fluorescence of acridine orange (FL1) and SSC, whereas the proteins do not stain green and form event populations lower on the FL1 scale.

The detection of bacteria in milk using flow cytometry is hampered by the highly refractile milk proteins and lipid globules that give milk its white color. To "clear" the milk of proteins, an enzymatic treatment with proteinase K is performed and the digested proteins along with the lipids are removed in the supernatant after centrifugation. This treatment may also require several wash steps to optimize the removal of protein debris; any residual lipid or protein molecules will lead to nonspecific binding of fluorescent stains used to detect the bacterial cells. It is therefore imperative to optimize the milk-clearing process prior to flow cytometric analysis.

To detect bacterial cells within the cleared milk, a suite of different nucleic acid stains are available. SYTO BC and SYTO 11-16 dyes are green fluorescent nucleic acid stains that will penetrate both gram-positive and gram-negative live and dead bacterial cells. SYTO dyes can be used in conjunction with dyes such as PI, which will only penetrate cells which have damaged cell membranes and are therefore generally considered nonviable. Cell uptake of PI produces an orange/red fluorescence and is therefore detected on the red fluorescence channel (FL3). Other possible stains include:

- 5-Cyanol-2,3- ditolyl tetrazolium chloride (CTC), which indicates live cells with active dehydrogenases (red fluorescence)

- Oxonol, which indicates cells with compromised membrane potential (green fluorescence)
- Hexidium iodide, which is selectively uptaken by gram-positive cells (red fluorescence)

Depending on the efficiency of the clearing method, the specificity of nucleic acid dyes can cause false-positive results. Initial validation of any flow cytometric analysis should be compared to more conventional culturing methods, for example, to support bacterial cell viability testing or existing methodologies (e.g., the Fossomatic instrument for somatic cell counts).

There are other more specific methods for bacterial cell detection within milk, such as fluorescein isothiocyanate (FITC)–labeled direct antibodies, which can label specific cells with FITC green fluorescence and then be detected by a flow cytometer. There are also fluorescent oligonucleotide-based techniques such as fluorescent in situ hybridization (FISH) to specifically probe for bacteria, thereby avoiding nonspecific binding of nucleic acid dyes to protein particles remaining in the cleared milk. However, it has been reported that FISH-based detection techniques correlate well with conventional methods only when the bacterial load is lower than 10^4 cells/mL. The major advantage of milk bacterial load analysis using flow cytometry is that an assay can be completed within 40 min, whereas FISH analysis takes 3 h and conventional culture methods require overnight incubation followed by lengthy microscopic analysis.

12.5.5 Brewing and Wine Production

Similar to the advantages realized within the milk analysis industry, the brewing industry is finding that flow cytometry can give valuable real-time results during the production process, enabling decisions such as on quality and yeast concentration to be made instantaneously and without critical delays. Dried yeast is used for inoculating fermentation processes during wine and beer production as well as baking. A percentage of yeast cells are rendered nonviable due to the drying and rehydration processes. The degree of damage and number of dead cells impact on the efficiency of the fermentation, and therefore it is necessary to have a quick and relatively simple method to detect the cell load and viability of the yeast within each fermentation batch.

Flow cytometry has been assessed as a method of monitoring the performance of yeast and bacteria within fermentation processes. The alcohol fermentation process is due to both yeast and malolactic bacteria activity, and flow cytometry has the capability to study viability and concentration of both cell populations simultaneously and in real time. Yeast and bacterial populations can be fluorescently stained using dyes such as Rhodamine 123, final concentration 5 μg/mL; calcein acetoxymethyl ester, 2 μM; 2′,7′-bis(carboxyethyl)-5(6)-carboxyfluorescein acetoxymethyl ester (BCECF-AM) 10 μM; and fluorescein diacetate (FDA), 0.01 mg/mL. As with the analysis of milk, a measurement of cell viability can be obtained when oxonol and PI are utilized. Such membrane integrity stains are key tools to indicate cell membrane damage to yeast cells during the drying process. Evidence has been presented in a number of careful studies indicating that cell damage during drying is primarily due to breaches in membrane permeability and structure. The detection limit for flow cytometric analysis of beer and wine depends largely on the quality of the sample preparation prior to analysis. Interference from debris within the fermentation limits the detection to 10^3 cells/mL; however, this causes few problems as generally the critical stages of fermentation require monitoring cell levels from 10^3 to 10^8 cells/mL. Samples can be cleaned and debris removed by simple washing and centrifugation methods.

12.5.6 Food Microbiology

The analysis of foods for bacterial contamination is another application suitable for flow cytometric analysis. With fluid samples, the preparation and separation of interfering particles are much the same as milk and beer products. The main issue with solid food samples is the presence of high levels of suspended material. Therefore, prior to flow analysis, it is necessary to extract or concentrate microorganisms from the food sample before an accurate enumeration of cell load can be made. Extraction methodologies would differ according to the food type; for example, fruit juices would be centrifuged at 12,000*g* for 10 min and then the bacteria-containing pellet removed and resuspended in phosphate-buffered saline (PBS); fatty foods such as meat and meat products such as paté would require a stomaching, or homogenizing, step to release the bacteria from the particulate food matter, a centrifugation wash step to remove the particulate matter, possibly a filtration step using coarse filters such as 80- and 25-μm nylon meshes, and then potentially a final chemical treatment such as 0.05% benzalkonium chloride to reduce cytometer background interference from the particulates and allow cells to be detected once stained. Following extraction, most methods rely upon the use of a mixture of fluorescent antibodies and viability stains such as PI. Species-specific antibodies label the organism for reliable detection while the proportion of dead cells is determined by the takeup of a viability dye by cells with damaged membranes. Immunofluorescent staining is the best method for detecting cells that are required to remain viable for sorting and culturing. Nucleic acid stains can effectively label cell populations to raise signal levels above background for efficient flow cytometry analysis. The disadvantage with nucleic acid stains is their toxic effect on bacterial cells, causing death or rendering them nonculturable. It is therefore advisable to ascertain what data will be required regarding viability before a staining approach is selected. Staining by both fluorescent antibodies and nucleic acid stains together is also possible, thereby providing highly specific detection in conjunction with a report on cell viability.

Flow cytometric analysis of food can also provide a rapid total-microorganism count through use of a nonspecific nucleic acid dye such as ethidium bromide. This technique provides a means of effectively screening a food product for microbial cells, which can be followed by single-cell sorting from populations of interest into growth media for further viability testing by traditional culture methodologies. The screening process is rapid and can give a same-day presumptive test result whereas traditional culture techniques require a minimum of 15 h.

The low-cost nature of the food microbiology testing industry precludes widespread application of the relatively expensive techniques of flow cytometry. Growth areas for flow cytometric analysis are in research and development (R&D) of new food processes and packaging and the challenge testing that occurs in this area.

12.5.7 Quality Control in Microbiological Testing in Various Industries

Over the past decade, new applications for flow cytometry have been steadily emerging. Flow cytometry and cell sorting are being used for the production of quality control standards that contain precise numbers of cells. These quality control standards are being used to spike samples to determine the detection efficiency of a test protocol. Such protocols were first reported at Thames Water in the United Kingdom, where quality control samples were prepared containing exactly 100 *Cryptosporidium* [11]. A suspension of *Cryptosporidium* oocysts was analyzed on a flow cytometer, light scatter properties were used to differentiate the oocysts from debris particles, and 100 of the *Cryptosporidium* oocysts were sorted into test tubes. These samples were then used to test and validate new methods for detecting *Cryptosporidium* oocysts in water. These samples proved so useful for monitoring the performance of testing that the U.S. Environmental Protection Agency (EPA) put in place regulations that required all water-testing laboratories in the United States to run one of these flow cytometry prepared standards whenever they analyzed water for *Cryptosporidium*. The U.K. Drinking Water Inspectorate then followed suite and insisted that all U.K. water laboratories used flow cytometry prepared standards on at least a daily basis. Many of the world's water-testing laboratories employing flow cytometers for the detection of *Cryptosporidium* have now switched to the use of prepared standards to validate their testing method. Bacterial testing also has moved to the use of these standards; precise numbers of bacteria are sorted by flow cytometry and collected into liquid nitrogen and then freeze dried into small 3-mm-diameter pellets. Within these pellets the bacteria remain viable and are stable for several years. The use of these standards has now been mandated in some areas of bacteriological testing. The advantage of using flow cytometry prepared standards is that there is very little variation between samples and between separate batches of samples. An example of this is given in Figure 12.10. The graph shows the quality control results from an Australian laboratory that tests water samples for the presence of *Escherichia coli*. Every day a sample of sterilized water is spiked with a low level of *E. coli* and this sample is processed through a standard *E. coli* test method. The graph shows the number of *E. coli* detected each day in the spiked sample. Initially the laboratory prepared the *E. coli* for spiking by diluting a culture; some time later it switched to using controls prepared by flow cytometry. Importantly, prior to the use of the flow cytometry prepared standards, the laboratory frequently failed to detect *E. coli* in the spiked sample. When this occurred, all test results for that day were invalidated. This problem cannot be solved by spiking with a high number of bacteria because it is important that the number of cells in the spike be close to the limit of sensitivity of the detection method. Clearly the use of flow cytometry prepared controls alleviates this problem.

A recent extension of the use of flow cytometry to dispense cells has been the application of this technology to the production of standards that contain a precise number of genes. By inserting a sequence of DNA into the chromosome of *E. coli* and then dispensing an exact number of these modified *E. coli*, it is possible to produce an exact number of genes. Recently the Australian National Measurement Institute has demonstrated the use of this technology to monitor the performance of PCR testing with samples spiked with a single copy of the target DNA sequence.

12.5.8 Cytometry: Where to Now?

There are few limitations to using flow cytometry for other applications. Key advantages of this technology arise from the rapidity of the test and the ability to selectively isolate (sort) cells or particles of interest. Applications such as monitoring for cells

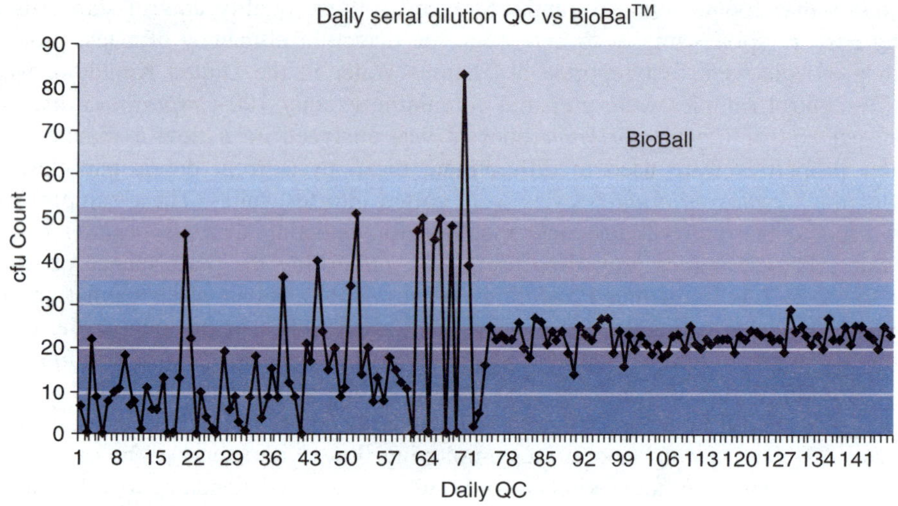

Figure 12.10 Routine quality control data from Australian official body involved in water testing. Water samples (100 mL) were spiked with *E. coli*. Initially the laboratory was spiking with *E. coli* prepared by serially diluting a culture. The graph highlights the reduction in variance after the laboratory switched to a new flow cytometry protocol that employed control samples (bioballs) containing exactly 30 colony-forming units of *E. coli*.

with particular gene expression traits rely solely on the availability of fluorescent antibodies for particular expressed proteins of choice. Therefore the use of flow cytometry is more limited by the availability of fluorescent markers to distinguish the particles of interest; the increased availability and range of such markers constantly open new avenues of flow cytometric exploration. A second front of major research activity is underway in the development of lab-on-chip microfluidic arrays that offer the promise of integrated fluidics together with excitation and detection optics for miniature flow cytometers at greatly reduced manufacturing costs.

REFERENCES

1. S. P. Perfetto, P. K. Chattopadhyay, and M. Roederer, "Innovation: Seventeen-color flow cytometry: Unraveling the immune system," *Nat. Rev. Immunol.* **4**(8), 648–655 (2004).
2. I. D. Goldberg, E. M. Rosen, H. M. Shapiro et al., "Isolation and culture of a tetraploid subpopulation of smooth muscle cells from the normal rat aorta," *Science* **226**(4674), 559–561 (1984).
3. G. Kohler and C. Milstein, "Continuous cultures of fused cells secreting antibody of predefined specificity," *Nature* **256**(5517), 495–497 (1975).
4. G. Valet, "Past and present concepts in flow cytometry: A European perspective," *J. Biol. Regul. Homeost. Agents* **17**, 213–222 (2003).
5. Toptica Photonics, Inc., Victor, NY, http://www.toptica.com.
6. G. C. Salzman, J. M. Crowell, J. C. Martin, et al., "Cell classification by laser light scattering: Identification and separation of unstained leukocytes," *Acta Cytol.* **19**(4), 374–377 (1975).

7. H. M. Shapiro, D. M. Feinstein, A. S. Kirsch, et al., "Multistation multiparameter flow cytometry: Some influences of instrumental factors on system performance," *Cytometry* **4**(1), 11–19 (1983).
8. U. Petrausch, D. Haley, W. Miller, et al., "Polychromatic flow cytometry: A rapid method for the reduction and analysis of complex multiparameter data," *Cytometry, Part A* **69A**(12), 1162–1173 (2006).
9. C. A. Morgan, P. Bigeni, N. Herman, M. Gauci, P. A. White, and G. Vesey, "Production of precise microbiology standards using flow cytometry and freeze drying," *Cytometry* **62**(2), 162–168 (2004).
10. P. L. Smith, C. R. WalkerPeach, R. J. Fulton, et al., "A rapid, sensitive, multiplexed assay for detection of viral nucleic acids using the FlowMetrix system," *Clin. Chem.* **44**, 2054–2056 (1998).
11. D. T. Reynolds, R. B. Slades, N. J. Sykes, A. Jonas, and C. R. Fricker, "Detection of *Cryptosporidium* oocysts in water: Techniques for generating precise recorvery data," *J. Appl. Microbiology* **50**, 78–85 (2002).

CHAPTER 13

Fluorescence in Diagnostic Imaging

MORRY SILBERSTEIN

Department of Medical Imaging and Radiation Sciences, Monash University,
Clayton, Victoria 3800, Australia

13.1 INTRODUCTION

Diagnostic imaging is a term that is applied to the application of imaging technologies to the diagnosis of disease in a clinical "whole-patient" setting. Regarded as a medical specialty, on a par with surgery, internal medicine, psychiatry, and so on, it is practiced by radiologists, employing a range of diagnostic techniques, including conventional X-ray imaging, computerized tomography (CT), ultrasound, and magnetic resonance imaging (MRI). It is only very recently that fluorescence imaging techniques have been applied to the diagnosis of clinical problems at a whole-patient level, with the first reports of breast tumor and brain imaging appearing in the literature.

In this chapter, we will review the principles of fluorescence that may be applied to clinical diagnosis and the specific imaging techniques that have been shown to potentially be beneficial in this situation. We will then describe specific clinical situations in which fluorescence imaging has been used to assist in making diagnoses and offer predictions for future expansion of the role of diagnostic fluorescence imaging.

13.2 PRINCIPLES OF FLUORESCENCE APPLIED TO MEDICAL DIAGNOSIS

13.2.1 Contrast Agents

While molecular biologists use the term *probes* for the agents used to induce fluorescence in tissues, radiologists are more familiar with the term *contrast agents* for substances which alter a tissue's characteristics so that it may be visualized with an imaging technique. Tissue visualization using optical imaging relies on either endogenous tissue contrast [20] or the introduction of fluorochromes, with or without molecular specificity.

The principal reasons for endogenous tissue contrast include absorption, scattering, and autofluorescence. The former may be observed by simply shining light across the tissue, where it is related to absorption, scattering, or both. This method was applied in

Fluorescence Applications in Biotechnology and Life Sciences, Edited by Ewa M. Goldys

optical mammography and it originally involved simple transillumination, with absorption dependent upon hemo/myoglobin content and scatter related to tissue architecture, including cellularity. A recent paper by Ntziachristos and colleagues [1] describes multispectral analysis of transmitted light as a potential tool for diagnosis in breast disease with potentially greater efficacy than traditional transillumination. Autofluorescence provides an additional mechanism for tissue contrast. All tissues contain intrinsic fluorophores, including nicotinamide adenine dinucleotide (NAD), flavins, collagen, and elastin. Disease results in changes in concentrations of these which potentially could be measured. Unfortunately, their concentrations are very low, and the difference in contrast between normal and diseased areas (in, e.g., cancer) means that it is very difficult to use these properties in clinical diagnosis. An endogenous precursor of a protoporphyrin [5-aminolevulinic acid (ALA)] can, however, be applied systemically in order to increase endogenous autofluorescence of malignant tissue. This technique has been successfully applied for the detection of dyplasia in Barrett's esophagus and colitis, as described below.

Nonspecific fluorochromes are often used as contrast agents. Cyanine dyes such as indocyanine green (ICG, cardiogreen) are examples of nonspecific fluorochromes, with ideal properties for in vivo imaging (Figure 13.1). ICG has been used clinically for many years for hepatic function testing, cardiac physiology tests, and ophthalmological fluorescence angiography, and experimental studies have proven the feasibility of tumor detection using nonspecific cyanine fluorochromes [24]. Moreover, in a clinical study on patients with various breast lesions, ICG-enhanced diffuse optical tomography (DOT) proved to be an efficient tool for lesion detection when compared with MRI [2]. Since ICG rapidly binds to albumin, ICG-enhanced DOT showed perfusion/accumulation effects with no additional molecular information on the tissue. The combination of optical tomography and novel contrast agents with molecular specificity holds promise to substantially increase the diagnostic potential for in vivo optical imaging.

Molecularly specific fluorochromes are a relatively new class of contrast agents [21]. The principal two classes are targeted and enzyme-activated fluorochromes. Fluorochromes can be tagged with various ligands which will bind to substances of interest. The cyanine dyes labeled with antibodies or peptides have been developed for diagnostic imaging. For example, both somatostatin and vasoactive intestinal polypeptide have been used as ligands with cyanine to detect mouse neuroendocrine tumors [22]. While not yet in widespread clinical use, this approach offers future potential, with another recent study using a fluorescent bisphosphonate to detect malignant osteoblastic activity [5]. Protease-sensing optical probes can also act as molecular contrast agents, with fluorescence resulting from enzymatic cleavage in tissues (Figure 13.2). These probes may be activated by lysosomal cystein or serin proteases such as cathepsin B or other enzymes such as matrix metalloproteinase 2, cathepsin D, or thrombin. In oncology, this approach has been tested in small-animal studies for detection of early colon and breast cancer, where there is an increase in protease activity [8]. There are also opportunities in imaging immunological and hemostatic disorders using this approach.

Another approach involves genetically engineered tissue fluorescence [1]. Rather than administering a contrast agent systemically, this approach employs modification of a tissue's genetic expression, resulting in variations in autofluorescence. This has been employed extensively in small-animal oncological imaging through insertion

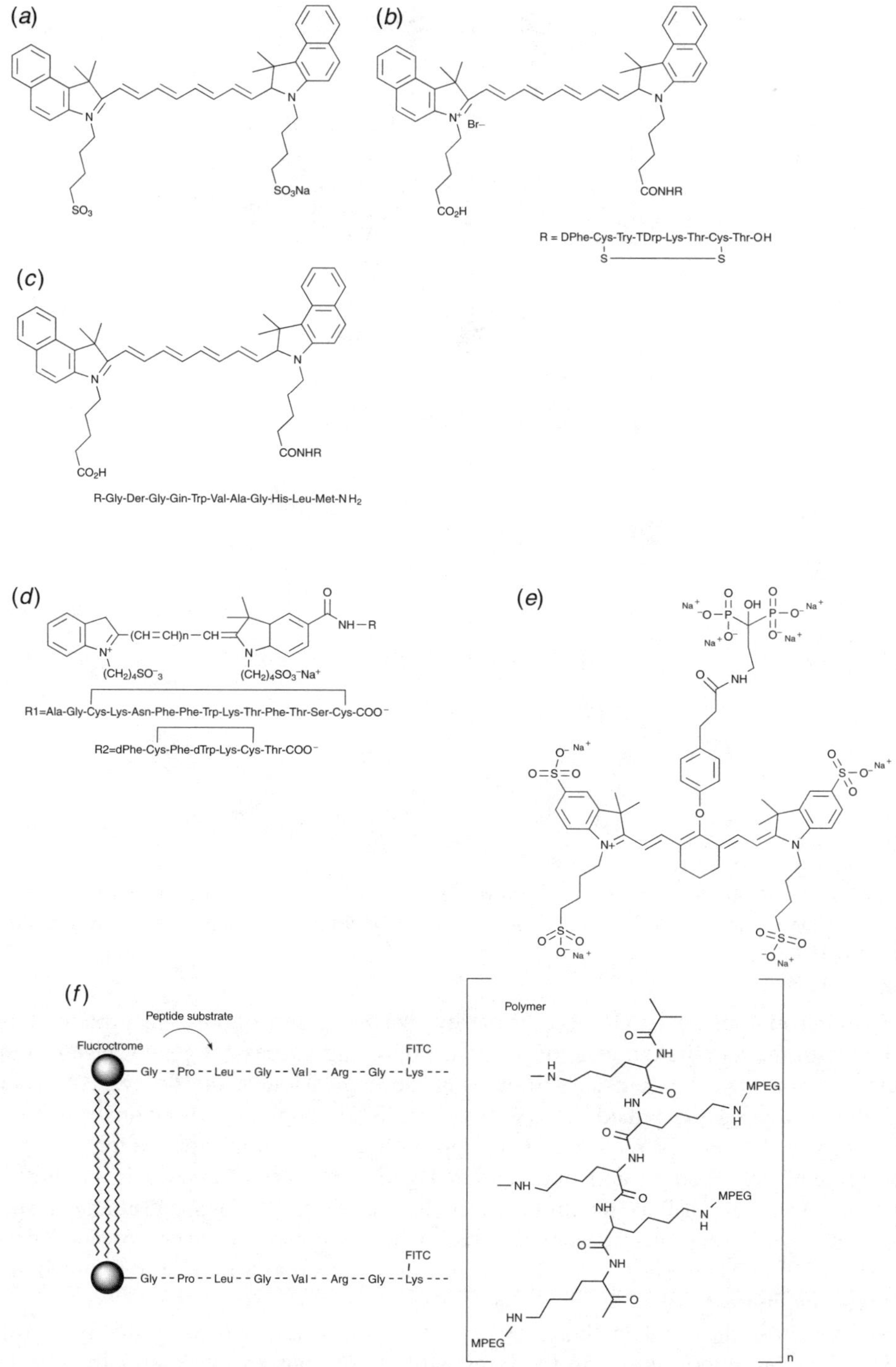

Figure 13.1 Molecular structures for (*a*) ICG; (*b*) cypate–octreotate, and (*c*) octreotate peptide complexes developed by Achilefu and co-workers; (*d*) indodicarbocyanine ($n = 2$) and indotricarbocyanine ($n = 3$) octreotate (R1) and somatostatin (R2) complexes developed by Becker and co-workers; (*e*) IRDye780–pamidronate complex developed by Frangioni and co-workers; (*f*) activateable quenching polymer complex developed by Weissleder and co-workers. (From [24].)

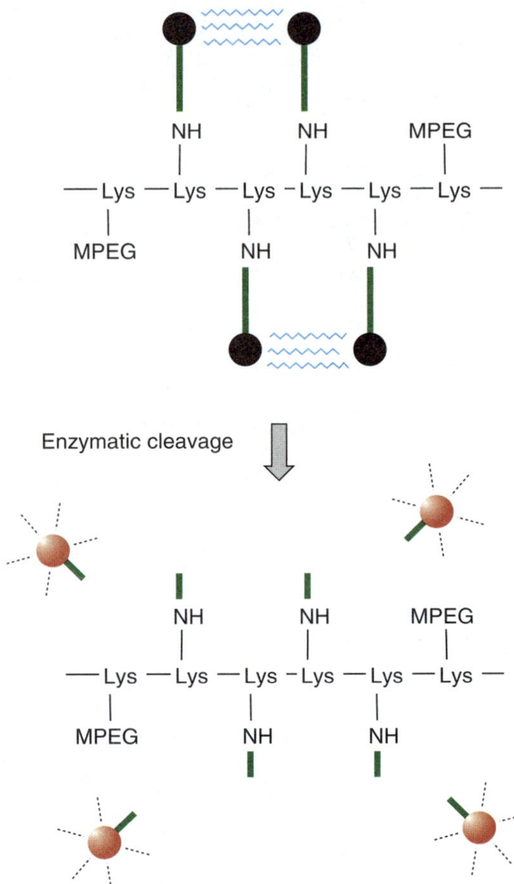

Figure 13.2 Example of activatable probe. These probes are dark in their native state, but after enzymatic cleavage of the backbone carrier they fluoresce when appropriately excited. (From [14].)

of imaging marker genes (IMGs), primarily that for green fluorescent protein (GFP) linked with the therapeutic gene of interest. Following successful gene transfer, transfected cells will start fluorescing, indicating the expression of the fluorescent protein and thus revealing the linked therapeutic gene. To be applicable for human imaging, local vector delivery is required. This approach has potential application for monitoring stem cell therapy and interventional gene transfer techniques in cardiology. One drawback of GFP is its fluorescence in the visible light spectrum in a spectral region with very little tissue penetration. More recent discovery of coral-based red-shifted fluorescing proteins offer much improved opportunities for future human in vivo imaging.

Other approaches and methods are as-yet experimental and are unlikely to offer human imaging opportunities in the foreseeable future but are of potential applicability in animal studies [8]. These include bioluminescence imaging, which exploits the emission of photons following luciferase reactions. Luciferase is an enzyme present in some organisms (e.g., bacteria, coral, and jellyfish), which is useful as a marker of energy consumption. Its absence in mammalian organisms and the fact that its substrate—luciferin—is not likely to be administered to humans make this currently inapplicable in the clinical setting. Another technology, molecular beacons, uses an oligonucleotide which, in the presence of a complementary (RNA) sequence, becomes fluorescent. This approach could potentially help answer the question as to whether a gene is activated and whether transcription of genetic information occurs. Defective or missing genetic information could be screened for with molecular beacons, but delivery issues to cells in vivo have yet to be conquered, currently making this an experimental technique only.

13.2.2 Delivery Issues

With the potential exception of imaging of endogenous tissue contrast, the use of fluorescence for diagnostic imaging requires the delivery of a specific compound (or biological agent, such as an IMG) to a cell or tissue. We shall not deal extensively with pharmacological issues such as biodistribution, nonspecific binding, metabolism, and excretion as these fall outside the scope of this text. However, biological delivery barriers, including vascular (im)permeability and transfer through interstitial space and cell walls, represent key challenges which must be overcome to enable contrast agents to reach their targets. This is opposite to most typical diagnostic imaging situations where exogenous enhancing agents are typically administered to enable luminal enhancement; for example, iodinated dyes are usually injected parenterally to visualize vascularity and the interstitial spaces. In some circumstances, regional localization of contrast-enhancing agents still enables intracellular consequences; for example, paramagnetic agents (such as Gd) result in effects on nearby protons irrespective of whether or not the agents are able to penetrate into cells.

To overcome cellular barriers in vivo, a number of strategies have been proposed, and preliminary data suggest that effective techniques may solve these issues. These include using peptide-derived membrane agents which actively pump compounds into cells, synthetic approaches to reduce immunogenicity, and pharmacological and physical synthetic approaches to enhance targeting. In addition, strategies to reduce the concentration of unbound compounds, which contribute to background noise, have also been described, such as introducing targeted tracers as “chasers” for the specific probe prior to the procedure. IMGs also have their own, different delivery issues, with the use of specific vectors required to ensure specific tissue delivery (e.g., neurotrophic viruses) [13].

Delivery to cells and tissues of contrast agents will always represent an area requiring novel solutions, but there are certainly existing strategies which can aid this process, and in the future newer methods are likely to improve outcomes. Additional opportunities incorporating nanoparticles and quantum dot technology offer positive directions for further investigation [15].

13.2.3 Amplification Strategies

A critical key to obtaining a satisfactory image of a tissue is high-enough signal-to-noise ratio (SNR), that is, the presence of sufficient signal in the tissue to enable an imaging system to visualize it over background “noise.” Amplification strategies are techniques which can be employed to enhance SNR from a contrast agent. For fluorescence imaging, useful strategies have included improving target concentration by administering

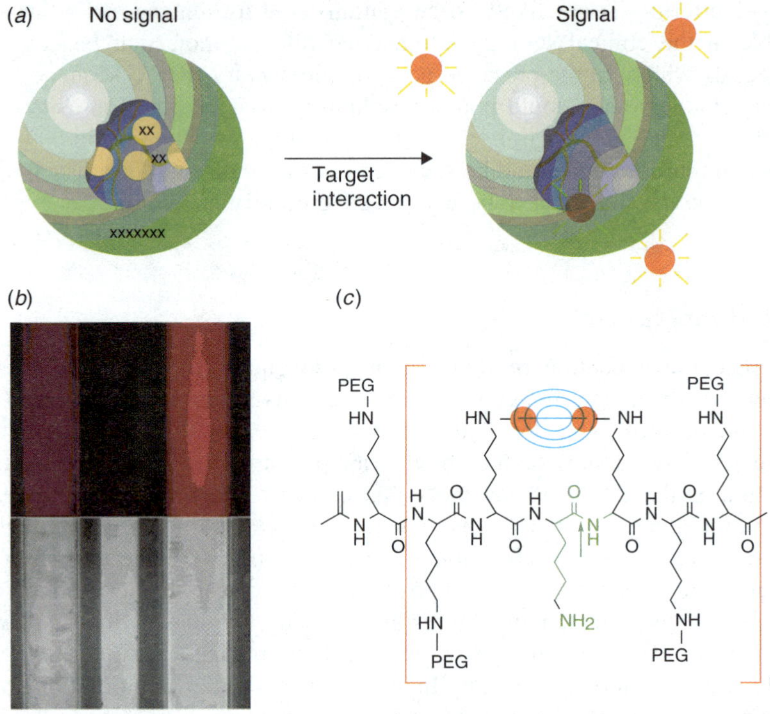

Figure 13.3 Schematic of probe activation. (*a*) Initial proximity of fluorochrome molecules to each other results in signal quenching. (*b*) Near infrared fluorescence (NIRF) image (top) and bright-light image (bottom) of nonactivated classical progastricsin (C-PGC) (also known as pepsinogen C) (left) and activated probe (right). Fluorochrome concentration, 0.17 μM; image acquisition time, 30 s; excitation, 670 nm; emission, 700 nm. Note the difference in signal intensity between enzyme-activated and enzyme-unactivated probe. (*c*) Chemical structure of repeating graft copolymer segment indicating quenching of Cy and enzymatic degradation site (green arrow). (From [22].)

pretargeting agents, making use of cell-specific functions (e.g., compound trapping), making use of physical changes in probes following interaction (e.g., fluorescence dequenching; Figure 13.3), and of course careful selection of the downstream target for gene expression when designing the probe or IMG to maximize specificity [14].

13.2.4 Introduction to Imaging Techniques

Irrespective of whether endogenous contrast or an introduced contrast agent is to be imaged, it is the imaging of emitted light that is required for the generation of data. There are two main approaches to capturing this light: reflectance imaging, where a source of light illuminates the area to be targeted and a sensor analyzes the reflected light (Figure 13.4), and tomographic imaging, where multiple projections are obtained and synthesized into one or more images. This is not dissimilar to the typical projection imaging techniques in radiology used, for example, in conventional radiography and sectional imaging in techniques such as CT and MRI. Each of these approaches will be described in detail in the next section.

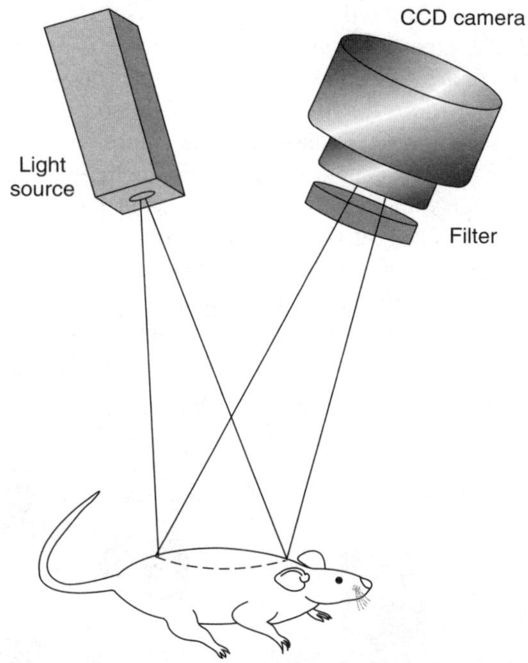

Figure 13.4 Typical fluorescence reflectance imaging (FRI) system for in vivo animal investigations. The illumination source and charge-coupled device (CCD) camera are on the same side of the animal imaged. The components shown are usually enclosed into a light-tight box. (From [14].)

13.3 OPTICAL FLUORESCENCE IMAGING TECHNIQUES IN VIVO

13.3.1 Near-Infrared Fluorescence Imaging

Near-infrared (NIR) fluorescence imaging has become feasible due to the development of fluorescence probes emitting in the NIR spectrum where tissue offers low absorption, the development of highly sensitive detectors, and monochomatic light sources (lasers) with safe levels of power per wavelength compared with white-light illuminators. While macroscopic fluorescence imaging in the visible has also been attempted using fluorescent proteins, the penetration depth is limited to only 1–2 mm, whereas it has been predicted that NIR fluorescent light can penetrate for several centimeters. Such an approach would enable investigations available currently only for in vitro studies to be used for in vivo human disease diagnosis and imaging of treatment response and enhance the field of molecular imaging. Imaging techniques that use the diffuse component of light for probing molecular events deep in tissue will now be described.

13.3.2 Fluorescence Reflective Imaging

Near-infrared fluorescence reflective imaging [14] employs light with a defined bandwidth as a source of photons that encounters a fluorescent molecule (*optical contrast agent* or *molecular probe*). The molecule then emits a light signal with specific spectral characteristics, generally different for different types of molecules, that can be resolved with an emission filter and captured by a high-sensitivity CCD camera. While filtered white light may be used as the light source, a laser source is preferred because it offers higher power delivery at narrower and better defined spectral windows (±3 nm for laser diodes against ±10 nm or more for filtered white-light sources). The reflected light is captured by a highly sensitive CCD camera since fluorescent signals are often weak (Figure 13.5). Two images are generated: an intrinsic light (simply, reflected visible light) image and an image obtained using a fluorescent bandpass filter. The intrinsic light image records the structure of the animal's surface and can yield high-resolution images after appropriate focusing, whereas the fluorescence (or luminescence) image records fluorescence signals emanating from under the surface and is by nature a low-resolution image that uses mainly the diffuse component of light. The side-by-side comparison or the superimposition of the two images into a single image yields a good visual effect since high resolution is retained (Figure 13.6).

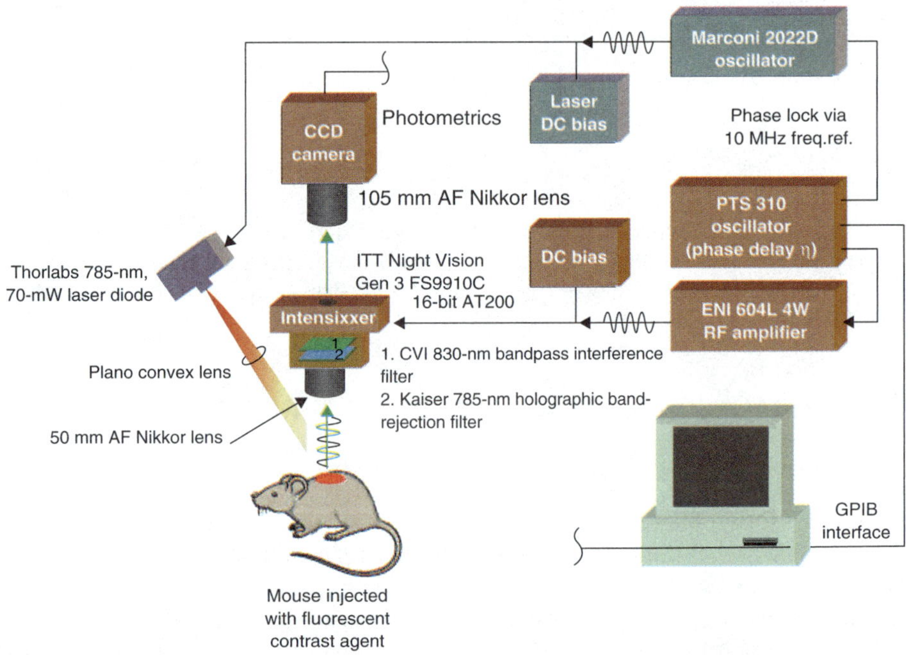

Figure 13.5 Experimental measurement involving whole-body illumination of small animal with area detection using a charge coupled or intensified charged coupled device (CCD or ICCD). CW measurements consist of whole-body illumination of animal with planar wave excitation light and registration of reemitted fluorescence from area detection using CCD or ICCD. Frequency domain photon migration (FDPM) techniques consist of modulating the incident planar excitation light and collecting the modulated emission light reemitted from the tissue surface. Detection of the amplitude is accomplished using homodyne techniques that involve modulating the multi-channel plate of the image intensifier with a radio frequency (RF) signal of the same frequency that is used to modulate the incident excitation light. The resulting steady image on the phosphor of the image intensifier is collected by the CCD chip and the phase between the gain modulation of the laser diode and the imaging intensifier is changed for consecutive acquisition of phase-sensitive images at the phosphor. The phase-sensitive images are collected and analyzed via fast Fourier transfer providing amplitude and phase of the reemitted fluorescence. (From [24].)

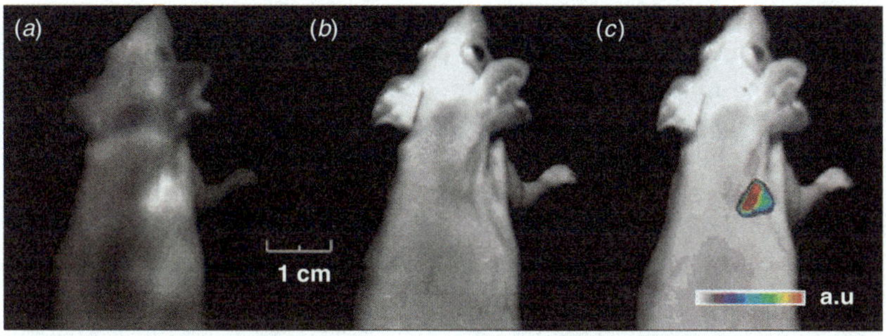

Figure 13.6 Example of typical images involved in FRI. (*a*) Fluorescence image obtained from the animal. In this example the image is obtained using a cathepsin B–sensitive fluorescent probe injected in an animal implanted with a HT1080 carcinoma in the upper posterior thorax. (*b*) Intrinsic light image obtained without the fluorescent bandpass filter. Such images are useful to outline with greater detail the animal investigated. (*c*) Superposition of (*a*) onto (*b*) improves the visual result. (From [14].)

Fluorescence reflective imaging has shown most promise for imaging surface fluorescent events in vivo or in excised tissues. It is simple to set up and is very sensitive to surface molecular events. Typical acquisition times range from a few seconds to a few minutes. Hardware development and implementation are straightforward and relatively inexpensive. Reflectance systems do not use ionizing radiation, employ safe laser powers, can be made portable, and have small space requirements.

However, reflective imaging has fundamental limitations as a clinical tool. First, the technique attains only small penetration depths (a few millimeters). The appearance of deeper lesions is significantly blurred and the signal detected is significantly attenuated as a function of lesion depth while the background noise remains constant in the reflectance mode, consisting of fluorescence signals from superficial layers and intrinsic light contaminating the fluorescence measurement due to imperfect filtering. This is in contrast to tomographic methods (discussed in the next section) where both signal and noise reduce so that the SNR remains significant for lesions that are much deeper than a few millimeters.

Second, reflective imaging is not capable of quantification. A small structure with high fluorochrome concentration that is deeper into tissue could yield the same appearance on the surface as a larger structure of low fluorochrome concentration that is closer to the surface. This is due to the nature of propagation of diffuse photon density waves into tissue. The photon count reading at a surface due to a lesion on or under the surface depends on the lesion depth, the lesion volume, and the optical properties of both the lesion and the surrounding tissue; therefore, images from different subjects or from the same subject at different time points are generally insufficient for yielding quantitative insights.

13.3.3 Fluorescence Molecular Tomography

Tomographic clinical imaging is now routine, with typical applications including ultrasound, CT, and MRI. Positron emission tomography (PET) is now widely used for molecular imaging. In optical tomography, multiple points on a tissue's boundary are illuminated and diffuse light patterns are collected around the boundary using a CCD camera. Each source–detector pair captures a different tissue projection. In order to perform fluorescence tomography (FMT) [11], tissue must be illuminated at different projections and multiple measurements are collected from the boundary of the tissue of investigation. This builds upon DOT, which uses multiple projections and measures light around the boundary of the illuminated body. It then effectively combines all measurements into an inversion scheme that takes into account the highly scattered photon propagation to deconvolute the effect of tissue on the propagating wave, even though high-frequency components are generally significantly attenuated and the resolution impaired. DOT has been used for quantitative imaging of absorption and scattering as well as concentration and fluorochrome lifetime measurements with simulated or phantom measurements. FMT, in its simplest implementation, needs only measurements of fluorescence and intrinsic light using constant-wave sources in order to resolve the single quantity being targeted, namely fluorochrome concentration. There are three optical domains for optical tomography called continuous wave (CW), time domain (TD), and frequency domain (FD). CW techniques involve a constant-intensity point source illuminating tissue at the excitation wavelength, with subsequent collection of fluorescent light emitted from a point or area on the surface. While SNR, depth penetration, and sensitivity are high, resolution is limited for CW imaging. TD techniques use a light source which delivers very short pulses of excitation light, resulting in varying areas of peak fluorescence intensity within tissues, enabling measurement of source depth. Resolution is high in this technique, but depth penetration may be limited, and this is a difficult technique to implement in practice. FD techniques offer a compromise, modulating intensity at a specified frequency, and measurements are directly related to TD through Fourier transform. Phase shifts within tissues enable depth resolution, offering similar advantages to TD techniques, but SNR is less than for CW techniques. Summarizing, commercial systems offering each of these techniques are available with selection dependent upon specific application. However, most reported studies for in vivo applications have used CW techniques.

There are three major advantages to FMT over fluorescence reflective imaging: First, FMT offers better resolution of structures at depth as tomographic imaging is superior for resolving deeper structures. Second, fluorochromes in tissues with varying background optical properties are resolved at higher contrast with FMT. Finally, fluorochromes in a highly absorbent background are better resolved with FMT. Hence, FMT is likely to be the technique of future choice for human clinical imaging subject to the challenges of designing tomographic systems able to cope with the depth of imaging large subjects in a tomographic environment. At present, however, most human imaging is performed using simple reflective techniques in the absence of dedicated human FMT "scanners." A recent report has described superimposition of NIR data on MRI images through a coupled system (Figure 13.7) as a potential direction for the future [10].

13.3.4 Superficial Confocal Imaging (Optical Coherence Tomography)

Optical coherence tomography performs high-resolution, cross-sectional tomographic imaging of the internal microstructure in materials and biological systems by measuring back-scattered or back-reflected light [19]. The OCT system performs multiple longitudinal scans at a series of lateral locations to provide a two- or three-dimensional map of reflection sites in the sample. In the original OCT system low-coherence light from

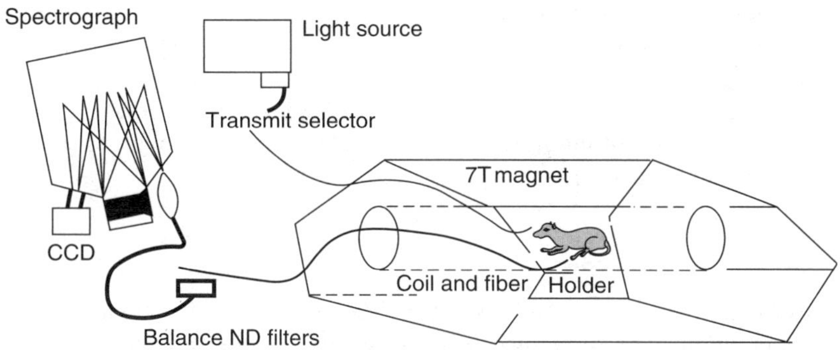

Figure 13.7 Schematic of MRI-coupled broadband NIR tomography system. It has eight source and eight detector fibers alternately surrounding the tissue in the magnet, yielding 64 attenuation spectra from 700 to 900 nm. (From [10].)

a broad-bandwidth superluminescent diode (SLD) centered at 830 nm was coupled into a single-mode fiber-optic Michelson interferometer. Light exiting the sample arm fiber is focused into the specimen being imaged. Light retroreflected from tissue structures is combined in the fiber-optic beamsplitter with light from a scanning reference mirror. Interference occurs at the detector only when the distance of the reflection from the sample is matched to the length of the reference arm to within the coherence length of the source. A longitudinal scan of the sample is then performed by scanning the reference mirror position and simultaneously recording the interferometric signal. The interferometric signal is demodulated using bandpass filtering and envelope detection, then digitized and stored on a computer for postprocessing. To acquire data for a two-dimensional image, a series of longitudinal scans are performed with the optical beam position translated laterally between scans. The data set is then displayed as either a false-color or gray-scale image (Figure 13.8). Both high-resolution structural images and spectroscopic data—dependent upon scatter from differing tissue properties—may be obtained.

External imaging systems were originally developed for superficial imaging applications, including the imaging of the ocular globe, including posterior segment and retinal pathology. Recent studies on imaging of skin pathology, including measurement of epidermal thickness have also been reported [18].

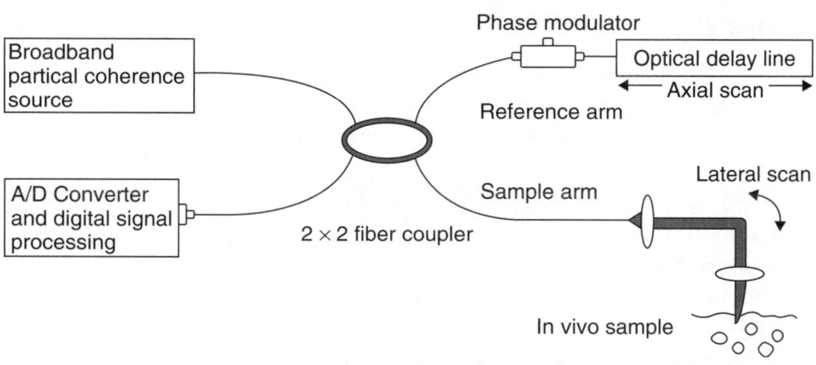

Figure 13.8 Schematic of OCT system. (From [25].)

Internal imaging systems involve coupling of the light source and detector to an endoscope for introduction into body cavities. Applications originally focused upon imaging of the gastrointestinal tract, from oral cavity to rectum [17], but there are also reports of this technique being used successfully for bladder imaging [16]. While initial studies employed autofluorescence, progress is anticipated with specific contrast agents for diagnosis of cancer.

13.3.5 Other Techniques

Bioluminescence tomography employs the bioluminescence property, mentioned under contrast agents, with a tomographic detection system. While offering opportunities in tissue and small-animal studies, no human applications are available as yet. Photoacoustic tomography measures acoustic waves produced by tissue expansion induced with short laser pulses. There is potential for this application to provide data on, for example, blood volume and tissue oxygenation in the future.

13.4 IMAGING OF WHOLE-BODY BIOLOGICAL SYSTEMS

Despite wide application of the techniques described thus far to cell and tissue imaging for research, these technologies have yet to be used widely in clinical diagnostic imaging. Whole-animal imaging has offered a vista for future potential clinical applications [1], where optical imaging may produce clinically relevant data in areas as diverse as oncology and cardiovascular, inflammatory, and neurovascular disorders. Fluorescence and bioluminescence do demonstrate certain advantages over existing diagnostic imaging techniques such as molecular specificity which is greater than that offered by, for example, PET and the absence of ionizing radiation and very high sensitivity provided by molecular optical target selection. They also have fewer problems with time-dependent decay of contrast agents and offer potential for multitarget imaging by spectral differentiation of contrast agents.

While reflective imaging and OCT are limited to superficial pathology, exogenous or intracavitary FMT offers similar potential to PET by generating data on deeper tissues. The following descriptions will review some published results of the application of techniques in pathology imaging.

13.4.1 Superficial Tumors

While, historically, reflective imaging was the first technique to offer potential for application to surface imaging of, for example, skin lesions, the lack of depth information has limited its application. In contrast, OCT has proven to be a robust technique for superficial imaging, offering cross-sectional information in addition to high-resolution data on the structure of cells and tissues. The most important application of this technique in a clinical setting has been in oncology, with the use of OCT for the endoscopic detection and monitoring (after treatment) of mucosal and submucosal lesions in the mouth, esophagus, and colon [12]. In a recent report describing the use of OCT in squamous cell carcinoma in the oral cavity (in a small-animal experimental model), epithelial and subepithelial structures were clearly discernible using OCT. OCT diagnosis agreed with the histopathological gold standard in 80% of readings (Figure 13.9). In the colon,

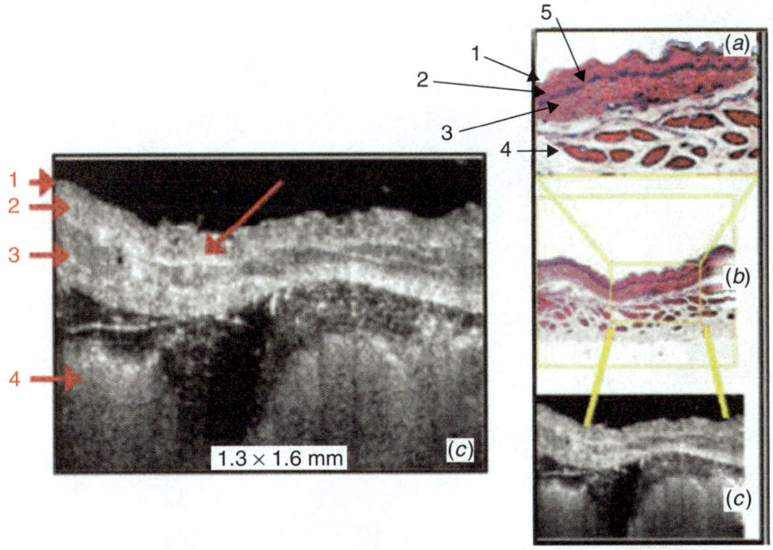

Figure 13.9 Healthy cheek pouch hematoxylin–eosin (H&E) stained image (*a*, 20×; *b*, 40×) and in vivo OCT (*c*) of same healthy cheek pouch tissues. Thin normal epithelial and thick subepithelial layers are visible: 1, keratinized surface layer; 2, flat stratified squamous epithelium; 3, submucosa, dense fibrous connective tissue; 4, longitudinal striated muscle fiber; 5, basement membrane.

confocal scanning has been successfully performed in living patients at 488 nm illumination for excitation of exogenously applied fluorophores (topical acriflavine and intravenous fluorescein), enabling imaging of cellular and subcellular structures (e.g., nuclei) of the gastrointestinal (GI) tract. The crypts of the colonic mucosa, the villi of the terminal ileum and duodenum, the gastric pits of the stomach, and the squamous epithelium of the distal esophagus are clearly visualized [12]. Acriflavine enhances the cell nuclei of the surface epithelium, including the absorptive epithelial cells and the mucus-secreting goblet cells. Fluorescein stains the extracellular matrix of the surface epithelium and also the subepithelial layers of the lamina propria. Images at increasing depth beneath the epithelium show the mucosal capillary network. Findings have been successfully correlated with the histology of biopsy specimens. Fluorescein-enhanced imaging of the esophagus has also yielded positive results, especially in the diagnosis of the clinically occult Barrett's esophagus and in monitoring the conversion of this premalignant condition into neoplasia [23]. Similar results have also been obtained in endoscopic imaging of bladder lesions and the diagnosis of transitional cell carcinoma at cystoscopy [16]. OCT certainly offers potential as an accompaniment to endoscopy and is set to enter routine clinical use in the foreseeable future.

13.4.2 Subsurface Tumors and Vascularity

Historically, subsurface imaging has yielded the most impressive images of tissue fluorescence obtained in vivo in whole animals, primarily in experimental studies. Most of these have involved the implantation of a tumor into a superficial (usually subcutaneous) location in a mouse or rat and subsequent reflective imaging after administration

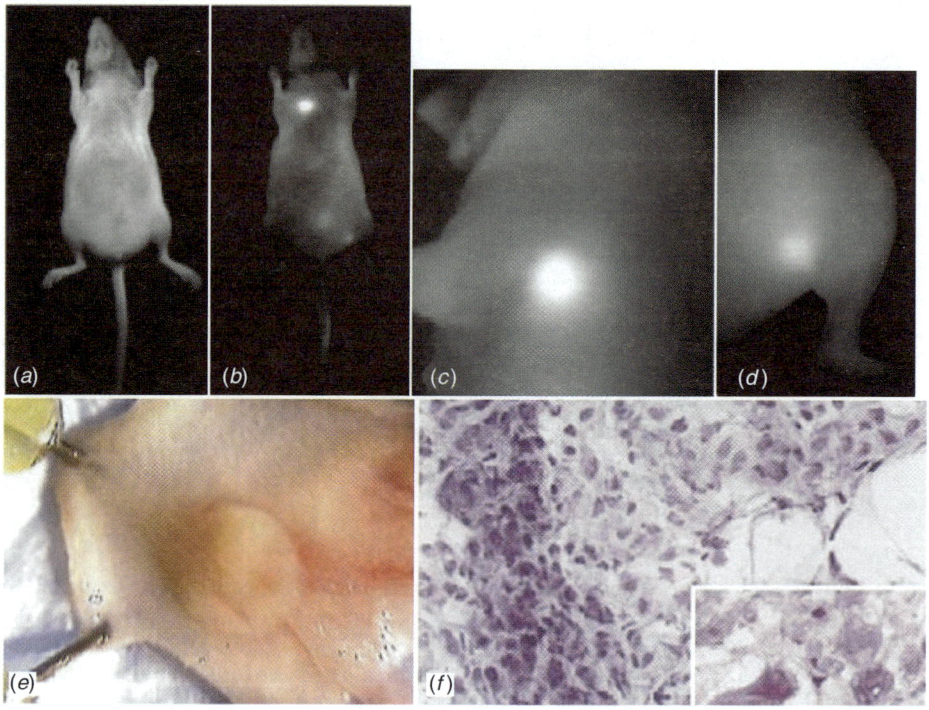

Figure 13.10 LX-1 tumor implanted into mammary fat pad of nude mouse: (*a*) light image; (*b*) raw NIRF image, note bright tumor in chest; (*c*) high-resolution NIRF images of chest wall tumor (2 mm); (*d*) high-resolution NIRF image of additional thigh tumor (<0.3 mm); (*e*) dissected tumor in mammary pad; (*f*) H&E section of NIRF positive tumor showing malignant and actively proliferating cells (magnification 200×; insert 400×). (From [22].)

of a protease-actived fluorophore (see Figures 13.10 and 13.6). In terms of human clinical applications, most published work has focused on imaging of breast tumors, either as a screening/primary diagnostic tool or for detection of spread and recurrence [9].

One of the first studies demonstrating the potential for breast imaging used MCT after the administration of ICG, correlating the resulting images with MRI in patients scheduled for excisional biopsy or surgery. The ICG-enhanced optical images coregistered accurately with gadolinium-enhanced magnetic resonance images validating the ability of MCT to image breast tissue, and both accurate localization and quantification of exogenous tissue fluorophore concentrations were obtained, indicating the potential to differentiate disease based on the fluorescent enhancement of suspicious lesions [2]. Real-time intraoperative detection of breast cancer axillary lymph node metastases following administration of a GFP-expressing herpes virus has also been recently reported in an experimental study in mice, with images obtained using a reflective system, and there is strong potential for the future application of this methodology to humans [7].

13.4.3 Lymphoreticular System

The application of the aforementioned techniques to the imaging of deeper tissues such as lymph nodes and bone marrow has been limited by both the lack of depth penetration of some of the imaging techniques that may be employed and the inherent physical limitations of some of the contrast agents used; for example, GFP fluorescence is extremely depth limited. A recent study has employed a red fluorescent protein for high-resolution noninvasive visualization of metastastatic breast cancer cells in the inguinal lymph nodes of mice, offering a potential direction for future investigation [3]. The use of an ICG-based probe bound to a lymphocytic monoclonal antibody for the imaging of lymphatic pathways has also been reported recently in a mouse experimental study [4].

Imaging of the lymph nodes is of critical importance in the staging and monitoring of chemotherapy in cancer, and there is a great deal of future potential for clinical fluorescence imaging in this area.

13.4.4 Bone

While there is no shortage of clinical imaging techniques for bone, ranging from X-ray-based radiography and CT through nuclear imaging and even MRI, functional imaging of cellular activity has been a deficiency, hindering early diagnosis of cancer spread to bone and osteoporosis. Fluorescence, by imaging cellular markers, offers the potential for monitoring osteoblastic activity in these settings. An early study used an ICG label to successfully track hydroxyapatite activity in mice using reflective imaging (Figure 13.11), and there is considerable promise for propagation of this and other techniques for functional imaging of bone growth and metabolism [5].

13.4.5 Brain

A range of potential clinical applications have shown promise in small-animal experimental studies, including brain tumor imaging [6], especially glioma and glioblastoma by, for example, NIR imaging of integrin receptors using a novel peptide–ICG conjugate arginine–glycine–aspartic acid (RGD)–Cy5.5; identification of radionecrosis, using autofluorescence; and assessment of tissue viability and prediction of the onset of apoptosis in vitro and in vivo. In addition, applications aimed at delineating anatomy and physiology have included attempts at detection of specific central nervous system (CNS) structures such as brain nuclei, identification of cell types by the presence of specific neurotransmitters, and the detection of optically labeled cells or drugs during therapeutic interventions. One recent study coupled magnetic resonance images for anatomical delineation to MCT images of NIR fluorescence as a marker for cerebral oxygenation in a rat based upon the endogenous tissue contrast effects of deoxyhemoglobin (Figure 13.12). Additionally, NIR contrast agents have also been described with specific affinity for amyloid plaques, a feature of Alzheimer's disease.

Brain imaging offers considerable potential for future clinical application of fluorescence, although, as yet, published results have only been limited to experimental animal models.

13.5 FUTURE DIRECTIONS

The field of clinical diagnostic fluorescence imaging offers an exciting future for application to the management of human disease. While, at present, there is virtually no

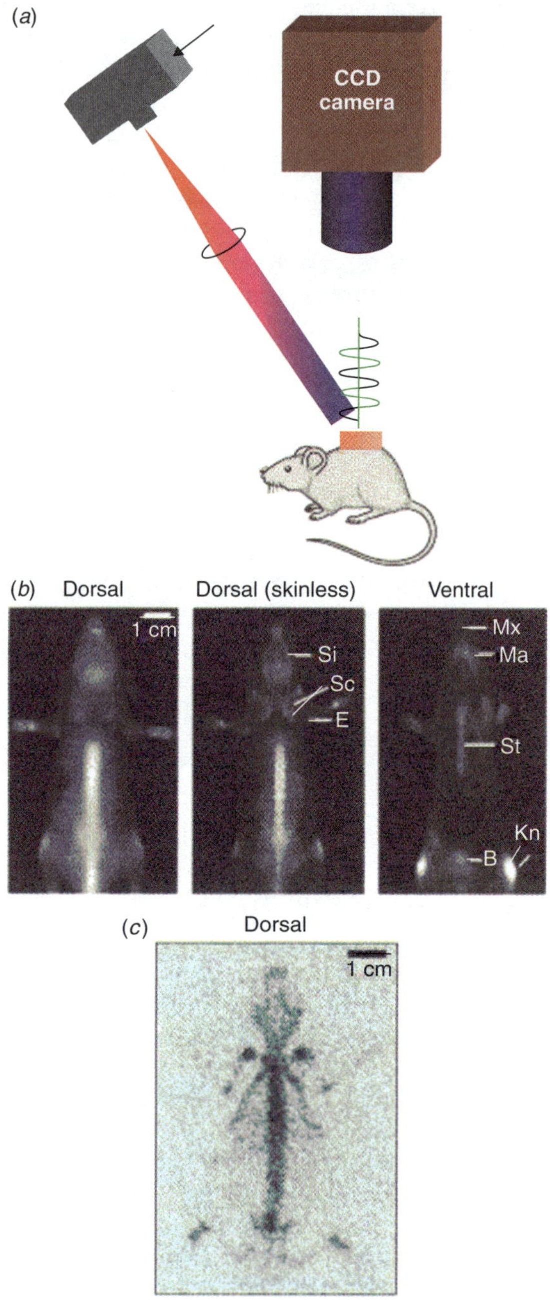

Figure 13.11 Comparison of in vivo NIR fluorescence imaging of hydroxyapatite in adolescent mouse using (*a*) area illumination and CCD detection following 2.6 nmol of IRDye conjugated to pamidronate following 500 ms CCD integration time in (*b*) dorsal, skinless dorsal, and ventral views. (*c*) standard radioscintigraphic imaging using 0.4 mCi of ^{99m}Tc-MDP with 30 min integration time is presented for comparison. (From [24].)

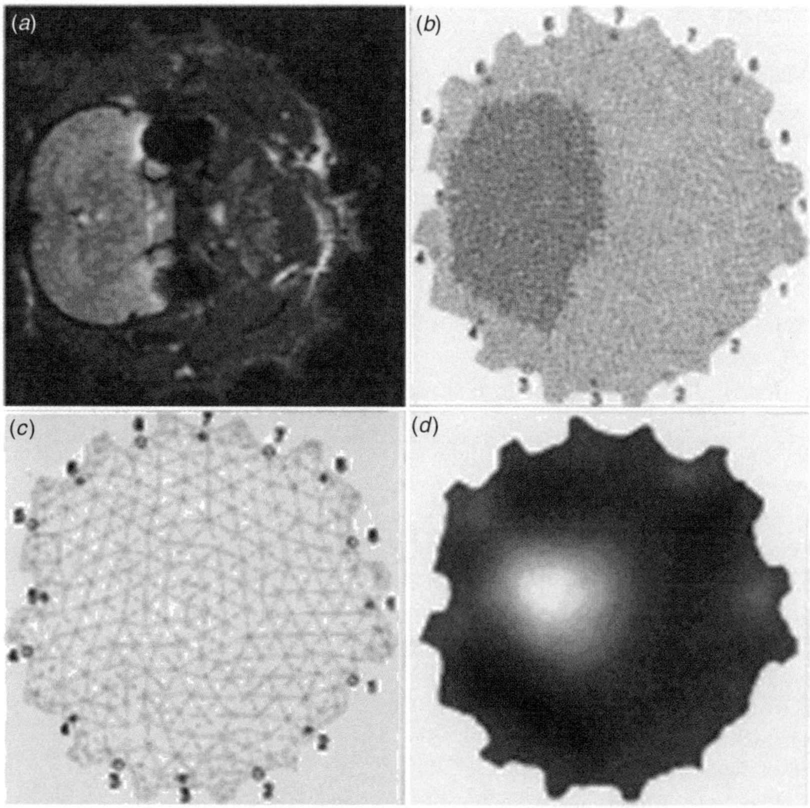

Figure 13.12 (*a*) Anatomically coronal T_2-weighted MRI slice of cranium with impressions caused by fibers all around periphery. (*b*) Two-region finite-element fine mesh with labeled source and detector locations as created from image (*a*). (*c*) Coarse mesh as used for reconstruction basis. (*d*) Reconstructed absorption image in initial resting state with animal breathing normal 30% oxygen. (From [10].)

general clinical application of fluorescence imaging techniques in in vivo human medical diagnosis, this situation is set to change dramatically in the very near future. It is likely that the first direct clinical applications will come in the broad field of oncology, with breast imaging the most likely application to incorporate regular—if not routine—use of fluorescence given the current lack of cellular specificity in existing imaging such as X-ray mammography, ultrasound, and MRI. Following from this application we expect widespread use of green and/or red fluorescent protein delivered by vectors to tumor cells to image spread prior to definitive treatment, an area that is currently not well addressed by other (e.g., nuclear imaging) techniques.

Key areas for future advances, these are likely to come in the use of fluorescence in imaging bone and brain. In the former, one can anticipate improved imaging of osteoporosis as well as tumor involvement of bone, while in the latter, visualization of specific cell types may offer improvements in diagnosis in cancer, stroke, and neurodegenerative diseases. Indeed, in terms of human diagnostic imaging with light, the future is shining bright.

REFERENCES

1. V. Ntziachristos, J. Ripoll, L. V. Wang, and R. Weissleder, "Looking and listening to light: The evolution of whole-body photonic imaging," *Nature Biotechnol.* **23**(3), 313–320 (2005).
2. V. Ntziachristos, A. G. Yodh, M. D. Schnall, and B. Chance, "MRI-guided diffuse optical spectroscopy of malignant and benign breast lesions," *Neoplasia* **4**(4), 347–354 (2002).
3. M. Dadiani, V. Kalchenko, A. Yosepovich, R. Margalit, Y. Hassid, H. Degani, and D. Seger, "Real-time Imaging of lymphogenic metastasis in orthotopic human breast cancer," *Cancer Res.* **66**(16), 8037–8041 (2006).
4. K. Licha, N. Debus, S. Emig-Vollmer, B. Hofmann, et al., "Optical molecular imaging of lymph nodes using a targeted vascular contrast agent," *J. Biomed. Opt.* **10**(4), 41205 (2005).
5. J. S. Souris, "Seeing the light in bone metabolism imaging," *Trends Biotechnol.* **20**(9), 364–366 (2002).
6. S. A. Toms, P. E. Konrad, W. C. Lin, and R. J. Weil, "Neuro-oncological applications of optical spectroscopy," *Technol. Cancer Res. Treat.* **5**(3), 231–238 (2006).
7. D. P. Eisenberg, P. S. Adusumilli, K. J. Hendershott, S. Chung, et al., "Real-time intraoperative detection of breast cancer axillary lymph node metastases using a green fluorescent protein-expressing herpes virus," *Ann. Surg.* **243**(6), 824–830 (2006).
8. E. R. McVeigh, "Emerging imaging techniques," *Circ. Res.* **98**(7), 879–886 (2006).
9. Y. Chen and X. Intes, "Development of high-sensitivity near-infrared fluorescence imaging device for early cancer detection," *Biomed. Instrum. Technol.* **39**(1), 75–85 (2005).
10. H. Xu, R. Springett, H. Dehghani, B. W. Pogue, K. D. Paulsen, and J. F. Dunn, "Magnetic-resonance-imaging-coupled broadband near-infrared tomography system for small animal brain studies," *Appl. Opt.* **44**(11), 2177–2188 (2005).
11. R. B. Schulz, J. Ripoll, and V. Ntziachristos, "Experimental fluorescence tomography of tissues with noncontact measurements," *IEEE Trans. Med. Imag.* **23**(4), 492–500 (2004).
12. R. S. Dacosta, B. C. Wilson, and N. E. Marcon, "Spectroscopy and fluorescence in esophageal diseases," *Best Pract. Res. Clin. Gastroenterol.* **20**(1), 41–57 (2006).
13. P. S. Adusumilli, B. M. Stiles, M. K. Chan, D. P. Eisenberg, Z. Yu, S. F. Stanziale, R. Huq, R. J. Wong, V. W. Rusch, and Y. Fong, "Real-time diagnostic imaging of tumors and metastases by use of a replication-competent herpes vector to facilitate minimally invasive oncological surgery," *FASEB J.* **20**(6), 726–728 (2006).
14. V. Ntziachristos, C. Bremer, and R. Weissleder, "Fluorescence imaging with near-infrared light: New technological advances that enable in vivo molecular imaging," *Eur. Radiol.* **13**(1), 195–208 (2003).
15. S. Santra, D. Dutta, G. A. Walter, and B. M. Moudgil, "Fluorescent nanoparticle probes for cancer imaging," *Technol. Cancer Res. Treat.* **4**(6), 593–602 (2005).
16. Z. G. Wang, D. B. Durand, M. Schoenberg, and Y. T. Pan, "Fluorescence guided optical coherence tomography for the diagnosis of early bladder cancer in a rat model," *J. Urol.* **174**(6), 2376–2381 (2005).
17. A. L. Polglase, W. J. McLaren, S. A. Skinner, R. Kiesslich, M. F. Neurath, and P. M. Delaney, "A fluorescence confocal endomicroscope for in vivo microscopy of the upper- and the lower-GI tract," *Gastrointest. Endosc.* **62**(5), 686–695 (2005).
18. C. Suihko, L. D. Swindle, S. G. Thomas, and J. Serup, "Fluorescence fibre-optic confocal microscopy of skin in vivo: Microscope and fluorophores," *Skin Res. Technol.* **11**(4), 254–267 (2005).
19. K. Hirano, Y. Ito, T. Suzuki, T. Kojima, S. Kachi, and Y. Miyake, "Optical coherence tomography for the noninvasive evaluation of the cornea," *Cornea* **20**(3), 281–289 (2001).

20. M. Hassan and B. A. Klaunberg, "Biomedical applications of fluorescence imaging in vivo," *Comp. Med.* **54**(6), 635–644 (2004).

21. C. Bremer, V. Ntziachristos, and R. Weissleder, "Optical-based molecular imaging: Contrast agents and potential medical applications," *Eur. Radiol.* **13**(2), 231–243 (2003).

22. R. Weissleder, C. H. Tung, U. Mahmood, and A. Bogdanov, Jr., "In vivo imaging of tumors with protease-activated near-infrared fluorescent probes," *Nat. Biotechnol.* **17**(4), 375–378 (1999).

23. R. Kiesslich, L. Gossner, M. Goetz, A. Dahlmann, et al., "In vivo histology of Barrett's esophagus and associated neoplasia by confocal laser endomicroscopy," *Clin. Gastroenterol. Hepatol.* **4**(8), 979–987 (2006).

24. E. M. Sevick-Muraca, J. P. Houston, and M. Gurfinkel, "Fluorescence-enhanced, near infrared diagnostic imaging with contrast agents," *Curr. Opin. Chem. Biol.* **6**(5), 642–650 (2002).

25. P. Wilder-Smith, W. G. Jung, B. Brenner, K. Osann, H. Beydoun, D. Messadi, and Z. Chen, "In vivo optical coherence tomography for the diagnosis of oral malignancy," *Lasers Surg. Med.* **35**(4), 269–275 (2004).

CHAPTER 14

Fluorescence in Clinical Diagnosis

WOUTER KALLE and PHILLIP BWITITI

School of Biomedical Sciences, Charles Sturt University, Wagga Wagga, New South Wales 2678, Australia

TODD WALKER

School of Science and Engineering, University of Ballarat, Ballarat, Victoria 3353, Australia

14.1 INTRODUCTION

An increasing number of technologies are now available to the pathologist and medical scientist to detect changes in the composition of body fluids and patient cells or tissues that are based on fluorescence. Because of the nature of the work of pathology, that is, routine diagnostic tests for the presence or absence of disease, these tests have to be relatively simple, cheap, and robust. Therefore, technologies that are at the forefront of current research and development will not be part of this chapter. This chapter provides a broad overview of the use of fluorescence-based technologies in the clinical biochemistry laboratory and other pathology laboratory units. It is set up to start with the detection of small molecules with spectrophotometric technologies and end with the detection of DNA molecules using fluorescence microscopy.

14.2 APPLICATIONS OF FLUORESCENCE IN CLINICAL BIOCHEMISTRY

Fluorescent molecules are sensitive to the environment (e.g., temperature, pH, polarity, and oxidation state) and the proximity of quenching groups can alter the quantum yield or wavelength of emitted light [1]. Such characteristics make fluorescence techniques ideal tools in measurement and also allow fluorescent compounds in tissues to be measured.

14.2.1 Advantages of Fluorescence Measurements

1. Fluorescence is characterized by very high sensitivity allowing concentrations of biomolecules to be measured down to as low as 10^{-18} M (attomole) and the measurements are also fast (e.g., a fraction of a second)

Fluorescence Applications in Biotechnology and Life Sciences, Edited by Ewa M. Goldys

2. The products of fluorescence and fluorescence itself are safe and hence there is no need for a licence in order to handle fluorescent molecules, as with radioactive compounds.
3. In most cases, there is little or no alteration in sample structure and hence fluorescence measurements are ideal for in vivo studies and studies of living tissues.
4. Fluorescence techniques are applicable to most types of specimens wet or dry and hence they are ideal for investigations such as forensics.
5. Fluorescence is affected by the chemistry (e.g., pH, ionic strength, and fluidity) of the environment and hence it can be applied to studies where a disease changes the chemistry of the environment.
6. Fluorescence can be induced by various types of radiation (e.g., ultraviolet, visible, and infrared), which are available in most laboratories.
7. The technique is versatile; for example, two different fluorescent dyes (probes) can be used in an experiment to increase sensitivity or to allow measurement of more that one molecule.
8. Fluorescence allows in situ studies, for example, binding of ligand such as a drug or hormone to a receptor.
9. Fluorescence is suitable for various types of studies (e.g., measurement of concentration of metabolites, study of structure, orientation, fluidity, and distances between molecules) and hence it is applicable to investigations of various disorders.
10. Measurement of extra- and intracellular levels of biomolecules can be carried out with fluorescence techniques, allowing a better understanding of extra- and intracellular changes in diseases.
11. There are several types of fluorescent molecules and hence it is easy to design assays.

14.2.2 Categories of Fluorescence Measurements

The categories of fluorescence measurements used in clinical biochemistry include the following:

1. Analysis of biomolecules that fluoresce to aid in the diagnosis and monitoring of disease:
   - Porphyrins in porphyrias
   - Glycosylated products in diabetes mellitus
   - Tumors that have different fluorescence characteristics to normal tissues
   - Various amino acids and drugs that fluoresce, allowing identification
2. Use of fluorescence or fluorescent molecules as analytical tools to measure biomolecules:
   - Coenzymes ($NADH_2$, $NADPH_2$, FAD, and FMN) that fluoresce
   - Enzymes that act on substrates causing fluorescence upon catalysis and the fluorescence is related to concentration of substrate
   - Enzyme-labeled antibodies or antigens that act on substrate causing fluorescence that is related to their concentration since the fluorescence changes upon antigen–antibody binding

- Antigens or antibodies labeled with fluorescence tags where the fluorescence changes upon antigen–antibody binding
- Large molecules, for example, antigen–antibody complexes that polarize fluorescence so that the magnitude of polarization is related to the antigen–antibody complex concentration
- Enzymes or cofactors labeled with fluorescence tags where fluorescence changes upon the enzyme binding to the substrate
- DNA or RNA labeled with fluorescent tags to locate complementary nucleic acids in the investigation of genetic diseases
- Substrates such as O_2 that can quench fluorescence and the magnitude of quenching is related to O_2 tension

14.2.3 Applications

Fluorescence measurements are applicable to most biological fluids such as blood, urine, and feces as well as to the analysis of nonfluid tissues such as nails. Fluorescence is used to detect or measure levels of exogenous compounds (e.g., drugs), endogenous compounds that are normally present in the body (e.g., hormones, vitamins), and endogenous compounds that are normally absent from the body or are present in minute levels but are present or elevated in concentration due to disease (e.g., some cancer markers).

We now discuss various examples of metabolites measured by fluorescence.

Autofluorescent Substances in Body The characterization of autofluorescence of organs is useful in diagnosis. For instance, normal bronchial tissue has intense, green autofluorescence but weak, reddish autofluorescence when cancerous, perhaps due to changes in metabolism cells by comparison with normal cells. Such autofluorescence can be observed through a bronchoscope allowing detection of lung cancers [2]. Advanced glycation end products (AGEs) are a heterogeneous group of compounds implicated in the pathogenesis of microvascular complications of diabetes mellitus. Some studies suggest that fluorescent AGEs are better associated with microvascular complications than nonfluorescent compounds and hence fluorescence of these products in serum has been used as a marker AGE modification [3].

Ions Ion-selective fluorescent probes or dyes are available to assay nonfluorescence ions such as Na^+, K^+, H^+, NH_4^+, Ca^{2+}, and Mg^{2+}. Such dyes have a high affinity for specific ions, and binding to an ion is accompanied by changes in fluorescent properties that are related to concentration of the ion [4]. Besides measuring minute levels of an ion, ion-selective fluorescent probes can measure the free fraction. There are cases when the level of free fraction is required since it is this fraction that mostly exerts biochemical activity. For instance, measurement of intra- or extracellular free calcium is useful in studying the role of calcium as a second messenger and in cell signaling and neural activity.

Some probes for measurement of metals incorporate porphyrins, which are fluorophores with high fluorescent quantum yields, large Stokes shifts, and flexible and tunable physiochemical properties [5]. Porphyrins and metalloporphyrins are also versatile in that they respond to electromagnetic fields, can interact with other chemical species, are thermally stable, and can act as shape- and size-selective catalysts [6]. Porphyrins and metalloporphyrins can be used as fluorescent carriers for determination of metal ions (e.g., iodine) [5, 7]. An optical fiber chemical sensor for mercury (Hg^{2+}) incorporating lipophilic porphyrin dimer is based on the fact that Hg^{2+} quenches fluorescence of the sensor and this is related to concentration of Hg^{2+} [8].

Some ion-selective electrodes contain ionophores that allow establishment of a gradient of activity of the ion across the membrane. Optodes measure changes in optical property due to the presence of an analyte, and such changes are a function of analyte concentration. In measurement of cations such as H^+ (pH), Na^+, and K^+, the sensors consist of ionophores and chromophores and interaction between these provides an optical signal. Migration of cations or protons in/out of the membrane is associated with protonation/deprotonation of the chromophore changing fluorescence that is quantified [9]. Porphyrin-derived chromophores have versatile photophysical properties [10] making them adaptable for measurement of biomolecules and ions.

A fluorescent probe, called cryptand, was developed for measuring K^+, and these bicyclic ionophores have better selectivity and affinity for cations than crown esters, which are also used to make fluorescent probes [11]. Another fluorescence fiber-optic sensor for measurement of K^+ concentration consists of hydrophobic indicator, ionophore valinomycin, and a fluorescent dye. The change in absorbance of hydrophobic indicator induced by K^+ is detected from quenching of fluorescence due to energy transfer [12]. Porphyrins have pH-dependent fluorescence spectra as well [5, 13], making them ideal for pH measurement.

Gases Measurement of partial pressures of CO_2 and O_2 is important in investigations of blood gases in animals. Fluorescence measurement of PCO_2 is based on the notion that CO_2 as an acid alters the pH of a buffer in a membrane, which can be sensed by a fluorescent pH indicator [14]. Unlike polarographic or amperometric PO_2 measurement, which measures current produced by O_2 as it is electrolytically reduced at the cathode, O_2 optodes, which are optical sensors, do not consume O_2 [15]. Polarographic analysis requires that O_2 is consumed, perhaps making this technique less suitable for detecting hypoxia, which is low O_2 tension in tissues, but such limitations are overcome by using fluorescence quenching. A probe that incorporates ruthenium is available and, when excited, ruthenium fluoresces and this fluorescence is quenched by O_2 [16, 17]. While measurement of PO_2 based on O_2 consumption at the cathode might not be sensitive at low PO_2, optodes for O_2 would be sensitive at low PO_2 since the intensity of fluorescence increases as PO_2 decreases [14].

Developments in fiber-optic sensors have included continuous and simultaneous determination of PO_2 and glucose. In such designs, the O_2 sensor allows O_2 permeability and also contains O_2-sensitive ruthenium dye while the glucose sensor is an O_2 sensor with an outer layer containing immobilized glucose oxidase. At the O_2-sensing site, Ru(II) complex fluorescence intensity is related to O_2 concentration in the sample, while at the glucose-sensing sites, glucose is catalyzed by glucose oxidase, causing depletion of O_2 and resulting in increase in fluorescence intensity. The levels of O_2 and glucose are therefore monitored simultaneously [18], which is important is some cases of diabetes mellitus that require glucose and blood gas levels to be monitored. Porphyrins and metalloporphyrins are also used as fluorescent carriers for the determination of PO_2 [5]. These compounds are versatile in that the heme can bind gases such as NO, CO_2, and O_2 and hence in theory are an ideal choice as sensors for detection of these important gases in medicine [12].

Porphyrins Not only are porphyrins used as analytical tools because of their fluorescence properties but such properties have also allowed diagnosis of porphyrias using porphyrins. Porphyrins are intermediates in the biosynthesis of heme and porphyrias are characterized by excessive production and excretion of porphyrins. When oxidized and subjected to ultraviolet light, porphyrins fluoresce [19]. Urine, feces, and red blood cells (RBCs) are used in the measurement of porphyrins in the diagnosis and management of porphyrias. Porphyrins emit fluorescence of specific wavelength when excited by light, and this phenomenon is also used to distinguish various porphyrias [20, 21].

Hemoglobin-Advanced Glycation End Products Protein glycosylation is critical to cell function and hence alterations in glycosylation are useful indicators of diseases. A method for detection of glycoproteins in gels and on blots involves oxidation of carbohydrate groups followed by conjugation with a fluorescent substrate or a tag [22]. Intrinsic fluorescence properties of these AGEs can be an index of long-term glycemic status due to their specificity and long half-lives [23]. Diabetic complications could also be consequences of AGEs, but measurement of these products is difficult due to low concentrations. Measurements using some of the chromatographic techniques are expensive and technically challenging while other methods only detect some of the AGEs, which are a small fraction of total AGEs in vivo. The intrinsic AGE-specific fluorescence can be monitored in serum and is associated with severity of diabetic complications such as nephropathy and retinopathy [24]. There is therefore a great potential for development of this type of measurement in the management of diabetic patients. Glycosylated hemoglobin measurement is used in the management of diabetes mellitus, and the principle of one of the methods is that emissions of certain fluorescent derivatives are quenched when bound to glycosylated hemoglobin. For instance, the fluorescence of an eosin–boronic acid derivative when mixed with hemolysates of erythrocytes is quenched in proportion to the level of glycosylated hemoglobin [25].

Glucose An area that has found wide application of fluorescence is glucose measurement. In one technique, boronic acid derivatives, which are fluorescent and also complex glucose rapidly and reversibly, are used as receptors in glucose sensing [26]. Contact lenses that monitor glucose levels in tears are being developed and incorporate a fluorescent probe that responds through color changes to glucose levels in tears [27]. An advantage of such fluorescent technology is noninvasiveness as it does not involve blood collection and hence avoids discomfort to the diabetic, and such a technique would offer continuous monitoring of glucose level, thereby optimizing diabetic management.

Another way of measuring glucose in biological fluids is by use of enzymes, and an enzyme commonly used is glucose oxidase, which oxidizes glucose. This reaction is accompanied by O_2 consumption, H_2O_2 production, and pH change, all which can be monitored and correlate with the level of glucose. Fluorescent technology has been adapted to glucose measurement using glucose oxidase, which has intrinsic fluorescence that changes during the reaction with glucose and also correlates with glucose level [26]. Modifications of the glucose oxidase method have included development of a reversible glucose oxidase fluorescent sensor using apo-glucose oxidase, resulting from removal of the cofactor flavin adenine dinucleotide (FAD). Glucose oxidase is still able to bind glucose with comparable affinity to that of the holo-enzyme, which is glucose oxidase plus the cofactor FAD [26]. An apo-enzyme (enzyme without cofactor) can bind substrate but cannot transform it, and in this case binding of enzyme to substrate results in enzymatic transformation that is detected by fluorescence [28], and since there is no catalysis involved, the reaction is reversible. A modification to this method involves apo-glucose oxidase interacting noncovalently with fluorophore ANS (8-anilino-1-napthalene sulfonic acid). The resulting fluorescence intensity and mean lifetime of ANS decrease as glucose concentration increases [26, 28]. The glucose oxidase method can again be modified by substituting ferrous sulfate for peroxidase to catalyze H_2O_2. This method couples oxidation of glucose with a Fenton reaction and ferrous ions react with H_2O_2 formed to yield hydroxyl radicals, which are scavenged by quinoline to form dihydroxylated products, which fluoresce [29]. Another assay for glucose oxidase activity via H_2O_2 is based on the response of europium (111) tetracycline probe to H_2O_2, forming europium tetracycline–H_2O_2, which is fluorescent [30]. In these cases, fluorescence is related to glucose level.

Another enzyme that is also used in analysis of glucose is hexokinase, which catalyzes the transfer of the phosphoryl group of adenosine triphosphate (ATP) to glucose, and like glucose oxidase, it has intrinsic fluorescence properties. The yeast hexokinase used has tryptophan residues that have fluorescence properties and are sensitive to the polarity of the microenvironment, being quenched by water, proximity of polar amino acids, and components of the solution such as O_2 and ions. Yeast hexokinase is a dimer with each monomer consisting of two lobes that have a cleft in the middle, and the binding of glucose in the cleft moves the two lobes closer. Therefore, when glucose is added to hexokinase, there is a decrease in intrinsic fluorescence consistent with the greater exposure of tryptophan residues to the aqueous environment in the closed form of hexokinase than in the open form, but the exact mechanism is not clear [31].

There are a number of binding proteins that interact with ligands, and these interactions have been utilized to develop biosensors. An example is the plant sugar–binding protein or lectin called concanavalin A (Con A), which binds mannose and glucose reversibly and is used in glucose sensing, utilizing fluorescence resonance energy transfer (FRET) and fluorescence intensity measurement for example [26]. Moschou et al (2004) gave a comprehensive review on fluorescence glucose detection [26]. A glucose binding protein (GBP) has been used as the recognition element in an energy transfer based sensor for glucose and this involves incorporating fluorescent reporters into GBP such that spatial separation between fluorescent moieties change when glucose binds thereby capitalising on FRET between fluorescent probes [32]. A ratiometric sensor based on GBP labelled with two fluorophores is also available. In this case the protein is labelled with a fluorophore e.g. acrylodan at one site and a metal ligand complex of ruthenium at the other terminal. The acrylodan emission is quenched in the presence of glucose while ruthenium emission remains constant, thereby serving as reference [33].

Another approach in glucose-sensing involves probing changes in glucose-induced cellular metabolism in cutaneous or sub-cutaneous tissue by measuring skin-surface auto-fluorescence. This detection is based on the hypothesis that glucose metabolism is related to auto-fluorescence, or can be tracked by fluorescent markers of various metabolic processes. Nicotinamide adenine dinucleotide NAD^+ and NAD^+ phosphate $NADP^+$, which are products of such metabolism, are used based on the fact that they are fluorescent when reduced. The skin fluoresces in regions attributed to tryptophan, protein crosslinks, and NAD(P)H and hence autofluorescence of skin component cells, fibroblast, and adipocytes is related to glucose concentration. Cell autofluorescence is a noninvasive measurement of glucose concentration and is detectable at the skin surface [34].

Hormones and Proteins Another area of clinical biochemistry where fluorescence has found wide application is in the measurement of hormones and proteins. Fluorescent techniques are incorporated in various immunoassays and fluorescence dyes are used to stain proteins (e.g., after protein separation). Examples of such uses of fluorescence are reviewed below.

Prostate-specific antigen, a marker for prostate cancer, can be assayed by enzyme immunoassay. This method incorporates alkaline phosphatase that hydrolyzes diflunisal phosphate (DFP) and the dephosphorylated form then reacts with Tb^{3+} (terbium) and ethylenediaminetetraacetic acid (EDTA) to form a fluorescent complex that is quantified in a time-resolved mode [35]. Capillary electrophoresis immunoassay has been carried out for analysis of estrone, an estrogenic hormone secreted by ovaries. In this assay, labeled and unlabeled antigen–antibody complexes are separated by capillary electrophoresis and detected by laser-induced fluorescence [36]. Qin, Peltola and Pettersson [37] described a FRET immunoassay for urine albumin. This assay uses albumin-specific monoclonal antibody labeled with fluorescent europium chelate as donor and albumin labeled with cyanine 5 as acceptor. The close proximity between the two labels allows energy transfer to take place between the pulse-excited europium chelate and the acceptor cyanine 5. As a result, the europium signal is quenched and the prolonged energy transfer signal is emitted from the sensitized cyanine 5. Addition of unlabeled albumin in urine dissociates the labeled antigen–antibody complex leading to reduced energy transfer and a lower signal, and the extent to which the energy transfer signal is reduced is dose dependent and related to the level of unlabeled albumin [37].

While some fluorescence assays measure concentration, fluorescence has also been used to measure binding. For instance, a body protein called p53 regulates cell cycle and is also a tumor suppressor. p53 is activated in response to DNA damage, resulting in cell cycle arrest or apoptosis. Another protein called murine double minute 2 (HDM2) binds to p53, thereby negatively regulating p53, and reports suggest that disruption or alteration of this binding may contribute to mechanisms by which chemotherapy mediates cell death. A homogenous time-resolved fluorescence assay has been developed to monitor p53/HDM2 binding. If the two proteins are fluorolabeled, then binding brings the fluorophores close, allowing FRET [38]. The applications and usefulness of such fluorescence techniques are wide and include assessment of the binding of a receptor to a ligand such as hormone or drug.

Kronick and Grossman (1983) cited in [39] described an immunoassay that uses fluorescent-colored dyes called phycobiliproteins, which exhibit high extinction coefficients and high quantum efficiency. Since phycobiliproteins are stable and hydrophilic, they can be linked to specific binding proteins, and assays for immunoglobulin G (IgG) have been developed [39]. Pregnancy-associated plasma protein A (PAPP-A) is found in human maternal serum and its concentration increases with gestational age in uncomplicated pregnancy. Decreased PAPP-A level in the first trimester is seen in Down syndrome and is therefore used as a marker for the disorder. A time-resolved immunofluorometric assay point-of-care test was developed for PAPP-A, utilizing fluorescent lanthanide chelate [40]. Adaptation of fluorescence measurements to point-of-care testing has obvious advantages in that such tests are fast allowing medical decisions to be made quickly, and these tests are simple and hence can be carried out by someone with little laboratory training. A light source with promising applications for fluorescence measurements is the light-emitting diode (LED), which has been used for analysis of various biomolecules in capillary electrophoresis, for example, riboflavin. A UV LED is also used as the excitation source for analysis of, for example, fluorescamine-derivatized bradykinin and lysine [41].

Peptides and proteins can also be analyzed using capillary electrophoresis and laser-induced fluorescence, and this is done by labeling with dyes that can be excited by a laser. A fluorogenic dye which is weakly fluorescent but fluoresces strongly after reacting with a primary amine of the N-terminus of a peptide is used and naphthalene-2,3-dicarboxaldehyde is one such dye used for quantitation of substance P, a neuropeptide and enterostatin, involved in regulation of appetite and insulin secretion. Fluorescein isothiocyanate has also been used for analysis of amino acids and insulin. Use of laser-induced fluorescence detection for proteins requires prior derivatization with a fluorescent dye, and to minimize the problems associated with this, noncovalent labeling is used. Indocyanine green is weakly fluorescent in the near-infrared (NIR) region in its unbound state in dilute aqueous solution, but when it is noncovalently bound to protein, its fluorescence is enhanced and hence it has been used as a label for ribonuclease A, transferrin, and cytochrome *c* [42].

Fluorescent dyes that bind noncovalently to proteins are popular in proteomic studies. SYPRO orange binds to proteins in sodium dodecyl sulfate–polyacrylamide gel electrophoresis (SDS–PAGE) with a detection limit in the nanogram-per-band range. A more sensitive fluorescence staining using SYPRO ruby can detect 1 ng/band of proteins on gels. Since the binding of these fluorescent dyes to protein bands is noncovalent, postgel protein characterization steps are not hampered by their presence. Fluorescein has low luminescence intensity in acidic aqueous media; however, when bound to proteins, an increase of intensity takes place, and this is used to visualize bands of protein in gel electrophoresis [43].

Drugs Chlorpromazine HCl, thioridazine HCl, clomipramine HCl, imipramine HCl, and desipramine HCl, which are psychoactive drugs, can be analyzed by spectrofluorimetric methods based on oxidation of the drugs using Ce(IV) in the presence of sulfuric acid and monitoring fluorescence of the formed Ce(III). Cerium (IV) is used as an oxidizing agent for spectrofluorometric determination of trimeprazine and trifluoperazine, reserpine, and macrolides [44]. Detection of dopamine in human urine using lipid films with incorporated resorcin-[4] arene receptor is also available. The lipid film without receptor fluoresces, and this is quenched by the receptor. Presence of dopamine "switches on'" the fluorescence, allowing detection of this stimulant [45]. The antihypertensive drug captopril can be analyzed using capillary electrophoresis laser-induced fluorescence after derivatization of captopril with fluorescent label 5-iodoacetamidofluorescein. There are also a variety of fluorochromes showing high affinity for the thiol group, such as fluorescein isothiocyanate, fluorescein-maleimides, and fluorescein-iodoacetamides, which are suitable for determination of various thiol compounds [46].

Fluorescence polarization is used to measure small molecules and is based on Brownian movement of a fluorochrome in solution, in which it tumbles rapidly and emits little light in the plane of polarization. If the fluorochrome is attached to an antibody that then reacts with an antigen, a large particle is produced which tumbles more slowly with restricted rotation and emits more light. This technique has been applied to measurement of various drugs such as phenytoin and phenobarbital, aminoglycoside antibiotics, theophylline, digoxin, and hormones, for example, human chorionic gonadotrophin [39].

Vitamins The name vitamin B refers to a collection of vitamins with a variety of structures. The activity of some of the B vitamins is attributed to structurally related compounds known as vitamers, which are believed to exhibit approximately equivalent or varying degrees of vitamin activity because of interconvertibility; B_2 and B_6 vitamins are examples. There are a variety of methods to quantitate B vitamins, but most do not offer quantitation of each vitamer, for which separation previous to determination is mandatory. Capillary electrophoresis–molecular fluorescence using a charge-coupled detector method was developed for simultaneous separation of B_2 and B_6 vitamers from human serum [47].

Amines, Amino Acids, and Lipids Catecholamines are neurotransmitters, and improper regulation of these compounds is associated with several neurological disorders. Laser-induced fluorescence detection is used in capillary electrophoresis for determination of catecholamines [48]. Detection of amino acids is important in the diagnosis of some metabolic disorders and in malnutrition. Cobalt (11) porphyrin displays selective affinity to histidine, and hence a porphyrin-dimer-based fluorescent sensor is available for histidine detection [5, 49]. There is evidence that oxidative modification of low-density lipoprotein (LDL) is important in the pathogenesis of atherosclerosis, and such modified LDL can be characterized by apo-B100 fluorescence to assess the level of modification [50].

14.3 FLUORESCENCE IN PATHOLOGY AND CANCER DIAGNOSTICS

Genetic abnormalities and cancer can be diagnosed many ways. The traditional path has been to implement a test of certain sensitivity to confirm a clinical symptom. The choice to select the appropriate test is usually left to the clinician investigating the patient. In most cases, the test involves staff and services from a pathology laboratory. Samples which may include tissue, cells, fluid, scrapings, aspirates, and excreted material are taken from the patient to be analyzed in various ways. In some circumstances, the pathology laboratory will implement its own testing regimes to either exclude or confirm a diagnosis. Among the armamentarium available to pathologists for reaching a diagnosis is fluorescence technology. This section will profile various applications of fluorescence technology in the diagnostics of genetic abnormalities and cancer.

14.3.1 Fluorescent In Situ Hybridization

Major advances in molecular techniques in the past decades have improved the diagnostic and prognostic value of medical cytogenetics. Especially the advent of fluorescence in situ hybridization (FISH), a technique which brings together molecular biology and cytogenetics, has increased the number of applications of cytogenetics. Some important features of the use of FISH in medical diagnosis are as follows:

- Diagnosis of congenital disorders
- Cancer diagnostics

- The ability to analyze single cells in the case of cancer research or prenatal diagnosis
- Single-cell research of normal cells and cell biology

In its most simple form, FISH uses known labeled DNA sequences or labeled probes to hybridize to cytological targets like chromosomes, cell nuclei, extended DNA fibers, and even DNA microarrays. FISH is based on the inherent capacity of two single-stranded lengths of nucleic acid (RNA or DNA) to hybridize according to the principle of complementary base pairing. This creates an extremely stable and specific bond between the labeled probe (the known sequence of nucleic acid) and its target on the sample to be studied. Probes can be labeled with either a fluorochrome or a molecule that can be detected later by immunological methods (hapten) like biotin or digoxigenin (see Figure 14.1). With the increase of the number of fluorochromes and fluorochrome-conjugated antibodies, it became possible to distinguish multiple probes in one sample. These advances in biological and physical possibilities held pace with

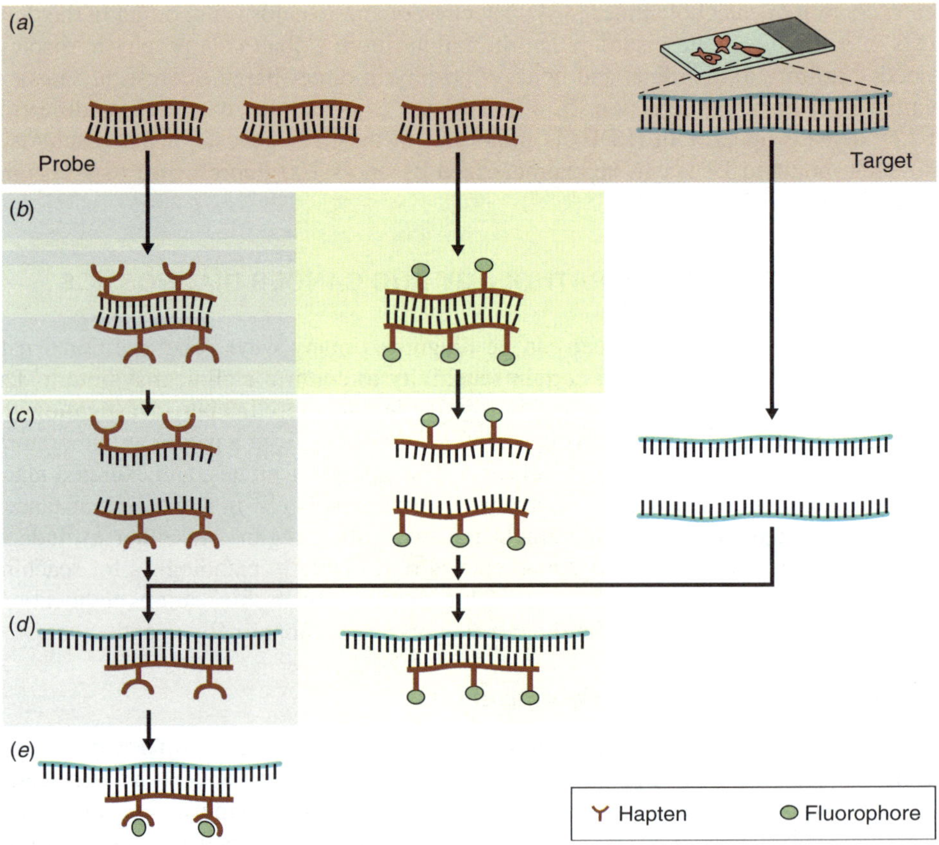

Figure 14.1 Principle of FISH. (*b*) The probe is labeled with either hapten or a fluorophore. (*c*) After denaturing of both probe and target DNA, (*d*) hybridization can take place. (*d*, *e*) The probe can then be detected by direct fluorescence or immunofluorescent detection of the hapten [51].

technological advances in fluorescence microscopy, fluorescence microscope filters, charge-coupled device (CCD), and computer technology.

One of the most important aims of FISH technology over the past years has been to increase the resolution with which chromosome rearrangements, gene order, and gene structure could be detected. This has been achieved by improvements in target pretreatment and probe quality. Target resolution has improved from using intact chromosomes (at a resolution of ~5 Mb) to the analysis of cell nuclei (50 kb–2 Mb) and finally to the level of DNA strands (5–500 kb) using FISH on DNA fibers or pretreated nuclei. Probe quality has increased considerably over the years. There is a larger choice of different probes with less background hybridization. Labeling procedures have also been optimized and fine tuned to provide high-quality labeled probes, reduce background hybridization, and give a large amount of detection options. The use of high-resolution microscopies like electron microscopy and scanning probe microscopy has been proposed as a way to increase the resolution of FISH studies. The difficulties in using these high-resolution microscopies lies in the fact that pretreatment of the samples is very difficult and sample turnover in these microscopes is very slow. Therefore these microscopies have never been used in routine diagnostics but are used only in a research setting.

There are many excellent review articles and books available on the development and applications of FISH in multiple areas [52–54].

FISH and Prenatal Diagnostics Conventional karyotyping (the arrangement of an individual's chromosomes according to length and position of the centromere) is an important tool in prenatal diagnostics for the identification of fetal changes in chromosome number (aneuploidy), transfer of chromosomal material from one chromosome to another (translocation), and the common autosomal trisomies 13 (Patau's syndrome), 18 (Edwards' syndrome), and 21 (Down's syndrome). The main drawback of this method is that fetal samples like amniotic fluid and chorionic villi have to be cultured before a karyotype can be produced. This means long delays of up to 14 days can easily occur before the result can be issued. This is a long interval and may cause great anxiety in parents. A further drawback is that the resolution of conventional cytogenetics is limited to chromosomal rearrangements that are larger than 5–10 million base pairs (Mb).

The use of FISH has multiple advantages over conventional karyotyping. First, using FISH with one or more chromosome-specific probes can give results within 24 to 48 h because there is no need for culturing the amniotic fluid or chorionic villi samples. In the normal situation, the FISH result will show up as two spots in the cell nucleus (see Figure 14.2*a*), representing the two homologue copies of the chromosome. If the FISH result shows one or three spots in the nucleus, this indicates a form of aneuploidy for that particular chromosome. By using differently labeled probes specific for chromosomes 13, 18, 21, X, and Y, a routine diagnostic procedure can detect the most common autosomal trisomies and the sex of the fetus in one test. Second, apart from using chromosome-specific probes that usually consist of tandemly repeated human DNA sequences such as centromeric DNA, unique sequences can be used when ultrasound imaging of the growing fetus raises the suspicion of the presence of microdeletion syndromes (e.g., when a fetal ultrasound shows a cardiac defect, FISH can be used to detect DiGeorge syndrome). These microdeletions can easily be missed by conventional karyotyping and show the increased resolution that can be obtained by using FISH.

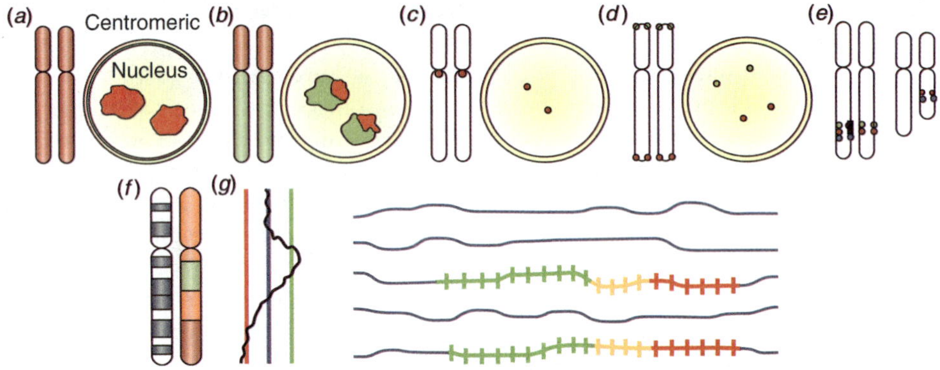

Figure 14.2 Examples of probes and their clinical uses. (*a*) Chromosome-painting probes stain specific chromosomes. In a normal diploid cell nucleus, two chromosome areas will be stained. In abnormal cases a different number of stained chromosome areas will be seen. (*b*) Specific part of chromosomes can be stained with regional painting probes. By using two probes with different labels, specific parts of the chromosomes and their location with respect to each other can be analyzed. (*c*) Centromeric probes are available for almost all human chromosomes. These probes are easy to use and have a very high signal-to-noise ratio. They can be used to analyze chromosome numbers in cells. (*d*) Clones are available for most genomic regions. (*d*) Large insert probes can be used to detect and analyze locations of specific genes on specific chromosomes. (*e*) Breakpoint analysis and its diagnosis can be analyzed using specifically designed probe sets that detect the breakpoint and two flanking genes. These sets can be used in interphase diagnostics to analyze structural rearrangements in samples. (*f*) Comparative genomic hybridization using test DNA (green label) and reference DNA (red label) to analyze gain or loss of DNA in tumor cells. Where there is no gain or loss, the chromosome will be fluorescing orange. Gain or loss will change fluorescence to either green or red. Computer software will produce a ratio profile of the two colors. (*g*) High-resolution analysis of deletions, duplications, exon–intron boundaries, and the order of specific genes on a chromosome can be performed using stretched DNA molecules. Red- and green-labeled probes are used and an orange color shows overlap between two probes. (Adapted from [51].)

A very exciting possibility is the use of FISH in preimplantation genetic diagnosis (PGD), which enables the determination of aneuploidies before implantation of the embryo after in vitro fertilization (IVF). Evidence has shown that a large number of preimplantation embryos are aneuploid. These aneuploid embryos can be detected before implantation and increase the success rate of IVF.

There are some major drawbacks for using FISH for prenatal diagnosis as well. FISH assays will only show abnormalities in the chromosomal/genomic areas which are targeted by the used probes. Furthermore, the technique is relatively labor intensive and requires highly trained staff. However, undoubtedly, FISH contributes substantially to the identification of chromosomal abnormalities in the unborn fetus. Review articles on the use of FISH in prenatal diagnostics include [53, 55–57].

FISH and Cancer Diagnostics Conventional karyotyping of solid tumors is often difficult because it is almost impossible to obtain suitable chromosomes from these tissues. As a consequence, information on the gross genetic aberrations in solid tumors was difficult to obtain. To overcome this problem, comparative genomic hybridization (CGH) was developed (see Figure 14.2*f*).

For CGH, DNA is extracted from the sample and mixed in a 1 : 1 ratio with a reference DNA sample. Both samples are differently labeled; for example, the test sample is labeled with a red fluorochrome and the reference DNA is labeled with a green fluorochrome. The resulting mixture is then hybridized to a normal metaphase spread and any DNA that is overrepresented in the test sample will show up as a green area in the metaphase while underrepresented DNA will show up as a red area in the metaphase spread. Deletions and amplifications of DNA in the test sample can then be identified and located on specific chromosomal areas. This creates an understanding and possible diagnostic tool for solid tumors and has the major advantage that it will identify regions of chromosomes often deleted or amplified in tumors. This will identify chromosomal areas which contain genes involved in cancer formation and also will provide a genetic signature for each tumor tested which will help with diagnosis and treatment [58]. New developments which combine CGH with microarray technology blur the boundaries between molecular biology and cytogenetics even more. These techniques can be considered more molecular than cytogenetic and fall outside the scope of this chapter.

One of the most exciting developments over the last decade has been the application of multicolor FISH technology to analyze whole sets of metaphase chromosomes for cytogenetic analysis. This approach enables the visualization of translocations without loss or gain of chromosomal material, something that is not possible with CGH. Two different approaches have been used to develop this type of technology. The first approach, spectral karyotyping (SKY), uses combinatorially labelled, chromosome-specific probes to differentiate the various chromosomes in a metaphase spread (reviewed in [52, 59]). Another approach, combined binary ratio fluorescence in situ hybridization (COBRA-FISH), uses a combination of differentially labeled chromosome probes and narrowband pass filters to reach the same effect, differential staining of all human chromosomes in a metaphase spread (reviewed in [60]). Both methods can be used as research tools and to visualize and analyze the complex karyotypes of solid tumors.

The main applications of the three techniques described above are in clinical and cancer diagnostics. All three techniques help in elucidating the often highly complex structural chromosomal abnormalities in cancer and therefore play a role in diagnosing the genetic basis of this disease.

In short, FISH has proven to be an incredibly versatile and useful technique. Starting as a reliable technique to determine chromosome number and gene localization, it has evolved into a complete genome-scanning technology which provides a combination of cell and whole-genome information. The future indeed looks promising for this technology.

14.3.2 Applications of Fluorescence in Clinical Cytology

Cytology pertains to the academic discipline of the studying cells. Diagnostic cytology (including cytopathology) narrows the definition to an application of studying cells to diagnose disease states (pathology). Modern diagnostic cytology encompasses a broad range of techniques from a varying array of human samples all with the common goal of aiding a quick and accurate diagnosis [61].

Sampling techniques for cytology collection can include retrieving cells from the body forcibly or collecting naturally exfoliated cells. Forcible removal of cells includes scraping (pap smears) or a needle (fine-needle aspiration), which involves using a thin-bore needle to target lesions [62].

The following sections take a systems approach to cancer diagnosis, which is a common way of reviewing cancer: Each section provides some comment on the applicability of fluorescent technology to the application of clinical cytology.

Lung Cancer Lung cancer is routinely diagnosed using a range of cytological investigations. These include noninvasive sputum collection, minimally invasive bronchoscopy, and fully invasive transthoracic fine-needle aspiration. Diagnostic specificity and sensitivity increase with the level of invasiveness. However, prognosis is strongly dependent on whether the carcinoma is of a large or small cell type.

There are few reports that indicate a potential utility of the FISH assay as an adjunct to bronchial washing cytology in routine clinical practice. These studies use a mixture of fluorescently labeled probes to the centromeric region of chromosome 1 and to the 5p15, 8q24 (site of the c-*myc* gene), and 7p12 (site of the *EGFR* gene) loci to assess cells in bronchial washing specimens for chromosomal abnormalities indicative of lung carcinoma [63]. In this study, the sensitivity of FISH for the detection of lung carcinoma was 82% compared with 54% sensitivity for routine cytology. This increase in sensitivity is significant, and there FISH as an adjunctive test should be strongly considered when lung cancer is suspected.

The most promising application of fluorescence occurs not in the laboratory but in the clinical setting. There are reports that suggest that using fluorescence bronchoscopy instead of white-light bronchoscopy aids in the clinical diagnosis of preinvasive lesions. Preinvasive bronchial lesions are small. They are difficult to detect and localize by white-light bronchoscopy. It has been shown that fluorescence bronchoscopy improves the detection rate from 40% using white-light bronchoscopy to 80% using fluorescence bronchoscopy [64].

Bladder Cancer In situ hybridization has been widely used as an investigative tool for diagnosing urothelial cancers [65, 66]. However, many studies compare FISH on routine urine samples to compare the relative sensitivities of urine cytology and FISH for detecting urothelial carcinoma. However, it has been clearly demonstrated that FISH has a greater sensitivity in detecting urothelial carcinoma when coupled with urine cytology, although it is not entirely clear at this time whether a positive FISH may indicate frank neoplastic urothelial transformation or merely be an indicator of unstable urothelium capable of malignant transformation. In this context, FISH might be useful at detecting patients at significant risk of developing urothelial carcinoma [65]. Nevertheless, basic light microscopy remains the staple modality for diagnosing bladder cancer.

Renal Cancer Unfortunately, there are little data to support the clinical diagnostic utility of fluorescence techniques for routine renal cancers. The reason for this is probably the lack of targeted research using fluorescence on renal cancers. Cytology of urine as it stands has a high specificity for diagnosing renal cancers, and these are augmented with other clinical tests: computerized axial tomography (CAT), magnetic resonance imaging (MRI), and intravenous pyelography. All reports to date focus on rare or benign tumors.

Chromophobe renal cell carcinoma (ChRCC) is characterized by a loss of chromosomes 1, 2, 6, 10, 13, 17, and 21). Iqbal et al. (2000) [67] have reported that FISH using probes for chromosomes 1, 2, 6, and 10 on smears from six histologically proven

ChRCCs demonstrated ranged from 48 to 88% (chromosome 1), 36 to 89% (chromosome 2), 26 to 98% (chromosome 6), and 64 to 99% (chromosome 10). These data suggest that FISH used on renal smears provides a useful adjunct to the diagnosis of ChRCC.

Another example involves the characterization of metanephric adenoma. This entity is a benign renal neoplasm with distinctive histologic features. Renshaw, Maurici, and Fletcher (1998) [68] presented the case study of a 48-year-old woman with a histologically confirmed tumor. They report the cytologic appearance and FISH studies of this tumor. Cytologically, the cells were arranged in tight, short papillae and loose sheets. The cells had scant cytoplasm, round monotonous nuclei with fine even chromatin, and rare small nucleoli. Immunohistochemistry revealed no reactivity for epithelial membrane antigen (EMA), keratins (AE1/AE3, callus, 34BE12), or primitive antigens associated with bowel cancer called carcinoembryonic antigen (CEA). FISH showed a distinctive pattern for chromosomes 7 and 17 and for the short arm of chromosome 3. The differential diagnosis includes Wilms' tumor, renal adenoma, papillary renal cell carcinoma, and metastatic tumors.

In clinically difficult diagnostic cases of suspected renal cancer a combined testing using immunohistochemistry and FISH may be of greater help than relying on either test alone.

Breast Cancer In Australia, 14,000 women are diagnosed with breast cancer each year. The human epidermal Growth factor receptor (HER2) gene will be amplified in 15–30% of these cases. HER2 amplification is associated with disease that is more aggressive. Detection of HER2 gene amplification can be by in situ hybridization (ISH) to identify the specific HER2 nucleic acid sequence within tissue sections or by immunohistochemistry (IHC) to detect the protein.

Detection of HER-2/neu alterations is increasingly used in breast cancer patients for therapeutic purposes. A study by Nizzoli et al. [69] examined the reliability of HER-2/neu immunocytochemical (ICC) assessment on 66 centrifuged prepared smears obtained by fine-needle aspiration biopsy from breast cancer patients. The results were compared with those obtained by both FISH on fine-needle aspirate (FNA) and IHC on matched histologic section targeting the same HER 2/neu genetic status. Concordance between immunocytochemistry and FISH was 78% and between ICC and IHC was 84%. Discordance mainly concerned seven cases that resulted positive by ICC and four cases scored negative by IHC but positive by ICC. Simultaneous assessment of HER-2/neu by ICC, IHC, and FISH was available in 24 cases; the concordance was 75%. In this study by Nizzoli et al. [69], the false positivity of immunocytochemical technique represents the major criticism. It can be concluded that FISH remains the most objective and powerful technique for HER-2/neu assessment on breast cancer FNAs. Because of the widespread use of IHC and ICC, this is a point that appears not to have reached most clinical pathologists.

In routine pathology laboratories chromogenic in situ hybridization (CISH) is a relatively new molecular technique used to detect and visualize in situ DNA or RNA nucleic acid sequences within a cell, within the tissue sample, or within a sample. This technique uses labeled DNA and RNA probes to localize the nucleic acid sequence of interest. CISH detection for the HER2 gene uses a double-stranded DNA probe in formalin-fixed paraffin-embedded specimens to detect the gene in the tissue. In this context, CISH provides a powerful testing modality for breast cancer since it has been shown to be a sensitive and specific method to determine the HER2/neu status of pathology specimens. Lin (2005) [70] reviewed 25 cases of fine-needle aspirate smears and smear preparations from infiltrating breast carcinomas. Both CISH and FISH were performed on each case using a digoxigenin-labeled HER2 DNA probe for CISH (Zymed) and both HER2 and chromosome 17 probes for FISH. Sixty tumor cells were evaluated in each case. Of the 25 cases analyzed, 23 (3 amplified and 20 nonamplified) showed similar results for both methods. Two cases were discordant. In these cases, low-level amplification was suggested by CISH but nonamplification by FISH. One of the cases can be explained by polysomy for chromosome 17 by FISH. These preliminary data suggest that CISH is a useful technique to determine HER2/neu oncogene status in cytologic specimens. In a case of low-level amplification, a CISH chromosome 17 probe should be used or FISH for confirmation of a suspected cancer. In reality, CISH has such low penetration in routine pathology that the value of the test is not fully realized; nevertheless there is strong mounting evidence to suggest it should be considered.

REFERENCES

1. G. Barnard, "The development of fluorescence immunoassays," *Prog. Clin. Biol. Res.* **285**, 15–37 (1988).
2. Y. Ueda and M. Kobayashi, "Spectroscopic studies of auto-fluorescence substances existing in human tissue: Influences of lactic acid and porphyrins," *Appl. Opt.* **43**(20), 3993–3998 (2004).
3. A. S. Januszewski, M. C. Thomas, J. S. Chung, C. S. Karschimkus, K. G. Rowley, C. Nelson, D. O'Neal, Z. Wang, J. D. Best, and A. J. Jenkins, "Plasma low-molecular weight fluorescence in Type 1 diabetes mellitus," *Ann. N.Y. Acad. Sci.* **1043**, 655–661 (2005).
4. G. Grynkiewicz, M. Poenie, and R. Y. Tsien, "A generation of Ca^{2+} indicators with greatly improved fluorescence properties," *J. Biol. Chem.* **260**, 3340–3350 (1985).
5. C-G. Niu, X-Q. Gui, G-M. Zeng, A-L. Guan, F-P. Gao, and p-Z. Qin, "Fluorescence ratiometric pH sensor prepared from covalently immobilised porphyrin and benzothioxanthene," *Anal. Bioanal. Chem.* **383**, 349–357 (2005).
6. K. S. Suslick, N. A. Rakow, M. E. Kosal, and J-H. Chou, "The materials chemistry of porphyrins and metalloporphyrins," *J. Porphyrins Phthalocyanines* **4**, 407–413(2000).
7. R-H. Yang, K-M. Wang, D. Xiao, and X-H. Yang, "Development of an iodine sensor based on fluorescence energy transfer," *Analyst* **125**, 1441–1445 (2000).
8. X-B. Zhang, C-C. Guo, Z-Z. Li, G-L. Shen, and R-Q. Yu, "An optical fiber chemical sensor for mercury ions based on a porphyrin dimer," *Anal. Chem.* **74**, 821–825 (2002).
9. J. S. Benco, H. A. Nienaber, and G. W. McGimpsey, "Optical sensors for blood gas analytes," *Spectrum* **14**(4), 1–18 (2001).
10. W. O'Neal and P. Jacobi, "Toward a general synthesis of chlorines," *J. Am. Chem. Soc.*, **130**(3), 1102–1108 (2008).
11. K. Golchini, M. Mackovic-Basic, S. Gharib, D. Masilamani, M. Lucas, and I. Kurtz, "Synthesis and characterisation of a new fluorescent probe for measuring potassium," *Am. J. Physiol.* **258**(27), (F438–F443) (1990).
12. J. N. Roe, F. C. Szoka, and A. S. Verkman, "Fiber optic sensor for the detection of potassium using fluorescence energy transfer," *Analyst* **115**, 353–358 (1990).

13. C-G. Niu, X-Q. Gui, G-M. Zeng, and X-Z. Yuan, "A ratiometric fluorescence sensor with broad dynamic range based on two pH-sensitive fluorophores," *Analyst* **130**, 1551–1556 (2005).

14. C. A. J. Bultzingslowen, Development of optical sensors (optodes) for carbon dioxide and their application to modified atmosphere packaging (MAD), Ph.D. thesis, University of Resensberg, Faculty of Chemistry and Pharmacy, 2004.

15. N. R. Glud, M. Kuhl, O. Kohls, and N. B. Ramsing, "Heterogeneity of oxygen production and consumption in a photosynthetic microbial mat as studied by planar optodes," *J. Phycol.* **35**, 270–279 (1999).

16. A. D. Shaw, Z. Li, Z. Thomas, and C. W. Stevens, "Assessment of tissue oxygen tension: Comparison of dynamic fluorescence quenching and polarographic electrode technique," *Crit. Care* **6**(1), 76–80 (2002).

17. W. Trettnak, W. Gruber, F. Reininger, P. O'Leary, and I. Klimant, "New instrument for optical measuring of oxygen in gas or dissolved in liquids," *Adv. Space Res.* **18**(4/5), 139–148 (1996).

18. L. Li and D. R. Walt, "Dual-analyte fibre-optic sensor for the simultaneous and continuous measurement of glucose and O_2," *Anal. Chem.* **67**(20), 3746–3752 (1995).

19. G. H. Elder, S. G. Smith, and S. J. Smyth, "Laboratory investigation of the porphyrias," *Ann. Clin. Biochem.* **27**, 395–412 (1990).

20. J. T. Hindmarsh, L. Oliveras, and D. C. Greenway, "Plasma porphyrins in the porphyrias," *Clin. Chem.* **45**(7), 1070–1076 (1999).

21. C. Lee, X. Qiao, D. E. Goeger, and K. E. Anderson, "Fluorometric measurement of 5-aminolevulinic acid in serum," *Clin. Chim. Acta* **347**, 183–188 (2004).

22. C. Hart, B. Schulenberg, T. H. Steinberg, W-Y. Leung, and W. F. Patton, "Detection of glycoproteins in polyacrylamide gels and on electroblots using Pro-Q Emerald 488 dye, a fluorescent periodate Schiff-base stain," *Electrophoresis* **24**(4), 588–598 (2003).

23. B. Gopalkrishnapillai, V. Nadanathangam, N. Karmakar, S. Anand, and A. Misra, "Evaluation of autofluorescent property of haemoglobin-advanced glycation end product as a long-term glycemic index of diabetes," *Diabetes* **52**, 1041–1046 (2003).

24. R. Sampathkumar, M. Balasubramanyam, M. Rema, C. Premanand, and V. Mohan, "A novel advanced glycation index and its association with diabetes and microangiopathy," *Metabolism Clin. Exp.* **54**, 1002–1007 (2005).

25. S. Blincko and R. Edwards, "Non-separation assay for glycohaemoglobin," *Endocrinol. Metab. Clin. Chem.* **44**(6), 1302–1308 (1998).

26. E. A. Moschou, B. V. Sharma, S. K. Deo, and S. Daunert, "Fluorescence glucose detection: Advances toward the ideal in vivo biosensor, *J. Fluorescence* **14**(5), 535–547 (2004).

27. R. Badugu, J. R. Lakowicz, and C. D. Geddes, "A glucose-sensing contact lens: From bench top to patient," *Curr. Opin. Biotechnol.* **16**, 100–107 (2005).

28. A. D'Auria and J. R. Lakowicz, "Enzyme fluorescence as a sensing tool: New perspectives in biotechnology," *Curr. Opin. Biotechnol.* **12**, 99–104 (2001).

29. J. Gao, J. Zhou, and X. Qu, "Fluorometric method for quantitative determination of glucose and its application to human serum," *Anal. Sci.* **21**, 409–412 (2005).

30. M. Wu, Z. Lin, M. Schaferling, A. Durkop, and O. S. Wolfbeis, "Fluorescence imaging of the activity of glucose oxidase using a hydrogen-peroxide-sensitive europium probe," *Anal. Biochem.* **340**(1), 66–73 (2005).

31. F. Hussain, D. J. S. Birch, and J. C. Pickup, "Glucose sensing based on the intrinsic fluorescence of sol-gel immobilised yeast hexokinase," *Anal. Biochem.* **339**(1), 137–143 (2005).

32. K. Ye and J. S. Schultz, "Genetic engineering of an allosterically based glucose indicator protein for continuous glucose monitoring by fluorescence resonance energy transfer," *Anal. Chem.* **75**, 3451–3459 (2003).

33. X. Ge, L. Tolosa, and G. Rao, "Dual-labelled glucose binding protein for ratiometric measurements of glucose," *Anal. Chem.* **76**, 1403–1410 (2004).

34. N. D. Evans, L. Gnudi, O. J. Rolinski, D. J. S. Birch, and J. C. Pickup, "Non-invasive glucose monitoring by NAD(P)H auto-fluorescence spectroscopy in fibroblasts and adipocytes: A model for skin glucose sensing," *Diabetes Technol. Ther.* **5**(5), 807–816 (2003).

35. H. Yu, E. P. Diamandis, A. F. Prestigiacomo, and T. A. Stamey, "Ultrasensitive assay of prostate-specific antigen used for early detection of prostate cancer relapse and estimation of tumour-doubling time after radical prostatectomy," *Clin. Chem.* **41**(3), 430–434 (1995).

36. P. Su, X-X. Zhang, and W-B. Chang, "Direct immunoassay of estrone by capillary electrophoresis with laser-induced fluorescence detection," *Electrophoresis* **24**(18), 3197–3201 (2003).

37. Q-P. Qin, O. Peltola, and K. Pettersson, "Time-resolved fluorescence resonance energy transfer assay for point-of-care testing of urinary albumin," *Clin. Chem.* **49**(7), 1105–1113 (2003).

38. S. A. Kane, C. A. Fleener, Y. S. Zhang, J. L. Davis, A. L. Musselman, and P. S. Huang, "Development of a binding assay for p53/HDM2 by using homogenous time-resolved fluorescence," *Anal. Biochem.* **278**(1), 29–38 (2000).

39. J. M. Hicks, "Fluorescence immunoassay," *Human Pathol.* **15**(2), 112–116 (1984).

40. Q-P. Qin, M. Christiansen, and K. Pettersson, "Point-of-care time-resolved immunofluorometric assay for human pregnancy-associated plasma protein A: Use in first-trimester screening for Down syndrome," *Clin. Chem.* **48**(3), 473–483 (2002).

41. C. Sluszny, Y. He, and E. S. Yeung, "Light-emitting diode-induced fluorescence detection of native proteins in capillary electrophoresis," *Electrophoresis* **26**, 4197–4203 (2005).

42. M. Lacroix, V. Poinsot, C. Fournier, and F. Couderc, "Laser-induced fluorescence detection schemes for the analysis of proteins and proteins using capillary electrophoresis (Review)," *Electrophoresis* **26**(13), 2608–2621 (2005).

43. C. Kang, H. J. Kim, D. Kang, D. Y. Jung, and M. Suh, "Highly sensitive and simple fluorescence staining of proteins in sodium dodecyl sulphate-polyacrylamide-based gels by using hydrophobic tail-mediated enhancement of fluorescein luminescence," *Electrophoresis* **24**(19/20), 3297–3304 (2003).

44. F. A. Mohamed, H. A. Mohamed, A. S. Hussein, and S. A. Ahmed, "A validated spectrofluorimetric method for determination of some psychoactive drugs," *J. Pharm. Biomed. Anal.* **39**, 139–146 (2005).

45. D. P. Nikolelis, D. A. Drivelos, M. G. Simantiraki, and S. Koinis, "An optical spot test for the detection of dopamine in human urine using stabilised in air lipid films," *Anal. Chem.* **76**, 2174–2180 (2004).

46. T. Perez-Ruiz, C. Martinez-Lozano, and R. Galera, "Development and validation of a capillary electrophoresis method with laser-induced fluorescence detection for the determination of captopril in human urine and pharmaceutical preparations," *Electrophoresis* **27**(12), 2310–2316 (2006).

47. F. Priego-Capote and M. D. Luque de Castro, "Determination of B_2 and B_6 vitamers in serum by capillary electrophoresis-molecular fluorescence-charge coupled detector," *Electrophoresis* **26**(12), 2376–2383 (2005).

48. I-T. Kuo, Y-F. Huang, and H-T. Chang, "Silica nanoparticles for separation of biologically active amines by capillary electrophoresis with laser-induced native fluorescence detection," *Electrophoresis* **26**(13), 2643–2651 (2005).

49. R. Yang, K. Wang, L. Long, D. Xiao, X. Yang, and W. Tan, "A selective optode membrane for histidine based on fluorescence enhancement of meso-meso-linked porphyrin dimer," *Anal. Chem.* **74**, 1088–1096 (2002).

50. U. Zorn, C. Haug, E. Celik, R. Wennauer, A. Schmid-Kotsa, M. G. Bachem, and A. Grunert, "Characterisation of modified low density lipoprotein subfractions by capillary isotachophoresis," *Electrophoresis* **22**(6), 1143–1149 (2001).

51. M. R. Speicher and N. P. Carter, "The new cytogenetics: Blurring the boundaries with molecular biology," *Nature Rev. Genet.* **6**, 782–792 (2005).

52. C. Lee, D. Gisselsson, C. Jin, A. Nordgren, D. O. Ferguson, E. Blennow, J. A. Fletcher, and C. C. Morton, "Limitations of chromosome classification by multicolor karyotyping," *Am. J. Hum. Genet.* **68**, 1043–1047 (2001).

53. Y-S. Fan, *Theory and Practice of Molecular Cytogenetics Applied to Medicine: Molecular Cytogenetics: Protocols and Applications*, Humana Press, Totowa, NJ, 2002.

54. T. Liehr (Ed.), *Multicolor FISH in Human Cytogenetics*, S. Karger, Basel, Switzerland, 2006.

55. M. A. Hulten, S. Dhanjal, and B. Pertl, "Rapid and simple prenatal diagnosis of common chromosome disorders: Advantages and disadvantages of the molecular methods FISH and QF-PCR," *Reproduction* **126**, 279–297 (2003).

56. L. Dudarewicz, W. Holzgreve, A. Jeziorowska, L. Jakubowski, and B. Zimmermann, "Molecular methods for rapid detection of aneuploidy," *J. Appl. Genet.* **46**(2), 207–215 (2005).

57. L. G. Shaffer and T. Bui, "Molecular cytogenetic and rapid aneuploidy detection methods in prenatal diagnosis," *Am. J. Med. Genet. Part C (Semin. Med. Genet.)* **145C**, 87–98 (2007).

58. A. M. Snijders, D. Pinkel, and D. G. Albertson, "Current status and future prospects of array-based comparative genomic hybridisation," *Briefings Funct. Genom. Proteom.* **2**, 37–45 (2003).

59. E. Schrock, P. Zschieschang, P. O'Brien, A. Helmrich, T. Hardt,, A. Matthaei, and K. Stout-Wieder, "Spectral karyotyping of human, mouse, rat and ape chromosomes—Applications for genetic diagnostics and research," *Cytogen. Genome Res.* **114**, 199–221 (2006).

60. A. K. Raap and H. J. Tanke, "COmbined Binary RAtio fluorescence in situ hybridiziation (COBRA-FISH): Development and applications," *Cytogen. Genome Res.* **114**, 227–239 (2006).

61. W. B. Marluce Bibbo (Ed.), *Comprehensive Cytopathology*, 2nd ed., Saunders, Philadelphia, 1997.

62. R. M. DeMay (Ed.), *The Art and Science of Cytopathology*, ASCP Press, Chicago, IL, 1996.

63. I. R. Sokolova, L. Bubendorf, A. O'Hare, M. S. Legator, K. Jacobson, B. S. Grilli, P. Dalquen, K. C. Halling, M. Tamm, S. A. Seelig, and L. E. Morrison, "A fluorescence in situ hybridization-based assay for improved detection of lung cancer cells in bronchial washing specimens," *Cancer Cytopathol.* **96**(5), 306–315 (2002).

64. S. Lam, C. MacAulay, J. C. leRiche, and B. Palcic, "Detection and localization of early lung cancer by fluorescence bronchoscopy," *Cancer* **89**(S11), 2468–2473 (2000).

65. R. Veeramachaneni, M. L. Nordberg, R. Shi, G. A. Herrera, and E. A. Turbat-Herrera, "Evaluation of fluorescence in situ hybridization as an ancillary tool to urine cytology in diagnosing urothelial carcinoma," *Diagnostic Cytopathol.* **28**(6), 301–307 (2003).

66. P. Jichlinski, M. Forrer, J. Mizeret, T. Glanzmann, D. Braichotte, G. Wagnières, G. Zimmer, L. Guillou, F. Schmidlin, P. Graber, H. van den Bergh, and H. Jürg Leisinger, "Clinical evaluation of a method for detecting superficial transitional cell carcinoma of the bladder by light-induced fluorescence of protoporphyrin IX following topical application of 5-aminolevulinic acid: Preliminary results," *Lasers Surg. Med.* **20**(4), 402–408 (1997).

67. M. A. Iqbal, M. Akhtar, C. Ulmer, F. Al-Dayel, and M. C. Paterson, "FISH analysis in chromophobe renal-cell carcinoma," *Diagnostic Cytopathol.* **22**(1), 3–6 (2000).

68. A. A. Renshaw, D. Maurici, and J. A. Fletcher, "Cytologic and fluorescence in situ hybridization (FISH) examination of metanephric adenoma," *Diagnostic Cytopathol.* **16**(2), 107–111 (1997).

69. R. Nizzoli, C. Bozzetti, P. Crafa, N. Naldi, A. Guazzi, B. Di Blasio, R. Camisa, and S. Cascinu, "Immunocytochemical evaluation of HER-2/neu on fine-needle aspirates from primary breast carcinomas," *Diagnostic Cytopathol.* **28**(3), 142–146 (2003).

70. F. Lin, T. Shen, and J. Prichard, "Detection of Her-2/neu oncogene in breast carcinoma by chromogenic in situ hybridization in cytologic specimens," *Diagnostic Cytopathol.* **33**(6), 376–380 (2005).

CHAPTER 15

Immunochemical Detection of Analytes by Using Fluorescence

EVGENIA G. MATVEEVA, IGNACY GRYCZYNSKI, and ZYGMUNT GRYCZYNSKI

University of North Texas, Health Science Center, Fort Worth, Texas 76107

EWA M. GOLDYS

Division of Information and Communication Sciences, Macquarie University, Sydney 2109, New South Wales, Australia

15.1 INTRODUCTION: DEFINITION AND GENERAL PRINCIPLES OF IMMUNOASSAYS

Immunoassay is a test that uses the binding of antibodies to antigens (target substances, also called analytes) to identify and measure such substances [1–5]. Immunoassays can also be used to identify and measure antibodies. The basic principle of immunoassays relies on the specificity of the antibody–antigen reaction. Immunoassays are very specific and sensitive and, at same time, easy to perform, which has resulted in their widespread use in analytical/clinical chemistry [3, 5–20].

The antibody is a protein (immunoglobulin) molecule produced by the immune system in humans and animals in response to a foreign substance (antigen). Antibodies belong to a type of protein called immunoglobulins; the most common one is immunoglobulin G (IgG). IgG is a Y-shaped large protein (molecular weight about 145–150 kDa) composed of two main structural and functional regions (Figure 15.1). The Fc region (fragment, crystallizable), located at the stem of the Y, is composed of two heavy chains. Its role involves binding to various cell receptors and complement proteins. The Fc region is a region of constant structure within an antibody class. The second, called the Fab region (fragment, antigen binding), which is located at each end of the forked portion of the Y on the antibody, is composed of one constant and one variable domain of each of the heavy and light chains. These domains shape the antigen-binding site at the amino terminal end of the monomer. The variable domains at the two chains bind the epitope on their specific antigens. It is important to note that Fab contains the antigen (Ag)–binding site that varies between different antibodies. Each antibody recognizes a particular foreign antigen and

Fluorescence Applications in Biotechnology and Life Sciences, Edited by Ewa M. Goldys

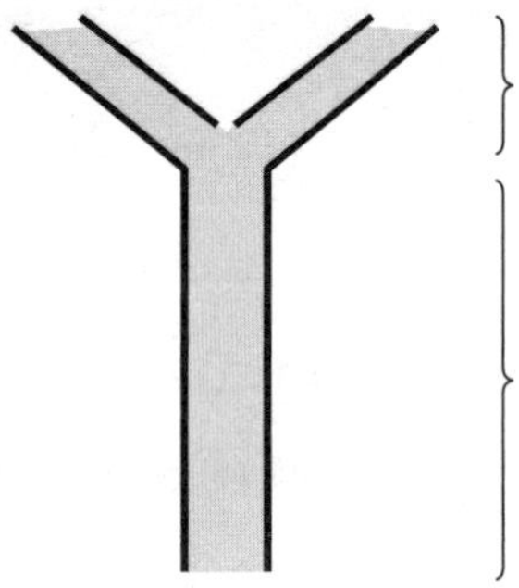

Figure 15.1 Structure and functional sites of the antibody: Fab region contains the antigen-binding site (it varies between different antibodies); Fc region has constant structure within an antibody class.

binds to it. Among different antigens we find relatively simple substances, including small molecules such as drugs or pesticides, or a complex ones such as proteins or viruses.

Although many types of immunoassays are available on the market, the fundamental principles and components of an immunoassay are common. In order to perform an immunoassay, we must carry out the calibration using appropriate standards, need to select an appropriate antibody, and choose the detection mode, which are described below.

1. *Standards and Calibration* Standards or calibrations are known concentrations of the analyte that are used to generate a standard curve [1, 2]. In order to produce such a standard curve, the "signal" detected from the assay is plotted versus the known "concentration" of the standard and a best-fit line or curve is drawn. The concentration of the analyte can then be determined by measuring the signal in an unknown sample and using the standard curve to deduce the concentration of the analyte.
2. *Antibody* Depending on the specific assay format, there may be one or more antibodies involved in binding to the analyte in the sample [1–5]. Antibodies are called polyclonal if produced by antigen injection into experimental animal and monoclonal if produced by cell fusion and cell culture techniques. Monoclonal antibodies have better specificity and more reproducible properties from batch to batch and are preferred in immunoassays.
3. *Detection Mode* The detection mode is defined by the character of the reporter label used in the immunoassay. All immunoassays require the use of labeling in order to visualize and measure the amount of antigen or antibody present. A label is a molecule that will react as part of the assay, so a change in signal can be measured in the solution. There are a number of different labels, such as substances that produce light (luminophores), radioactive isotopes, or enzymes producing color or fluorescence, used for quantification of a sample's response. Depending on the assay format, these labels can be located on the antigen or the antibody. Here we will focus on immunoassays utilizing fluorescent labels.

15.2 IMMUNOASSAY TYPES AND FORMATS

15.2.1 Competitive and Sandwich Immunoassays

In a "competitive" immunoassay, the antigen (analyte) in the sample competes with the labeled antigen (tracer) for a limited number of antibody-binding sites (Figure 15.2). The bound antigen is separated from the excess analyte, which did not bind to the antibody. The amount of the analyte in the unknown sample is inversely proportional to the amount of labeled antigen, which can be measured in a fluorometer or spectrophotometer. In the one-step competitive format (Figure 15.2), both the labeled antigen reagent (Ag*) and the unlabeled specimen or test sample analyte Ag compete for a limited amount of antibody. In the two-step competitive format, the antibody is first incubated with specimen containing antigens of interest; then, in the second step, labeled antigen is added. Two-step competitive assay formats usually provide improved assay sensitivity by a factor of severalfold compared to one-step assay formats.

In noncompetitives, or "sandwich," immunoassays, the analyte is sandwiched between two antibodies, the capture antibody and the detection antibody (Figure 15.3). Typically, the capture antibody is coated to a solid phase (such as a well), and the detection antibody (which should be present in excess) is labeled with a fluorophore, radioactive label (such as I-125), or an enzyme. As the amount of analyte antigen is increased, the amount of labeled antibody–antigen complex also increases. Thus, the amount of analyte in an unknown sample is directly proportional to the amount of labeled detection antibody measured by the detection system. Noncompetitive assay formats can also utilize either one-step or two-step methods, as with the competitive assay. The two-step assay format employs washing steps in which the sandwich-binding complex is isolated and washed to remove excess unbound labeled reagent and any other interfering substances. These steps are omitted in one-step assays. The two-step noncompetitive format usually offers the highest specificity and sensitivity of all the assay formats discussed here.

15.2.2 Homogeneous and Heterogeneous (Solid-Phase) Immunoassays

Immunoassays which do not require separation are referred to as homogeneous immunoassays. An example of a homogeneous immunoassay is given in Figure 15.4, where antigen (Ag) is binding to a labeled antibody (Ab*) and the resulting Ag–Ab* complex is being detected in solution. In this case, in order to be detected, the fluorescence properties of the label in the complex with antigen should be different from the fluorescent properties of the free labeled antibody. This difference, resulting from Ag binding (such as fluorescence quenching, polarization, or shift in the spectral maxima), is proportional to the Ag concentration. It is also worthwhile to mention

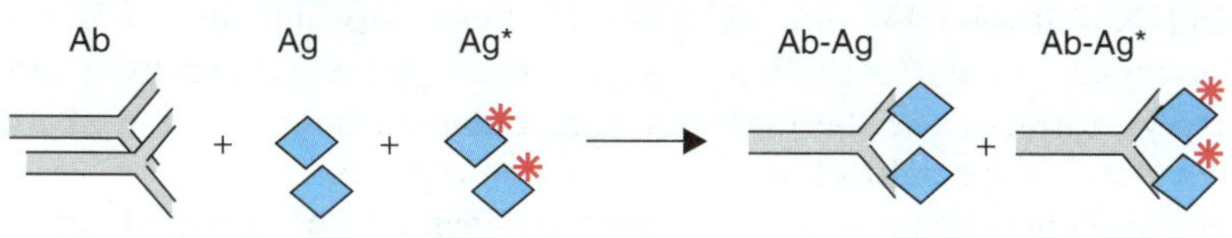

Figure 15.2 One-step competitive immunoassay format.

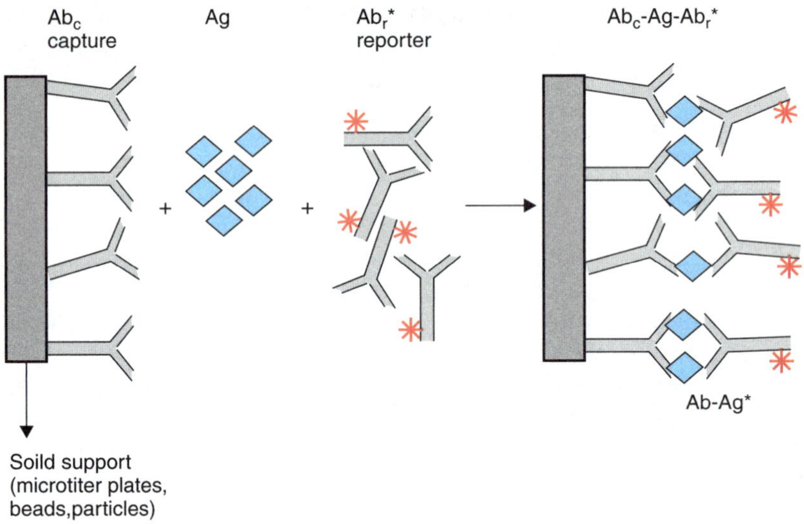

Figure 15.3 One-step noncompetitive sandwich immunoassay format.

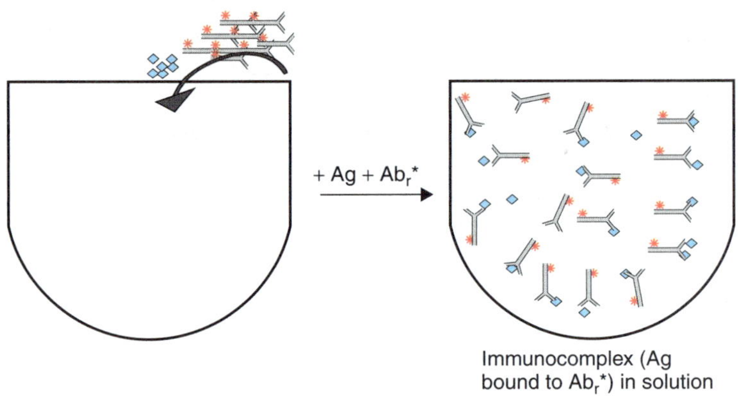

Figure 15.4 Homogeneous immunoassay.

homogeneous methods which do not require the separation of the bound Ab–Ag* from the free Ag*. These immunoassays are generally easy and fast to perform. Homogeneous methods have been generally applied to the measurement of small analytes such as pesticides and drugs. Immunoassay methods that require separation of bound Ab–Ag* complex are referred to as heterogeneous immunoassays, or "solid-phase" assays (Figure 15.5). These assays are often performed on a surface coated with antibody or antigen. The immunological binding takes place on the surface and is followed by one or more washing steps to achieve separation of Ab–Ag* complex from free reactants. As the solid phase utilized by heterogeneous immunoassays, one can use the inner surface of immunoassay plate wells, tubes, the surface of a slide, or specialized reagents including magnetic particles or plastic beads. Since heterogeneous immunoassays require the separation of unbound complexes, no change in fluorescent properties of the label is needed in this case, and the signal (usually fluorescence intensity on the surface) is proportional to the Ag concentration.

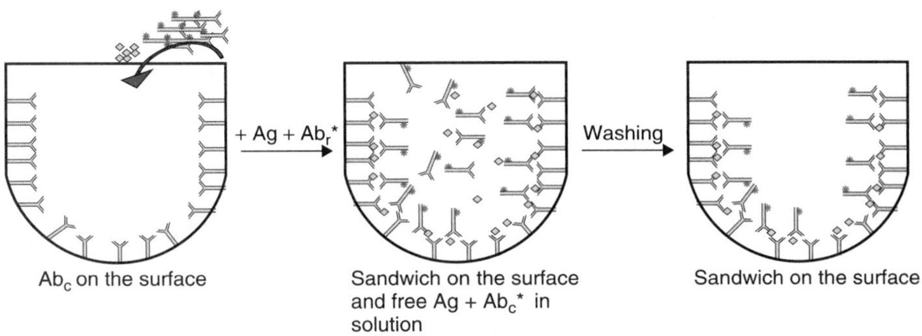

Figure 15.5 Heterogeneous immunoassay.

15.2.3 Types of Labels Used in Immunoassays with Fluorescence Detection (Fluorophores, Enzymes with Fluorogenic Substrates)

Immunoassays are usually named after the detection type, which also defines the type of label used. For example, RIAs (radioimmunoassays) [20–22], enzyme immunoassays like ELISA (enzyme-linked immunosorbent assays) [4, 5], LIA (luminescent immunoassays), and FIA (fluorescent immunoassays) are widely used in research, drug discovery, and diagnostics for highly specific and cost-efficient detection of analytes not detectable with other techniques. The antibodies are labeled with radioisotopes, fluorescent dyes [e.g., fluorescein isothiocyanate (FITC)], or enzymes [e.g., horseradish peroxidase (HRP) or alkaline phosphate (AP)], which catalyze fluorogenic or luminogenic reactions.

15.3 TYPES OF ANALYTES

An analyte is anything measured by a laboratory test. In immunoassay testing, the analyte may be either an antibody or an antigen (such as a large protein, a small molecule, or even an ion).

15.3.1 Cations, Metal Ions, and Anions

Immunoassays are rarely used for detection of ions, such as metal ions. Mostly, other techniques are used to measure trace metals in natural materials, for example, plasma atomic emission spectroscopy. Antibody-based immunoassays are an alternative approach, with some advantages over other instrument-intensive methods. However, very few antibodies have been available for the analysis of metal ions. The development of such antibodies requires converting of the metal ion into some type of complex or other derivative. Examples of competitive immunoassays using EDTA (ethylenediaminetetraacetic acid) or DTPA (diethylenetriaminepentaacetic acid) metal complexes for detections of heavy metal ions in water samples have been described [23, 24]. In some cases, the complexes of metal ions are used as labels in immunoassays, for example, DTPA complexes of heavy metals [25–27] or criptate complexes of rare earth metals [28].

15.3.2 Small-Molecule Analytes (Pesticides, Toxins, and Biomarkers)

Small molecules (<5 kDa), such as pesticides, toxins, and some biomarkers, often do not have enough epitopes for antibody recognition. Such molecules can often bind to only one antibody molecule, so small analytes are detected using a competitive immunoassay format with various types of detection. Among those fluorescence polarization is widely used for small-molecule detection [14–16].

15.3.3 Proteins

Large molecules, such as proteins, mostly have several epitopes and are capable of binding to at least two antibodies simultaneously, so a wide variety of immunoassay formats is available for proteins. Since competitive assays have limited sensitivity, sandwich-type assay format is normally used for protein detection.

Immunoassays also can be designed to detect antibodies themselves. They provide information on antibody activity rather than antibody concentration. Since circulating antibodies are very heterogeneous in terms of their epitope affinity, the results of such antibody assay can vary if antigens of varying quality/purity are used. Another concern for the antibody immunoassays in clinical sample is that circulating antibodies may be partially already bound to the appropriate antigens and hence their activity will not show up in the assay.

15.4 STEADY-STATE FLUORESCENCE IMMUNOASSAYS

15.4.1 Intensity-Based (Quenching, Enhancement) Assays: Environmentally Sensitive Probes

Most homogeneous immunoassays are based on some change occurring after antigen–antibody binding: for example, it may be a change in the fluorescence intensity of the label conjugated with antigen or antibody or fluorescence of the antigen itself (quenching or enhancement of the fluorescence) or variations in fluorescence polarization. Several types of immunoassays have been conceived which rely on such changes. For example, a quenching fluoroimmunoassay (QFIA) is based on the detection of the difference of fluorescence intensity between fluorescence-labeled antigen and its immunocomplex [9, 29–32]. The fluorescence intensity of the fluorescein-labeled antigen (small molecule, hapten) is quenched after binding to specific antibodies. This quenching may be caused by the change of the fluorescein microenvironment to a more hydrophobic one (due to the fact that fluorescein becomes located more closely to the hydrophobic active site of the antibody). The addition of a free, nonlabeled hapten (e.g., from the standard or sample), which competes with a labeled hapten for binding sites of antibodies, leads to a partial restoration of the initial fluorescence intensity (Figure 15.6). A similar quenching effect can be observed if antigen itself is also a fluorophore (Figure 15.7), for example, for binding of coproporphyrin to specific anti-coproporphyrin antibodies [33]. Examples of the dose–response curves are given in Figure 15.8.

A variation of QFIA is so-called indirect quenching fluoroimmunoassay [9, 34–36]. In this case the system includes the fluorescein–hapten conjugate together with a fluorescence-quenching antifluorescein antibody and an antianalyte antibody. Due to

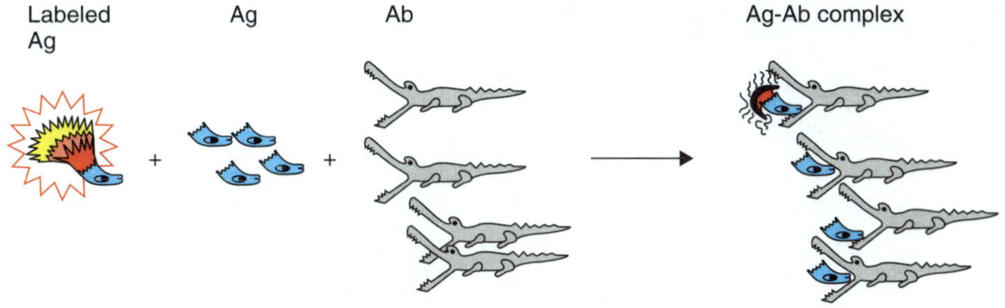

Figure 15.6 Fluorescence-quenching immunoassay: free analyte competes with labeled analyte. Fluorescence is quenched after fluorophore is binding to the antibody.

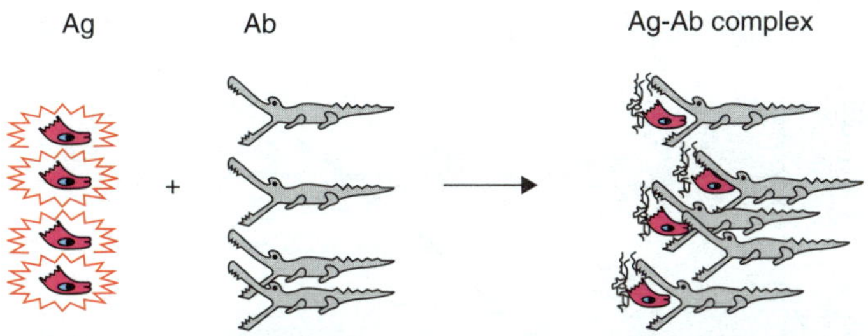

Figure 15.7 Fluorescence-quenching immunoassay: analyte itself is fluorescent. Fluorescence is quenched after fluorophore is binding to the antibody.

steric hindrance, simultaneous binding of both antibodies to the conjugate is not possible. This equilibrium can be easily shifted by adding free hapten, which competes with the conjugate to bind to the antianalyte antibody.

15.4.2 Energy Transfer Assays

Another variation of the quenching assay is excitation transfer assay [9, 37, 38]. The system includes the fluorescently labeled hapten donor (hapten conjugate) together with a fluorescence-quenching acceptor (anti-analyte antibody labeled with the quencher). When hapten–antibody binding occurs, dipole–dipole-coupled excitation energy transfer takes place within the antigen–antibody complex. The resulting quenching of fluorescence can be inhibited by competitive binding with unlabeled hapten. Alternatively, separate antibody samples can be labeled with fluorescing label and quencher, respectively. Unlabeled antigen causes aggregation of the separately labeled components, which produces quenching.

15.4.3 Chemiluminescence Assays: Enzyme Immunoassays Utilizing Fluorescent Substrates

Chemi- and bioluminescent systems have been extensively used for in vitro diagnostic immunoassays [3, 7, 13, 22]. Bioluminescence is a luminescent process mediated by an enzyme or other biological system. An example of an enzyme immunoassay utilizing luminescing substrates is given in Figure 15.9. This is a competitive immunoassay

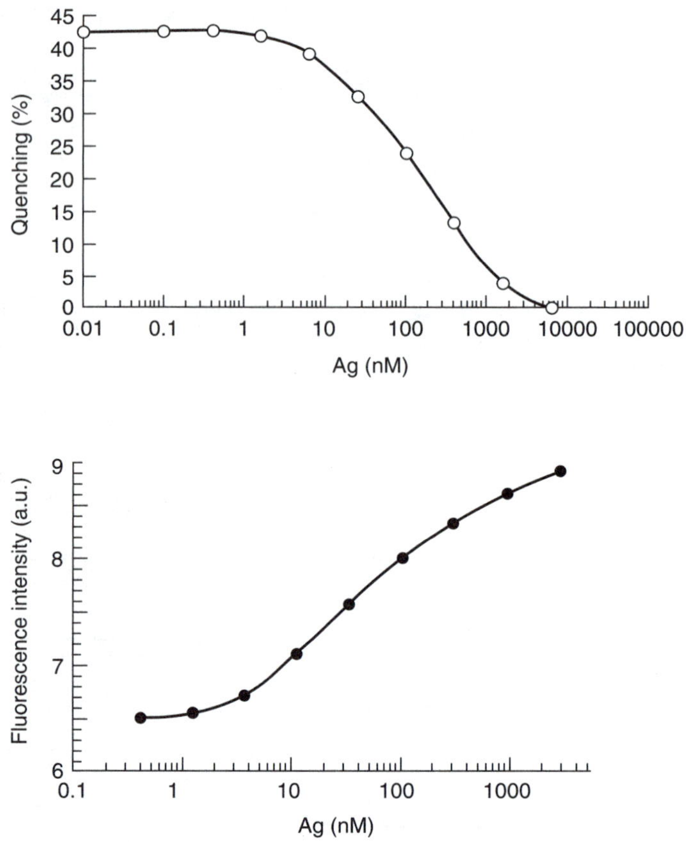

Figure 15.8 Fluorescence-quenching immunoassay: examples of dose–response curves. Fluorescence is quenched after fluorophore is binding to the antibody.

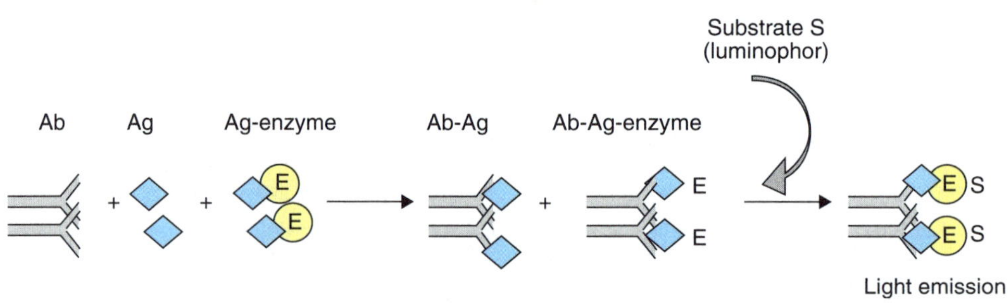

Figure 15.9 Enzyme immunoassay utilizing luminescing substrates: scheme of the competitive immunoassay involving antigen labeled with an enzyme (peroxidase, alkaline phosphatase) and a substrate (luminol or acridine based) emitting light when reacting with the enzyme.

involving an antigen (small molecule, such as hormone) labeled with an enzyme (peroxidase, or alkaline phosphatase). When a substrate (luminol or acridine-based) is added, it reacts with the enzyme leading to light emission. The amount of the emitted light is proportional to the enzyme label and inversely proportional to the amount of competing free analyte (see typical standard curve in Figure 15.10).

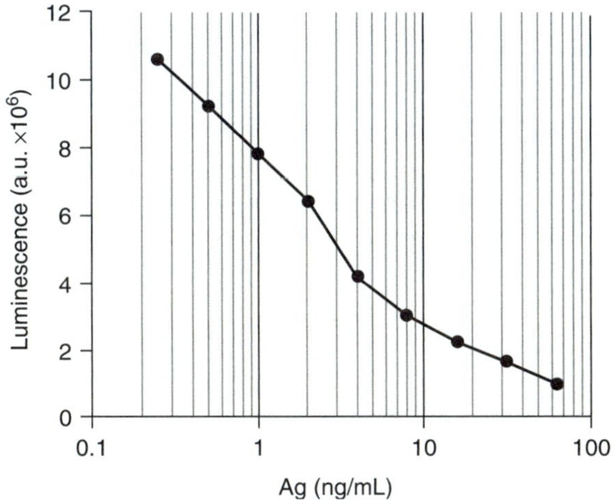

Figure 15.10 Enzyme immunoassay utilizing luminescing substrates—typical standard curve.

Similarly, enzyme labels and luminescing substrates can be utilized to set up a sandwich immunoassay (ELISA). In such immunoassays the first antibody is immobilized on the bottom of an immunoplate well and "captures" the analyte. A second antibody that recognizes a different epitope is used to detect the captured analyte. This antibody is coupled to an enzyme which reacts with a substrate to produce a luminescent signal. In this case the signal is proportional to the amount of analyte present in the standard or sample.

15.4.4 Polarization Assays

The method of polarization fluoroimmunoassay (PFIA) is widely used for rapid determination of small molecules, such as pesticides and drugs [14–16, 39]. PFIA is a homogeneous competition method based on detection of the difference of fluorescence polarization between a small fluorescently labeled hapten (where quick rotation of the molecule ensures low polarization) and its immunocomplex with specific antibody (where slow rotation of the large immunocomplex leads to high level of polarization) (Figure 15.11). The observed fluorescence polarization of a fluorescently labeled hapten

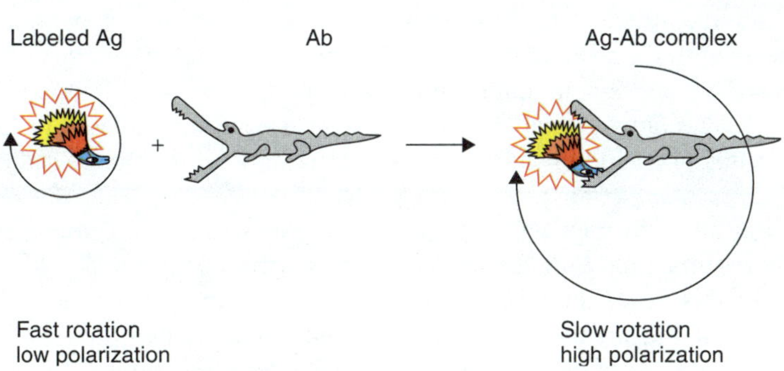

Figure 15.11 Fluorescence polarization immunoassay.

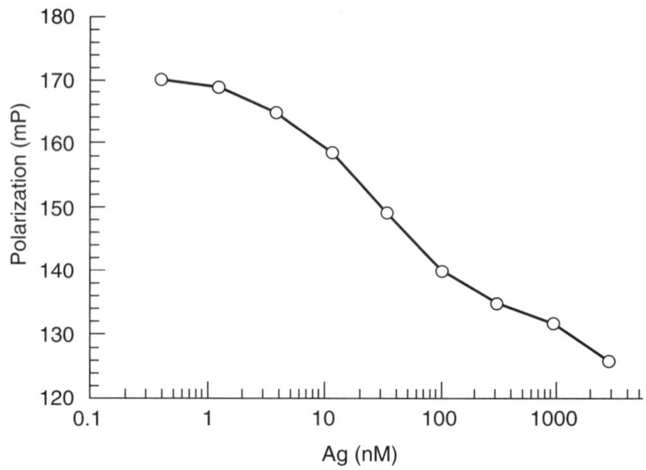

Figure 15.12 Fluorescence polarization immunoassay; example of dose–response curve.

(tracer) is inversely related to the free hapten concentration (Figure 15.12). The level of hapten (such as pesticide or drug) in a given sample therefore can be determined by comparison with a calibration curve.

15.5 TIME-RESOLVED AND KINETIC APPROACHES AS TOOLS FOR ELIMINATION OF FLUORESCENCE BACKGROUND

15.5.1 Kinetic Approach, Stopped-Flow Immunoassays, Time-Gated Detection, and Lifetime Assays

Homogeneous methods of immunoanalysis are simple and fast; however, the detection limits obtained in homogeneous immunoassays are frequently affected by matrix effects. Although these effects can be relatively insignificant in environmental analysis where samples are usually water suspensions which are simple as a matrix, the minimization of the matrix effect becomes more important when immunoassay is applied to clinical or food analysis where the sample matrices are far more complex. One of the approaches involves a kinetic methodology which uses the initial rate of the antibody–antigen reaction as the analytical parameter, measured in only 4–5 s. [14]. The sample matrix affects the static fluorescence intensity or polarization signal but not its variation with time (Figure 15.13). The antigen–antibody interaction in solution is usually very fast, and kinetic data can be obtained by the using stopped-flow mixing technique [14]. The antigen–antibody binding on the surface takes a longer time, up to tens of minutes [40], and in such a case the reaction kinetics can be monitored more easily.

If excitation is performed using pulsed light, the subsequent emission by different fluorophores may have different decay rates, depending on the lifetime of the fluorophore. In this case, fluorescence from long-lived fluorophores can be detected selectively by delaying the measurement until some time ("gated time") after the excitation pulse, when all short-lived components have decayed (Figure 15.14). This type of detection is called "time gated" or "time resolved" and requires using a long-lived

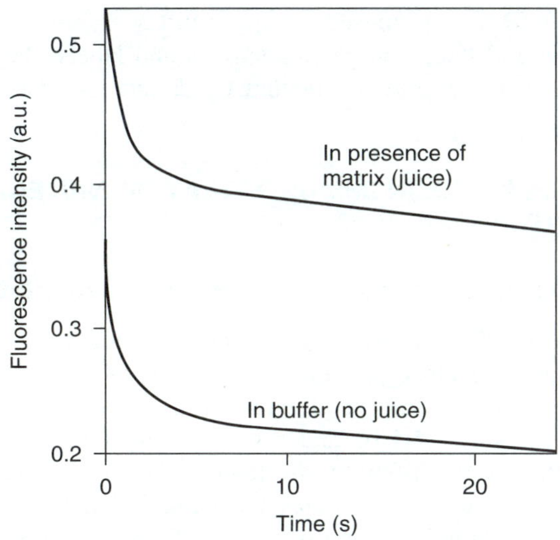

Figure 15.13 Kinetic approach to immunoassay detection, stopped-flow mixing—example of dose–response curve.

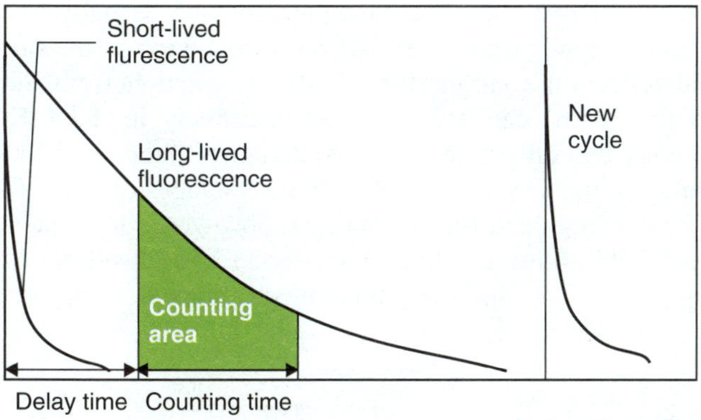

Figure 15.14 Kinetic approach to immunoassays—time-gated detection.

luminescent label (half-life microseconds to milliseconds) [41]. A typical background in most biological/clinical samples is caused by organic fluorophores which are short-lived (half-life of a few nanoseconds) and these can be easily eliminated by this technique.

15.5.2 Near-Infrared Fluorophores

The near-infrared (NIR) region of the spectrum (650–1100 nm) offers advantages over the traditional ultraviolet (UV) visible region for bioanalytical applications such as immunoassays [42, 43]. Using luminescence detection in the NIR region results in reduced background signals since only a few species happen to fluoresce in the NIR. Another reason for using the NIR region is its lower background absorption of the biological (tissue) samples in the NIR optical window between the water absorption band and the absorption of hemoglobin. The required instrumentation includes simple and inexpensive red diode lasers.

Examples of the NIR dyes proposed for applications in immunoassays include new long-wave absorbing and fluorescing cyanine dyes and labels; they are water soluble and have high absorbances and their quantum yields increase if bound to proteins.

15.6 RECENT ADVANCES IN IMMUNOASSAY SIGNAL ENHANCEMENT AND THROUGHPUT

15.6.1 Metal-Particle-Enhanced Immunoassays: Nanoparticles as Labels

Recently a significant fluorescence signal enhancement was demonstrated when fluorophores are placed in close proximity to a layer of metallic particles [44–47]. This is due to two factors: enhanced local field, which enhances the excitation rate (dotted line in Figure 15.15), and radiative rate enhancement (dashed line), which is responsible for the lifetime shortening. At close proximity to the metal (Figure 15.15), below 5 nm, fluorophores are strongly quenched (solid black line). The effective brightness (solid red line in Figure 15.15) is a combination of all three effects: the strongest enhancement values are observed at approximately 10 nm from the metal particle surface [48]. This phenomenon of metal-enhanced fluorescence (MEF) observed, for example, with silver island films (SIFs) can be used to improve signal-to-noise level for quantitative bioanalyte detection. Usually MEF is performed with front-face optical configuration (excitation from the top of the sample). However, the total internal reflection configuration (TIRF) (excitation from the bottom of the sample through the prism) can also be used effectively in the MEF-based assays. TIRF is a technology that allows selective excitation of fluorescent molecules in close (200-nm) proximity to the surface [49, 50]. The advantages of TIRF for surface-based bioassays have been recognized for many years; however, confinement and formation of the evanescent field above the highly scattering and absorbing layer of metallic particles as an application for surface immunoassays have been reported only recently

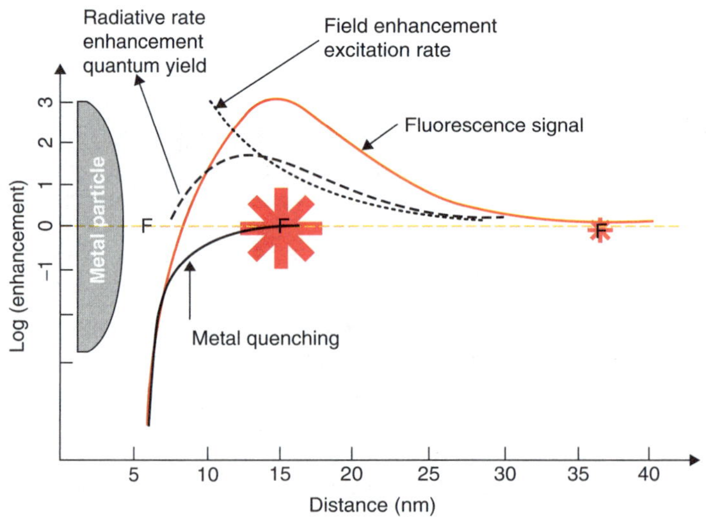

Figure 15.15 Fluorescence enhancement as function of fluorophore to metal particle distance.

[51–53]. The evanescent wave excitation confines the excitation volume to the assay surface, eliminating the need for washing the solution from above the assay surface. Enhancement in the brightness of the fluorophores near the silvered surface facilitates easy measurements of kinetic binding. MEF also significantly decreases the lifetimes of the fluorophores, which in turn increases the photostability.

Nanoparticles (e.g., quantum dots, metal nanoparticles, dye-doped nanoparticles) are currently widely used also as immunoassay labels [54–56]. Various types of nanoparticles, both organic and inorganic, are being detected by electromagnetic or optical techniques, including static and time-resolved luminescence, one- and two-photon absorption, Raman and Rayleigh scattering, and surface plasmon resonance. The application of nanoparticles makes it possible to achieve lowering of detection limits (if possible, down to single-molecule level), parallel integration of multiple signals (multiplexing), and signal amplification by several orders of magnitude. The photobleaching effects are also prevented while maintaining antigen-binding specificity and sensitivity.

15.6.2 Surface Plasmon–Coupled Emission-Based Immunoassays

Thin metal films (approximately 50 nm thick, typically, silver or gold) support collective oscillations of free electrons called surface plasmons. These surface plasmons are induced by excited fluorophores located near a thin-film surface. The plasmons then radiate into the glass substrate at the surface plasmon angle for the emission wavelength (θ_F) (Figure 15.16). The plasmons radiate at the plasmon angle because such an angle is required to match the light and plasmon wave vectors [57]. This phenomenon is called surface plasmon–coupled emission (SPCE). The optical properties of surface plasmons and the applications of surface plasmon resonance (SPR) to measurement of bioaffinity reactions have been described in detail [58–61]. Surface plasmons cannot be excited from air by incident light; SPR occurs when light is incident on a metal through a higher refractive index medium such as glass. The surface plasmons are only excited at a specific angle of incident (θ_{SP}) where the reflectivity decreases (Figure 15.16).

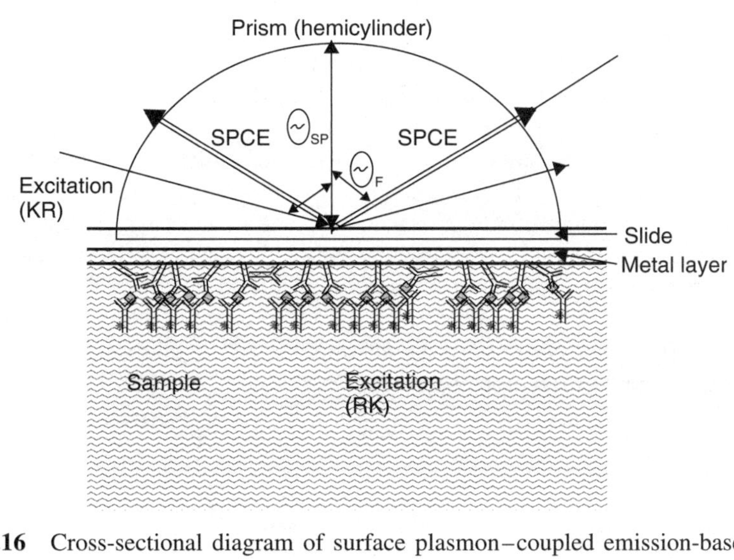

Figure 15.16 Cross-sectional diagram of surface plasmon–coupled emission-based immunoassay.

There are two possible configurations for SPCE measurements. The sample can be illuminated from the sample side in the reverse Kretschmann (RK) configuration. This excitation cannot create surface plasmons in the metal surface. The excited fluorophores near the metal couple and create plasmons which emit SPCE into the glass prism. In the RK configuration fluorophores are excited almost uniformly across the sample. However, only the excitation energy from the near field (up to about 200 nm) couples to the surface plasmons. The far-field radiation is effectively reflected from the metal mirror film.

The sample can also be illuminated through the prism at the plasmon angle (θ_{SP}), which is called the Kretschmann (KR) configuration (shown in Figure 15.16). KR illumination results in a strong selective excitation near the metal surface. The enhanced field makes it possible for the illumination intensity to be decreased, further reducing the background.

A diagram of a model SPCE immunoassay is shown in Figure 15.16. The sample (protein-coated silver slide) assembled in a cuvette is illuminated in the KR configuration. When fluorophore-labeled antiprotein antibody solution is added to the cuvette, this antibody binds to the surface-immobilized protein, producing an SPCE signal which is being observed on the prism side of the sample, at the plasmon resonance angle. The intensity observed through the prism is strongly directional and sharply concentrated near the θ_F angle. The spectrum of the SPCE is characteristic of the fluorophore probe used in the assay and is not affected by scattered light at the excitation wavelength, even in the presence of optically dense sample matrices (serum, whole blood). The SPCE-based immunoassays [62, 63] are ultrasensitive and easy to perform and can be carried out in the presence of a dense matrix background, such as a whole blood. They do not require washing steps and are fast.

15.6.3 Assay Miniaturization (Arrays, Microchips)

The miniaturization of immunoassays [19, 64–68] is particularly relevant to diagnostic applications because the reduction of sample volume is of great importance when only minimal amounts of samples are available. In addition, immunoassay miniaturization makes it possible to develop rapid and multiplexed assays which are more sensitive than macroscopic ones. Historically, simple low-throughput multiplex immunoassays were first developed; these were followed by low-level multiplexing and high-throughput array-based immunoassays. Recently, two types of high-level multiplexing and high-throughput diagnostic methods using microspot arrays and bead arrays have been introduced to complement single-analyte assays [19]. Nanoanalytical devices applicable to immunoassays include nanochips, nanoparticles, nanotiter plates [65, 66], and nanobiosensors. Immunosensing microfluidic devices fabricated in glass, silicon, and polymers are reviewed in [67], with fluorescence being the most common detection method. Novel detection methods such as SPCE allow minimization of the detection volume down to 1–2 aL [68].

REFERENCES

1. J. P. Gosling (Ed.), *Immunoassays: A Practical Approach*, Practical Approach Series 228, Oxford University Press, New York, 2000.

2. P. Englebienne (Ed.), *Immune and Receptor Assays in Theory and Practice*, CRC Press, Boca Raton, FL, 2000.

3. A. Ronald and W. H. Stimson, "The evolution of immunoassay technology," *Parasitology* **117**, S13–27 (1998).

4. E. Ishikawa, "Ultrasensitive and rapid enzyme immunoassay," in *Laboratory Techniques in Biochemistry and Molecular Biology*, S. Pillai and P. C. van der Vliet (Eds.), Elsevier, Amsterdam, 1999, pp. 1–334.

5. J. R. Crowther, *The ELISA Guidebook*, Methods in Molecular Biology, Vol. 149, Humana Press, Totowa, NJ, 2001.

6. R. E. Curry, H. Heitzman, D. H. Riege, R. V. Sweet, and M. G. Simonsen, "A systems approach to fluorescent immunoassay: General principles and representative applications," *Clin. Chem.* **25**, 1591–1595 (1979).

7. T. P. Whitehead, L. J. Kricka, T. J. Carter, and G. H. Thorpe, "Analytical luminescence: Its potential in the clinical laboratory," *Clin. Chem.* **25**, 1531–1546 (1979).

8. J. F. Place, R. M. Sutherland, and C. Dahne, "Opto-electronic immunosensors: A review of optical immunoassay at continuous surfaces," *Biosensors* **1**, 321–353 (1985).

9. I. Hemmila, "Fluoroimmunoassays and immunofluorometric assays," *Clin. Chem.* **31**, 359–370 (1985).

10. S. S. Gazzaz, B. A. Rasco, and F. M. Dong, "Application of immunochemical assays to food analysis," *Crit. Rev. Food Sci. Nutr.* **32**, 197–229 (1992).

11. D. P. Herzog, *Immunoassays for Environmental Contaminants (Pesticides) in Food and Water*, Ohmicron, Newtown, PA, 1993.

12. P. B. Luppa L. J. Sokoll, and D. W. Chan, "Immunosensors—Principles and applications to clinical chemistry," *Clin. Chim. Acta* **314**, 1–26 (2001).

13. L. J. Kricka, "Chemiluminescent and bioluminescent techniques," *Clin. Chem.* **37**, 1472–1481 (2003).

14. A. Gomez-Hens and M. P. Aguilar-Caballos, "Stopped-flow fluorescence polarization immunoassay," *Comb. Chem. High Throughput Screen.* **6**, 177–182 (2003).

15. S. A. Eremin and D. S. Smith, "Fluorescence polarization immunoassays for pesticides," *Comb. Chem. High Throughput Screen.* **6**, 257–266 (2003).

16. T. J. Burke, K. R. Loniello, J. A. Beebe, and K. M. Ervin, "Development and application of fluorescence polarization assays in drug discovery," *Comb. Chem. High Throughput Screen.* **6**, 183–194 (2003).

17. U. Bilitewski, M. Genrich, S. Kadow, and G. Mersal, "Biochemical analysis with microfluidic systems," *Anal Bioanal. Chem.* **377**, 556–569 (2003).

18. G. D. Grothaus, M. Bandla, T. Currier, R. Giroux, G. R. Jenkins, M. Lipp, G. Shan, J. W. Stave, and V. Pantella, "Immunoassay as an analytical tool in agricultural biotechnology," *J AOAC Int.* **89**, 913–928 (2006).

19. M. M. Ling, C. Ricks, and P. Lea, "Multiplexing molecular diagnostics and immunoassays using emerging microarray technologies," *Expert Rev. Mol. Diagn.* **7**, 87–98 (2007).

20. S. G. Johansson, "Radioimmunoassay of IgE and IgE antibody and its clinical application," *J. Clin. Pathol. Suppl. (Assoc. Clin. Pathol.)* **6**, 33–37 (1975).

21. D. S. Skelley, L. P. Brown, and P. K. Besch, "Radioimmunoassay," *Clin. Chem.* **19**, 146–186 (1973).

22. R. F. Schall, Jr. and H. J. Tenoso, "Alternatives to radioimmunoassay: Labels and methods," *Clin. Chem.* **27**, 1157–1164 (1981).

23. D. A. Blake, R. M. Jones, R. C. Blake II, A. R. Pavlov, I. A. Darwish, and H. Yu, "Antibody-based sensors for heavy metal ions," *Biosens. Bioelectron.* **16**, 799–809 (2001).

24. D. K. Johnson (2003), "Fluorescence polarization immunoassays for metal ions," *Comb. Chem. High Throughput Screen.* **6**, 245–255 (2003).

25. F. J. Hayes, H. B. Halsall, and W. R. Heineman, "Simultaneous immunoassay using electrochemical detection of metal ion labels," *Anal. Chem.* **66**, 1860–1865 (1994).

26. F. Lu, K. H. Wang, and Y. Lin, "Rapid, quantitative and sensitive immunochromatographic assay based on stripping voltammetric detection of a metal ion label," *Analyst* **130**, 1513–1517 (2005).

27. A. K. Das, R. Chakraborty, M. L. Cervera, and M. de la Guardia, "Determination of thallium in biological samples," *Anal. Bioanal. Chem.* **385**, 665–670 (2006).

28. G. Mathis, "Rare earth cryptates and homogeneous fluoroimmunoassays with human sera," *Clin. Chem.* **39**, 1953–1959 (1993).

29. E. J. Shaw, R. A. Watson, J. Landon, and D. S. Smith, "Estimation of serum gentamicin by quenching fluoroimmunoassay," *J. Clin. Pathol.* **30**(6), 526–531 (1977).

30. Y. Kobayashi, N. Tsubota, K. Miyai, and F. Watanabe, "Fluorescence quenching immunoassay of serum cortisol," *Steroids* **36**, 177–183 (1980).

31. E. G. Matveeva, N. S. Melik-Nubarov, P. Miethe, and A. V. Levashov, "Antigen–antibody interactions in the reverse micellar system: Quenching of the fluorescence of fluorescein-labeled atrazine by antibodies against atrazine," *Anal. Biochem.* **234**, 13–18 (1996).

32. J. Feng, G. Shan, B. D. Hammock, and I. M. Kennedy, "Fluorescence quenching competitive immunoassay in micro droplets," *Biosens. Bioelectron.* **18**, 1055–1063 (2003).

33. E. G. Matveeva, A. P. Savitsky, and A. Gómez-Hens, "Determination of corproporphyrin in urine by using stopped-flow fluoroimmunoassay," *Anal. Chim. Acta* **361**, 27–32 (1998).

34. R. D. Nargessi, J. Landon, and D. S. Smith DS, "Use of antibodies against the label in non-separation non-isotopic immunoassay: 'Indirect quenching' fluoroimmunoassay of proteins," *J. Immunol. Methods* **26**, 307–313 (1979).

35. R. F. Zuk, G. L. Rowley, and E. F. Ullman, "Fluorescence protection immunoassay: A new homogeneous assay technique," *Clin. Chem.* **25**, 1554–1560 (1979).

36. F. Sellrie, A. Warsinke, and B. Micheel, "Homogeneous indirect fluorescence quenching immunoassay for the determination of low molecular weight substances," *Anal. Bioanal. Chem.* **386**, 206–210 (2006).

37. E. F. Ullman, M. Schwarzberg, and K. E. Rubenstein, "Fluorescent excitation transfer immunoassay. A general method for determination of antigens," *J. Biol. Chem.* **251**, 4172–4178 (1976).

38. M. Lee, D. R. Walt, and P. Nugent, "Fluorescent excitation transfer immunoassay for the determination of spinosyn A in water," *J. Agric. Food Chem.* **47**, 2766–2770 (1999).

39. M. S Nasir and M. E. Jolley, "Fluorescence polarization: An analytical tool for immunoassay and drug discovery," *Comb. Chem. High Throughput Screen.* **2**, 177–190 (1999).

40. A. Sadana and A. M. Beelaram, "Antigen-antibody diffusion-limited binding kinetics of biosensors: A fractal analysis," *Biosens. Bioelectron.* **10**, 301–316 (1995).

41. E. F. Dickson, A. Pollak, and E. P. Diamandis, "Ultrasensitive bioanalytical assays using time-resolved fluorescence detection," *Pharmacol. Ther.* **66**, 207–235 (1995).

42. R. J. Williams, J. M. Peralta, V. C. W. Tsang, N. Narayanan, G. A. Casay, M. Lipowska, L. Strekowski, and G. Patonay, "Near-infrared heptamethine cyanine dyes: A new tracer for solid-phase immunoassays," *Appl. Spectrosc.* **51**, 836–843 (1997).

43. B. Oswald, M. Gruber, M. Bohmer, F. Lehmann, M. Probst, and O. S. Wolfbeis, "Novel diode lascr-compatible fluorophores and their application to single molecule detection, protein labeling and fluorescence resonance energy transfer immunoassay," *Photochem. Photobiol.* **74**, 237–245 (2001).

44. N. Stich, A. Gandhum, V. Matushin, C. Mayer, G. Bauer, and T. Schalkhammer, "Nanofilms and nanoclusters: Energy sources driving fluorophores of biochip bound labels," *J. Nanosci. Nanotechnol.* **1**, 397–405 (2001).
45. J. R.Lakowicz, "Radiative decay engineering: Biophysical and biomedical applications," *Anal. Biochem.* **298**, 1–24 (2001).
46. J. R. Lakowicz, Y. Shen, S. D'Auria, J. Malicka, J. Fang, Z. Gryczynski, and I. Gryczynski, "Radiative decay engineering 2: Effects of silver island films on fluorescence intensity lifetimes and resonance energy transfer," *Anal. Biochem.* **301**, 261–277 (2002).
47. N. Lochner, C. Lobmaier, M. Wirth, A. Leitner, F. Pittner, and F. Gabor, "Silver nanoparticle enhanced immunoassays: One step real time kinetic assay for insulin in serum," *Eur. J. Pharm. Biopharm.* **56**, 469–477 (2003).
48. J. Malicka, I. Gryczynski, Z. Gryczynski, and J. R. Lakowicz, "Effects of fluorophore-to-silver distance on the emission of cyanine-dye-labeled oligonucleotides," *Anal. Biochem.* **315**, 57–66 (2003).
49. D. Axelrod, E. H. Hellen, and R. M. Fulbright, "Total internal reflection fluorescence," in *Topics in Fluorescence Spectroscopy*, Volume 3: Biochemical Applications, J. R. Lakowicz (Ed.), Plenum, New York, 1992, pp. 289–343.
50. D. Axelrod, "Total internal reflection fluorescence microscopy," *Methods Cell Biol.* **30**, 245–270 (1989).
51. E. Matveeva, Z. Gryczynski, J. Malicka, I. Gryczynski, and J. R. Lakowicz, "Metal-enhanced fluorescence immunoassays using total internal reflection and silver island-coated surfaces," *Anal. Biochem.* **334**, 303–311 (2004).
52. E. Matveeva, Z. Gryczynski, and J. R. Lakowicz, "Myoglobin immunoassay based on metal particle-enhanced fluorescence," *J. Immunol. Methods* **302**(1/2), 26–35 (2005).
53. E. G. Matveeva, I. Gryczynski, A. Barnett, Z. Leonenko, J. R. Lakowicz, and Z. Gryczynski, "Metal particle-enhanced fluorescent immunoassays on metal mirrors," *Anal. Biochem.* **363**, 239–245 (2007).
54. M. Seydack, "Nanoparticle labels in immunosensing using optical detection methods," *Biosens. Bioelectron.* **20**, 2454–2469 (2005).
55. S. Santra, J. Xu, K. Wang, and W. Tan, "Luminescent nanoparticle probes for bioimaging," *J. Nanosci. Nanotechnol.* **4**, 590–599 (2004).
56. K. K. Jain, "Nanodiagnostics: Application of nanotechnology in molecular diagnostics," *Expert Rev. Mol. Diagn.* **3**, 153–161 (2003).
57. J. R. Lakowicz, "Radiative decay engineering 3. Surface plasmon-coupled directional emission," *Anal. Biochem.* **324**, 153–169 (2004).
58. H. Raether, "Surface plasmon oscillations and their applications" in *Physics of Thin Films, Advances in Research and Development*, Vol. 9, G. Hass, M. H. Francombe, and R. W. Hoffman (Eds.), Academic, New York, 1977, pp. 145–261.
59. H. Raether, *Surface Plasmons on Smooth and Rough Surfaces and on Gratings*, Springer-Verlag, New York, 1988.
60. P. Englebienne, A. Van Hoonacker, and M. Verhas, "Surface plasmon resonance: Principles, methods and applications in biomedical sciences," *Spectroscopy* **17**, 255–273 (2003).
61. D. A. Stuart, A. J. Haes, C. R. Yonzon, E. M. Hicks, and R. P. Van Duyne, "Biological applications of localised surface plasmonic phenomenae," *Nanobiotechnol. IEEE Proc.* **152**, 13–32 (2005).
62. E. Matveeva, Z. Gryczynski, I. Gryczynski, and J. R. Lakowicz, "Immunoassays based on directional surface plasmon-coupled emission," *J. Immunol. Methods* **286**, 133–140 (2004).
63. E. Matveeva, Z. Gryczynski, I. Gryczynski, J. Malicka, and J. R. Lakowicz, "Myoglobin immunoassay utilizing directional surface plasmon-coupled emission," *Anal. Chem.* **76**, 6287–6292 (2004).

64. M. Magliulo, E. Michelini, P. Simoni, M. Guardigli, and A. Roda, "Ultrasensitive and rapid nanodevices for analytical immunoassays," *Anal. Bioanal. Chem.* **384**, 27–30 (2006).

65. U. Schobel, I. Coille, A. Brecht, G. M. Steinwand, and G. Gauglitz, "Miniaturization of a homogeneous fluorescence immunoassay based on energy transfer using nanotiter plates as high-density sample carriers," *Anal Chem.* **73**, 5172–5179 (2001).

66. M. Seidel, D. M. Dankbar, and G. Gauglitz, "A miniaturized heterogeneous fluorescence immunoassay on gold-coated nano-titer plates," *Anal. Bioanal. Chem.* **379**, 904–912 (2004).

67. A. Bange, H. B. Halsall, and W. R. Heineman, "Microfluidic immunosensor systems," *Biosens. Bioelectron.* **20**, 2488–2503 (2005).

68. Z. Gryczynski, J. Borejdo, N. Calander, E. G. Matveeva, and I. Gryczynski, "Minimization of detection volume by surface-plasmon-coupled emission," *Anal. Biochem.* **356**, 125–131 (2006).

CHAPTER 16

Membrane Organization

ASTRID MAGENAU, CARLES RENTERO, and KATHARINA GAUS

Centre for Vascular Research, School of Medical Sciences, University of New South Wales, Sydney 2052, Australia

16.1 CONCEPTS OF ORGANIZATION OF BIOLOGICAL MEMBRANES

16.1.1 Bilayer

Biological membranes are two-dimensional fluids comprised of a plethora of lipids and proteins. In most cell membranes, these components are organized into a bilayer with asymmetrical leaflets and lateral heterogeneities. In eukaryotic cells, membranes are sites for many fundamental functions and play an important role in defining cell shape and movement, trafficking and transport of lipids and proteins, cell signaling, and many other specialized tasks. The plasma membrane separates the extracellular space from the intracellular cytoplasm and forms a protective layer around the cell and its organelles. Since the majority of the cellular machinery is embedded into membranes, the underlying organization of the membrane critically influences cellular responses. Yet with over 1000 lipids identified and about one-third of the human genome encoding integral membrane proteins, the enormous complexity of cell membranes has made it difficult to unravel the underlying organizational principles. The membrane bilayer consists of two leaflets with a hydrophobic core and hydrophilic groups on either side facing the aqueous medium. The three main lipid classes in eukaryotic membranes are glycerophospholipids, sphingolipids, and sterols that are all amphipathic. Phospholipids (glycerophospholipids and phosphate-containing sphingolipids) are the most abundant lipid type in most cells, but the exact composition varies greatly between cell types. Phospholipids have a hydrophilic phosphate head group and a hydrophobic lipid tail, the fatty acid moiety. The fatty acid chain consists of 14–24 carbons, with 16- and 18-carbon fatty acids being the most common. Fatty acids contain both saturated and unsaturated carbon chains.

Glycerophospholipids and sphingolipids self-assemble into an $\sim$5 nm-thick bilayer when fully hydrated. Hydrophobic forces orientate amphipathic lipids in such a way that a shell of hydrophilic heads protects the hydrophobic lipid tails. Van der Waals forces, hydrogen bonds, and electrostatic attractions further stabilize the membrane bilayer. Cholesterol, the most abundant sterol, plays an important role as a determinant

Fluorescence Applications in Biotechnology and Life Sciences, Edited by Ewa M. Goldys

of membrane fluidity. Its hydroxyl group places itself close to the polar head of phospholipids. The steroid ring interacts with the part of the fatty acid chain that is closest to the polar head group. This configuration causes partial immobilization of the hydrocarbon chains, rendering membranes less fluid and therefore preventing possible phase transition as well as increasing mechanical stability. These interactions are discussed in more detail in Section 16.3.

16.1.2 Conceptual Models of Membrane Organization

In 1972, Singer and Nicolson put forward the idea that biological membranes resemble a "lipid sea" with integral membrane proteins floating in it like icebergs [26]. Using techniques such as electron microscopy and nuclear magnetic resonance spectroscopy, Singer and Nicolson observed that the membrane bilayer behaves more like a fluid than a solid. They discovered that proteins are embedded in a discontinuous lipid bilayer and proposed a model in which lipids and proteins are able to diffuse freely within the plane of the membrane. This model is known as the *fluid mosaic model* (Figure 16.1*a*). The packing of lipids and proteins within the membrane allows rapid lateral diffusion. Heterogeneities in cell membranes lead to the identification of membrane domains with distinct morphologies and physical or biochemical features that distinguish them from the surrounding membrane. Examples of such distinct regions are membrane protrusions, cell–cell junctions, and coated pits, each of which specializes in a particular function such as cell polarization, cell communication, or endocytosis. One notable feature of membrane domains is that they differ in their molecular composition from that of the surrounding membrane. How this compartmentalization of the membrane occurs forms the basis of new models, which have emerged since the early 1990s. The models distinguish between (i) lipid domains, (ii) domains whose composition is mainly derived from specific protein–protein interactions, and (iii) membrane compartments that are created by the underlying membrane skeleton. The existence of lipid domains was first suggested by the discovery that glycosphingolipids cluster in the Golgi apparatus before being sorted to the apical membrane of polarized epithelial cells. In 1988, Simons and van Meer postulated the lipid raft hypothesis of sphingolipid- and cholesterol-enriched assemblies into which proteins can partition to function in processes such as signaling and trafficking [24] (Figure 16.1*b*). A definition of lipid rafts emerged at the 2006 Keystone Symposium on Lipid Rafts and Cell Function: "Membrane rafts are small (10–200 nm), heterogeneous, highly dynamic, sterol- and sphingolipid-enriched domains that compartmentalize cellular processes. Small rafts can sometimes be stabilized to form larger platforms through protein-protein and protein-lipid interactions." Because of the tight association between predominantly saturated sphingolipids and cholesterol, lipid rafts are viewed as condensed and highly ordered compared to their more fluid surroundings. Conflicting data obtained from biochemical raft assays and observations made in intact cells by microscopy have questioned the extent to which lipid rafts contribute to the compartmentalization of cellular membranes. In particular, variations in lipid raft size proposed that other lipid domains may exist, such as lipid shells, condensed complexes, and nanodomains, which do not exceed a few nanometers in size [12]. In the lipid shell model, raft-favoring proteins, usually a single protein, are encased in a shell of cholesterol and sphingolipid. Similarly, lipid complexes of cholesterol and phospholipids form clusters of only ~15–30 molecules, making them significantly

(a)
(b)
(c)

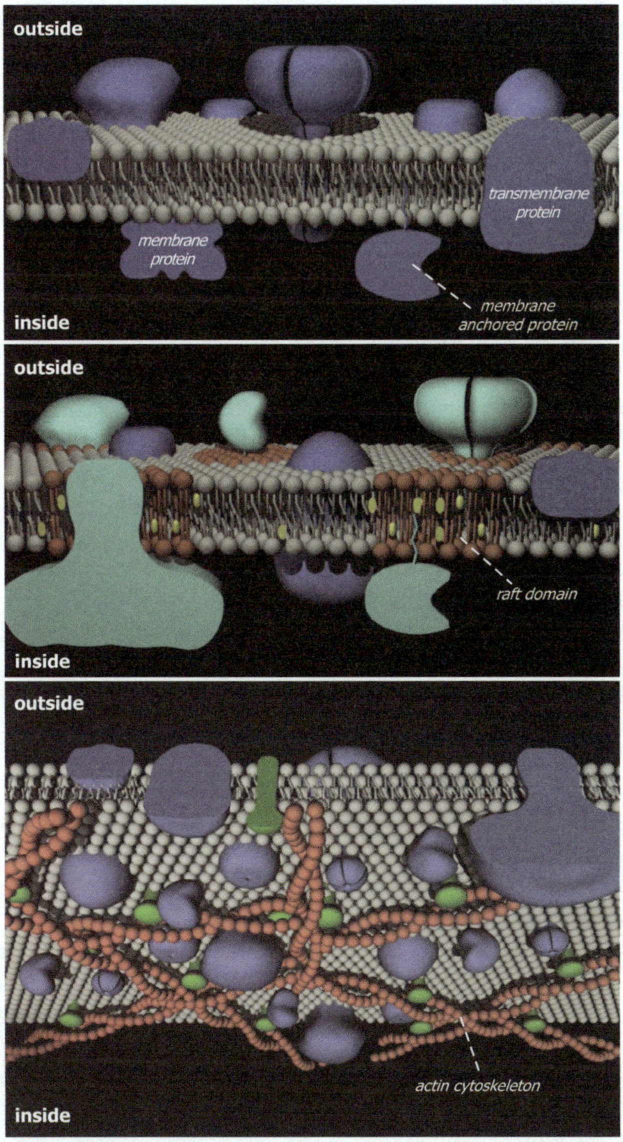

Figure 16.1 Cell membrane models. (*a*) Singer and Nicolson fluid mosaic membrane model. This model proposes that phospholipids (grey) form a fluid membrane bilayer, into which membrane proteins are embedded or attached. Both lipids and proteins diffuse freely within the plane of the membrane. (*b*) Lipid raft model proposed by Simons and van Meer. Raft domains (red) are enriched in sphingolipids and cholesterol (yellow) to form highly ordered platforms. Proteins with specific lipid anchors preferentially associate with lipid rafts. It has been suggested that lipids and proteins diffuse slower within lipid rafts facilitating their interactions and thus signaling. (*c*) Picket-fence model proposed by Kusumi. In this model, the membrane cytoskeleton of actin filaments (red) forms a “fence” that compartmentalizes the membrane. Transmembrane proteins anchored to the cytoskeleton form pickets (green). Lipids and protons diffuse freely within the membrane domain surrounded by the fence but need to hop across the fence for long-range diffusion.

smaller domains than lipid rafts. The dynamic nature of these small entities makes their detection extremely difficult and hence their existence controversial. Proteins that collect at certain membrane sites do so because they contain a specific "address tag" for that site. For example, a number of transmembrane receptors are targeted to coated pits, which mediate their uptake in a process called endocytosis. The targeting of these receptors to coated pits occurs when a binding site in their cytoplasmic tail recognizes one or more coat proteins directly or recognizes an adaptor protein, which then interacts with the coat proteins. Modification of the targeting motif in the receptor protein (e.g., by phosphorylation) can dynamically regulate the location of the receptor. Equally dynamic is the formation and maintenance of the coated pit itself, which requires the peripheral association of the structural protein clathrin and clathrin adaptors to form a polygonal pit. Coated pits are an example of protein-driven membrane domains whose composition is determined both by their structure as well as the molecules they attract. Kusumi and colleagues have observed that the lateral diffusion of individual proteins and lipids closely mirrors the meshwork of the underlying membrane skeleton made of actin filaments, found 2–3 nm below the cell membrane bilayers [18]. They proposed a "picket-fence" model in which membrane corrals are defined by transmembrane proteins either colliding with the membrane skeleton (creating "fences") or anchored to the skeleton ("pickets") (Figure 16.1*c*). Lipids and proteins within a membrane compartment diffuse freely, while transitions between compartments are infrequent, giving rise to characteristic trajectories, which Kusumi described as "hop diffusion" [31]. The approach of single-particle tracking using fluorescence was instrumental in the development of the hop diffusion concept and is described in more detail in Section 16.2.6.

16.2 FLUORESCENCE METHODS TO STUDY MEMBRANE ORGANIZATION

Fluorescence is the method of choice to visualize, quantify, and elucidate the functions of biochemically diverse domains [19] as it allows domain characterization of intact membranes in live cells. However, the characterization of membrane microdomains is complicated by the dynamic nature of cell membranes, meaning that domains can vary greatly in size and lifetime. Hence the spatial and temporal resolution of the microscope must be considered before settling on a specific fluorescence approach. Here, we present a brief summary of the different fluorescence approaches available and the insights they can provide into membrane organization.

16.2.1 Fluorescence Intensity Imaging and Membrane Probes

Fluorescence intensity imaging of a number of different protein and lipid "raft markers" have been used to image membrane domains. This straightforward approach relies on the nonuniform distribution of fluorescently labeled or tagged markers. The key to this approach lies in the choice of marker. We will discuss the most commonly used membrane probes and markers and briefly summarize their advantages and disadvantages. This list is not exhaustive and further approaches can be found in Section 16.3. In Section 16.4 we take a closer look at protein motifs that target proteins to specific domains. A summary of all the probes discussed can be found in Table 16.1.

TABLE 16.1 Summary of Fluorescent Membrane Probes

Probes	Type	Specificity
Carbocyanine (DiI and DiO)	Lipophilic fluorophore attached to alkyl tail	Nonspecific membrane dye
FM 1-43	Lipophilic styryl probe	Nonspecific outer leaflet dye; not fluorescent in water
Laurdan (6-dodecanoyl-2-dimethylaminonaphthalene)	Lipophilic naphthalene probe	Polarity-sensitive membrane dye to assess acyl chain packing
Di-4-ANEPPDHQ	Lipophilic styryl dye	Polarity-sensitive membrane dye to assess lipid rigidity; not fluorescent in water
Nitrobenzoxadiazole (NBD)–cholesterol	Cholesterol analogue	Environment-sensitive fluorophore of cholesterol
Dehydroergosterol (DHE)	Cholesterol analogue	Fluorescent sterol probe
Filipin	Antibiotic and antifungal agent	Binds specifically to cholesterol
Perfringolysin O	Toxin	Binds specifically to cholesterol
BODIPY-GM1	Fluorophore coupled to ganglioside GM1	GM1-enriched raft domains
Cholera toxin subunit B	Toxin	Pentavalent binding of ganglioside GM1
Headgroup-labeled phospholipids (e.g., F1-DPPE)	Fluorophore coupled to lipid analogue	Localization in membrane according to chain length
Aerolysin	Toxin	Binds to GPI–AP
Fusion Proteins	**Origin**	**Specificity**
Glycosylphospatidylinositol (GPI)–GFP	Protein analogue	Fluorescent-labeled outer leaflet protein; localizes to lipid rafts
PH-PLCδ	Pleckstrin homology domain of PLCδ	Binds to PI (4,5) P2
PH-GRP	Pleckstrin homology domain of GRP	Binds to PI (3,4,5) P3
PH-GRP	Pleckstrin homology domain of GRP	Binds to PI (3,4,5) P3
PH-Akt	Pleckstrin homology domain of Akt	Binds to PI (3,4,5) P3
C1-PKC	C-terminal domain of PKC	Binds to DAG
Lyn-13N-mCFP/mYFP	N-terminal 13aa of Lyn coupled to a fluorophore	Binds to inner leaflet to assess lipid raft clustering
CAAX-Rho-mCFP/mYFP	CAAX box of Rho coupled to a fluorophore	Binds to inner leaflet to assess protein clustering
Lck-13N-GFP	N-terminal 13aa of Lck coupled to a fluorophore	Binds to inner leaflet to assess protein clustering in lipid rafts

Using intensity imaging to characterize membrane heterogeneity requires carefully controlled experiments, particularly in cell membranes. Since heterogeneous staining in cells can also arise from membrane folding, the "amount" of membrane per imaged area has to be independently measured. There are common dyes such as carbocyanine or FM 1-43, which are lipophilic probes that stain membranes independently of their compositions and are essentially nonfluorescent in water. Hence their fluorescence intensity can be used to assess membrane morphology.

When imaging membrane organization, it is logical to assume that fluorescent analogues of membrane components will localize to the domains in which these components are enriched. However, this is not necessarily the case. Due to the fluidity of the membrane, attaching a fluorophore to a membrane constituent often changes the partitioning of that molecule. For example, nitrobenzoxadiazole (NBD)–cholesterol and BODIPY-GM1 do not associate with lipid raft domains in model membranes, although cholesterol and the sphingolipid GM1 without the fluorescent tags do so in identical membranes. This is probably due to the bulkiness of the NBD and BODIPY groups. Dehydroergosterol (DHE) and the antibiotic agent filipin that stains cholesterol-rich membranes are less disruptive, but their low quantum yield and ultraviolet (UV) absorption mean that high concentrations are often necessary. In some cases, cytotoxicity caused by these agents has been reported. A popular alternative is perfringolysin O, a toxin that binds to cholesterol-rich membranes with high affinity. While this agent identifies membrane regions with higher levels of cholesterol, it does not give detailed information about the molecular composition or physical properties of these domains. As well as fluorescent cholesterol analogues, phospholipids are also available with covalently coupled fluorophores. Most commonly, the head group of the phospholipid is derivatized with a fluorescent dye to minimize the disruption in the fatty acid packing order in the bilayers of the analogue. To which extent these phospholipid analogues perturb the organization of a membrane largely depends on their concentration in the membrane. Concentration-dependent effects on the packing orders of the lipid bilayer, however, have to be determined independently.

The nontoxic subunit B of cholera toxin (CTB) binds specifically to the sphingolipid GM1. Hence CTB tagged with a fluorophore accurately determines the location of this lipid in model and cellular membranes. However, CTB is pentavalent and as such can introduce a degree of crosslinking that affects membrane organization, particularly of small and highly mobile domains.

The green fluorescent protein (GFP) revolutionized cell biology, and its variants are now commonly used to image proteins in live cells. To overcome the tendency of some of these fluorescent proteins to oligomerize, monomeric versions are now available. We will discuss modifications of GFP below, for example, various lipid anchors, which target GFP to the plasma membrane and specific domains.

16.2.2 Fluorescence Recovery After Photobleaching

Fluorescence recovery after photobleaching (FRAP) has been frequently used in vivo to elucidate the mobility of fluorescent proteins or lipids within the plasma membrane [16]. A high-intensity pulse is used to photobleach the fluorophores in a small and defined area. Subsequently, unbleached fluorophores diffuse into the photobleached area. The recovery of fluorescence intensity in the bleached area gives insight into two parameters: (i) The rate of recovery relates to the diffusion coefficient D, for example, the rate at which a molecule moves within the two-dimensional plane of the membrane and (ii) the percentage of recovery, termed "mobile fractions," contains information about diffusion barriers.

The detection of lipid domains with FRAP, particularly lipid rafts, has been controversial. For example, FRAP has been used to investigate the lateral mobility of Ras proteins which are attached to the inner leaflet of the plasma membrane. Different types of membrane anchors (discussed below) affected the lateral mobility of Ras in a cholesterol-dependent manner. While these data were initially interpreted as Ras interacting with lipid rafts, Kenworthy and colleagues demonstrated that the apparent diffusion coefficient over large areas does not match raft association [17]. Difficulties in comparing FRAP data arise due to limitations of this technique: (i) Fluorescence recovery depends on the size and geometry of the bleached area. In fact, it has been suggested that measurements over a range of bleached spot sizes should be carried out to distinguish between shorter and longer range diffusion. (ii) FRAP is an intrinsically macroscopic measurement which makes it difficult to interpret information regarding small, submicrometer, and highly dynamic rafts. (iii) Lateral diffusion may not be dramatically influenced by lipid raft domains (see Section 16.3) but instead may depend on the size of the fluorescent molecules, their interactions with the cytoskeleton and other proteins, molecular crowding, membrane folding, vesiculation, and other factors.

16.2.3 Fluorescence Correlation Spectroscopy and Image Correlation Spectroscopy

Fluorescence correlation spectroscopy (FCS) measures and analyzes fluctuations in fluorescence intensity at a defined and fixed spot [17]. The fluctuations arise from the diffusion of fluorophores moving in and out of the illumination spot (typically 1 fL volume). In order to monitor the fluctuation over time, sensitive detectors are used to observe just a small number of fluorescent molecules. Fluorescence fluctuations are observed in time from which the autocorrelation function is calculated. The key to FCS is to fit autocorrelation functions to appropriate models. From the fit, one can derive the diffusion coefficient over five orders of magnitude as well as the number of fluorescence molecules in the illumination spot. In the dual-color version of FCS, the cross correlation between two fluctuating fluorescent molecules provides information about the molecular interactions between these two molecules as well as their relative concentrations, and thus this technique is particularly suited for studying ligand–receptor binding.

Diffusion coefficients are more accurately determined with FCS than FRAP. Nevertheless, FCS data are only as good as the model to which the data are fitted. This requires precise knowledge of the size and geometry of the illumination spot, which must be determined by calibration. FCS also requires a low concentration of fluorophores, which has its own advantages (less perturbation to the native membrane) and disadvantages (some expression systems in cells cannot be used). Additionally, FCS only detects mobile species, as immobile ones do not fluctuate in time. Similarly, slowly diffusing fluorescent molecules are likely to be photobleached, confounding results. Recently, Lenne and collaborators investigated FCS-derived diffusion coefficients as a function of spot size. By doing so, they could distinguish between fluorescent molecules whose diffusion is affected by cholesterol-dependent lipid rafts from proteins whose diffusion is limited by the actin membrane skeleton [20]. This landmark study was one of the first to reconcile the lipid raft with the picket-fence model.

Image correlation spectroscopy (ICS) is the spatial "cousin" of FCS. While in FCS the temporal fluctuations are recorded and correlated, ICS explores fluctuation in space by correlating pixels within single images or in time through pixels in an image time series. As discussed above, FCS is ideally suited for fast diffusion and low concentrations. In contrast, ICS measures slower dynamics or even immobile molecules and is independent of the overall intensity. By analyzing intensity fluctuation in single images, protein clustering and density can be determined. By applying ICS to a time series of images, diffusion coefficients or transport speeds of a protein can be calculated. As with FCS, cross-correlation ICS can be used to study interactions between proteins that are labeled with different fluorophores.

To date, both FCS and ICS are highly specialized techniques due to difficulties in implementation, sample preparation, and image analysis. Nevertheless, given the suitability of these approaches for the study of membrane domains both in model and cell membranes, the increasing use of these techniques in the field of membrane biology is eagerly anticipated.

16.2.4 Fluorescence Resonance Energy Transfer and Fluorescence Lifetime Imaging Microscopy

In fluorescence resonance energy transfer (FRET), the energy of an excited donor fluorophore transfers to an acceptor molecule. Importantly for membrane domains, the energy transfer depends on the distance between the donor and acceptor. Typically, the donor–acceptor distance for a 50% energy transfer is 1–10 nm. Thus FRET is ideal to measure clustering of membrane components well below the limits of optical resolution. There are a number of approaches one can take to characterize membrane domains with FRET. The simplest method is to probe the decrease in donor fluorescence or increase in acceptor fluorescence as FRET occurs. Examining the effect of acceptor photobleaching, which increases donor intensity and lifetime if FRET occurred prior to quenching, enhances the accuracy of the measurement. We further distinguish between homotransfer, in which donor and acceptor have the same molecular structure, and heterotransfer, in which donor and acceptor are different. In homotransfer FRET, the fluorescence emission is depolarized and this depolarization can be detected by steady-state or time-resolved measurements.

To detect molecular clusters, it is assumed that energy transfer efficiencies are independent of the acceptor and donor density. However, the degree to which energy transfer occurs also depends on other factors, such as the relative orientation of the donor and acceptor dipole moments, the rotational freedom of the donor and the acceptor, which particularly affects fluorescence depolarization measurements in homotransfer FRET, and the potential photodamage when acceptor bleaching is employed. To overcome some of the technical issues, fluorescence lifetime imaging microscopy (FLIM) has proven to be extremely powerful. Unlike intensity, the lifetime of a fluorophore strongly depends on the local environment affecting the fluorescence quantum efficiency. If FRET occurs, the lifetime of the donor is reduced. FLIM can be used to measure homo- and hetero-FRET between fluorescent proteins and fluorescently labeled phospholipids. This gives insights in interactions between proteins and lipids in cellular membranes.

A number of studies have used FRET to investigate clustering of putative markers for lipid rafts in cells (summarized in Table 16.1). These include heterotransfer between different glycosylphosphatidylinositol-anchored green fluorescent proteins (GPI–GFPs) by acceptor emission, between different lipid-anchored proteins attached to the inner leaflet of the plasma membrane, and between different GPI-anchored proteins and the sphingolipid GM1 labeled with CTB by increased donor intensity after acceptor bleaching and homotransfer between GPI-anchored proteins detected by fluorescence anisotropy. The results of these studies are seemingly contradictory with some concluding that raft proteins are randomly distributed and others suggesting that they are clustered. A recent study by Sharma et al. combined theoretical modeling with both homo- and heterotransfer FRET between GPI-anchored proteins detected by time-resolved imaging [22]. They concluded that the majority of GPI-anchored proteins are present as a monomer with a minor fraction (20–40%) being localized in small, cholesterol-dependent domains. Differences in membrane anchorage, cell type, and activation status may account for some of the observed discrepancies between studies. However, the important contribution of these FRET studies to our view of cell membrane organization should not be underestimated. Studies of this type lead to the consensus that lipid rafts are small (10–200 nm) and highly dynamic.

16.2.5 Total Internal Reflection Fluorescence Microscopy

The fluorescence approaches discussed so far all suffer from a lack of axial resolution; therefore any illumination spot or pixel contains signals from the plasma membrane as well as the cytoplasm. The use of total internal reflection fluorescence microscopy (TIRFM) partially overcomes this limitation. The excitation light in TIRFM is directed to the glass–sample interface at an angle that is greater than the critical angle and thus reflected back by the glass and is unable to penetrate the sample. This creates an evanescent field, that is, a nonpropagating, exponentially decaying wave of the same wavelength as the reflected light that is used to excite fluorophores. Because of the exponential decay of the evanescent field, only fluorophores within ~100 nm of the glass interface are excited. Hence, if cells are plated onto glass surfaces, the fluorophores in the cell body are not excited, resulting in an excellent signal-to-noise ratio of membrane-associated fluorescence. Because of the enhanced contrast and unprecedented axial resolution, studies of membrane organization combine the use of TIRFM with single-particle tracking.

16.2.6 Single-Particle Tracking

Single-particle tracking (SPT) is the ability to record the trajectories of individual molecules within the plane of the membrane. The molecule of interest is labeled with a probe, such as a fluorescent moiety, bead, or gold particle, and the location of the probe, defined by the centroid of the imaged diffraction pattern, is recorded in time. By plotting the position of the probe from all time points in a single graph, the trajectory of the probe's movement can be visualized. The mean-square displacement (MSD) versus time provides a measure of the average distance the tagged molecule travels in a given time window and can illustrate nonrandom modes of motion, such as confinement. Analysis of SPT trajectories and MSD graphs gives information about diffusion coefficients, particle confinement, and the size of confinement areas, for example, regions in which the observed particle resides for a brief period of time and the residence times, or lifetimes, in confinement areas. One of the great challenges of SPT is to ensure that just a single molecule is observed at a time. In other words, the probe attached to the molecule of interest has to be strictly monovalent. In addition, the size of the bead or particle can also influence the movement of the molecules. The relative small size of fluorophores compared to beads and particles offers a distinct advantage. SPT has thus been applied to fluorescent lipid analogues, GFP fusion proteins, and monovalent Fab antibody fragments conjugated to fluorescent dyes and is referred to as single molecular fluorescence tracking (SMFT). SPT and SMFT have the ability to monitor complex movements of proteins or lipids, one molecule at a time, revealing details often missed using other approaches such as FRAP or ICS. For example, temporal confinement to a membrane domain for a short period of time can only be directly observed with SPT. Herein also lies the disadvantage—because only a few molecules are observed in each experiments, this approach is time consuming. The group led by Kusumi has revolutionized SPT by introducing sampling frequencies of 40,000 Hz equivalent to a spatial resolution of ~20 nm [18]. Tracking a large range of lipids and proteins, the group identified confinement areas of 30–230 nm with residence times of 1–25 ms for phospholipids and 3 ms–1 s for transmembrane proteins. Within each confinement area, molecules could diffuse freely whereas long-range diffusion was significantly lower because of the transition barriers that dictated confinement. These compartments were found to be dependent on the actin membrane skeleton but not on the cholesterol levels in the membrane. These observations led Kusumi to propose the picket-fence model of membrane organization (see above).

Clustering of proteins, for example, with multivalent particles, greatly reduces the hop rate. Clusters of approximately six CD59 molecules, a GPI-anchored receptor, undergo frequent but transient immobilization [27]. Using simultaneous single-molecule tracking of two proteins, the authors demonstrated that CD59 clusters recruit other proteins via both protein–protein and lipid–lipid (raft) interactions and thus induce signaling. The temporal arrest of the cluster is possibly mediated by transient anchorage to the actin cytoskeleton mediated by the recruited kinases. Previously, Jacobson and co-workers observed transient confinement zones (TCZs) also using single-particle tracking [12]. TCZs are distinctly different from the corrals defined by the picket-fence model [18] and resemble more closely the transient immobilization of CD59 clusters.

SPT data have made an important contribution to our understanding of membrane organization, as it is the only technique to date able to identify the complex diffusion of proteins and lipids and the temporal variations in diffusion. It allows membrane biologists to distinguish between membrane domains in native, unstimulated membranes and activated membranes that contained ligated receptors and crosslinked proteins. As discussed in Section 16.4.3, protein clusters can induce the formation of membrane domains that have distinct biochemical and biophysical properties.

16.3 MODEL MEMBRANES

The proposal of the existence of lipid-based membrane domains, particularly lipid rafts in biological membranes, has triggered a dramatic rise in biophysical studies exploring lateral heterogeneity in synthetic membranes. Artificial membranes can be created as supported bilayers and monolayers that form on flat surfaces such as glass slides. To alleviate the effect of the support on lipid behavior, complementary studies are performed in giant unilamellar vesicles (GUVs) whose large size (>40 μm) easily allows the visualization of lipid domains. Model membranes have the distinct advantage that they can be composed of a specific lipid mixture. By systematically varying the membrane composition, differential interactions between components have been discovered which can drive membrane segregation. Such forces include mismatches between the hydrophobic thickness of molecular components, cohesive forces (van der Waals interactions), and lipid chain entropy. Favored interactions between components can lead to domain formation overcoming entropy forcing a homogeneous distribution of components. The line tension or edge energy between chemically different parts of the membrane is minimized when larger but fewer domains are formed rather than smaller but more abundant domains. This results in a phase separation at equilibrium where immiscible components form two separate regions that are homogeneous within themselves.

Phase separation has been observed in model membranes containing sufficient amounts of cholesterol and order-preferring phospholipids such as sphingomyelin. The separation into a liquid-ordered (l_o) and liquid-disordered (l_d) phase supports the lipid raft hypothesis of spontaneous self-assembly of ordered domains [25]. The l_o state remains fluid (unlike gel-like or solid ordered, s_o, phases) allowing rapid lateral diffusion (known as low translational order). However, conformational order, which relates to the packing of the acyl chains of the phospholipids, is higher in l_o phases than in liquid-disordered regions and is more similar to gel phases. Biological membranes can thus exhibit liquid–liquid immiscibility. Critically, the separation of the membrane into l_o/l_d phases is driven by the greater tendency of phospholipids with unsaturated fatty acids, such as sphingomyelin, to associate with cholesterol. Cholesterol has a flat, rigid structure, which increases conformational order of the neighboring aliphatic chain without imposing a drastic reduction of the lateral mobility of that lipid. In s_o phases, on the other hand, cholesterol does not pack perfectly into the crystalline lattice and so disrupts and reduces the translational order to a fluid state. Hence, the level of cholesterol in the membrane is critical in the regulation of membrane order by reducing the fluidity of gel phases and increasing the fluidity of liquid-ordered phases. Thus the cholesterol concentration can regulate the formation of l_o phases.

Liquid–liquid phase separation has been observed with a number of fluorescence approaches. London [21] and Wang et al. [28] pioneered a fluorescence quenching approach by mixing quencher lipids (bromines or nitroxide groups attached to the lipid head group) with an appropriate membrane-bound fluorescent probe. In bilayers with a random mixture, the fluorescence is low due to the close proximity of quencher-containing lipids to the fluorophore. In bilayers with lipid immiscibility, regions of high and low quencher concentration exist, and if the fluorescent probe associates with quencher-depleted domains, the fluorescence intensity is significantly higher. These studies have been extremely useful to elucidate the type of lipids which cholesterol associates with to induce lipid domains. Importantly, London and Wang and colleagues demonstrated that membranes containing a mixture of fluid-favoring phospholipids (low lipid melting temperature, T_m), such as 1-palmityl-2-oleoyl-phosphatidylcholine (POPC) and at least 20 mol% of high-T_m lipids, such as sphingomyelin or 1,2-dipalmitoyl-phosphatidulcholine (DPPC), promote the formation of an l_o phase in the presence of 33 mol% of cholesterol [21]. These concentrations are of physiological relevance, indicating that l_o raft domains may exist in cell membranes.

Fluorescence quenching studies were also used to determine the affinity of molecules for l_o phases since the fluorescence intensity depends on the relative partition of the fluorophore into quencher-rich and quencher-poor domains [28]. Association with l_o domains is strongest for fluorescent lipids that are long and saturated and gradually decreases with decreasing chain length and increasing unsaturation. These observations made use of fluorescent lipids as l0 markers popular in model membranes, but their usefulness in cell membranes is limited. A commonly used pair of markers is fluorescein–dipalmitoylphosphatidylethanolamine (Fl–DPPE) and the glycosphingolipid GM1. While Fl-DPPE associates with liquid-disordered domains, GM1 has a strong preference for liquid-ordered and gel phases. Hence simple fluorescence imaging allows the visualization of domain formation in artificial membranes. This further opened the door to assess translational diffusion within membrane domains using FRAP approaches. These experiments clearly indicated that both l_o and l_d phases are distinctly fluid.

A different fluorescence approach to study lipid-phase behavior was taken by Bagatolli and colleagues [1]. Instead of relying on the preferential association of lipids with a specific phase, they probed membrane order using environmentally sensitive dyes. They defined generalized polarization (GP) analogously to polarization and anisotropy. While the latter measures rotational diffusion, GP measurements assess membrane order in terms of lipid packing or configurational order rather than diffusion or translational order. Particularly, the lipid probe lauroyl-2-dimethylaminonaphthalene (Laurdan) has proven to be useful in assessing acyl chain packing. Laurdan contains a naphthalene moiety on a fatty acid tail and hence aligns itself with phospholipids in a bilayer (Figure 16.2).

It does not preferentially associate with any lipid phases. In closely packed bilayers, the fluorescence is derived from the intrinsic fluorescence of the naphthalene group (known as the locally excited state, LE). However, in more fluid membranes, when water molecules partially penetrate the membrane, an internal charge transfer (ICT) is created by the larger dipole moment. In other words, the emission peak of Laurdan is shifted from ~500 nm in fluid membranes to ~445 nm in ordered ones. By recording the intensity of two emission regions simultaneously, the emission ratio, defined by the GP, gives a measure of lipid order [7]. The attraction of this approach is that it is independent of the lipid composition. For example, Dietrich et al. used lipids extracted from brush border membranes, which are highly enriched in cholesterol, to demonstrate that cell lipids form domains with the hallmarks of l_o phases: fluid with low translational order but condensed lipid packing due to high configurational order [3]. It is possible to incorporate peptides and proteins into model membranes, particular GUVs. Again fluorescent imaging methods, not least fluorescence quenching studies, were instrumental in determining the affinity of peptides for l_o and l_d phases. Peptides with prenylated (see Section 16.4.2) or unsaturated acyl anchors associate much more weakly with l_o phases than peptides anchored by multiple saturated acyl chains [28]. The study of transmembrane domains is technically more challenging, but even acylated peptides mimicking the transmembrane section of the T-cell signaling protein LAT (linker for activation for T cells, see below) are largely excluded from l_o phases [23].

Two recent observations using the model membrane systems have attracted the attention of cell biologists. The first one assessed the location and diffusion of a GPI-anchored protein, placental alkaline phosphatase (PLAP), using FCS [14]. This

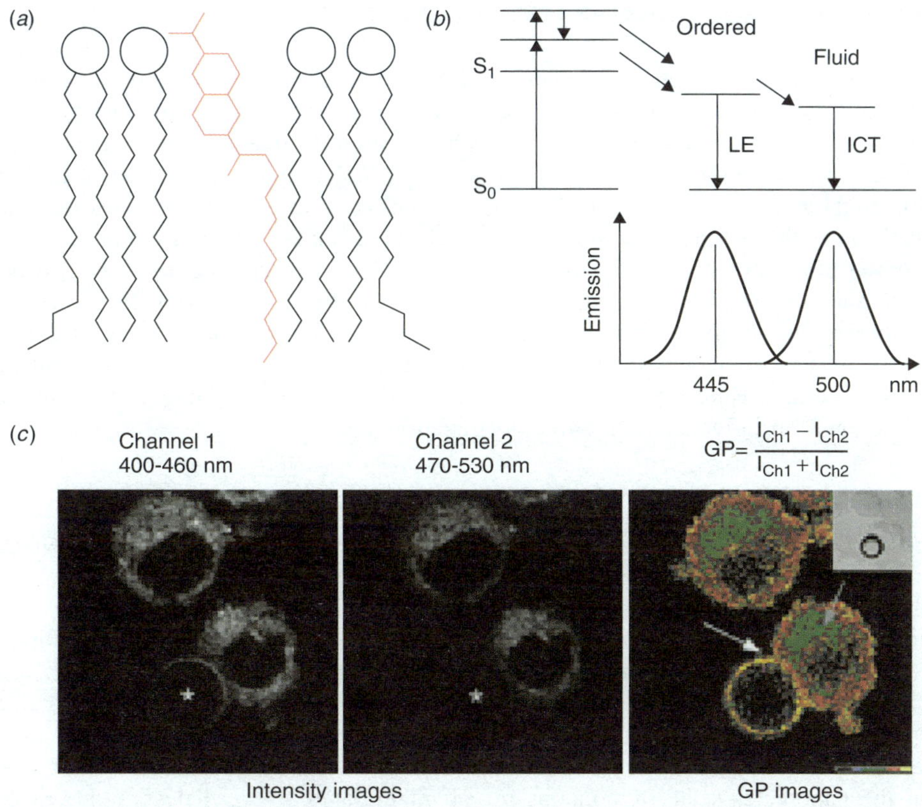

Figure 16.2 Laurdan two-photon microscopy. Laurdan (*a*) aligns parallel to the phospholipids and (*b*) undergoes a shift in its peak emission wavelength from 500 nm in fluid membranes to 440 nm in ordered membranes caused by partial penetration of water molecules into more fluid membranes; a polar environment favors an ICT state of the probe with an energetically lower excited state and hence a longer emission wavelength. A less polar environment favors an LE state with an energetically higher excited state and hence a shorter emission wavelength. (*c*) Intensity images of a macrophage recorded simultaneously between 400–460 nm and 470–530 nm with a two-photon microscope. A normalized ratio of the two emission regions, given by the GP, provides a relative measure of lipid order in cell membranes. GP values range from −1 to +1, with fluid domains ranging from 0.05 to 0.25 and ordered domains from 0.25 to 0.55. GP images were pseudocolored, so that ordered, raftlike domains are yellow or red (white arrow) and fluid membranes green (grey arrow). The asterisks mark the position of the 6.7-μm IgG-coated polystyrene bead, which is phagocytosed by a J774 mouse macrophage.

monomeric protein partitioned only weakly into ordered phases in GUVs with coexisting l_d/l_o phases. However, external crosslinking of PLAP with an antibody strongly increased the partitioning of PLAP clustered in the liquid-ordered phase. In the second study, the order-favoring ganglioside GM1 was incorporated close to the phase boundary in GUVs with a single liquid-disordered phase [10]. When the pentavalent cholera toxin subunit B was added to the uniform GUV, a dramatic large-scale separation in l_o and l_d phases occurred. Together, these observations indicate that domain formation can be dynamically regulated by crosslinking of order-favoring ("raftophilic") lipids or proteins.

16.4 MEMBRANE ORGANIZATION IN CELLS

Cell membranes are clearly different from the artificial membranes discussed above. First, cell membranes contain more numerous and varied proteins than are generally introduced into artificial membranes. It has been estimated that cell membranes contain 20,000–35,000 proteins/μm^2. This crowding and the resultant interaction of proteins with lipids and other proteins can induce formation of membrane domains that vary greatly in both spatial and temporal range. Second, unlike artificial membranes, cell membranes are not at a thermodynamic equilibrium. With continuous arrival of new membrane components and endocytosis of others, the composition of the largest cell membrane, the plasma membrane is constantly in flux. Membrane domains can therefore not only be characterized on the basis of their composition, fluidity, or size but also on their lifetime. Here we discuss how lipid–lipid, lipid–protein, and protein–protein interactions can influence membrane organization.

16.4.1 Lipid Organization in Cell Membrane

The spatial organization of lipids within membranes has a major impact on cell function. The lipid raft hypothesis originally described lipid rafts as cholesterol–and sphingolipid–membrane domains in order to explain protein sorting in polarized epithelial cells. While model membranes elucidated the biophysical framework to account for liquid–liquid immiscibility, phase separation in liquid-ordered (l_o) and liquid-disordered (l_d) phases has not yet been reported in cell membranes. This can be explained either by the existence of a continuous gradient of membrane order, rather than discrete phases, or by the limitations in spatial resolution fluorescence microscopy and the nanometer scale of domains in cell membranes. Nevertheless, lipids in cell membranes may organize membrane proteins even without complete phase separation between raft and nonraft domains. The lipid raft hypothesis suggested that proteins with appropriate lipid anchors and affinities, such as signaling proteins, prefer to partition into lipid rafts. Therefore the lipid–lipid interactions of raft components can organize, for example, signaling processes, in space and time.

While fluorescence methodologies have been used to accurately quantify the nature and extent of lipid interactions in model systems, the translation of these approaches to cell membranes has proven difficult. For example, fluorescence quenching assays require high concentrations of fluorophores and quencher lipids that will perturb the native lipid organization. Similarly, fluorescent lipid analogues can alter cell membranes (as discussed in Section 16.2.1) due to the bulkiness of the fluorophore. In addition, these probes do not completely segregate in the plasma membrane, making quantification of domain size and abundance difficult. A routinely used marker to identify lipid rafts is CTB, which binds to the glycosphingolipid ganglioside GM1. GM1 associates not only with liquid-ordered (l_o) domains in model membranes but also with detergent-resistant membranes (DRMs) in biochemical assays of raft isolation. Hence CTB labeled with a fluorophore reveals the distribution of lipid rafts in the cell membrane. However, as mentioned above, CTB has five binding sites and therefore crosslinks multiple GM1 molecules, which may lead to an artificial increase in membrane organization. In particular, this poses problems for the study of small and dynamic domains and thus allows visualization but not quantification of raft domains.

We have successfully used Laurdan to image and quantify membrane order in both live and fixed cells [6]. As described above, Laurdan is an environmentally sensitive probe whose peak emission depends on the polarity of the membrane. By calculating the GP of the intensities of the two different emissions, we gain insights into the membrane order. Two issues should be kept in mind when using this approach. First, the spatial limitation of the microscope does not allow for visualization of individual lipid rafts but gives the overall membrane order in a defined region of interest (ROI). The ROI can be defined by a confocal immunofluorescence image. In this case fluorophore-conjugated antibodies with an emission wavelength outside the emission region of Laurdan are used. This approach allowed us to characterize the membrane order of focal adhesions and the dependency of focal adhesion order on the structural protein caveolin 1 [7]. The second issue to keep in mind is that Laurdan GP values determine the overall packing density of the membrane to which both lipids as well as proteins contribute. To date, we have not found any proteins or protein complexes that directly affect Laurdan's spectral properties and thus could lead to an imprecise determination of membrane order. However, the extent to which protein crowding influences the packing density of lipids and thus Laurdan is not yet known and requires further investigation.

Recently, a new dye, di-4-ANEPPDHQ, has become available with similar properties to Laurdan [13]. Di-4-ANEPPDHQ is a styryl membrane dye that is derived from voltage-sensitive fluorophores. Similar to Laurdan, di-4-ANEPPDHQ is blue shifted in condensed membrane domains when compared to fluid membranes. While Laurdan responds to lipid packing, di-4-ANEPPDHQ senses lipid rigidity that stretches the charged groups of the probe further apart. It has been effectively employed to measure membrane phases in liposomes and fluidity differences in cell membranes by shifts in emission or lifetime of the dye. It should also be noted that, unlike Laurdan, di-4-ANEPPDHQ senses cholesterol independently from lipid packing, possibly because cholesterol directly interacts with this probe [13]. The advantage of di-4-ANEPPDHQ over Laurdan is that it can be excited at 488 nm while Laurdan requires two-photon excitation due to photoinstability under single-photon excitation. Nevertheless, the broad emission spectrum of di-4-ANEPPDHQ makes it difficult to combine it with immunofluorescence. In contrast to Laurdan, di-4-ANEPPDHQ exhibits very low internalization and is therefore not useful for studies of intracellular membranes. Given the complexity of cell membranes, two structurally unrelated dyes that quantify membrane order based on different physical properties complement each other perfectly and can independently confirm fluidity differences in cell membranes.

16.4.2 Protein–Lipid Interactions

The lipid raft hypothesis suggested that proteins have differential preferences for ordered and fluid domains. Some proteins can directly bind to a specific lipid species. As an example we discuss the interactions of peripheral actin-remodeling proteins with phosphatidylinositols. Partitioning of proteins into lipid domains in model systems is dependent on the lipid modification of the protein. In the second part of this section, posttranslational lipid modifications of proteins and how this affects targeting of proteins to membrane domains are discussed. Further information can be found in the excellent review by Deborah Brown outlining the interactions of peripheral and transmembrane proteins with lipid rafts and detergent-resistant membranes [2].

Lipid-Recruiting Proteins: Role of Phosphoinositides The actin skeleton plays a major role not only in compartmentalization of the membrane, as suggested by

Kusumi's single-particle tracking studies (see Section 16.2.6), but also in defining cell shape and cell motility, in endocytosis and exocytosis, as well as in the signal transduction process. Numerous studies have linked actin remodeling to changes in phosphatidylinositol metabolism. The distribution of certain phosphoinositides has a major impact on the recruitment of signaling pathways to specific membrane sites. One example is phosphatidylinositol-mediated actin polymerization during phagocytosis, which is the engulfment of foreign particles or bacteria by macrophages. Binding of actin-associated proteins to phosphatidylinositols, specifically to phosphatidylinositol 4,5-biphosphate [PtdIns(4,5)P_2], is believed to link the filaments of the membrane skeleton to the lipid bilayer. Actin-associated proteins such as gelsolin and cofilin contain a short motif with alternating hydrophobic and cationic residues, called a KR domain. This domain binds to PtdIns(4,5)P_2 and therefore influences the localization and distribution of the protein containing the KR domain. Other signaling and catalytic proteins such as phospholipase Cδ (PLCδ) contain a more complex structure, that is, the pleckstrin homology (PH) domain that also binds to PtdIns(4,5)P_2. However, not all PH domains bind to the same lipid. The PH domain of the general receptor for phosphoinositides isoform 1 (GRP1) or of a signaling protein of the PI3 kinase pathway, Akt, specifically recognizes phosphatidylinositol 3,4,5-triphosphate (PtdIns(3,4,5)P_3), which is itself a product of PI3 kinase. The C1 domain of protein kinase Cδ (PKCδ) recognizes diacylglycerol (DAG), a product of PLC. By constructing chimeric proteins containing these lipid recognition sequences and a fluorescent protein such as GFP, one can probe for the location of specific lipids and their effect on protein recruitment.

Expression of GFP fusion proteins containing the PH or C1 domains of PLCδ, Akt, or GRP1 in macrophages allowed Yeung and colleagues to image the dynamic association of phosphoinositides with phagocytic membranes [29]. Their work demonstrates that first PtdIns(4,5)P_2 levels increase during the formation of the phagocytic cup, which is the extension of the membrane around the particle or bacteria. Once the phagocytic cup closes around the particle, PtdIns(4,5)P_2 levels drop and PtdIns(3,4,5)P_3 and subsequently DAG levels increase sharply. This is the time period of intense signaling leading to the recruitment of small Rho GTPases, which are master regulators of actin filament polymerization. Finally the concentration of PtdIns(3,4,5)P_3 drops, partly due to the enzymatic action of PLC, terminating the activation of the GTPases and resulting in internalization of the particle. Inhibition of the lipid conversions also inhibits actin restructuring around the engulfed particle and thus the phagocytic process, indicating that phosphoinositides play an organizational role during phagocytosis.

Lipid-Modified Proteins Posttranslational protein modifications are key regulators of protein activity and subcellular location. Covalent attachment of lipids (long-chain fatty acids, prenyl groups, sterols, and glycosylated derivates of phosphatidylinositol) to proteins modulates protein interaction with membranes and membrane microdomains as well as signal transduction processes. There are different lipid modifications of proteins which determine the strength of membrane interaction of the modified protein as well as the specificity of membrane targeting. Some of these lipid modifications require the synergized action of basic residue clusters to create electrostatic interactions with acidic membrane phospholipids and promote membrane binding and targeting.

Lipid-Modified Proteins in Inner Leaflet of Plasma Membrane The covalent modifications of proteins by attachment of lipophilic moieties, which are located in the inner leaflet of the plasma membrane, can be classified as follows:

1. *Fatty Acylation of Proteins* Fatty acid protein modification occurs with a wide variety of proteins by the addition of a myristic acid, palmitic acid, or both. N-myristoylation is the covalent attachment of a 14-carbon, saturated fatty acid (myristate) to the amino acidic sequence Met–Gly in the protein N-terminus by *N*-myristoyl transferases (NMT). The initial Met is removed and myristate is then linked to the N-terminal glycine via an amide bond. Of all proteins in the human genome, 15% contain the amino acids Met–Gly at their N-termini. However, only 0.5% of all proteins are N-myristoylated, indicating that other additional features are involved in the substrate recognition by NMT. Protein palmitoylation involves the covalent attachment of a 16-carbon, saturated fatty acid (palmitate) to a cysteine residue via thio-ester linkage. Unlike N-myristoylation, there is no consensus sequence or predictive algorithm for palmitoylation resulting in a wide variety of palmitoylated proteins. There are few reports of nonenzymatic incorporation of palmitate into peptides.
2. *Protein Prenylation* Many proteins, particularly small G proteins, are prenylated via thio-ester linkage of a farnesyl or geranylgeranyl moieties to cysteine residues at or near the C-terminus. The CAAX motif is the common consensus sequence for prenylation. This sequence is recognized by farnesyl transferases (X = Met or Ser) or geranylgeranyl transferase I (X = Leu). Examples of prenylated proteins include the Rab proteins.

All of these lipid modifications determine the association with and specificity for the plasma membrane. Palmitate or geranylgeranyl moieties are hydrophobic enough to strongly attach the modified protein to membranes. In contrast, neither myristate nor farnesyl modifications are strong enough to provide stable membrane association. A second signal, such as a cluster of basic amino acid residues or other lipid modification, is then required to enhance membrane association. An overview of lipid modifications can be found in Figure 16.3.

These lipid motifs not only associate the proteins with the plasma membrane but also partition them into plasma membrane subdomains. FRET is a powerful tool to study this partitioning, allowing the detection of protein compartmentalization in clusters smaller than the resolution limit of the light microscope. Zacharias and collaborators have described the differential partitioning of fluorescent proteins with different types of lipid anchors using in vivo FRET measurements [30]. Fusing the 13 NH_2-terminus amino acids of kinase Lyn (both myristoylated and palmitoylated, Lyn-N13) to monomeric mutants of cyan and yellow-fluorescent proteins (mCFP and mYFP) enabled the imaging of lipid raft clustering. Similarly, clustering occurred between caveolin 1, a lipid raft protein that is naturally tripalmitoylated, and both the Lyn-N13-mCFP and a dipalmitoylated NH_2-terminal 20 residue of GAP-43 fused to mYFP (GAP-43–N20–mYFP). In contrast, the effectiveness of prenyl modifications in protein targeting to lipid rafts was investigated. To do so, the prenylation motif of the small G protein Rho was fused to the COOH-terminus of mCFP or mYFP (GerGer–Rho–mCFP), causing the addition of a single geranylgeranyl moiety to the fluorescent proteins. Although these fluorescent fusion proteins clustered, they did so in a cholesterol-independent manner,

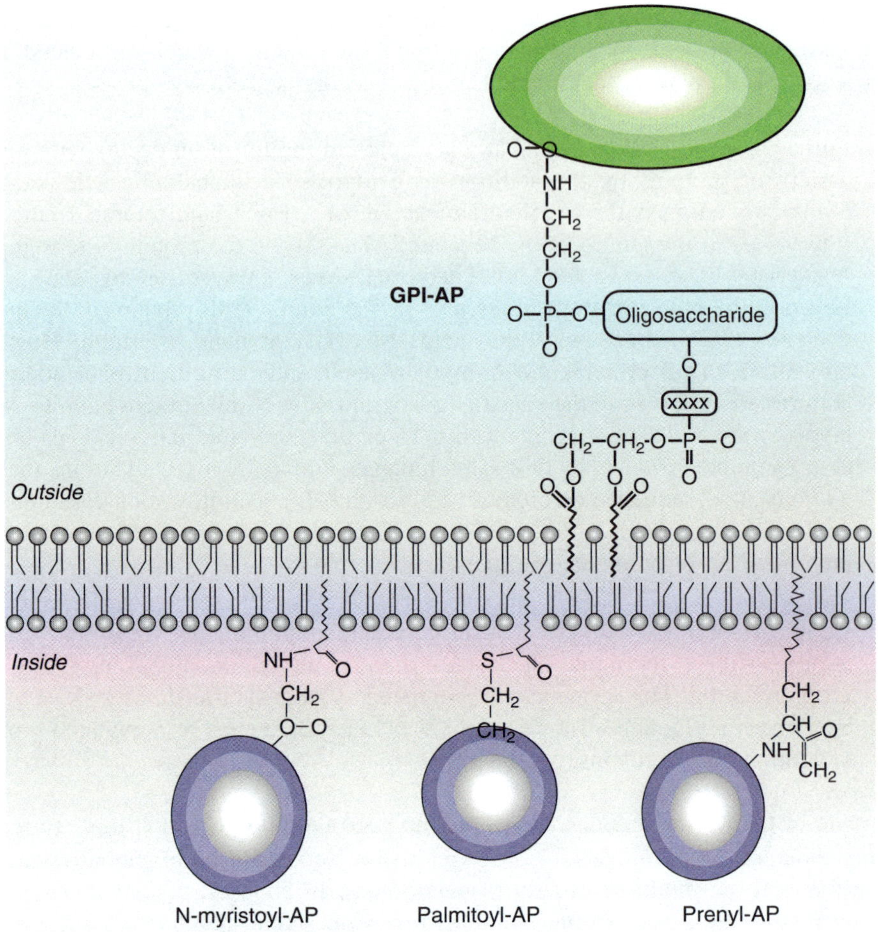

Figure 16.3 Lipid modification of membrane APs. Different lipid modifications anchor proteins to the inner leaflet of the plasma membrane. The *N*-myristoyl moiety is bound to an amino-terminal glycine, whereas a palmitoyl moiety is attached to an internal cysteine. Farnesyl and geranyl–geranyl (C_6H_5-groups) modify carboxyl-terminal cysteine. The GPI anchor attaches to the carboxyl-terminal residue of a protein to anchor the protein (GPI–AP) to the outer leaflet of the plasma membrane.

coclustering with neither caveolin-1 nor the Lyn–N13–mCFP construct. In conclusion, these FRET studies revealed that acylation (myristoylation and palmitoylation) but not prenylation promotes clustering of proteins in lipid rafts. Although geranylgeranylation also promotes clustering, these domains are not identical to raft domains.

GPI-Anchored Proteins Glycosylated derivates of GPI-anchored proteins form a special group of lipid-modified proteins. GPI is a derivate of phosphatidylinositol in which the inositol holds a short oligosaccharide that may be covalently joined to the carboxyl-terminal residue of the protein through a phosphoethanolamine (Figure 16.3). GPI-anchored proteins are located exclusively on the outer leaflet of the plasma membrane and are confined within clusters. Approximately 0.5% of eukaryotic proteins are GPI anchored, a lipid modification that occurs in the luminal side of the endoplasmic reticulum through the action of a GPI transamidase and other enzymes. These lipid-modified proteins, together with myristoylated and palmitoylated proteins, are preferentially localized to lipid raft domains in the outer leaflet. This raftophilic behavior is presumably a consequence of their more stable association with the cholesterol and long acyl groups in lipid rafts than with the surrounding phospholipids.

FRET and SPT have been used to study the relationship between GPI-anchored proteins and lipid rafts with contradictory results. Glebov and Nichols used a FRET approach to show that GPI-anchored fluorescent proteins are mostly present in a random distribution on the plasma membrane, with a similar distribution as non-raft, transmembrane proteins [9]. In contrast, using homo- and hetero-FRET-based experiments, Sharma et al. suggested that 20–40% of GPI-anchored fluorescent proteins are present in nanoscale cholesterol-sensitive clusters [22]. These studies also suggest a weak lipid-dependent organization of GPI-anchored proteins. Recent studies by Suzuki and collaborators using ultrahigh-speed imaging and single-molecule tracking provided further evidence that GPI-anchored protein clusters recruit signaling molecules through both cholesterol-dependent lipid–lipid (e.g., lipid raft-mediated) interactions and protein–protein interactions [27].

16.4.3 Protein–Protein Interactions

Protein–protein interactions are the most frequently studied molecular binding events in cell biology. Since many signaling pathways are multimolecular assemblies, clustering and recruitment of receptors and other membrane-associated proteins define signaling pathways. Signaling proteins are modular structures that contain one or more motifs or domains which recognize other proteins. Some of the best understood motifs include the Src homology (SH2) and phosphotyrosine-binding (PTB) domains that allow protein binding to a phosphotyrosine motif. Others are able to bind to phosphoserine and/or phosphothreonine residues. Different domains such as the Src homology 3 (SH3) domain recognize and bind proline-rich regions on the effector protein. Multiple combinations of these binding domains together with lipid-binding and catalytic domains generate a large variety of proteins involved in cellular signaling and allow the fine tuning of signaling pathways.

How such a multitude of protein–protein interactions can affect membrane segregation is demonstrated by the T-cell receptor (TCR) signaling pathway (see Figure 16.4). The recognition of a specific antigen on the surface of an antigen-presenting cell (APC) triggers the activation of T cells. In terms of molecular interactions, ligation of the TCR leads to the formation of the TCR/CD3 complex that recruits signaling molecules such as Lck/Fyn and ZAP70 kinases. Lck is a lipid raft-associated Src family kinase that, enhanced by co-receptors CD4 or CD8, phosphorylates both CD3 subunits and the kinase ZAP70. ZAP70, recruited by phosphorylated CD3ζ and activated by Lck, phosphorylates the transmembrane scaffolding protein LAT, enhancing the formation of an activation microcluster. LAT is crucial for the organization of the TCR signaling machinery involved in recruiting and complexing adaptor proteins like Grb2 and SLP76 and enzymes like phospholipase Cγ (PLCγ) via phosphotyrosine-based docking motifs. This forms a cooperative network of multiple downstream effector molecules that couple TCR activation to the induction of Ca^{2+} fluxes (via PLCγ), activation of the

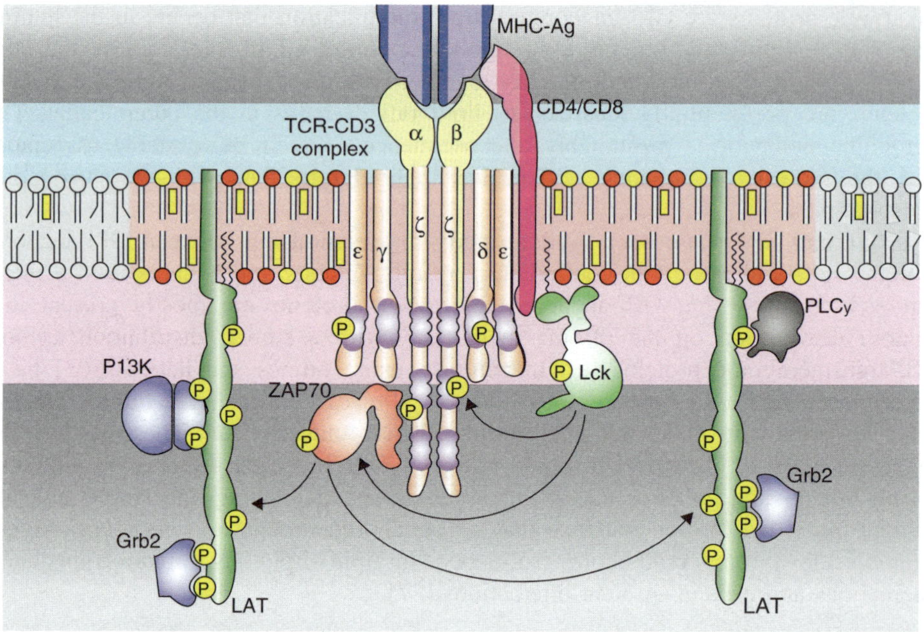

Figure 16.4 Early TCR signaling events. The TCR–CD3 complex is a large transmembrane protein structure that is ligated by the major histocompatibility complex (MHC) conjugated to an Ag on an antigen-presenting cell. Upon engagement of the TCR–CD3 complex by the MHC–antigen complex, Lck kinase is recruited to the complex by CD4 or CD8 coreceptors. Lck phosphorylates specific CD3 domains, which recruit the kinase ZAP70. After activation by Lck, ZAP70 phosphorylates tyrosine residues of the transmembrane scaffolding protein LAT. The enzymes and adaptor proteins binding to phosphorylated LAT enhance the formation of activation clusters, which act as a platform for T-cell activation. Raft domains (in red) play an important role in TCR activation facilitating clustering of proteins and thus mediate signaling.

PI3 kinase (PI3K), Ras/MAPK (via Grb2/Sos1) pathways, and actin nucleation. Thus it executes T-lymphocyte functions from signal transduction to cytokine secretion.

A number of fluorescence approaches have been employed to elucidate not only TCR protein interactions but also the contribution of TCR signaling complexes to membrane organization [11]. The myristoylated and palmitoylated Lyn-GFP fusion protein (Lyn–N13–GFP, see above) accumulates at T-cell activation sites indicating enhanced lipid raft accumulation upon TCR triggering. The same fusion protein was used in a single-particle tracking study that also indicated that this lipid raft marker preferentially partitions into the T-cell activation site. However, a FRET study conducted by Glebov and Nichols concluded that for different raft marker GPI-anchored fluorescent proteins are not enriched at the T-cell activation site [9]. Douglass and Vale combined TIRF microscopy with SPT to follow T-cell-signaling clusters [4]. Using GFP-tagged signaling proteins Lck and LAT, as well mutants that are not myristoylated and palmitoylated (Lck mutant) or dual palmitoylated [LAT(C-S)–GFP], they observed that protein–protein interactions and not lipid anchors are the driving force for the recruitment of these signaling proteins to the activated TCR. The latter study is in agreement with our own work using Laurdan fluorescence (see above) to quantify membrane order at T-cell activation sites [5]. We observed that upon TCR triggering the membrane at the activation sites condensed to form highly ordered domains—a hallmark of lipid raft accumulation. This receptor-mediated membrane condensation required Lck kinase activation as well as LAT expression and phosphorylation. In other words, ordered raft domains formed in response to protein–protein interactions at the T-cell activation site. To what extent the membrane order facilitates the recruitment of raft-favoring proteins such as Lck–13N–GFP requires further investigation. Only by combining various fluorescence approaches will we be able to gain greater insight into how proteins and lipids interact to form functional membrane domains.

REFERENCES

1. L. A. Bagatolli, S. A. Sanchez, T. Hazlett, and E. Gratton, "Giant vesicles, Laurdan, and two-photon fluorescence microscopy: Evidence of lipid lateral separation in bilayers," *Methods Enzymol.* **360**, 481–500 (2003).
2. D. A. Brown, "Lipid rafts, detergent-resistant membranes, and raft targeting signals," *Physiol. (Bethesda)* **21**, 430–439 (2006).
3. C. Dietrich, L. A. Bagatolli, Z. N. Volovyk, N. L. Thompson, M. Levi, K. Jacobson, and E. Gratton, "Lipid rafts reconstituted in model membranes," *Biophys. J.* **80**(3), 1417–1428 (2001).
4. A. D. Douglass and R. D. Vale, "Single-molecule microscopy reveals plasma membrane microdomains created by protein-protein networks that exclude or trap signalling molecules in T cells," *Cell* **121**(6), 937–950 (2005).
5. K. Gaus, E. Chklovskaia, B. Fazekas de St Groth, W. Jessup, and T. Harder, "Condensation of the plasma membrane at the site of T lymphocyte activation," *J. Cell Biol.* **171**(1), 121–131 (2005).
6. K. Gaus, E. Gratton, E. P. Kable, A. S. Jones, I. Gelissen, L. Kritharides, and W. Jessup, "Visualizing lipid structure and raft domains in living cells with two-photon microscopy," *Proc. Natl. Acad. Sci. U.S.A.* **100**(26), 15554–15559 (2003).
7. K. Gaus, S. Le Lay, N. Balasubramanian, and M. A. Schwartz, "Integrin-mediated adhesion regulates membrane order," *J. Cell Biol.* **174**(5), 725–734 (2006).
8. K. Gaus, T. Zech, and T. Harder, "Visualizing membrane microdomains by Laurdan 2-photon microscopy," *Mol. Membr. Biol.* **23**(1), 41–48 (2006).
9. O. O. Glebov and B. J. Nichols, "Lipid raft proteins have a random distribution during localized activation of the T-cell receptor," *Nat. Cell. Biol.* **6**(3), 238–243 (2004).
10. A. T. Hammond, F. A. Heberle, T. Baumgart, D. Holowka, B. Baird, and G. W. Feigenson, "Crosslinking a lipid raft component triggers liquid ordered-liquid disordered phase separation in model plasma membranes," *Proc. Natl. Acad. Sci. U.S.A.* **102**(18), 6320–6325 (2005).
11. T. Harder, C. Rentero, T. Zech, and K. Gaus, "Plasma membrane segretation during T cell activation: Probing the order of domains," *Curr. Opin. Immunol.*, **19**(4), 470–475 (2007).
12. K. Jacobson, O. G. Mouritsen, and R. G. Anderson, "Lipid rafts: At a crossroad between cell biology and physics," *Nat. Cell Biol.* **9**(1), 7–14 (2007).
13. L. Jin, A. C. Millard, J. P. Wuskell, H. A. Clark, and L. M. Loew, "Cholesterol-enriched lipid domains can be visualized by di-4-ANEPPDHQ with linear and nonlinear optics," *Biophys. J.* **89**(1), L04–L06 (2005).
14. N. Kahya, D. A. Brown, and P. Schwille, "Raft partitioning and dynamic behavior of human placental alkaline phosphatase in giant unilamellar vesicles," *Biochemistry* **44**(20), 7479–7489 (2005).

15. N. Kahya and P. Schwille, "Fluorescence correlation studies of lipid domains in model membranes," *Mol. Membr. Biol.* **23**(1), 29–39 (2006).
16. A. K. Kenworthy, "Imaging protein-protein interactions using fluorescence resonance energy transfer microscopy," *Methods* **24**(3), 289–296 (2001).
17. A. K. Kenworthy, B. J. Nichols, C. L. Remmert, G. M. Hendrix, M. Kumar, J. Zimmerberg, and J. Lippincott-Schwartz, "Dynamics of putative raft-associated proteins at the cell surface," *J. Cell Biol.* **165**(5), 735–746 (2004).
18. A. Kusumi, I. Koyama-Honda, and K. Suzuki, "Molecular dynamics and interactions for creation of stimulation-induced stabilized rafts from small unstable steady-state rafts," *Traffic* **5**(4), 213–230 (2004).
19. B. C. Lagerholm, G. E. Weinreb, K. Jacobson, and N. L. Thompson, "Detecting microdomains in intact cell membranes," *Annu. Rev. Phys. Chem.* **56**, 309–336 (2005).
20. P. F. Lenne, L. Wawrezinieck, F. Conchonaud, O. Wurtz, A. Boned, X. J. Guo, H. Rigneault, H. T. He, and D. Marguet, "Dynamic molecular confinement in the plasma membrane by microdomains and the cytoskeleton meshwork," *EMBO J.* **25**(14), 3245–3256 (2006).
21. E. London, "Insights into lipid raft structure and formation from experiments in model membranes," *Curr. Opin. Struct. Biol.* **12**(4), 480–486 (2002).
22. P. Sharma, R. Varma, R. C. Sarasij, Ira, K. Gousset, G. Krishnamoorthy, M. Rao, and S. Mayor, "Nanoscale organization of multiple GPI-anchored proteins in living cell membranes," *Cell* **116**(4), 577–589 (2004).
23. H. Shogomori, A. T. Hammond, A. G. Ostermeyer-Fay, D. J. Barr, G. W. Feigenson, E. London, and D. A. Brown, "Palmitoylation and intracellular domain interactions both contribute to raft targeting of linker for activation of T cells," *J. Biol. Chem.* **280**(19), 18931–18942 (2005).
24. K. Simons and G. van Meer, "Lipid sorting in epithelial cells," *Biochem. J.* **27**(17), 6197–6202 (1988).
25. K. Simons and W. L. Vaz, "Model systems, lipid rafts, and cell membranes," *Annu. Rev. Biophys. Biomol. Struct.* **33**, 269–295 (2004).
26. S. J. Singer and G. L. Nicolson, "The fluid mosaic model of the structure of cell membranes," *Science* **175**(4023), 720–731 (1972).
27. K. G. Suzuki, T. K. Fujiwara, F. Sanematsu, R. Iino, M. Edidin, and A. Kusumi, "GPI-anchored receptor clusters transiently recruit Lyn and G alpha for temporary cluster immobilization and Lyn activation: Single-molecule tracking study 1," *J. Cell Biol.* **177**(4), 717–730 (2007).
28. T. Y. Wang, R. Leventis, and J. R. Silvius, "Fluorescence-based evaluation of the partitioning of lipids and lipidated peptides into liquid-ordered lipid microdomains: A model for molecular partitioning into "lipid rafts," *Biophys. J.* **79**(2), 919–933 (2000).
29. T. Yeung, B. Ozdamar, P. Paroutis, and S. Grinstein, "Lipid metabolism and dynamics during phagocytosis," *Curr. Opin. Cell Biol.* **18**(4), 429–437 (2006).
30. D. A. Zacharias, J. D. Violin, A. C., Newton and R. Y. Tsien, "Partitioning of lipid-modified monomeric GFPs into membrane microdomains of live cells," *Science* **296**(5569), 913–916 (2002).
31. A. Kusumi, C. Nakada, K. Ritchie, K. Murase, K. Suzuki, H. Murakoshi, R. S. Kasai, J. Kondo, and T. Fujiwara, "Paradigm shift of the plasma membrane concept from the two-dimensional continuum fluid to the partitioned fluid: High-speed single-molecule tracking of membrane molecules," *Ann. Rev. Biophys. and Biomol. Sci* **34**(1), 351–378 (2005).

CHAPTER 17

Probing Kinetics of Ion Pumps via Voltage-Sensitive Fluorescent Dyes

RONALD J. CLARKE

School of Chemistry, University of Sydney, Sydney, New South Wales 2006, Australia

17.1 INTRODUCTION: VOLTAGE-DEPENDENT PHYSIOLOGICAL PROCESSES, ION PUMPS, AND CHANNELS

Ion pumps, many of which are driven by adenosine triphosphate (ATP) hydrolysis, play a critical role in the physiology of plant and animal cells [1, 2]. The H^+,K^+–ATPase, for example, of stomach epithelial cells is responsible for the acidification of the stomach and hence for digestion but also for stomach ulcers in diseased individuals. The Ca^{2+}–ATPase of the sarcoplasmic reticulum membrane is responsible for reducing Ca^{2+} levels in the cytoplasm of muscle cells and hence allows muscle relaxation. The plasma membrane H^+–ATPases of plants provide the driving force for nutrient uptake. In humans (and all other animals), the Na^+,K^+–ATPase plays a variety of crucial roles in processes such as nutrient reabsorption in the kidney, maintenance of the resting potential and generation of the action potential in nerves, heart function, and maintenance of cell volume. The development of a greater understanding of the functions of these important enzymes, their regulation, and the roles they play in disease requires detailed investigations of their kinetics and the elucidation of their mechanisms. In this chapter we describe one approach to that goal: the utilization of voltage-sensitive fluorescent membrane probes.

All of the ion pumps mentioned above have the common characteristic that they transport ions across a membrane against a concentration or electrochemical potential gradient. For that reason they require a source of energy, commonly ATP; but ion pumps also exist which are light driven (e.g., bacteriorhodopsin) or driven by the energy released by a redox reaction (e.g., the cytochrome *c* oxidase). Because the ions are transported against an electrochemical potential gradient (termed *active transport*), the enzymes' ion-binding sites cannot be open to both sides of the membrane simultaneously. The ions must first be bound from one side of the membrane, then occluded within the protein via a conformational change, and then released to the other side of the membrane via a further protein conformational change. This is in contrast to the mechanism of ion channels, which have their ion-binding sites open to both sides

Fluorescence Applications in Biotechnology and Life Sciences, Edited by Ewa M. Goldys

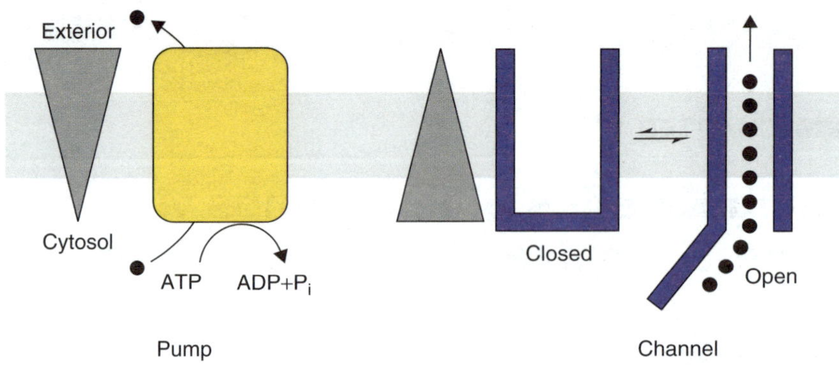

Figure 17.1 Ion-transporting membrane proteins. Channels can exist in an open state, in which ions move *down* an electrochemical potential gradient. No energy is required. The transport is termed facilitated diffusion. Pumps transport ions *against* an electrochemical potential gradient. The ion-binding sites are open alternately to the cytosol and the exterior. Energy is required. The transport is termed active transport. In the example shown the energy is derived from ATP hydrolysis.

of the membrane at once (see Figure 17.1). Ion transport through a channel therefore requires no source of energy. It is merely driven by diffusion, with the channel providing a pathway for the ions to follow. Ion transport through a channel is thus termed *facilitated diffusion*.

Because of these differences in mechanism, the timescales of ion pumps and ion channels are very different. A channel open to both sides of the membrane at once allows a rapid flux of ions across the membrane. For example, open Na^+ channels of the nerve membrane allow a flux of 10^7 ions/s, which corresponds to an average time for the transport of a single ion of 0.1 μs. Ion channels are thus ideally studied by electrophysiological techniques, for example, single channel patch-clamp measurements, because of the relatively large currents they produce, typically in the picoampere range. Ion pumps, on the other hand, function on a much slower timescale. In this case ion transport requires significant conformational changes to drive the ions across the membrane. These conformational changes, because of the large number of amino acid side chains involved and the number of intermolecular interactions which need to be broken and formed, typically have rate constants on the order of 100 s^{-1}. The overall turnover of an ion pump then usually occurs on a timescale of milliseconds to seconds, that is, four to six orders of magnitude slower than that of ion channels. Single ion pumps thus produce only very small currents across membranes which are not measurable by electrophysiological means.

One approach to investigating the activity of ion pumps is to measure the current due to many ion pump molecules simultaneously, that is, by inhibiting the pumps with a specific inhibitor (e.g., ouabain in the case of the Na^+,K^+–ATPase) and measuring the change in current. This can be done via the whole-cell patch-clamp technique. Another approach is to synchronize the pumps. One way of doing this is to have them in a medium lacking one of the essential substrates (e.g., ATP) and then rapidly adding it to the medium. This could be done via the stopped-flow method or by photochemically releasing a caged substrate via a laser flash. Another way of synchronizing many pumps is to perturb their steady-state activity by a rapid change in temperature, pressure, or membrane voltage, that is, utilize a relaxation kinetic method. Whichever method one chooses, one also requires a detection method to follow pump activity. As mentioned above, the detection of ion pump–induced current is a possible means. Many ion pumps exchange ions across the membrane. For example, the Na^+,K^+–ATPase pumps three Na^+ ions from the cytoplasm into the extracellular fluid and two K^+ from the extracellular fluid into the cytoplasm per hydrolyzed ATP molecule. Thus, the Na^+,K^+-ATPase produces a net current from the cytoplasm to the extracellular space, which builds up a voltage across the entire membrane. Ion pumps which do this are termed *electrogenic*. For electrogenic ion pumps the voltage across the membrane is also an observable quantity which could be used to follow its kinetics.

However, not all ion pumps are electrogenic. Under physiological conditions the H^+,K^+–ATPase pumps one H^+ ion into the stomach from the stomach epithelial cell cytoplasm and one K^+ ion out of the stomach into the cell's cytoplasm per hydrolyzed ATP. Hence, there is no net current across the membrane and no change in electrical membrane potential produced. However, even in the case of such nonelectrogenic pumps, individual reactions of the entire pump cycle do involve charge transport. If the ion transport is sequential or ping-pong (as it generally seems to be) and not synchronous, then the transport of the H^+ ions alone or the K^+ ions alone are electrogenic reactions. Furthermore, conformational changes of the proteins which are associated with the ion transport must involve the movement of charged amino acid residues of the protein within the membrane. These then produce changes in local electric field strength within the membrane, which are also experimentally detectable. Therefore, methods are available for observing the kinetics of both electrogenic and nonelectrogenic ion pumps.

The current and voltage signals produced by ion pumps can be observed directly by electrical means, that is, by the use of electrodes. An alternative approach, which is the topic of this chapter, is to convert these electrical signals into an optical signal which can be observed spectroscopically. This can be done via the application of voltage-sensitive membrane probes. These undergo changes in their ultraviolet (UV) visible absorption spectrum, their fluorescence excitation spectrum, or their fluorescence emission spectrum when either the transmembrane electrical potential or the intramembrane electric field strength changes. The major advantage of using voltage-sensitive probes is that they can be used on small cells, cell organelles, vesicles, or in some cases even open membrane fragments, into which electrodes are difficult or impossible to insert. They therefore represent a valuable complement to more standard electrophysiological techniques.

17.2 VOLTAGE-SENSITIVE DYES: MECHANISMS, RESPONSE TIMES, AND THEIR RELEVANCE FOR KINETIC STUDIES

Voltage-sensitive dyes respond to changes in the membrane electric potential and electric field strength by a variety of different mechanisms with widely varying response times depending on their chemical structure and their interaction with the membrane. An understanding of the mechanisms of dye response and their response times is important for an appropriate choice of a probe for a particular application. The purpose of this section is therefore to provide a very brief overview of the dyes presently available and how they respond to voltage changes. More detailed reviews of dye mechanisms can be found elsewhere [3–7].

The development of voltage-sensitive fluorescence probes has been concentrated in a relatively small number of laboratories, notably in those of Cohen [8, 9] (Yale University), Waggoner [10–12] (Amherst College), Grinvald and Hildesheim [13] (Weizmann Institute, Israel), Loew [3, 6] (University of Connecticut), and more recently Fromherz [5, 4] (Max-Planck-Institute for Biochemistry, Germany). Many of the dyes synthesized have been screened for the magnitude of their fluorescent response to voltage pulses on squid axons. From this screening process and from theoretical calculations, several classes of dyes have been identified which give measurable responses. Normally the dyes are grouped into two categories based on their response times:

1. Fast-response probes (response times less than milliseconds): styrylpyridinium and annellated hemicyanine dyes and merocyanine dyes
2. Slow-response probes (response times greater than milliseconds): cationic carbocyanine and rhodamine dyes and anionic oxonol dyes

The basis for the different response times of these probes is their response mechanism. In order to produce a change in fluorescence, a change in electric field must induce some movement either of the dye molecule as a whole or of its electrons. The degree of movement determines the speed of the fluorescence response.

In the case of the fast-response probes a major voltage-sensing mechanism appears to be electrochromism. The styrylpyridinium and the annellated hemicyanine dyes belong to this category. These dyes undergo a significant charge shift on excitation; that is, the electron distribution is very different in the excited state than in the ground state. Any local electric field within the membrane hence causes a different degree of stabilization or destabilization of the ground and excited states of membrane-bound probes. This causes a shift in the dye's fluorescence excitation spectrum, which is then evident as either an increase or decrease in fluorescence intensity depending on the wavelength of fluorescence excitation. Because this mechanism only involves a redistribution of the probe's electrons, its response mechanism is expected to be very fast, that is, femtoseconds.

It is possible, however, that the electrochromic response of some styrylpyridinium probes (e.g., RH421) (see Figure 17.2) is enhanced by a reorientation of the dye molecule as a whole within the membrane. There is a steep gradient in polarity on going from the aqueous environment across the lipid headgroup region and into the hydrocarbon interior of a lipid membrane. Therefore, any small reorientation of a probe within the membrane is likely to lead to a change in its local polarity and hence a solvatochromic shift of its fluorescence excitation spectrum. Such a reorientation could easily come about because of the altered electronic distribution of the probe caused by the electrochromic mechanism. The observed fluorescence change of any particular probe could thus be the result of a combination of more than one overlapping voltage response mechanism. A reorientation mechanism would be expected to have a much slower response time than a purely electrochromic mechanism. Intramembrane reorientation would most likely occur on the nanosecond timescale. Merocyanine dyes (e.g., merocyanine 540) (see Figure 17.2) also respond via a reorientation mechanism, either with or without an electrochromic component to the response. These dyes have a dipolar fluorophore, which would be expected to reorient itself along the electric field lines within the membrane on the application of a membrane potential or on a change in intramembrane electric field strength. Upon reorientation it has been suggested that merocyanine 540 also undergoes a change in its state of aggregation within

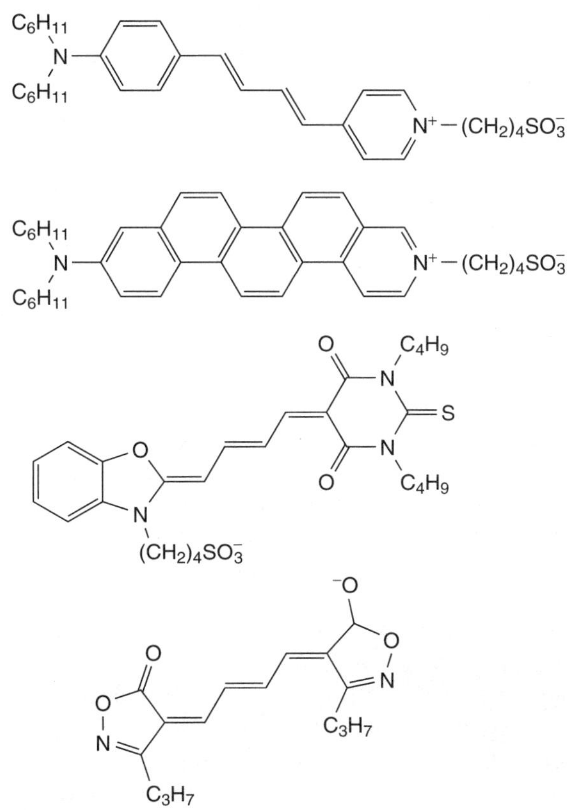

RH421

ANNINE 5

Merocyanine 540

Oxonol VI

Figure 17.2 Examples of structures of a few voltage-sensitive fluorescent dyes.

the membrane. If a probe dimerizes, then the interaction between two adjacent fluorophore's electronic systems would also be expected to result in a change in the probe's fluorescence excitation or emission spectrum.

In contrast to the fast-response probes discussed so far, which respond via electronic or molecular movement *within* the membrane, the slow-response probes, that is, carbocyanine, rhodamine, and oxonol dyes (see Figure 17.2), respond via a movement of the dye across the entire membrane. These dyes have a net charge (positive in the case of the carbocyanine and rhodamine dyes; negative in the case of the oxonol dyes). When the membrane potential changes, this therefore perturbs the equilibrium distribution of the dyes across the membrane. For example, if the electrical potential of the cytoplasm of a cell becomes more negative relative to the extracellular fluid, this would cause a positively charged probe to accumulate within the cell, whereas a negatively charged probe would favor the extracellular fluid. Because the total volumes of the cytoplasm and the extracellular fluids are generally very different, such a perturbation of the distribution of probe across the membrane would also perturb the partition (or binding) equilibrium between the membrane and aqueous phases on each side of the membrane. For example, a redistribution of dye into the cytoplasm would be expected to increase the proportion of membrane-bound dye because the cytoplasmic volume is generally much smaller than that of the extracellular fluid. The quantum yield of voltage-sensitive probes is normally much higher when they are membrane bound. Therefore, an increase in the proportion of membrane-bound dye would be expected to cause an increase in fluorescence at low dye concentrations. At high dye concentrations, however, increased dye accumulation within the membrane can cause a decrease in fluorescence because of the proximity of dye molecules within the membrane and fluorescence quenching via fluorophore–fluorophore interactions (either an inner filter effect or energy transfer). However, regardless of the direction of the fluorescence response, the rate-determining step for such slow-response probes is the movement of dye across the membrane from one leaflet of the membrane to the other. This is a relatively slow process and dye response times are generally in the millisecond–second timescale.

Although slow-response probes are much slower than fast-response probes, if kinetic resolution is not an issue, they do have the advantage that the magnitude of the change in fluorescence intensity observed is generally much greater than in the case of fast-response probes. This is because the change in the probe's environment produced by the membrane potential is much greater. For slow-response probes there is a net movement of probe between the aqueous and the membrane environments, whereas the fast-response dyes remain in the membrane phase. Based on measurements on squid axons, fast-response dyes typically show a 2–10% fluorescence change per 100-mV change in membrane potential, whereas for slow-response probes the fluorescence response is typically 100% per 100 mV. For equilibrium monitoring of the membrane potential, therefore, slow-response probes are preferred.

Another important factor in the choice of a dye and in its experimental application is its photochemical stability. Styrylpyridinium dyes in particular have been found to undergo a photochemical reaction causing a change in fluorescence unrelated to their voltage sensitivity [15]. This is most likely due to their trans double bonds, which are prone to photoisomeristion. For this reason Kuhn and Fromherz [14] have recently produced a series of derivatives of the styrylpyridinium dyes with rigid polycyclic structures. These are the annellated hemicyanine (ANNINE) dyes (see Figure 17.2). For application in fluorescence microscopy with high-intensity illumination a high degree of photochemical stability would certainly be desirable. Otherwise, for kinetic measurements it is necessary to carry out careful control experiments to know what the timescales of any photochemical reaction and voltage response are, so that they can be distinguished and if necessary suppress the photochemical reaction by the use of neutral density filters and low-light-intensity excitation.

For the measurement of the kinetics of ion pumps (i.e., the topic of this chapter), it is important to consider what kinetic information one is after when choosing a probe. From the preceding discussion of mechanisms, it is clear that slow-response probes only respond to changes in the total membrane potential. Therefore, they are normally used on electrogenic ion pumps which produce a net ion transport and hence a change in membrane potential. Furthermore, the change in membrane potential that electrogenic pumps produce is a consequence of their entire pumping cycle. For example, in the case of the Na^+,K^+–ATPase three Na^+ ions are pumped out of the cell and two K^+ ions in per turnover, giving a net positive current out. Therefore, slow-response probes cannot be used to observe the kinetics of individual partial reactions of an electrogenic pump. They can only be used to measure the overall kinetics of the buildup or change of a membrane potential due to the steady-state activity of the pump's entire enzymatic cycle. In contrast, fast-response probes, because they detect changes in intramembrane electric field strength, can be used to observe the kinetics of any ion pump reaction or conformational change which causes a movement of charge (either an ion or a charged amino acid residue) within the membrane. Therefore, fast-response probes offer the ability of obtaining much more detailed kinetic information and hence mechanistic information about the function of an ion pump. Although they have a lower sensitivity to membrane potential than slow-response probes, this fact is not really relevant when resolving ion pump partial reactions, since these can produce very large changes in local electric field strength within the membrane, which results in changes of fluorescence intensity of up to 100%. In order to observe such large responses, however, every dye molecule must be relatively close to an ion pump molecule in order to detect the local changes in intramembrane electric field strength it produces. Therefore, such measurements are limited to preparations of ion pumps that are present in a high density within the membrane.

17.3 STEADY-STATE ION PUMP ACTIVITY

From the discussion of voltage-sensitive probe mechanisms in the previous section it is clear that, because of the magnitude of their fluorescence response, the most appropriate dyes for following the steady-state activity of ion pumps are slow-response probes, that is, carbocyanine, rhodamine, and oxonol dyes. Because these dyes detect changes in the total transmembrane electrical potential, they can only be used to follow the kinetics of ion pumps when the ion-pumping activity causes a change in the electrical membrane potential. This is the case for electrogenic ion pumps, which cause a net current across the membrane. However, it could also be the case for nonelectrogenic ion pumps, which cause only a change in the concentration of ions across the membrane, because the membrane normally has varying ion permeabilities and any change in concentrations across the membrane would then change the steady-state diffusion potential.

If one wishes to perform a quantitative measurement of ion pump activity using voltage-sensitive probes, the fluorescence change observed on activating the ion pump must be mathematically converted into its corresponding voltage change and, based on the ion pump's stoichiometry, this can then be converted into a turnover or activity. The first step is therefore to calibrate the dye's fluorescence response. If one is using large cells such as squid axons, this could be done directly by using electrodes via the voltage-clamp technique. Voltage changes and fluorescence changes could then be directly compared and any fluorescence level could be associated with an absolute value of the membrane potential. If one is using smaller cells, cell organelles, or vesicles, however, such an approach is not appropriate. Under such conditions the calibration is normally carried out by adding the cells or vesicles into solutions of known K^+ concentration and then adding valinomycin, a K^+ carrier, to make the membrane selectively permeable to K^+ ions [11, 16]. If the intracellular or intravesicular K^+ concentration is known, the transmembrane electrical potential V_m can be calculated theoretically from the Nernst equation:

$$V_m = \frac{RT}{F} \ln \frac{c_K^{\text{in}}}{c_K^{\text{out}}} \tag{17.1}$$

where R is the gas constant, T is the absolute temperature, and F is Faraday's constant. If the fluorescence levels of dye in the presence of cells or vesicles of known values of V_m are recorded, a calibration curve for the fluorescence probe can be constructed. Once the fluorescent dye has been calibrated, any voltage change recorded on activation of an ion pump, for example, by the addition of ATP in the case of an ATP-driven pump, is related to the current it produces across the membrane by the expression

$$\frac{dV_m}{dt} = -\frac{I}{AC_m} \tag{17.2}$$

where I is the current across the membrane, A is the membrane surface area, and C_m is the specific membrane capacitance, that is, the capacitance per unit area. A typical value for C_m is 1 μF/cm^2. If the membrane's passive permeability to ions was absolutely zero, Eq. 17.2 predicts a continuous increase in membrane potential until the potential of dielectric breakdown of the membrane is reached and the membrane bursts. In practice, however, a membrane would have some passive permeability which would cause a leakage current opposing the pump current. Therefore, after a certain time period from initiation of pumping, a membrane potential would be reached where the rates of ion pumping and the rates of the passive leak are equal and opposite. At this point the membrane potential and the fluorescence level would level off. The fluorescence would then stay at this level until the source of energy for the ion pump (e.g., ATP) was exhausted. The fluorescence would then decay back to its initial level prior to pump activation via leakage pathways with a time constant τ determined by the product of the specific membrane capacitance and the specific membrane resistance R_m. This is based on the equivalent circuit model of a lipid membrane as a resistor and capacitor in parallel, where $1/\tau = RC$. The decay of the fluorescence signal thus allows an estimation of the specific membrane resistance [17]. An example of this behavior is shown in Figure 17.3. Here the voltage across the membrane was generated by the Na^+,K^+–ATPase reconstituted into lipid vesicles and the kinetics of changes in voltage across the membrane were followed using the slow voltage-sensitive fluorescent dye oxonol VI (see Figure 17.2).

If the membrane's passive permeability is low, the initial rate of increase of V_m allows the ion pump current I_p to be estimated from Eq. 17.2. To relate this to a pumping rate of the enzyme, ν (in s^{-1}), the number of pump molecules per cell or per vesicle, n, needs to be known as well as the stoichiometry of the pump. If, as in the case of the Na^+,K^+–ATPase, it is known that there is only one net charge transported per pump cycle, then $I_p = n\nu$. This is the simplest possible case. If there is a significant passive permeability, the situation becomes much more complicated.

To account for passive ion permeability, if there is more than one ion making a significant contribution to the passive leak, the leakage current $I_{i,l}$ of each ion can be accounted for by the Goldman equation:

$$I_{i,l} = z_i e_0 P_i A u \frac{c_i^{\text{in}} \exp(z_i u) - c_i^{\text{out}}}{\exp(z_i u) - 1} \tag{17.3}$$

where $u = FV_m/RT$, z_i is the valence of the ion, e_0 is the electronic charge, and P_i is the permeability of the membrane for the ion. The Goldman expressions for the passive current of each of the permeable ions must be added to the pump current and substituted into Eq. 17.2 for the total current in order to calculate the rate of change of the membrane potential. If one is only interested in the initial rate of voltage generation, this is sufficient. However, if one wishes to describe the complete time

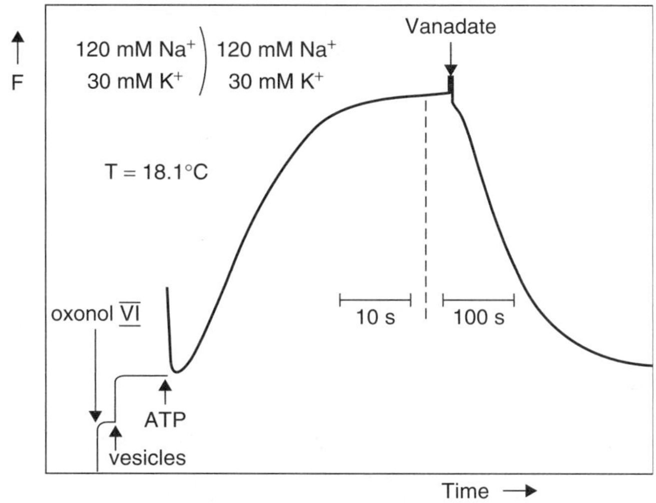

Figure 17.3 Fluorescence signal associated with generation of inside-positive membrane potential after activation of Na^+,K^+–ATPase by the addition of ATP [17]. 30 nM oxonol VI, vesicles (8 μg/mL dioleoylphosphatidylcholine), 250 μM ATP, and 2 mM vanadate were successively added to buffer containing 60 mM Na_2SO_4, 15 mM K_2SO_4, 30 mM imidazole, 1 mM L-cysteine, 1 mM ethylenediaminetetraacetic acid (EDTA), and 5 mM $MgSO_4$. The pH of the buffer was adjusted to pH 7.2 with H_2SO_4. The vesicles were prepared in the same buffer. F is the fluorescence intensity. The temperature was 18.1°C. In the fluorescence signal shown the Na^+,K^+–ATPase was inhibited before the ATP was exhausted by the addition of vanadate, which is an analogue of phosphate that binds to the phosphorylation site of the enzyme and inhibits ion pumping by the enzyme.

course of the development of the voltage, one also has to take into account the fact that the intracellular or intravesicular concentrations of the ions, c_i^{in}, are changing with time due to the ion-pumping process and the leakage currents. The extracellular or extravesicular ion concentrations can generally be assumed to be constant, because the volume would be much greater than that of the cytoplasm or the intravesicular space. If c_i^{in} changes with time, then, according to Eq. 17.3, $I_{i,l}$ is also time dependent. The change in c_i^{in} with time for any particular ion is given by

$$\frac{dc_i^{\text{in}}}{dt} = -\frac{I_i}{z_i e_0 V} \tag{17.4}$$

where I_i represents the total current (defined to be positive when directed outward) due to pumping plus passive leak, that is, $I_i = I_{i,p} + I_{i,l}$. Thus, Eqs. 17.2–17.4 represent a coupled series of differential equations which must be solved numerically if one wishes to either fit or simulate the entire time course of the voltage change [17]. The situation can be simplified greatly, however, if one works under conditions where the membrane has a much higher permeability for one particular ion over all others. This can be achieved by adding an ion carrier to the system, for example, valinomycin in the case of K^+. Under such conditions the high K^+ permeability short circuits the membrane, compensating any pumping current by passive K^+ diffusion across the membrane. The only voltage change which is then observed is that due to the K^+

concentration difference across the membrane, which is given by the Nernst equation (Eq. 17.1). Differentiating the Nernst equation then yields

$$\frac{dV_m}{dt} \approx -\frac{RT}{Fc_K^{\text{in}}}\frac{dc_K^{\text{in}}}{dt} \tag{17.5}$$

In order then to relate dc_K^{in}/dt to a pumping rate of the enzyme, the stoichiometry of the pump must be known. If the pump is electrogenic, then the passive flow of K^+ ions producing the change in c_K^{in} has to be exactly equal in magnitude and opposite in direction to any net electrogenic pumping of the enzyme.

17.4 KINETICS OF ION PUMP PARTIAL REACTIONS

If the aim is to obtain kinetic information about the partial reactions of an ion pump, slow-response dyes are not appropriate. This is not only because they are slow but also because they respond to the total membrane potential. Ion pumps produce a change in membrane potential as a consequence of their entire pump cycle. Therefore, slow-response dyes will only yield kinetic information about the overall steady-state activity of an ion pump. If one wishes to detect individual partial reactions, one must use one of the fast-response dyes, which respond to local electric field strength changes within the membrane, for example, a sytrylpyridinium dye such as RH421. Such local electric field strength changes come about via charge movement within the membrane by the protein, of either ions or charged amino acid residues. It is worthwhile pointing out here, however, that reactions which involve no charge movement can also be kinetically followed by fast-response dyes. In order to observe a fluorescence change, it is only necessary that for any reaction to be observed it must either itself involve charge translocation or be directly coupled to a preceding or subsequent reaction involving charge translocation.

As in the case of slow-response dyes, the fluorescence response of fast-response probes to changes in membrane potential have been calibrated using voltage clamp or by applying the method of inducing a K^+ diffusion potential via valinomycin [16]. For the purposes of investigating the kinetics of ion pumps, however, this has little value. Fast-response dyes detect intramembrane electric field strength. Any transmembrane potential present will cause an intramembrane electric field strength, but this is likely to very different and much smaller than the local electric fields around ion pumps, which without a crystal structure cannot even be theoretically calculated. Therefore, the prime application of fast-response probes to the study of ion pumps is not to gain information on electrical behavior of the pump, but to use them as a means for converting their electrical activity into an optical signal which one can follow and thus resolve the pump's kinetics and its mechanism.

The fact that these dyes detect intramembrane electric field strength also means that it is not necessary to have a closed cell or vesicle. Although an open membrane fragment surrounded by electrolyte can never have a transmembrane electrical potential, if it contains an active ion pump, local changes in the electric field will still occur within the membrane when the pump is activated. These can be detected by a fast-response probe if it is located within the membrane close enough to the ion pump. In fact, many studies of ion pump kinetics using fast-response probes have involved open membrane fragments [18]. In Figure 17.4 an example of the use of the

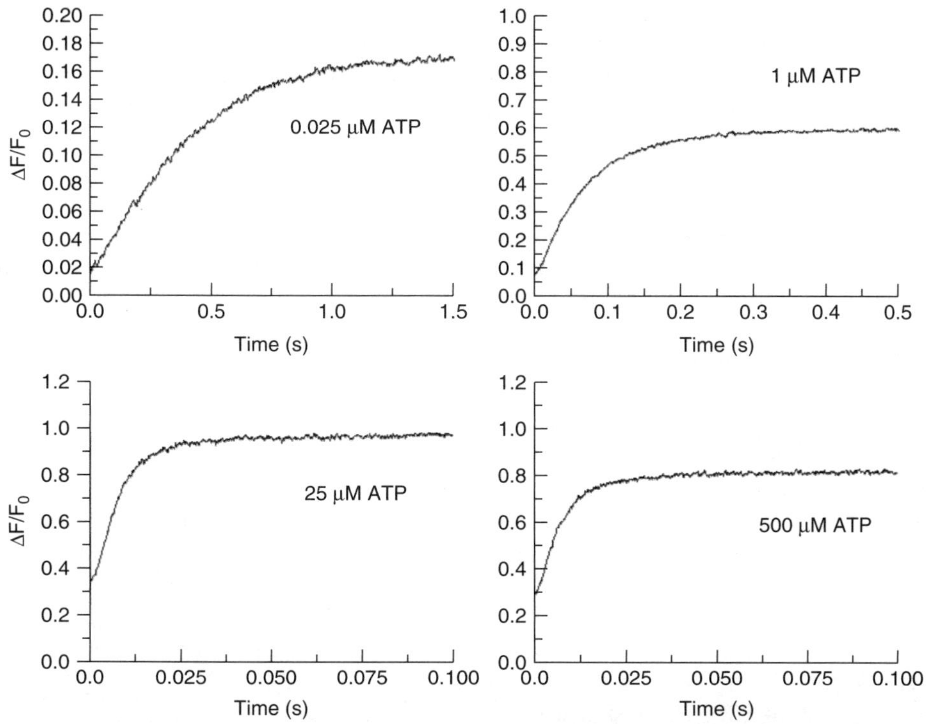

Figure 17.4 Stopped-flow fluorescence transients of Na^+,K^+–ATPase-containing membrane fragments from pig kidney noncovalently labeled with RH421 (75 nM, after mixing) [19]. Na^+,K^+–ATPase (10 μg/mL or 68 nM, after mixing) was rapidly mixed with an equal volume of a solution containing varying concentrations of Na_2ATP. Both the enzyme suspension and the Na_2ATP solutions were prepared in a buffer containing 130 mM NaCl, 30 mM imidazole, 5 mM $MgCl_2$, and 1 mM EDTA (pH 7.4, 24°C). The fluorescence of membrane-bound RH421 was measured at an excitation wavelength of 577 nm at emission wavelengths of ≥665 nm (RG665 glass cutoff filter). The calculated observed rate constants (or reciprocal relaxation times) were (*a*) 0.025 μM ATP, 2.57 (± 0.03) s^{-1}; (*b*) 1 μM ATP, 6.51 (± 0.04) s^{-1}; (*c*) 25 μM ATP, 138 (±2) s^{-1} (96% of the total amplitude) and 12 (± 3) s^{-1} (4%); and (*d*) 500 μM ATP, 179 (±6) s^{-1} (89%) and 41 (± 6) s^{-1} (11%).

styrylpyridinium probe RH421 is shown [19]. Here the kinetics of the phosphorylation reaction of the Na^+,K^+–ATPase was followed in a stopped-flow apparatus. The observed rate constant of the fluorescence change was found to increase with increasing ATP concentration until it reached a saturating value of around 180 s^{-1}. This indicates that the phosphorylation reaction is preceded by a fast ATP binding equilibrium.

In principle, fast-response probes allow the kinetics of ion pump partial reactions to be followed down to the nanosecond timescale. Up to now, however, the kinetic studies that have been carried out using fast-response dyes have been limited to the timescale of milliseconds and longer. This has been due not to the probes but to the methods used to activate the ion pumps, that is, stopped-flow mixing, photolytic release of caged substrates, and flash photolysis. Once other experimental procedures are used, fast-response dyes could potentially provide kinetic information over a much wider timeframe.

The application of fast-response dyes, in particular styrylpyridinium and annellated hemicyanine dyes, to the investigation of ion pumps is not straightforward. In order to gain fluorescence signals with a large signal-to-noise ratio, care must be taken in the selection of the experimental conditions. First, the mechanism of their response is at least partly due to electrochromism, which causes a shift in the fluorescence excitation spectrum. The percentage change in probe absorption is therefore much less in the middle of the absorbance band than on its flanks. Therefore, if one is using fixed wavelengths for excitation and emission, care must be taken in the selection of the excitation wavelength. For the best signal-to-noise ratio and the greatest percentage change in fluorescence, it is advisable to excite on the red edge of the visible absorbance band of the dye.

Another important experimental consideration is the concentration of the probe. In order to sense a change in local electric field strength arising from an ion pump, any fast-response dye must itself be either charged or dipolar. Therefore, these probes themselves cause changes in local electric field strength within the membrane. If the probes can detect fields coming from an ion pump, then it is only logical that ion pumps should detect fields coming from the probes. Therefore, the electric fields induced by fast-response probes could in principle affect the kinetics of charge-translocating partial reactions of ion pumps. In fact, inhibition of the Na^+,K^+–ATPase at micromolar concentrations of the voltage-sensitive probe RH421 has been observed [20, 21]. In order to avoid any perturbation of the system being studied, it is therefore important to keep the probe concentration as low as possible. In the case of RH421 a typical total concentration of 100–200 nM is used.

A limitation on the application of fast-response probes in studying ion pumps is that, in order to detect local electric field strength changes, a probe must be relatively close to a pump molecule. The electric field strength changes caused by an individual pump molecule within the membrane would show an exponential radial decay in all directions from the molecule. The situation is thus very different to that when the total transmembrane potential is being monitored via slow-response probes, where the transmembrane potential causes a constant electric field strength throughout the whole membrane matrix of a cell or vesicle. Because of the radial decay of field strength around pump molecules, any voltage-sensitive probe molecules which are located at a large distance from a pump molecule would detect little or no change in field strength. Thus, these probe molecules would represent a constant background fluorescence signal. In order to observe a large signal-to-noise ratio, it is then desirable to have all probe molecules close to a pump molecule so as to minimize the background of nonresponsive probes. The only way that this can be achieved is by having a high density of pump molecules in the membrane. Many membrane preparations of ion pumps are not appropriate for kinetic measurements via fast-response probes. The studies that have been performed have concentrated on specialized tissues where a high density of pumps is naturally present. These include the kidney outer medulla, the rectal salt gland of shark, and the electric organ of electric eel, which are all rich sources of the Na^+,K^+–ATPase; the purple membrane of *Halobacterium halobium*, which has a high density of bacteriorhodopsin; and muscle sarcoplasmic reticulum membranes, in which there is a high level of expression of the Ca^{2+}–ATPase.

17.5 FUTURE DIRECTIONS

In terms of probing the kinetics of ion pumps, it would appear to the author that the most interesting future developments in the application of voltage-sensitive probes are most likely to lie in the development and use of fast-response probes rather than slow-response probes. This is predominantly because of the higher temporal resolution that fast-response probes offer and the more detailed mechanistic information that they can provide. However, another reason is that there is probably less scope for improvement in slow-response probes. The voltage sensitivities of the slow-response probes currently available are already quite large, and because the kinetics of production of transmembrane potentials via ion pumps occur on the timescale of milliseconds and slower, there is no reason to try and improve their time resolution beyond the millisecond range.

In the case of fast-response probes, however, although much valuable research has already been carried out on a number of ion pumps, there are still good reasons to invest time and money in the development of further dyes with improved voltage sensitivity and photostability. The restriction on the use of fast-response dyes to ion pumps occurring in high densities is a major hurdle. If dyes with greater voltage sensitivity could be synthesized, these could perhaps find a wider application to ion pumps which are present in lower concentrations than those so far studied. In order to improve signal-to-noise ratios, it would also be advantageous if one could use high light intensities. Many of the most sensitive dyes currently available suffer, however, from the disadvantage that they are photochemically unstable and even phototoxic to cells. This therefore restricts the intensity of the illumination that can be used. If dyes could be found which were as near as possible to being photochemically inert, this would certainly be a significant improvement and open up a wider field of application. The new ANNINE dyes [14], which have recently been synthesized, appear promising in this respect.

Even without the development of new probes, however, many interesting new applications of the currently available fast-response probes remain to be discovered or developed. It appears that the potential of fast-response probes still has not been fully exploited. For example, although they in principle allow a time resolution down to the nanosecond range, up to now they have only been applied in the millisecond–second range in ion pump research. If other kinetic methods were applied, for example, relaxation kinetic techniques, the fast-response probes still offer the possibility of gaining much more kinetic information over a much wider time range. One reason that the fast-response probes still have not been used to their full potential is probably that it is still not entirely clear what they are detecting. Certainly they are detecting changes in intramembrane local electric field strength. However, there are a number of possible origins of the field strength changes, that is, translocation of transported ions, movement of charged or dipolar amino acid residues, and changes in protein surface hydration. Because of this uncertainty in what the probes are responding to, some researchers have probably preferred to stick to more traditional electrophysiological approaches. However, one might rather see the present uncertainty as a challenge for future research. If the time range of measurement using fast-response probes were extended toward the nanosecond range, this could allow the actual partial reactions of an ion pump which are responsible for the field strength changes detected by the probe to be conclusively identified. Apart from providing valuable kinetic information, the probes could then be utilized as a tool for identifying in which steps of an ion pump's reaction cycle charge is actually being transported.

REFERENCES

1. P. Läuger, *Electrogenic Ion Pumps*, Sinauer Associates, Sunderland, MA, 1991.
2. M. G. Palmgren, "Plant plasma membrane H^+-ATPases: Powerhouses for nutrient uptake," *Annu. Rev. Plant Physiol. Mol. Biol.* **52**, 817–845 (2001).
3. L. M. Loew, "How to choose a potentiometric membrane probe" in *Spectroscopic Membrane Probes*, Vol. **2**, L. M. Loew (Ed.), CRC Press, Boca Raton, FL, 1988, pp. 139–151.
4. J. C. Smith, "Potential-sensitive molecular probes in membranes of bioenergetic relevance," *Biochim. Biophys. Acta* **1016**, 1–28 (1990).
5. P. Fromherz, K. H. Dambacher, H. Ephardt, A. Lambacher, C. O. Müller, R. Neigl, H. Schaden, O. Schenk, and T. Vetter, "Fluorescent dyes as probes of voltage transients in neuron membranes: Progress report," *Ber. Bunsenges. Phys. Chem.* **95**, 1333–1345 (1991).
6. L. M. Loew, "Characterization of potentiometric membrane dyes," in *Biomembrane Electrochemistry*, M. Blank and I. Vodyanoy (Eds.), American Chemical Society, Washington, DC, 1994. pp. 151–173.
7. J. Plášek and K. Sigler, "Slow fluorescent indicators of membrane potential: A survey of different approaches to probe response analysis," *J. Photochem. Photobiol. B: Biol.* **33**, 101–124 (1996).
8. W. N. Ross, B. M. Salzberg, L. B. Cohen, A. Grinvald, H. V. Davila, A. S. Waggoner, and C. H. Wang, "Changes in absorption, fluorescence, dichroism and birefringence in stained giant axons: Optical measurement of membrane potential," *J. Membr. Biol.* **33**, 141–183 (1977).
9. M. Zochowski, M. Wachowiak, C. X. Falk, L. B. Cohen, Y-W. Lam, S. Antic, and D. Zecevic, "Imaging membrane potential with voltage-sensitive dyes," *Biol. Bull.* **198**, 1–21 (2000).
10. A. Waggoner, "Optical probes of membrane potential," *J. Membr. Biol.* **27**, 317–334 (1976).
11. A. S. Waggoner, "Dye indicators of membrane potential," *Ann. Rev. Biophys. Bioeng.* **8**, 47–68 (1979).
12. A. S. Waggoner, "Dye probes of cell, organelle, and vesicle membrane potentials," in *The Enzymes of Biological Membranes*, 2nd ed., Vol. **3**, A. N. Martonosi (Ed.), Plenum, New York, 1985, pp. 313–331.
13. A. Grinvald, R. D. Frostig, E. Lieke, and R. Hildesheim, "Optical imaging of neuronal activity," *Physiol. Rev.* **68**, 1285–1366 (1988).
14. B. Kuhn and P. Fromherz, "Anellated hemicyanine dyes in a neuron membrane: Molecular Stark effect and optical voltage recording," *J. Phys. Chem. B* **107**, 7903–7913 (2003).
15. S. Amoroso, V. V. Agon, T. Starke-Peterkovic, M. D. McLeod, H.-J. Apell, P. Sebban, and R. J. Clarke, "Photochemical behaviour and Na^+,K^+-ATPase sensitivity of voltage-sensitive styrylpyridinium fluorescent membrane probes," *Photochem. Photobiol.* **82**, 495–502 (2006).
16. V. Montana, D. L. Farkas, and L. M. Loew, "Dual-wavelength ratiometric measurements of membrane potential," *Biochemistry* **28**, 4536–4539 (1989).
17. R. J. Clarke, H.-J. Apell, and P. Läuger, "Pump current and Na^+/K^+ coupling ratio of Na^+/K^+-ATPase in reconstituted lipid vesicles," *Biochim. Biophys. Acta* **981**, 326–336 (1989).

18. E. Bamberg, R. J. Clarke, and K. Fendler, "Electrogenic properties of the Na^+,K^+-ATPase probed by presteady state and relaxation studies," *J. Bioenerg. Biomembr.* **33**, 401–405 (2001).

19. R. J. Clarke and D. J. Kane, "Two gears of pumping by the sodium pump," *Biophys. J.* **93**, 4187–4196 (2007).

20. J. Frank, A. Zouni, A. van Hoek, A. J. W. G. Visser, and R. J. Clarke, "Interaction of the fluorescent probe RH421 with ribulose-1,5-bisphosphate carboxylase/oxygenase and with Na^+,K^+-ATPase membrane fragments," *Biochim. Biophys. Acta* **1280**, 51–64 (1996).

21. D. J. Kane, K. Fendler, E. Grell, E. Bamberg, K. Taniguchi, J. P. Froehlich, and R. J. Clarke, "Stopped-flow kinetic investigations of conformational changes of pig kidney Na^+,K^+-ATPase," *Biochemistry* **36**, 13406–13420 (1997).

INDEX

Fluorescence Applications in Biotechnology and Life Sciences, Edited by Ewa M. Goldys